GRAY'S

BASIC
ANATOMY

THIRD EDITION

GRAY'S

BASIC
ANATOMY

Richard L. Drake, PhD, FAAA
Professor Emeritus of Surgery
Cleveland Clinic Lerner College of Medicine
Case Western Reserve University
Cleveland, Ohio

A. Wayne Vogl, PhD, FAAA
Professor of Anatomy and Cell Biology
Department of Cellular and Physiological Sciences
Faculty of Medicine
University of British Columbia
Vancouver, British Columbia

Adam W.M. Mitchell, MBBS, FRCS, FRCR
Consultant Radiologist
Director of Radiology
Fortius Clinic
London, United Kingdom

Illustrations by
Richard Tibbitts and **Paul Richardson**

Photographs by
Ansell Horn

ELSEVIER

Elsevier
1600 John F. Kennedy Blvd.
Ste 1800
Philadelphia, PA 19103-2899

GRAY'S BASIC ANATOMY, THIRD EDITION   ISBN: 978-0-323-83442-1

Copyright © 2023 by Elsevier, Inc. All rights reserved.

First Edition copyrighted 2012 by Churchill Livingstone, an imprint of Elsevier, Inc.

Notice

Practitioners and researchers must always rely on their own experience and knowledge in evaluating and using any information, methods, compounds or experiments described herein. Because of rapid advances in the medical sciences, in particular, independent verification of diagnoses and drug dosages should be made. To the fullest extent of the law, no responsibility is assumed by Elsevier, authors, editors or contributors for any injury and/or damage to persons or property as a matter of products liability, negligence or otherwise, or from any use or operation of any methods, products, instructions, or ideas contained in the material herein.

Previous editions copyrighted 2018 and 2012.

Publisher: Jeremy Bowes
Director, Content Development: Rebecca Gruliow
Publishing Service Manager: Shereen Jameel
Senior Project Manager: Beula Christopher
Design Direction: Amy Buxton

Printed in India

9 8 7 6 5 4 3 2 1

www.elsevier.com • www.bookaid.org

To my parents who guide me,
To my wife who supports me,
To my students who challenge me
RLD

To my family, my colleagues, my mentors, and my students
AWV

To all my family, Cathy, Max and Elsa, and my colleagues
AWMM

Acknowledgments

Any book, no matter the size, is a major undertaking, and we want to thank all of the individuals who have helped move this project to completion. These include William Schmitt and Rebecca Gruliow, who both helped in initially evaluating the need for this type of concise textbook and in moving the first edition forward to completion. Jeremy Bowes and Rebecca Gruliow guided the third edition through to completion. We also appreciate the contributions of our illustrators, Richard Tibbitts and Paul Richardson, who did all of the artwork.

We'd also like to thank Professor Richard A. Buckingham of the Abraham Lincoln School of Medicine, University of Illinois, for Fig. 8.100B; Dr. Murray Morrison, Dr. Joanne Matsubara, Dr. Brian Westerberg, Laura Hall, and Jing Cui for contributing images for the head and neck chapter; and Dr. Bruce Crawford and Logan Lee for help with images for the surface anatomy of the upper limb. We also want to thank Dr. Bradley Little and Dr. Arlo Adams for contributing non-binary and transgender elements to the text and Clinical Apps to make the book more inclusive.

Finally, we are very appreciative of the numerous individuals, anatomists, and educators who provided feedback on the first and second editions and whose suggestions were included in this third edition.

Richard L. Drake
A. Wayne Vogl
Adam W.M. Mitchell

Preface

Gray's Basic Anatomy was developed in response to students and colleagues from around the world who requested a more concise description of anatomy than that presented in *Gray's Anatomy for Students*. To accomplish this goal, we reworked the material to focus mainly on regional anatomy and integrated the clinical material, imaging, and surface anatomy information directly into the text as:

- **Clinical apps**, which give students context for why a strong anatomical background helps facilitate the solving of clinical problems;
- **Imaging apps,** which offer students a great introduction to the different techniques and modalities available for imaging relevant anatomy; and
- **Surface anatomy boxes,** which help students visualize the relationship between anatomical structures and surface landmarks necessary for any kind of patient examination.

In addition, at the beginning of each chapter students are directed to additional learning resources available on Student Consult (Elsevier's online educational website).

Summarizing, *Gray's Basic Anatomy* uses a regional approach, similar to *Gray's Anatomy for Students,* with eight chapters: The Body, Back, Thorax, Abdomen, Pelvis and Perineum, Lower Limb, Upper Limb, and Head and Neck. The artwork presents the same familiar illustrations from *Gray's Anatomy for Students*, but they have been resized to fit within a smaller format while retaining a close physical location to the text with which each figure is associated. Finally, while some verbiage has been sacrificed in keeping with the goal of presenting a concise textbook of anatomy (e.g., muscle descriptions have for the most part been incorporated into tables with no loss of content), additional clinical and imaging material has been added to enhance learning in context.

This third edition includes numerous edits resulting from reader feedback, some new and revised figures, and revisions based on current research in the field of the anatomical sciences.

We hope you will continue to find this new edition a useful and valuable resource whether you are an educator or a student.

Richard L. Drake
A. Wayne Vogl
Adam W.M. Mitchell

Index of Clinical Apps, Imaging Apps, and Surface Anatomy Boxes

1 The Body

CLINICAL APPS

Bone marrow transplants   10
Bone fractures   11
Avascular necrosis   11
Osteoporosis   11
Epiphyseal fractures   11
Joint replacement   13
Degenerative joint disease   14
Arthroscopy   15
The importance of fascias   15
Muscle paralysis   16
Muscle atrophy   16
Muscle injuries and strains   16
Atherosclerosis   17
Varicose veins   17
Anastomoses and collateral circulation   17
Lymph nodes   19
Dermatomes and myotomes   23
Referred pain   33

IMAGING APPS

Determination of skeletal age   10

2 Back

CLINICAL APPS

Spina bifida   43
Vertebroplasty   43
Scoliosis   44
Kyphosis   44
Lordosis   44
Variation in vertebral numbers   44
The vertebrae and cancer   44

Osteoporosis   44
Back pain   45
Herniation of intervertebral discs   45
Joint diseases   46
Ligamenta flava   47
Vertebral fractures   47
Pars interarticularis fractures   48
Surgical procedures on the back   48
Nerve injuries affecting superficial back
    muscles   49
Lumbar cerebrospinal fluid tap   59
Anesthesia within the vertebral
    canal   60
Herpes zoster   60

IMAGING APPS

Typical cervical vertebrae   36
Typical thoracic vertebrae   37
Typical lumbar vertebrae   37
Articulation between atlas and axis   40

SURFACE ANATOMY

How to identify specific vertebral spinous processes   41
Primary and secondary curvatures in the sagittal plane   43
Visualizing the inferior ends of the spinal cord and
    subarachnoid space   58

3 Thorax

CLINICAL APPS

Axillary process of breast   65
Breast cancer   66
Thoracic outlet syndrome   67
Cervical ribs   72
Rib fractures   72
Collection of sternal bone marrow   73

The manubriosternal joint as reference   75
Surgical access to the chest   82
Thoracostomy (chest) tube insertion   82
Intercostal nerve block   83
The arrangement of pleural cavities is clinically significant   85
Innervation of parietal and visceral pleura   86
Pleural recesses   87
Pleural effusion   88
Pneumothorax   88
Inhaled objects   94
Lung cancer   101
Pneumonia   101
Pericardial innervation   104
Pericarditis   104
Pericardial effusion   105
Constrictive pericarditis   105
Valve disease   116
Common congenital heart defects   117
Cardiac auscultation   117
Clinical terminology for coronary arteries   120
Cardiac conduction system   121
Heart attack   124
Classic symptoms of heart attack   124
Referred pain   125
Are heart attack symptoms the same in men and women?   125
Ectopic parathyroid glands in the thymus   127
Left brachiocephalic vein   129
Venous access for central and dialysis lines   130
Using the superior vena cava to access the inferior vena cava   130
Coarctation of the aorta   131
Traumatic injury to the aorta   131
Aortic dissection   132
Aortic arch and its anomalies   132
Abnormal origin of great vessels   133
The vagus nerves, recurrent laryngeal nerves, and hoarseness   134
Esophagus constrictions   136
Esophageal cancer   137
Esophageal rupture   137

IMAGING APPS

Visualizing the pulmonary trunk by computed tomography   96
Visualizing the lungs   98
Plain chest radiograph   100
Visualizing the heart   108
Visualizing the chambers of the heart   110
Visualizing the left atrium and pulmonary veins   113

Visualizing structures in the superior mediastinum   128
Visualizing structures at the TIV vertebral level   132
Visualizing the mediastinum in the axial plane   141

SURFACE ANATOMY

The breast in women   67
How to count ribs   76
Visualizing structures at the TIV/V vertebral level   76
Visualizing the pleural cavities and lungs, pleural recesses, and lung lobes and fissures   91
Where to listen for lung sounds   93
Visualizing the margins of the heart   110
Where to listen for heart sounds   116
Visualizing structures in the superior mediastinum   134

4   *Abdomen*

CLINICAL APPS

Preperitoneal vs. retroperitoneal   153
Surgical incisions   160
Cremasteric reflex   161
Masses around the groin   161
Inguinal hernias   162
Indirect inguinal hernias   162
Direct inguinal hernias   162
Femoral hernias   162
Umbilical hernias   163
Incisional hernias   163
Sportsmen's groin/sportsmen's hernia   163
Other hernias   163
Potential problem of hernias   163
The peritoneum   164
Innervation of peritoneum   164
Ventriculoperitoneal shunts   164
Hemodialysis and peritoneal dialysis   164
Peritoneal spread of disease   164
Perforated bowel   165
The greater omentum   166
Epithelial transition between the abdominal esophagus and stomach   171
Surgery for obesity   172
Duodenal ulceration   172
Examination of the bowel lumen   172
Meckel's diverticulum   172
Carcinoma of the stomach   172

Appendicitis 175

Congenital disorders of the gastrointestinal
tract 178

Bowel obstruction 178

Diverticular disease 178

Ostomies 182

Segmental anatomy of the liver 182

Anular pancreas 184

Pancreatic cancer 185

Gallstones 186

Jaundice 186

Spleen disorders 187

Vascular supply to the gastrointestinal
system 193

Portosystemic anastomosis 195

Hepatic cirrhosis 195

Psoas muscle abscess 205

Diaphragmatic hernias 205

Hiatal hernia 206

Urinary tract stones 210

Urinary tract cancer 210

Kidney transplant 210

Abdominal aortic stent graft 213

Inferior vena cava filter 215

Retroperitoneal lymph node surgery 217

IMAGING APPS

Visualizing the stomach 169

Visualizing the jejunum and ileum 171

Visualizing the large intestine 173

Endoscopic examination of the abdominal gastrointestinal
tract 179

Visualizing the liver 181

Visualizing the pancreas 184

Visualizing the diaphragm 205

Investigation of the urinary tract 211

SURFACE ANATOMY

Using abdominal quadrants to locate major viscera 147

Defining surface regions to which pain from the gut is
referred 147

How to find the superficial inguinal ring 161

Visualizing the position of major blood vessels 215

5 *Pelvis and Perineum*

CLINICAL APPS

Bone marrow biopsy 226

Common problems with the sacro-iliac joints 228

Pelvic fracture 230

Pelvic measurements in obstetrics 232

Defecation 234

Episiotomy 236

Digital rectal examination 237

Carcinoma of the colon and rectum 237

Bladder cancer 239

Bladder stones 240

Suprapubic catheterization 240

Bladder infection 241

Urethral catheterization 241

Undescended testes 242

Hydrocele of the testis 243

Testicular tumors 243

Vasectomy 243

Prostate problems 244

Ovarian cancer 245

Hysterectomy 246

Tubal ligation 246

Carcinoma of the cervix and uterus 247

The recto-uterine pouch 250

Pudendal block 254

Prostatectomy and impotence 258

Hemorrhoids 262

Abscesses in the ischio-anal fossae 265

Urethral rupture 271

IMAGING APPS

Visualizing the male pelvic cavity and perineum in the axial
plane 276

Visualizing the female pelvic cavity and perineum in the
sagittal plane 279

Visualizing the female pelvic cavity and perineum in the
coronal plane 281

Visualizing the female pelvic cavity and perineum in the axial
plane 282

SURFACE ANATOMY

Defining the margins of the perineum   264
Superficial features of the external genitalia in women   267
Superficial features of the external genitalia in men   269

6 Lower Limb

CLINICAL APPS

Pelvic fractures   290
Femoral neck fractures   292
Intertrochanteric fractures   293
Femoral shaft fractures   293
Varicose veins   298
Deep vein thrombosis   298
Harvesting veins for grafts   299
Vascular access in the lower limb   303
Trendelenburg's sign   305
Intramuscular injection in the gluteal region: avoiding the sciatic nerve   307
Shin splints   313
Quadriceps injury   315
Hamstring injuries   317
Compartment syndrome   317
Peripheral vascular disease   320
Soft tissue injuries to the knee   328
Clinical tests for tears in the cruciate ligaments   328
Arthroscopy   328
Foot drop   340
Fracture of the talus   342
Calcaneal (Achilles) tendon rupture   343
Ankle injuries   348
Bunions   350
Morton's neuroma   361
Dermatomes and myotomes in the lower limb   362
Testing sensory innervation carried by major peripheral nerves in the lower limb   363
Tendon taps in the lower limb   364
Gait and gait defects   364

IMAGING APPS

Visualizing the hip joint   296
Visualizing the knee joint   328
Visualizing the bones of the foot   344
Visualizing the ankle joint   347

SURFACE ANATOMY

Finding the femoral artery in the femoral triangle   303
Visualizing the contents of the popliteal fossa   331
Finding the tarsal tunnel—the gateway to the foot   352
Finding the dorsalis pedis artery   359
Pulse points   365

7 Upper Limb

CLINICAL APPS

Fracture of the proximal humerus   372
Fractures of the clavicle and dislocations of the acromioclavicular and sternoclavicular joints   376
Dislocations of the glenohumeral joint   377
Rotator cuff disorders   377
Quadrangular space syndrome   380
"Winging" of the scapula   384
Trauma to the arteries in and around the axilla   389
Central venous access via the subclavian/axillary vein   389
Damage to long thoracic nerve   393
Injuries to the brachial plexus   397
Lymphatic drainage and breast cancer   398
Rupture of biceps tendon   401
Median nerve injury in the arm   402
Radial nerve injury in the arm   403
Supracondylar fracture of the humerus   407
Pulled elbow   407
Fracture of the head of radius   407
"Tennis" and "golfer's" elbow (epicondylitis)   407
Ulnar nerve injury at the elbow   408
Construction of a dialysis fistula   409
Blood pressure measurement   409
Fractures of the radius and ulna   412
Fracture of the scaphoid and avascular necrosis of the proximal scaphoid   426
Knuckle cracking   426
De Quervain syndrome   427
Carpal tunnel syndrome   428
Tenosynovitis   429
Trigger finger   429
Allen's test   435
Ulnar nerve injury   436
Radial nerve injury   439
Dermatomes and myotomes in the upper limb   439
Tendon taps in the upper limb   439
Testing sensory innervation carried by major peripheral nerves in the upper limb   440

IMAGING APPS

Visualizing the sternoclavicular joint   373
Visualizing the acromioclavicular joint   374
Visualizing the glenohumeral joint   375
Visualizing the rotator cuff muscles   376
Developmental changes in the elbow joint   406
Visualizing the elbow joint   407
Visualizing the forearm   411
Visualizing the hand and wrist joint   424

SURFACE ANATOMY

Locating the brachial artery in the right arm   404
Identifying tendons and locating major vessels and nerves in the distal forearm   421
Position of the flexor retinaculum and the recurrent branch of the median nerve   427
Motor function of the median and ulnar nerves in the hand   438
Pulse points   441

8   *Head and Neck*

CLINICAL APPS

Medical imaging of the head   461
Fractures of the skull vault   461
Cerebrospinal fluid leak   466
Hydrocephalus   466
Meningitis   466
Endarterectomy   468
Stroke   468
Intracerebral aneurysms   468
Emissary veins   472
Head injury   472
Concussion   472
Types of intracranial hemorrhage   473
Scalp and meninges   474
Cranial nerve lesions   481

Overview of cranial nerves   481
Parotid gland—tumors and stones   490
Trigeminal neuralgia   491
Facial nerve [VII] palsy (Bell's palsy)   496
Scalp laceration   500
Orbital fracture   502
Full and partial ptosis   505
Horner's syndrome   505
The H–test   514
Ophthalmoscopy   519
Glaucoma   520
Cataracts   520
Swimmer's ear   524
Surfer's ear   524
Examination of the ear   525
Mastoiditis   528
Temporomandibular joint disorders   539
Lingual nerve injury   546
Anesthesia of the inferior alveolar nerve   546
Middle meningeal artery and extradural hematoma   550
Spread of infection from the pterygoid plexus into the cranial cavity   550
Dry eye   555
Spread of neck infections   560
Central venous access   561
Tracheobronchial injury   569
Thyroidectomy   571
Goiter   572
Hyperparathyroidism   572
Ectopic parathyroid glands   572
Recurrent laryngeal nerve palsy   580
Clinical lymphatic drainage of the head and neck   584
Laryngoscopy   593
Cricothyrotomy   597
Exogenous testosterone and vocal cord mass   601
Tracheostomy   603
Deviated nasal septum   606
Surgical approach to the pituitary gland   609
Epistaxis   614
Oral cancer   617
Test for cranial nerve XII   624
Test for cranial nerve X   631

Index of Clinical Apps, Imaging Apps, and Surface Anatomy Boxes

IMAGING APPS

Visualizing the skull—anterior view   447

Visualizing the skull—lateral view   449

Visualizing the internal carotid and vertebral arteries   468

Visualizing the muscles of the eyeball   512

Visualizing the nasal cavities and paranasal sinuses   608

SURFACE ANATOMY

Anatomical position of the head and major landmarks   450

Estimating the position of the middle meningeal artery   461

Major features of the face   497

The eye and lacrimal apparatus   506

How to outline the anterior and posterior triangles of the neck   558

How to find the thyroid gland   572

How to locate the cricothyroid ligament   597

Pulse points   639

Contents

1 The Body

What is anatomy? 2
How can gross anatomy be studied? 2
Important anatomical terms 2
Imaging 3
Diagnostic imaging techniques 3
Image interpretation 7
  Plain radiography 7
  Computed tomography 8
  Magnetic resonance imaging 8
  Nuclear medicine imaging 8
Safety in imaging 8
Body systems 9
Skeletal system 9
  Cartilage 9
  Bone 9
  Joints 11
Skin and fascias 15
  Skin 15
  Fascia 15
Muscular system 15
Cardiovascular system 16
Lymphatic system 18
  Lymphatic vessels 18
  Lymph nodes 18
  Lymphatic trunks and ducts 19
Nervous system 20
  Central nervous system 20
  Functional subdivisions of the CNS 21
Other systems 33

2 Back

Regional anatomy 36
Skeletal framework 36
  Vertebrae 36
  Intervertebral foramina 40
  Posterior spaces between vertebral
      arches 41
  Curvatures of vertebral column 41

Joints 42
  Joints between vertebrae in the back 42
Ligaments 46
  Anterior and posterior longitudinal ligaments 46
  Ligamenta flava 46
  Supraspinous ligament and ligamentum nuchae 46
  Interspinous ligaments 47
Back musculature 48
  Superficial group of back muscles 48
  Intermediate group of back muscles 50
  Deep group of back muscles 51
  Thoracolumbar fascia 53
Spinal cord 55
  Vasculature 56
  Meninges 57
  Arrangement of structures in the vertebral canal 58
  Spinal nerves 58

3 Thorax

Regional anatomy 64
Pectoral region 64
  Breast 64
  Muscles of the pectoral region 66
Thoracic wall 66
  Superior thoracic aperture 67
  Inferior thoracic aperture 67
  Skeletal framework 68
  Intercostal spaces 75
Diaphragm 81
  Venous drainage 83
  Innervation 83
Movements of the thoracic wall and diaphragm during
      breathing 84
Pleural cavities 84
  Pleura 84
  Lungs 88
Mediastinum 97
  Anterior mediastinum 102
  Middle mediastinum 102
  Superior mediastinum 126
  Posterior mediastinum 135

Contents

4 Abdomen

Regional anatomy   146
Surface topography   146
   Four-quadrant pattern   146
   Nine-region pattern   146
Abdominal wall   147
   Superficial fascia   148
   Anterolateral muscles   149
   Extraperitoneal fascia   152
   Peritoneum   153
   Innervation   153
   Arterial supply and venous drainage   155
   Lymphatic drainage   155
Groin   156
   Inguinal canal   157
Abdominal viscera   163
   Peritoneum   163
   Peritoneal cavity   164
   Organs   167
   Arterial supply to the gastrointestinal tract   187
   Venous drainage   193
   Lymphatics   196
   Innervation   196
Posterior abdominal region   201
   Posterior abdominal wall   201
   Viscera   206
   Vasculature   212
   Lymphatic system   216
   Nervous system in the posterior abdominal region   217
   Sympathetic trunks and splanchnic nerves   217

5 Pelvis and Perineum

Regional anatomy   224
Pelvis   224
   Bones   224
   Joints   227
   Orientation   229
   Differences between men and women   229
   True pelvis   230
   Viscera   236
   Fascia   247
   Peritoneum   248
   Nerves   251
   Blood vessels   258
   Lymphatics   262

Perineum   262
   Borders and ceiling   263
   Ischio-anal fossae and their anterior recesses   264
   Anal triangle   265
   Urogenital triangle   265
   Somatic nerves   271
   Visceral nerves   271
   Blood vessels   272
   Veins   274
   Lymphatics   274

6 Lower Limb

Regional anatomy   286
The hip   287
   Bony pelvis   287
   Proximal femur   290
   Hip joint   292
   Gateways to the lower limb   295
   Nerves   297
   Arteries   297
   Veins   298
   Lymphatics   299
   Deep fascia and the saphenous opening   300
   Femoral triangle   301
Gluteal region   303
   Muscles   303
   Nerves   305
   Arteries   308
   Veins   308
   Lymphatics   308
Thigh   309
   Bones   309
   Muscles   313
   Arteries   317
   Veins   321
   Nerves   321
   Knee joint   323
   Tibiofibular joint   329
   Popliteal fossa   329
Leg   331
   Bones   331
   Joints   333
   Posterior compartment of leg   333
   Lateral compartment of leg   337
   Anterior compartment of leg   338
Foot   340
   Bones   340
   Joints   344

Tarsal tunnel, retinacula, and arrangement of major
structures at the ankle 351
Arches of the foot 352
Plantar aponeurosis 353
Fibrous sheaths of toes 353
Extensor hoods 354
Intrinsic muscles 355
Arteries 357
Veins 359
Nerves 359

7 Upper Limb

Regional anatomy 368
Shoulder 370
Bones 370
Joints 372
Muscles 377
Posterior scapular region 379
Gateways to the posterior scapular region 379
Nerves 380
Arteries and veins 381
Axilla 381
Axillary inlet 382
Anterior wall 382
Medial wall 383
Lateral wall 384
Posterior wall 384
Gateways in the posterior wall 386
Floor 386
Contents of the axilla 386
Arm 398
Bones 398
Muscles 401
Nerves 401
Arteries and veins 403
Elbow joint 405
Cubital fossa 408
Forearm 410
Bones 410
Joints 412
Anterior compartment of the forearm 414
Muscles 414
Arteries and veins 414
Nerves 417
Posterior compartment of the forearm 418
Muscles 418
Arteries and veins 418
Nerves 421

Hand 422
Bones 423
Joints 425
Carpal tunnel and structures at the wrist 426
Palmar aponeurosis 427
Anatomical snuffbox 428
Fibrous digital sheaths 429
Extensor hoods 429
Muscles 430
Arteries and veins 432
Nerves 435

8 Head and Neck

Regional anatomy 445
Head 446
Neck 446
Skull 446
Anterior view 446
Lateral view 448
Posterior view 451
Superior view 451
Inferior view 452
Cranial cavity 454
Roof 455
Floor 455
Meninges 462
Cranial dura mater 462
Arachnoid mater 465
Pia mater 465
Meningeal spaces 465
Brain and its blood supply 466
Brain 466
Blood supply 467
Venous drainage 469
Cranial nerves 475
Olfactory nerve [I] 475
Optic nerve [II] 475
Oculomotor nerve [III] 477
Trochlear nerve [IV] 478
Trigeminal nerve [V] 478
Ophthalmic nerve [V₁] 478
Maxillary nerve [V₂] 479
Mandibular nerve [V₃] 479
Abducent nerve [VI] 479
Facial nerve [VII] 479
Vestibulocochlear nerve [VIII] 479
Glossopharyngeal nerve [IX] 480
Vagus nerve [X] 480

Contents

Accessory nerve [XI]   480
Hypoglossal nerve [XII]   484
Face   484
Muscles   484
Parotid gland   487
Innervation   489
Vessels   492
Scalp   496
Layers   496
Innervation   498
Vessels   499
Lymphatic drainage   500
Orbit   501
Bony orbit   501
Eyelids   502
Lacrimal apparatus   505
Sensory innervation   506
Fissures and foramina   507
Fascial specializations   509
Muscles   510
Vessels   513
Innervation   515
Eyeball   519
Ear   522
External ear   522
Middle ear   526
Internal ear   530
Temporal and infratemporal fossae   535
Bony framework   536
Temporomandibular joints   538
Masseter muscle   540
Temporal fossa   540
Infratemporal fossa   541
Pterygopalatine fossa   550
Skeletal framework   551
Gateways   551
Contents   552
Neck   557
Fascia   558
Superficial venous drainage   560
Anterior triangle of the neck   561
Posterior triangle of the neck   572
Root of the neck   577
Pharynx   584
Skeletal framework   585
Pharyngeal wall   586
Fascia   587
Gaps in the pharyngeal wall and structures passing through them   587
Nasopharynx   588
Oropharynx   590

Laryngopharynx   590
Tonsils   590
Vessels   590
Nerves   591
Larynx   592
Laryngeal cartilages   593
Extrinsic ligaments   595
Intrinsic ligaments   596
Laryngeal joints   597
Cavity of the larynx   598
Intrinsic muscles   600
Function of the larynx   601
Vessels   602
Nerves   603
Nasal cavities   604
Lateral wall   605
Regions   605
Skeletal framework   606
External nose   606
Paranasal sinuses   607
Walls, floor, and roof   609
Nares   611
Choanae   611
Gateways   611
Vessels   613
Innervation   614
Oral cavity   616
Skeletal framework   617
Walls: the cheeks   620
Floor   621
Salivary glands   627
Roof—palate   629
Oral fissure and lips   633
Oropharyngeal isthmus   634
Teeth and gingivae   634

9 Neuroanatomy (e-only)

Jennifer M. McBride, PhD
Cleveland Clinic, Cleveland Clinic Lerner College of Medicine

To access this BONUS chapter PLUS the complete enhanced eBook - see the inside front cover for instructions + your unique PIN code.

Index   641

1

The Body

What is anatomy? 2

How can gross anatomy be studied? 2
Important anatomical terms 2

Imaging 3

Diagnostic imaging techniques 3
Image interpretation 7
    Plain radiography 7
    Computed tomography 8
    Magnetic resonance imaging 8
    Nuclear medicine imaging 8
Safety in imaging 8

Body systems 9

Skeletal system 9
    Cartilage 9
    Bone 9
    Joints 11
Skin and fascias 15
    Skin 15
    Fascia 15
Muscular system 15
Cardiovascular system 16
Lymphatic system 18
    Lymphatic vessels 18
    Lymph nodes 18
    Lymphatic trunks and ducts 19
Nervous system 20
    Central nervous system 20
    Functional subdivisions of the CNS 21
Other systems 33

What is anatomy?

Anatomy includes those structures that can be seen grossly (without the aid of magnification) and microscopically (with the aid of magnification). Typically, when used by itself, the term *anatomy* tends to mean gross or macroscopic anatomy—that is, the study of structures that can be seen without using a microscope. Microscopic anatomy, also called histology, is the study of cells and tissues using a microscope.

Observation and visualization are the primary techniques a student should use to learn anatomy. Anatomy is much more than just memorization of lists of names. Although the language of anatomy is important, the network of information needed to visualize the position of physical structures in a patient goes far beyond simple memorization. Knowing the names of the various branches of the external carotid artery is not the same as being able to visualize the course of the lingual artery from its origin in the neck to its termination in the tongue. An understanding of anatomy requires an understanding of the context in which the terminology can be remembered.

HOW CAN GROSS ANATOMY BE STUDIED?

The term *anatomy* is derived from the Greek word *temnein,* meaning "to cut." Clearly, at its root, the study of anatomy is linked to dissection. Dissection of cadavers by students is now augmented, or even in some cases replaced, by viewing prosected (previously dissected) material and plastic models or using computer teaching modules, virtual and augmented reality experiences, and other learning aids.

Anatomy can be studied following either a regional or a systemic approach.

- With a **regional approach,** each *region* of the body is studied separately and all aspects of that region are studied at the same time. For example, if the thorax is to be studied, all of its structures are examined. This includes the vasculature, nerves, bones, muscles, and all other structures and organs located in the region of the body defined as the thorax. After studying this region, the other regions of the body (i.e., the abdomen, pelvis, lower limb, upper limb, back, head, and neck) are studied in a similar fashion.
- In contrast, in a **systemic approach,** each *system* of the body is studied and followed throughout the entire body. For example, a study of the cardiovascular system looks at the heart and all of the blood vessels in the body. This approach continues for the whole body until every system, including the nervous, skeletal, muscular, gastrointestinal, respiratory, lymphatic, and reproductive systems, has been studied.

IMPORTANT ANATOMICAL TERMS

The anatomical position

The anatomical position is the standard reference position of the body used to describe the location of structures (Fig. 1.1). The body is in the anatomical position when standing upright with feet together, hands by the side, and face looking forward. The mouth is closed and the facial expression is neutral. The rim of bone under the eyes is in the same horizontal plane as the top of the opening to the ear, and the eyes are open and focused on something in the distance. The palms of the hands face forward with the fingers straight and together and with the pad of the thumb turned 90° to the pads of the fingers. The toes point forward.

Anatomical planes

Three major groups of planes pass through the body in the anatomical position (Fig. 1.1).

- **Coronal planes** are oriented vertically and divide the body into anterior and posterior parts.

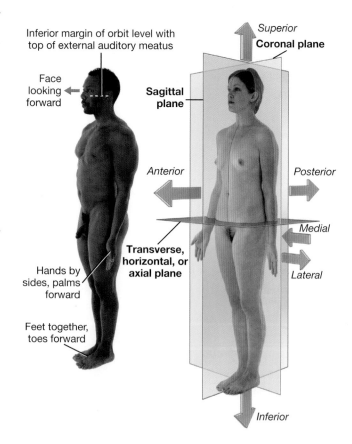

Fig. 1.1 The anatomical position, planes, and terms of location and orientation.

- **Sagittal planes** also are oriented vertically, but are at right angles to the coronal planes and divide the body into right and left parts. The plane that passes through the center of the body dividing it into equal right and left halves is termed the **median sagittal plane.**
- **Transverse, horizontal,** or **axial planes** divide the body into superior and inferior parts.

Terms to describe location

Anterior (ventral) and posterior (dorsal), medial and lateral, superior and inferior

Three major pairs of terms are used to describe the location of structures relative to the body as a whole or to other structures (Fig. 1.1).

- **Anterior** (or **ventral**) and **posterior** (or **dorsal**) describe the position of structures relative to the "front" and "back" of the body. For example, the nose is an anterior (ventral) structure, whereas the vertebral column is a posterior (dorsal) structure.
- **Medial** and **lateral** describe the position of structures relative to the median sagittal plane and the sides of the body. For example, the thumb is lateral to the little finger.
- **Superior** and **inferior** describe structures in reference to the vertical axis of the body. For example, the head is superior to the shoulders.

Proximal and distal, cranial and caudal, and rostral

Other terms used to describe positions include proximal and distal, cranial and caudal, and rostral.

- **Proximal** and **distal** are used with reference to being closer to or farther from a structure's origin, particularly in the limbs. For example, the hand is distal to the elbow joint. These terms are also used to describe the relative positions of branches along the course of linear structures, such as airways, vessels, and nerves. For example, distal branches occur farther away toward the ends, whereas proximal branches occur closer to and toward the origin.
- **Cranial** (toward the head) and **caudal** (toward the tail) are sometimes used instead of superior and inferior, respectively.
- **Rostral** is used, particularly in the head, to describe the position of a structure with reference to the nose. For example, the forebrain is rostral to the hindbrain.

Superficial and deep

Two other terms used to describe the position of structures in the body are **superficial** and **deep.** These terms are used to describe the relative positions of two structures with respect to the surface of the body. For example, the sternum is superficial to the heart.

Trans/Non-Binary Anatomical Terminology

While anatomy is classically discussed in binary terms (female and male), many individuals do not fit into these models. These can include intersex individuals or non-binary/transgender individuals who may undergo various degrees of gender-affirming care (e.g., hormones, surgery). Clinically, the anatomical terminology preferred by the patient should be used, which may include non-binary terms for classically gendered anatomy. In general, it is appropriate to use gender inclusive anatomical language when engaging with non-binary/transgender patients. Some common examples are as follows:

Preferred term	Instead of
Upper body	Chest/breast
Erectile tissue	Penis/clitoris
Gonads	Testes/ovaries

Clinicians should not assume, based on an individual's gender presentation, which anatomical features are present. In the clinic, acquiring a history of the patient's relevant anatomy should be considered including the patient's preferred terminology to guide appropriate and sensitive care. Clinicians should proceed to screen and treat patients based on the anatomy present if the criteria to do so are met.

Imaging
DIAGNOSTIC IMAGING TECHNIQUES

In 1895 Wilhelm Röntgen used the X-rays from a cathode ray tube to expose a photographic plate and produce the first radiographic exposure of his wife's hand. Over the past 35 years there has been a revolution in medical imaging that has been paralleled by developments in computer technology.

Plain radiography

X-rays are photons (a type of electromagnetic radiation) and are generated from a complex X-ray tube, which is a type of cathode ray tube (Fig. 1.2). The X-rays are then collimated (i.e., directed through lead-lined shutters to stop them from fanning out) to the appropriate area of the body. As the X-rays pass through the body they are attenuated (reduced in energy) by the tissues. Those X-rays that pass through the tissues interact with the photographic film.

In the body:

- Air attenuates X-rays a little.
- Fat attenuates X-rays more than air but less than water.
- Bone attenuates X-rays the most.

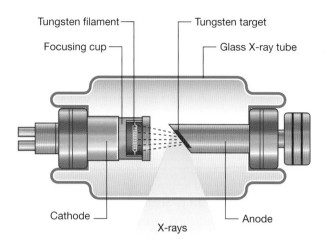

Fig. 1.2 Cathode ray tube for the production of X-rays.

Fig. 1.4 Barium sulfate follow-through.

Fig. 1.3 Fluoroscopy unit.

These differences in attenuation result in differences in the level of exposure of the film. When the photographic film is developed, bone appears white on the film because this region of the film has been exposed to the least amount of X-rays. Air appears dark on the film because these regions were exposed to the greatest number of X-rays. Modifications to this X-ray technique allow a continuous stream of X-rays to be produced from the X-ray tube and collected on an input screen to allow real-time visualization of moving anatomical structures, barium studies, angiography, and fluoroscopy (Fig. 1.3).

Contrast agents

To demonstrate specific structures, such as bowel loops or arteries, it may be necessary to fill these structures with a substance that attenuates X-rays more than bowel loops or arteries do normally. It is, however, extremely important that these substances are nontoxic. Barium sulfate, an insoluble salt, is a nontoxic, relatively high-density agent that is extremely useful in the examination of the gastrointestinal tract. When a **barium sulfate suspension** is ingested it attenuates X-rays and can therefore be used to demonstrate the bowel lumen (Fig. 1.4).

For some patients it is necessary to inject contrast agents directly into arteries or veins. In this case, iodine-based molecules are suitable contrast agents. **Iodine** is chosen because it has a relatively high atomic mass and so markedly attenuates X-rays, but also, importantly, it is naturally excreted via the urinary system. Intra-arterial and intravenous contrast agents are extremely safe and are well tolerated by most patients. These agents not only help in visualizing the arteries and veins, but, because they are excreted by the urinary system, they can also be used to visualize the kidneys, ureter, and bladder in a process known as **intravenous urography.**

Subtraction angiography

During angiography it is often difficult to appreciate the contrast agent in the vessels through the overlying bony structures. To circumvent this, the technique of subtraction angiography has been developed. Simply, one or two images are obtained before the injection of contrast media. These images are inverted (such that a negative is created from the positive image). After injection of the contrast media into the vessels, a further series of images are obtained,

Fig. 1.5 Digital subtraction angiogram.

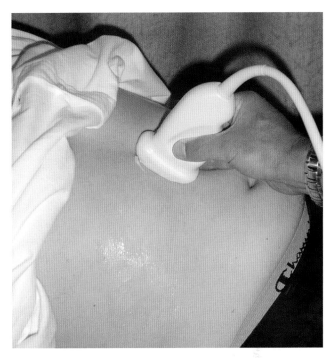

Fig. 1.6 Ultrasound examination of the abdomen.

demonstrating the passage of the contrast through the arteries and into the veins. By adding the "negative pre-contrast image" to the positive post-contrast images, the bones and soft tissues are subtracted to produce a solitary image of contrast only (Fig. 1.5).

Ultrasound

Ultrasonography of the body is widely used for all aspects of medicine (Fig. 1.6).

Ultrasound is a very high frequency sound wave (not electromagnetic radiation) generated by piezoelectric materials, such that a series of sound waves is produced. Importantly, the piezoelectric material can also receive the sound waves that bounce back from the internal organs. The sound waves are then interpreted by a powerful computer, and a real-time image is produced on the display panel.

Developments in ultrasound technology, including the size of the probes and the frequency range, mean that a broad range of areas can now be scanned.

Traditionally ultrasound is used for assessing the abdomen (Fig. 1.6) and the fetus in pregnant women. Ultrasound is also widely used to assess the eyes, neck, soft tissues, and peripheral musculoskeletal system. Probes have been placed on endoscopes, and endoluminal ultrasound of the esophagus, stomach, and duodenum is now routine. Endocavity ultrasound is carried out most commonly to assess the genital tract in women using a transvaginal or transrectal route. In men, transrectal ultrasound is the imaging method of choice to assess the prostate in those with suspected prostate hypertrophy or malignancy.

Doppler ultrasound

Doppler ultrasound enables determination of flow, its direction, and its velocity within a vessel using simple ultrasound techniques. Sound waves bounce off moving structures and are returned. The degree of frequency shift determines whether the object is moving away from or toward the probe and the speed at which it is traveling.

Computed tomography

A computed tomography (CT) scanner obtains a series of images of the body (slices) in the axial plane. The patient lies on a bed, an X-ray tube passes around the body (Fig. 1.7), and a series of images are obtained. A computer carries out a complex mathematical transformation on the multitude of images to produce the final image (Fig. 1.8).

Magnetic resonance imaging

The process of magnetic resonance imaging (MRI) is dependent on the free protons in the hydrogen nuclei in molecules of water (H_2O). Because water is present in almost all biological tissues, the hydrogen proton is ideal. The protons within a patient's hydrogen nuclei should be regarded

Fig. 1.7 Computed tomography scanner.

Fig. 1.8 Computed tomography scan of the abdomen at vertebral level L2.

as small bar magnets, which are randomly oriented in space. The patient is placed in a strong magnetic field, which aligns the bar magnets. When a pulse of radio waves is passed through the patient the magnets are deflected, and as they return to their aligned position they emit small radio pulses. The strength and frequency of the emitted pulses and the time it takes for the protons to return to their pre-excited state produces a signal. These signals are analyzed by a powerful computer, and an image is created (Fig. 1.9).

Fig. 1.9 A T2-weighted MR image in the sagittal plane of the pelvic viscera in a woman.

By altering the sequence of pulses to which the protons are subjected, different properties of the protons can be assessed. These properties are referred to as the "weighting" of the scan. By altering the pulse sequence and the scanning parameters, T1-weighted images (Fig. 1.10A) and T2-weighted images (Fig. 1.10B) can be obtained. These two types of imaging sequences provide differences in image contrast, which accentuate and optimize different tissue characteristics.

From the clinical point of view:

- Most T1-weighted images show dark fluid and bright fat—for example, within the brain the cerebrospinal fluid (CSF) is dark.
- T2-weighted images demonstrate a bright signal from fluid and an intermediate signal from fat—for example, in the brain the CSF appears white.

MRI can also be used to assess flow within vessels and to produce complex angiograms of the peripheral and cerebral circulation.

Nuclear medicine imaging

Nuclear medicine involves imaging using gamma rays, which are another type of electromagnetic radiation. The important difference between gamma rays and X-rays is that gamma rays are produced from within the nucleus of an atom when an unstable nucleus decays, whereas X-rays are produced by bombarding an atom with electrons.

For an area to be visualized, the patient must receive a gamma-ray emitter, which must have a number of

Fig. 1.10 T1-weighted **(A)** and T2-weighted **(B)** MR images of the brain in the coronal plane.

properties to be useful, including a reasonable half-life (e.g., 6 to 24 hours); an easily measurable gamma ray; and an energy deposition in as low a dose as possible in the patient's tissues.

The most commonly used radionuclide (radioisotope) is technetium-99m. This may be injected as a technetium salt or combined with other complex molecules. For example, by combining technetium-99m with methylene diphosphonate (MDP), a radiopharmaceutical is produced. When injected into the body this radiopharmaceutical specifically binds to bone, allowing assessment of the skeleton. Similarly, combining technetium-99m with other compounds permits assessment of other parts of the body; for example, the urinary tract and cerebral blood flow.

Images obtained using a gamma camera are dependent on how the radiopharmaceutical is absorbed, distributed, metabolized, and excreted by the body after injection.

Positron emission tomography

Positron emission tomography (PET) is an imaging modality for detecting positron-emitting radionuclides. A positron is an anti-electron, which is a positively charged particle of antimatter. Positrons are emitted from the decay of proton-rich radionuclides. Most of these radionuclides are made in a cyclotron and have extremely short half-lives.

The most commonly used PET radionuclide is fluorodeoxyglucose (FDG) labeled with fluorine-18 (a positron emitter). Tissues that are actively metabolizing glucose take up this compound, and the resulting localized high concentration of this molecule compared to background emission is detected as a "hot spot."

PET has become an important imaging modality in the detection of cancer and the assessment of its treatment and recurrence.

IMAGE INTERPRETATION

Plain radiography

Plain radiographs are undoubtedly the most common form of image obtained in a hospital or local practice. Before interpretation, it is important to know about the imaging technique and the standard views obtained.

In most instances (apart from chest radiography), the X-ray tube is 1 m away from the X-ray film. The object in question, for example a hand or a foot, is placed upon the film. When describing subject placement for radiography, the part closest to the X-ray tube is referred to first and that closest to the film is referred to second. For example, when positioning a patient for an anteroposterior (AP) radiograph, the more anterior part of the body is closest to the tube and the posterior part is closest to the film.

When X-rays are viewed on a viewing box, the right side of the patient is placed to the observer's left; therefore the observer views the radiograph as though looking at a patient in the anatomical position.

Chest radiograph

The chest radiograph is one of the most commonly requested plain radiographs. An image is taken with the patient erect and placed posteroanteriorly (PA chest radiograph); that is, with the patient's back closest to the X-ray tube.

Occasionally, when patients are too unwell to stand erect, films are obtained on the bed in an AP position. These films are less standardized than PA films, and caution should always be taken when interpreting AP radiographs.

A good quality chest radiograph will demonstrate the lungs, cardiomediastinal contour, diaphragm, ribs, and peripheral soft tissues.

Abdominal radiograph

Plain abdominal radiographs are obtained in the AP supine position. From time to time an erect plain abdominal radiograph is obtained when small bowel obstruction is suspected.

Gastrointestinal contrast examinations

High-density contrast medium is ingested to opacify the esophagus, stomach, small bowel, and large bowel. The bowel is insufflated with air (or carbon dioxide) to provide a double-contrast study. In many countries, endoscopy has superseded upper gastrointestinal imaging, but the mainstay for imaging the large bowel is the double-contrast barium enema. Typically the patient needs to undergo bowel preparation in which powerful cathartics are used to empty the bowel. At the time of the examination a small tube is placed into the rectum and a barium suspension is run into the large bowel. The patient undergoes a series of twists and turns so that the contrast passes through the entire large bowel. The contrast is emptied and air is passed through the same tube to insufflate the large bowel. A thin layer of barium coats the normal mucosa, allowing mucosal detail to be visualized (see Fig. 1.4).

Urological contrast studies

Intravenous urography is the standard investigation for assessing the urinary tract. Intravenous contrast medium is injected, and images are obtained as the medium is excreted through the kidneys. A series of films are obtained during this period from immediately after the injection up to approximately 20 minutes later, when the bladder is full of contrast medium.

This series of radiographs demonstrates the kidneys, ureters, and bladder and enables assessment of the retroperitoneum and other structures that may press on the urinary tract.

Computed tomography

CT is the preferred terminology rather than computerized tomography, though physicians use both terms interchangeably.

Most images are acquired in the axial plane and viewed such that the observer looks from below and upward toward the head (from the foot of the bed). By implication:

- the right side of the patient is on the left side of the image; and
- the uppermost border of the image is anterior.

Many patients are given oral and intravenous contrast media to differentiate bowel loops from other abdominal organs and to assess the vascularity of normal anatomical structures. When intravenous contrast is given, the earlier the images are obtained, the greater the likelihood of arterial enhancement. As the time is delayed between injection and image acquisition, a venous phase and an equilibrium phase are also obtained.

The great advantage of CT scanning is the ability to extend and compress the gray scale to visualize the bones, soft tissues, and visceral organs. Altering the window settings and window centering provides the physician with specific information about these structures.

Magnetic resonance imaging

There is no doubt that MRI has revolutionized the understanding and interpretation of the brain and its coverings (Fig. 1.10). Furthermore, it has significantly altered the practice of musculoskeletal medicine and surgery. Images can be obtained in any plane and in most sequences. Typically the images are viewed using the same principles as CT. Intravenous contrast agents are also used to further enhance tissue contrast. Typically, MRI contrast agents contain paramagnetic substances (e.g., gadolinium and manganese).

Nuclear medicine imaging

Most nuclear medicine images are functional studies. Images are usually interpreted directly from a computer, and a series of representative films are obtained for clinical use.

SAFETY IN IMAGING

Whenever a patient undergoes an X-ray or nuclear medicine investigation, a dose of radiation is given (Table 1.1). As a general principle, it is expected that the dose given is as low as reasonably possible for a diagnostic image to be obtained. Numerous laws govern the amount of radiation exposure that a patient can undergo for a variety of procedures, and these are monitored to prevent any excess or additional dosage.

Imaging modalities such as ultrasound and MRI are ideal because they do not impart significant risk to the patient.

Table 1.1 The approximate dosage of radiation exposure as an order of magnitude

Examination	Typical effective dose (mSv)	Equivalent duration of background exposure
Chest radiograph	0.02	3 days
Abdomen	1.00	6 months
Intravenous urography	2.50	14 months
CT scan of head	2.30	1 year
CT scan of abdomen and pelvis	10.00	4.5 years

Moreover, ultrasound imaging is the modality of choice for assessing the fetus.

Body systems

SKELETAL SYSTEM

The skeleton can be divided into two subgroups, the axial skeleton and the appendicular skeleton. The axial skeleton consists of the bones of the skull (cranium), vertebral column, ribs, and sternum, whereas the appendicular skeleton consists of the bones of the upper and lower limbs (Fig. 1.11).

The skeletal system consists of cartilage and bone.

☐ Axial skeleton

☐ Appendicular skeleton

Fig. 1.11 The axial skeleton and the appendicular skeleton.

Cartilage

Cartilage is an avascular form of connective tissue consisting of extracellular fibers embedded in a matrix that contains cells localized in small cavities. The amount and kind of extracellular fibers in the matrix vary depending on the type of cartilage. In heavy weight-bearing areas or areas prone to pulling forces, the amount of collagen is greatly increased and the cartilage is almost inextensible. In contrast, in areas where weight-bearing demands and stress are less, cartilage containing elastic fibers and fewer collagen fibers are common. The functions of cartilage are to:

- support soft tissues,
- provide a smooth, gliding surface for bone articulations at joints, and
- enable the development and growth of long bones.

There are three types of cartilage:

- hyaline—most common; matrix contains a moderate amount of collagen fibers (e.g., articular surfaces of bones);
- elastic—matrix contains collagen fibers along with a large number of elastic fibers (e.g., external ear);
- fibrocartilage—matrix contains a limited number of cells and ground substance amidst a substantial amount of collagen fibers (e.g., intervertebral discs).

Cartilage is nourished by diffusion and has no blood vessels, lymphatics, or nerves.

Bone

Bone is a calcified, living, connective tissue that forms the majority of the skeleton. It consists of an intercellular calcified matrix, which also contains collagen fibers, and several types of cells within the matrix. Bones function as:

- supportive structures for the body,
- protectors of vital organs,
- reservoirs of calcium and phosphorus,
- levers on which muscles act to produce movement, and
- containers for blood-producing cells.

There are two types of bone, compact and spongy (trabecular or cancellous). Compact bone is dense bone that forms the outer shell of all bones and surrounds spongy bone. Spongy bone consists of spicules of bone enclosing cavities containing blood-forming cells (marrow). Classification of bones is by shape.

- Long bones are tubular (e.g., humerus in the upper limb; femur in the lower limb).
- Short bones are cuboidal (e.g., bones of the wrist and ankle).
- Flat bones consist of two compact bone plates separated by spongy bone (e.g., skull).
- Irregular bones are bones with various shapes (e.g., bones of the face).
- Sesamoid bones are round or oval bones that develop in tendons.

Bones are vascular and are innervated. Generally, an adjacent artery gives off a nutrient artery, usually one per bone, which directly enters the internal cavity of the bone and supplies the marrow, spongy bone, and inner layers of compact bone. In addition, all bones are covered externally, except in the area of a joint where articular cartilage is present, by a fibrous connective tissue membrane called the periosteum, which has the unique capability of forming new bone. This membrane receives blood vessels whose branches supply the outer layers of compact bone. A bone stripped of its periosteum will not survive. Nerves accompany the vessels that supply the bone and the periosteum. Most of the nerves passing into the internal cavity with the nutrient artery are vasomotor fibers that regulate blood flow. Bone itself has few sensory nerve fibers. On the other hand, the periosteum is supplied with numerous sensory nerve fibers and is very sensitive to any type of injury.

Developmentally, all bones come from mesenchyme by either intramembranous ossification in which mesenchymal models of bones undergo ossification, or endochondral ossification in which cartilaginous models of bones form from mesenchyme and undergo ossification.

Fig. 1.12 A developmental series of radiographs showing the progressive ossification of carpal (wrist) bones from 3 (**A**) to 10 (**D**) years of age.

Imaging app

Determination of skeletal age

Throughout life the bones develop in a predictable way to form the skeletally mature adult at the end of puberty. In western countries, skeletal maturity tends to occur between the ages of 20 and 25 years.

Up until the age of skeletal maturity, bony growth and development follow a typically predictable ordered state, which can be measured through either ultrasound, plain radiographs, or MRI scanning. Typically, the nondominant (left hand) is radiographed and is compared with a series of standard radiographs. From these images the bone age can be determined (Fig. 1.12).

Clinical app

Bone marrow transplants

There are two types of bone marrow, red marrow (otherwise known as myeloid tissue) and yellow marrow. Red blood cells, platelets, and most white blood cells arise from within red marrow. In yellow marrow a few white cells are made; however, this marrow is dominated by large fat globules (producing its yellow appearance).

From birth most of the body's marrow is red; however, as the subject ages, more red marrow is converted into yellow marrow within the medulla of the long and flat bones.

There are a number of diseases that may involve the bone marrow, including infection and malignancy. In patients who develop a bone marrow malignancy (e.g., leukemia), it may be possible to harvest nonmalignant cells from the patient's bone marrow or cells from another person's bone marrow. The patient's own marrow can be destroyed with chemotherapy or radiation and the new cells infused. This treatment is referred to as a bone marrow transplant.

Clinical app

Bone fractures

Fractures occur in normal bone because of abnormal load or stress in which the bone gives way. Fractures may also occur in bone that is of poor quality (osteoporosis). In these cases, a normal stress is placed upon a bone that is not of sufficient quality to withstand this force and subsequently fractures.

In children whose bones are still developing, fractures may occur across the growth plate or across the shaft. These shaft fractures typically involve partial cortical disruption, similar to breaking a branch of a young tree; hence they are termed *greenstick* fractures.

Clinical app

Avascular necrosis

Avascular necrosis is cellular death of bone resulting from a temporary or permanent loss of blood supply to that bone. A typical site for avascular necrosis is a fracture across the femoral neck in an elderly patient. In these patients blood flow to the femoral head is compromised. It subsequently undergoes necrosis and collapses. In these patients it is necessary to replace the femoral head with a prosthesis.

Clinical app

Osteoporosis

Osteoporosis is a disease in which the bone mineral density is significantly reduced. This renders the bone significantly more at risk of fracture. Typically, osteoporotic fractures occur in the femoral necks, the vertebrae, and the wrists. Although osteoporosis may occur in men, especially elderly men, the typical patients are postmenopausal women. However, transgender or gender-diverse patients who undergo gender-affirming gonadectomy or those who are hypogonadal as part of gender-affirming hormonal therapy are also at risk.

Clinical app

Epiphyseal fractures

As the skeleton develops, there are stages of intense growth typically around the ages of 7 to 10 years and later in puberty. These growth spurts are associated with increased cellular activity around the growth plate and the metaphyseal region. This increase in activity renders the growth plates and metaphyseal regions more vulnerable to injuries such as dislocation across a growth plate or fracture through a growth plate. Occasionally an injury may result in growth plate compression, destroying that region of the growth plate, which may result in asymmetric growth.

Joints

The sites where two skeletal elements come together are termed *joints*. The two general categories of joints (Fig. 1.13) are those in which:

- the skeletal elements are separated by a cavity (i.e., **synovial joints**); and
- there is no cavity and the components are held together by connective tissue (i.e., **solid joints**).

Blood vessels that cross over a joint and nerves that innervate muscles acting on a joint usually contribute articular branches to that joint.

Synovial joints

Synovial joints are connections between skeletal components where the elements involved are separated by a narrow articular cavity. In addition to containing an articular cavity, these joints have a number of characteristic features (Fig. 1.14).

First, a layer of cartilage, usually **hyaline cartilage,** covers the articulating surfaces of the skeletal elements. In other words, bony surfaces do not normally contact one another directly. As a consequence, when these joints are viewed in normal radiographs, a wide gap seems to separate the adjacent bones because the cartilage that covers the articulating surfaces is more transparent to X-rays than bone.

A second characteristic feature of synovial joints is the presence of a **joint capsule** consisting of an inner **synovial membrane** and an outer **fibrous membrane.**

- The synovial membrane attaches to the margins of the joint surfaces at the interface between the cartilage and bone and encloses the articular cavity. The synovial

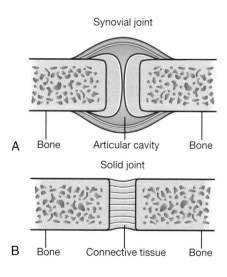

Fig. 1.13 Joints. **A.** Synovial joint. **B.** Solid joint.

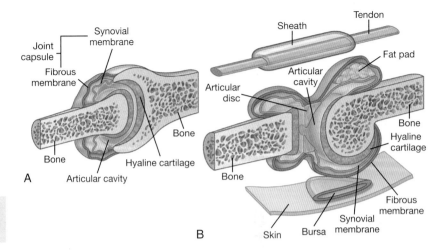

Fig. 1.14 Synovial joints. **A.** Major features of a synovial joint. **B.** Accessory structures associated with synovial joints.

membrane is highly vascular and produces synovial fluid, which percolates into the articular cavity and lubricates the articulating surfaces. Closed sacs of synovial membrane also occur outside joints where they form synovial bursae or tendon sheaths. Bursae often intervene between structures, such as tendons and bone, tendons and joints, or skin and bone, and reduce the friction of one structure moving over the other. Tendon sheaths surround tendons and also reduce friction.

■ The **fibrous membrane** is formed by dense connective tissue and surrounds and stabilizes the joint. Parts of the fibrous membrane may thicken to form ligaments, which further stabilize the joint. Ligaments outside the capsule usually provide additional reinforcement.

Another common but not universal feature of synovial joints is the presence of additional structures within the area enclosed by the capsule or synovial membrane:

■ **Articular discs** (usually composed of fibrocartilage) absorb compression forces, adjust to changes in the contours of joint surfaces during movements, and increase the range of movements that can occur at joints.
■ **Fat pads** occur between the synovial membrane and the capsule and move into and out of regions as joint contours change during movement.
■ **tendons.**

Descriptions of synovial joints based on shape and movement

Synovial joints are described based on shape and movement:

■ Based on the shape of their articular surfaces, synovial joints are described as plane (flat), hinge, pivot, bicondylar (two sets of contact points), condylar (ellipsoid), saddle, and ball and socket (Fig. 1.15).

■ Based on movement, synovial joints are described as uni-axial (movement in one plane), bi-axial (movement in two planes), and multi-axial (movement in three planes).

Hinge joints are uni-axial, whereas ball-and-socket joints are multi-axial.

Specific types of synovial joints (Fig. 1.15)

■ Plane joints—allow sliding or gliding movements when one bone moves across the surface of another (e.g., acromioclavicular joint)
■ Hinge joints—allow movement around one axis that passes transversely through the joint; permit flexion and extension (e.g., elbow [humeroulnar] joint)
■ Pivot joints—allow movement around one axis that passes longitudinally along the shaft of the bone; permit rotation (e.g., atlanto-axial joint)
■ Bicondylar joints—allow movement mostly in one axis with limited rotation around a second axis; formed by two convex condyles that articulate with concave or flat surfaces (e.g., knee joint)
■ Condylar (ellipsoid) joints—allow movement around two axes that are at right angles to each other; permit flexion, extension, abduction, adduction, and circumduction (limited) (e.g., wrist joint)
■ Saddle joints—allow movement around two axes that are at right angles to each other; the articular surfaces are saddle shaped; permit flexion, extension, abduction, adduction, and circumduction (e.g., carpometacarpal joint of the thumb)
■ Ball-and-socket joints—allow movement around multiple axes; permit flexion, extension, abduction, adduction, circumduction, and rotation (e.g., hip joint)

Solid joints

Solid joints are connections between skeletal elements where the adjacent surfaces are linked together either by

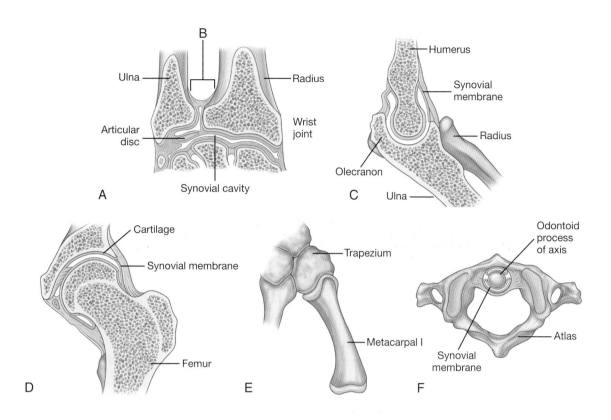

Fig. 1.15 Various types of synovial joints. **A.** Condylar (wrist). **B.** Gliding (radioulnar). **C.** Hinge or ginglymus (elbow). **D.** Ball and socket (hip). **E.** Saddle (carpometacarpal of thumb). **F.** Pivot (atlanto-axial).

fibrous connective tissue or by cartilage, usually fibrocartilage (Fig. 1.16). Movements at these joints are more restricted than at synovial joints.

Fibrous joints include sutures, gomphoses, and syndesmoses.

- **Sutures** occur only in the skull where adjacent bones are linked by a thin layer of connective tissue termed a *sutural ligament*.
- **Gomphoses** occur only between the teeth and adjacent bone. In these joints, short collagen tissue fibers in the periodontal ligament run between the root of the tooth and the bony socket.
- **Syndesmoses** are joints in which two adjacent bones are linked by a ligament. Examples are the ligamentum flavum, which connects adjacent vertebral laminae, and an interosseous membrane, which links, for example, the radius and ulna in the forearm.

Cartilaginous joints include synchondroses and symphyses.

- **Synchondroses** occur where two ossification centers in a developing bone remain separated by a layer of cartilage, for example, the growth plate that occurs between the head and shaft of developing long bones. These joints allow bone growth and eventually become completely ossified.

- **Symphyses** occur where two separate bones are interconnected by cartilage. Most of these types of joints occur in the midline and include the pubic symphysis between the two pelvic bones and intervertebral discs between adjacent vertebrae.

Clinical app

Joint replacement

Joint replacement is undertaken for a variety of reasons. These predominantly include degenerative joint disease and joint destruction. Joints that have severely degenerated or lack their normal function are painful. In some patients, the pain may be so severe that it prevents them from leaving the house and undertaking even the smallest of activities without discomfort.

Large joints are commonly affected, including the hip, knee, and shoulder. However, with ongoing developments in joint replacement materials and surgical techniques, even small joints of the fingers can be replaced.

Typically, both sides of the joint are replaced. In the hip joint the acetabulum will be reamed, and a plastic or metal cup will be introduced. The femoral component will be fitted precisely to the femur and cemented in place (Fig. 1.17).

Fig. 1.16 Solid joints.

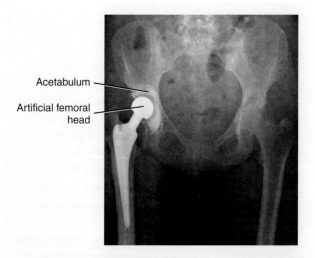

Fig. 1.17 This is a radiograph, anterior–posterior view, of the pelvis after a right total hip replacement. There are additional significant degenerative changes in the left hip joint, which will also need to be replaced.

Clinical app

Degenerative joint disease

Degenerative joint disease is commonly known as osteoarthritis or osteoarthrosis. The disorder is related to aging but not caused by aging. Typically, there are decreases in water and proteoglycan content within the cartilage. The cartilage becomes more fragile and more susceptible to mechanical disruption. As the cartilage wears, the underlying bone becomes fissured and also thickens. Synovial fluid may be forced into small cracks that appear in the bone's surface, which produces large cysts. Furthermore, reactive juxta-articular bony nodules are formed (osteophytes). As these processes occur, there is slight deformation, which alters the biomechanical forces through the joint. This, in turn, creates abnormal stresses, which further disrupt the joint (Fig. 1.18).

Osteophytes

Fig. 1.18 This radiograph demonstrates the loss of joint space in the medial compartment and presence of small spiky osteophytic regions in the joint.

Loss of joint space

Clinical app

Arthroscopy

Arthroscopy is a technique of visualizing the inside of a joint using a small camera placed through a tiny incision in the skin. Arthroscopy can be performed in most joints, including the elbow and wrist joints. However, it is most commonly performed in the knee, shoulder, ankle, and hip joints.

Arthroscopy allows the surgeon to view the inside of the joint and its contents. Notably, in the knee, the menisci and the ligaments are easily seen, and it is possible using separate puncture sites and specific instruments to remove the menisci and repair the cruciate ligaments. The advantages of arthroscopy are that it is performed through small incisions, it enables patients to quickly recover and return to normal activity, and it only requires either a light anesthetic or regional anesthesia during the procedure.

SKIN AND FASCIAS

Skin

The skin is the largest organ of the body. It consists of the epidermis and the dermis. The epidermis is the outer cellular layer of stratified squamous epithelium, which is avascular and varies in thickness. The dermis is a dense bed of vascular connective tissue.

The skin functions as a mechanical and permeability barrier and as a sensory and thermoregulatory organ. It also can initiate primary immune responses.

Fascia

Fascia is connective tissue containing varying amounts of fat that separates, supports, and interconnects organs and structures, enable movement of one structure relative to another, and allow the transit of vessels and nerves from one area to another. There are two general categories of fascia: superficial and deep.

- Superficial (subcutaneous) fascia lies just deep to and is attached to the dermis of the skin. It is made up of loose connective tissue, usually containing a large amount of fat. The thickness of the superficial fascia (subcutaneous tissue) varies considerably, both from one area of the body to another and from one individual to another. The superficial fascia allows movement of the skin over deeper areas of the body, acts as a conduit for vessels and nerves coursing to and from the skin, and serves as an energy (fat) reservoir.

- Deep fascia usually consists of dense, organized connective tissue. The outer layer of deep fascia is attached to the deep surface of the superficial fascia and forms a thin fibrous covering over most of the deeper region of the body. Inward extensions of this fascial layer form intermuscular septa that compartmentalize groups of muscles with similar functions and innervations. Other extensions surround individual muscles and groups of vessels and nerves, forming an investing fascia. Near some joints the deep fascia thickens, forming retinacula. These fascial retinacula hold tendons in place and prevent them from bowing during movements at the joints. Finally, there is a layer of deep fascia separating the membrane lining the abdominal cavity (the parietal peritoneum) from the fascia covering the deep surface of the muscles of the abdominal wall (the transversalis fascia). This layer is referred to as **extraperitoneal fascia**. A similar layer of fascia in the thorax is termed the **endothoracic fascia.**

Clinical app

The importance of fascias
Clinically, fascias are extremely important because they often limit the spread of infection and malignant disease. When infection or malignant diseases cross a fascial plane, a primary surgical clearance may require a far more extensive dissection to render the area free of tumor or infection.

MUSCULAR SYSTEM

The muscular system is generally regarded as consisting of one type of muscle found in the body—skeletal muscle. However, there are two other types of muscle tissue found in the body, smooth muscle and cardiac muscle, which are important components of other systems. These three types of muscle can be characterized by whether they are controlled voluntarily or involuntarily, whether they appear striated (striped) or smooth, and whether they are associated with the body wall (somatic) or with organs and blood vessels (visceral).

- Skeletal muscle forms the majority of the muscle tissue in the body. It consists of parallel bundles of long, multinucleated fibers with transverse stripes, is capable of powerful contractions, and is innervated by somatic and branchial motor nerves. This muscle is used to move bones and other structures, provides support, and gives form to the body. Individual skeletal muscles are often named on the basis of shape (e.g., rhomboid major muscle), attachments (e.g., sternohyoid muscle), function (e.g., flexor pollicis longus muscle), position (e.g., palmar interosseous muscle), or fiber orientation (e.g., external oblique muscle).
- Cardiac muscle is striated muscle found only in the walls of the heart (myocardium) and in some of the large vessels close to where they join the heart. It consists of a branching network of individual cells linked electrically and mechanically to work as a unit. Its contractions are less powerful than those of skeletal muscle, and it is resistant to fatigue. Cardiac muscle is innervated by visceral motor nerves.
- Smooth muscle (absence of stripes) consists of elongated or spindle-shaped fibers capable of slow and sustained contractions. It is found in the walls of blood vessels (tunica media), associated with hair follicles in the skin, located in the eyeball, and found in the walls of various structures associated with the gastrointestinal, respiratory, genitourinary, and urogenital systems. Smooth muscle is innervated by visceral motor nerves.

Clinical app

Muscle paralysis
Muscle paralysis is the inability to move a specific muscle or muscle group and may be associated with other neurologic abnormalities, including loss of sensation. Paralysis may be due to abnormalities in the brain, the spinal cord, and the nerves supplying the muscles. Major causes include stroke, trauma, poliomyelitis, and iatrogenic factors. Paralysis may also be caused by drugs that affect the neurotransmitters at the nerve endings and their action on the muscle themselves.

In the long term, muscle paralysis will produce secondary muscle wasting and overall atrophy of the region due to disuse.

Clinical app

Muscle atrophy
Muscle atrophy is a wasting disorder of muscle. It can be produced by a variety of causes, which include nerve damage to the muscle and disuse.

Muscle atrophy is an important problem in patients who have undergone long-term rest or disuse, requiring extensive rehabilitation and muscle-building exercises to maintain normal activities of daily living.

Clinical app

Muscle injuries and strains
Muscle injuries and strains tend to occur in specific muscle groups and usually are related to a sudden exertion and muscle disruption. They typically occur in athletes.

CARDIOVASCULAR SYSTEM

The cardiovascular system consists of the heart, which pumps blood throughout the body, and the blood vessels, which are a closed network of tubes that transport the blood. There are three types of blood vessels:

- arteries, which transport blood away from the heart;
- veins, which transport blood toward the heart; and
- capillaries, which connect the arteries and veins, are the smallest of the blood vessels and are where oxygen, nutrients, and wastes are exchanged within the tissues.

The walls of the blood vessels of the cardiovascular system usually consist of three layers or tunics:

- tunica externa (adventitia)—the outer connective tissue layer,
- tunica media—the middle smooth muscle layer (may also contain varying amounts of elastic fibers in medium and large arteries), and
- tunica intima—the inner endothelial lining of the blood vessels.

Arteries are usually further subdivided into three classes according to the variable amounts of smooth muscle and elastic fibers contributing to the thickness of the tunica media, the overall size of the vessel, and its function.

- Large elastic arteries contain substantial amounts of elastic fibers in the tunica media, allowing expansion and recoil during the normal cardiac cycle. This helps maintain a constant flow of blood during diastole. Examples of large elastic arteries are the aorta and the brachiocephalic trunk.
- Medium muscular arteries are composed of a tunica media that contains mostly smooth muscle fibers. This characteristic allows these vessels to regulate their diameter and control the flow of blood to different parts of the body. Examples of medium muscular arteries are most of the named arteries, including the femoral, axillary, and radial arteries.
- Small arteries and arterioles control the filling of the capillaries and directly contribute to the arterial pressure in the vascular system.

Veins also are subdivided into three classes.

- Large veins contain some smooth muscle in the tunica media, but the thickest layer is the tunica externa. Examples of large veins are the superior vena cava, the inferior vena cava, and the portal vein.
- Small and medium veins contain small amounts of smooth muscle, and the thickest layer is the tunica externa. Examples of small and medium veins are superficial veins in the upper and lower limbs and deeper veins of the leg and forearm.
- Venules are the smallest veins and drain the capillaries.

Although veins are similar in general structure to arteries, they have a number of distinguishing features.

- The walls of veins, specifically the tunica media, are thin.
- The luminal diameters of veins are large.
- There often are multiple veins (venae comitantes) closely associated with arteries in peripheral regions.
- Valves often are present in veins, particularly in peripheral vessels inferior to the level of the heart. These are usually paired cusps that facilitate blood flow toward the heart.

More specific information about the cardiovascular system and how it relates to the circulation of blood throughout the body will be discussed, where appropriate, in each of the succeeding chapters of the text.

Clinical app

Atherosclerosis
Atherosclerosis is a disease that affects arteries. There is a chronic inflammatory reaction in the walls of the arteries, with deposition of cholesterol and fatty proteins. This may in turn lead to secondary calcification, with reduction in the diameter of the vessels impeding distal flow. The plaque itself may be a site for attraction of platelets that may "fall off" (embolize) distally. Plaque fissuring may occur, which allows fresh clots to form and occlude the vessel.

Clinical app

Varicose veins
Varicose veins are tortuous dilated veins that typically occur in the legs, although they may occur in the superficial veins of the arm and in other organs.

In normal individuals the movement of leg muscles pumps the blood in the veins to the heart. Blood also moves from the superficial veins through the investing layer of fascia of the leg into the deep veins. Valves in these perforating veins may become damaged, allowing blood to pass in the opposite direction. This increased volume and pressure produces dilatation and tortuosity of the superficial veins (Fig. 1.19).

Varicose veins

Fig. 1.19 Photograph demonstrating varicose veins.

Clinical app

Anastomoses and collateral circulation
All organs require a blood supply from the arteries and drainage by veins. Within most organs there are multiple ways of perfusing the tissue such that if the main vessel feeding the organ or vein draining the organ is blocked, a series of smaller vessels (collateral vessels) continue to supply and drain the organ.

Some organs have more than one vessel perfusing them, such as the hand, which is supplied by the radial and ulnar arteries. Loss of either the radial or the ulnar artery may not produce any symptoms of reduced perfusion to the hand. The brain also has multiple vessels supplying it, dominated by the carotid arteries and the vertebral arteries. However, vessels within the brain are end arteries and have a poor collateral circulation; hence any occlusion will produce long-term cerebral damage.

Normal vascular anastomoses associated with an organ are important. Some organs, such as the duodenum, have a dual blood supply arising from the branches of the celiac trunk and from the branches of the superior mesenteric artery. Should either of these vessels be damaged, blood supply to the organ will be maintained.

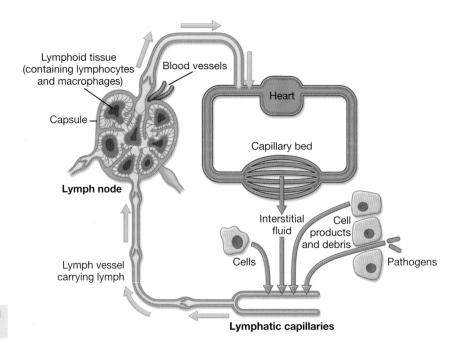

Fig. 1.20 Overview of the structure and function of the lymphatic system.

LYMPHATIC SYSTEM

Lymphatic vessels

Lymphatic vessels form an extensive and complex inter-connected network of channels, which begins as "porous" blind-ended lymphatic capillaries in tissues of the body and converges to form a number of larger vessels, which ultimately connect with large veins in the root of the neck.

Lymphatic vessels mainly collect fluid lost from vascular capillary beds during nutrient exchange processes and deliver it back to the venous side of the vascular system (Fig. 1.20). Also included in this interstitial fluid that drains into the lymphatic capillaries are pathogens, cells of the lymphocytic system, cell products (such as hormones), and cell debris.

In the small intestine, certain fats absorbed and processed by the intestinal epithelium are packaged into protein-coated lipid droplets (**chylomicrons**), which are released from the epithelial cells and enter the interstitial compartment. Together with other components of the interstitial fluid, the chylomicrons drain into lymphatic capillaries (known as **lacteals** in the small intestine) and are ultimately delivered to the venous system in the neck. The lymphatic system is therefore also a major route of transport for fat absorbed by the gut.

The fluid in most lymphatic vessels is clear and colorless and is known as **lymph.** That carried by lymphatic vessels from the small intestine is opaque and milky because of the presence of chylomicrons and is termed **chyle.**

There are lymphatic vessels in most areas of the body, including associated with the central nervous system (CNS).* Exceptions include bone marrow and avascular tissues such as epithelia and cartilage.

The movement of lymph through the lymphatic vessels is generated mainly by the indirect action of adjacent structures, particularly by contraction of skeletal muscles and pulses in arteries. Unidirectional flow is maintained by the presence of valves in the vessels.

Lymph nodes

Lymph nodes are small (0.1 to 2.5 cm long), encapsulated structures that interrupt the course of lymphatic vessels and contain elements of the body's defense system, such as clusters of lymphocytes and macrophages. They act as elaborate filters that trap and phagocytose particulate matter in the lymph that percolates through them. In addition, they detect and defend against foreign antigens that are also carried in the lymph.

Because lymph nodes are efficient filters and flow through them is slow, cells that metastasize from (migrate away from) primary tumors and enter lymphatic vessels often lodge and grow as secondary tumors in lymph nodes. Lymph nodes that drain regions that are infected or contain other forms of disease can enlarge or undergo certain physical changes, such as becoming "hard" or "tender." These changes can be used by clinicians to detect pathological changes or to track spread of disease.

---

*Louveau A et al. *Nature* 2015;523:337; Aspelund A et al. *J Exp Med* 2015;212:991; Absinta M et al. *eLIFE* 2017;6:e29738.

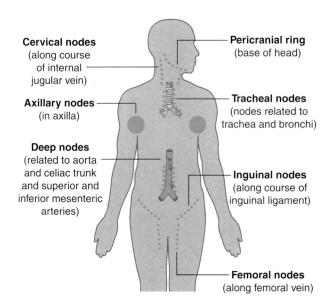

Cervical nodes
(along course
of internal
jugular vein)

Pericranial ring
(base of head)

Axillary nodes
(in axilla)

Tracheal nodes
(nodes related to
trachea and bronchi)

Deep nodes
(related to aorta
and celiac trunk
and superior and
inferior mesenteric
arteries)

Inguinal nodes
(along course of
inguinal ligament)

Femoral nodes
(along femoral vein)

Fig. 1.21 Regions associated with clusters or a particular abundance of lymph nodes.

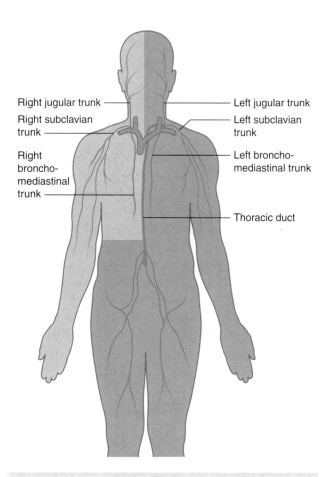

Right jugular trunk

Right subclavian trunk

Right broncho-mediastinal trunk

Left jugular trunk

Left subclavian trunk

Left broncho-mediastinal trunk

Thoracic duct

Fig. 1.22 Major lymphatic vessels that drain into large veins in the neck.

A number of regions in the body are associated with clusters or a particular abundance of lymph nodes (Fig. 1.21). Not surprisingly, nodes in many of these regions drain the body's surface, the digestive system, or the respiratory system. All three of these areas are high-risk sites for the entry of foreign pathogens.

Lymph nodes are abundant and accessible to palpation in the axilla, the groin and femoral region, and the neck (Fig. 1.21). Deep sites that are not palpable include those associated with the trachea and bronchi in the thorax and with the aorta and its branches in the abdomen.

Lymphatic trunks and ducts

All lymphatic vessels coalesce to form larger trunks or ducts, which drain into the venous system at sites in the neck where the internal jugular veins join the subclavian veins to form the brachiocephalic veins (Fig. 1.22):

- Lymph from the right side of the head and neck, the right upper limb, and the right side of the thorax is carried by lymphatic vessels that connect with veins on the right side of the neck.
- Lymph from all other regions of the body is carried by lymphatic vessels that drain into veins on the left side of the neck.

Specific information about the organization of the lymphatic system in each region of the body is discussed in the appropriate chapter.

Clinical app

Lymph nodes

Lymph nodes are efficient filters and have an internal honeycomb of reticular connective tissue filled with lymphocytes. These lymphocytes act on bacteria, viruses, and other bodily cells to destroy them. Lymph nodes tend to drain specific areas, and if infection occurs within a drainage area, the lymph node will become active. The rapid cell turnover and production of local inflammatory mediators may cause the node to enlarge and become tender. Similarly, in patients with malignancy, the lymphatics may drain metastasizing cells to the lymph nodes. These can become enlarged and inflamed and will need to be removed if clinically symptomatic.

Lymph nodes may become diffusely enlarged in certain systemic illnesses (e.g., viral infection), or local groups may become enlarged with primary lymph node malignancies, such as lymphoma.

NERVOUS SYSTEM

The nervous system can be separated into parts based on structure and on function:

- Structurally, it can be divided into the CNS and the peripheral nervous system (PNS) (Fig. 1.23).
- Functionally, it can be divided into somatic and visceral parts.

The CNS is composed of the brain and spinal cord, both of which develop from the neural tube in the embryo.

The PNS is composed of all nervous structures outside the CNS that connect the CNS to the body. Elements of this system develop from neural crest cells and as outgrowths of the CNS. The PNS consists of the spinal and cranial nerves, visceral nerves and plexuses, and the enteric system. The detailed anatomy of a typical spinal nerve is described in Chapter 2, as is the way spinal nerves are numbered. Cranial nerves are described in Chapter 8. The details of nerve plexuses are described in chapters dealing with the specific regions in which the plexuses are located.

Central nervous system

Brain

The parts of the brain are the cerebral hemispheres, the cerebellum, and the brainstem. The cerebral hemispheres consist of an outer portion, or the **gray matter,** containing cell bodies; an inner portion, or the **white matter,** made up of axons forming tracts or pathways; and the **ventricles,** which are spaces filled with CSF.

The cerebellum has two lateral lobes and a midline portion. The components of the brainstem are classically defined as the diencephalon, midbrain, pons, and medulla. However, in common usage today, the term *brainstem* usually refers to the midbrain, pons, and medulla.

A further discussion of the brain can be found in Chapter 8.

Spinal cord

The spinal cord is the part of the CNS in the superior two-thirds of the vertebral canal. It is roughly cylindrical in shape, and is circular to oval in cross-section with a central canal. A further discussion of the spinal cord can be found in Chapter 2.

Meninges

The meninges (Fig. 1.24) are three connective tissue coverings that surround, protect, and suspend the brain and spinal cord within the cranial cavity and vertebral canal. They consist of:

- the dura mater, which is the thickest and most external of the coverings;

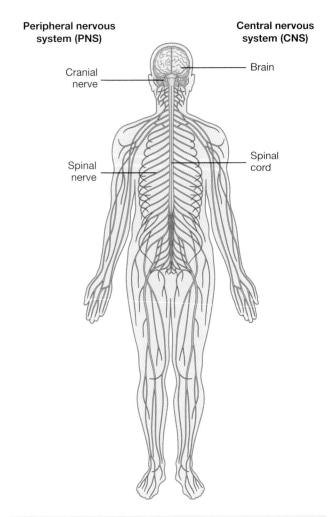

Fig. 1.23 CNS and PNS.

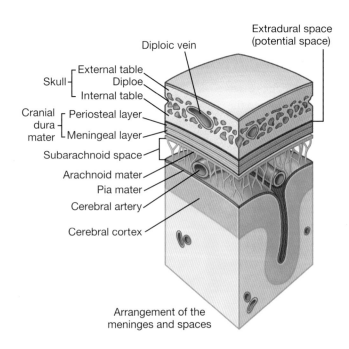

Fig. 1.24 Arrangement of meninges in the cranial cavity.

- the arachnoid mater, which is against the internal surface of the dura mater; and
- the pia mater, which is adherent to the brain and spinal cord.

Between the arachnoid and pia mater is the subarachnoid space, which contains CSF.

A further discussion of the cranial meninges can be found in Chapter 8 and of the spinal meninges in Chapter 2.

Functional subdivisions of the CNS

Functionally, the nervous system can be divided into somatic and visceral parts.

- The **somatic part** (*soma,* from the Greek for "body") innervates structures (skin and most skeletal muscle) derived from somites in the embryo and is mainly involved with receiving and responding to information from the external environment.
- The **visceral part** (*viscera,* from the Greek for "guts") innervates organ systems in the body and other visceral elements, such as smooth muscle and glands, in peripheral regions of the body. It is concerned mainly with detecting and responding to information from the internal environment.

Somatic part of the nervous system

The somatic part of the nervous system consists of:

- nerves that carry conscious sensations from peripheral regions back to the CNS, and
- nerves that innervate voluntary muscles.

Somatic nerves arise segmentally along the developing CNS in association with **somites,** which are themselves arranged segmentally along each side of the neural tube. Part of each somite (the **dermatomyotome**) gives rise to skeletal muscle and the dermis of the skin. As cells of the dermatomyotome differentiate, they migrate into posterior (dorsal) and anterior (ventral) areas of the developing body.

- Cells that migrate anteriorly give rise to muscles of the limbs and trunk (**hypaxial muscles**) and to the associated dermis.
- Cells that migrate posteriorly give rise to the intrinsic muscles of the back (**epaxial muscles**) and the associated dermis.

Developing nerve cells within anterior regions of the neural tube extend processes peripherally into posterior and anterior regions of the differentiating dermatomyotome of each somite (Fig. 1.25).

Simultaneously, derivatives of neural crest cells (cells derived from neural folds during formation of the neural tube) differentiate into neurons on each side of the neural tube and extend processes both medially and laterally (Fig. 1.25).

- Medial processes pass into the posterior aspect of the neural tube.
- Lateral processes pass into the differentiating regions of the adjacent dermatomyotome.

Neurons that develop from cells within the spinal cord are **motor neurons,** and those that develop from neural crest cells are **sensory neurons.**

Fig. 1.25 Somatic sensory and motor neurons. *Blue lines* indicate motor neurons and *red lines* indicate sensory neurons.

Somatic sensory and somatic motor fibers that are organized segmentally along the neural tube become parts of all spinal nerves and some cranial nerves.

The clusters of sensory nerve cell bodies derived from neural crest cells and located outside the CNS form sensory ganglia.

Generally, all sensory information passes into the posterior aspect of the spinal cord, and all motor fibers leave anteriorly.

Somatic sensory fibers carry information from the periphery into the CNS and are also called **somatic sensory afferents** or **general somatic afferents (GSAs).** The modalities carried by these nerves include temperature, pain, touch, and proprioception. Proprioception is the sense of determining the position and movement of the musculoskeletal system detected by special receptors in muscles and tendons.

Somatic motor fibers carry information away from the CNS to skeletal muscles and are also called **somatic motor efferents** or **general somatic efferents (GSEs).** Like somatic sensory fibers that come from the periphery, somatic motor fibers can be very long. They extend from cell bodies in the spinal cord to the muscle cells they innervate.

Dermatomes

Because cells from a specific somite develop into the dermis of the skin in a precise location, somatic sensory fibers originally associated with that somite enter the posterior region of the spinal cord at a specific level and become part of one specific spinal nerve (Fig. 1.26). Each spinal nerve therefore

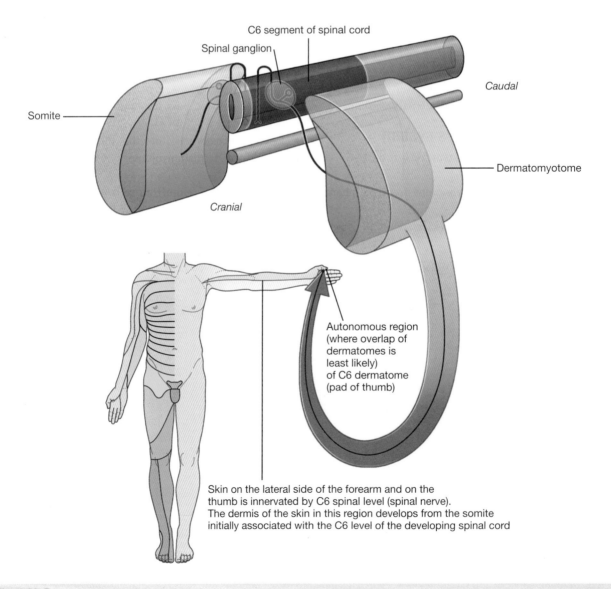

C6 segment of spinal cord

Spinal ganglion

Caudal

Somite

Dermatomyotome

Cranial

Autonomous region (where overlap of dermatomes is least likely) of C6 dermatome (pad of thumb)

Skin on the lateral side of the forearm and on the thumb is innervated by C6 spinal level (spinal nerve). The dermis of the skin in this region develops from the somite initially associated with the C6 level of the developing spinal cord

Fig. 1.26 Dermatomes.

carries somatic sensory information from a specific area of skin on the surface of the body. A **dermatome** is that area of skin supplied by a single spinal cord level or, on one side, by a single spinal nerve.

There is overlap in the distribution of dermatomes, but usually a specific region within each dermatome can be identified as an area supplied by a single spinal cord level. Testing touch in these autonomous zones in a conscious patient can be used to localize lesions to a specific spinal nerve or to a specific level in the spinal cord.

Myotomes

Somatic motor nerves that were originally associated with a specific somite emerge from the anterior region of the spinal cord and, together with sensory nerves from the same level, become part of one spinal nerve. Therefore each spinal nerve carries somatic motor fibers to muscles that originally developed from the related somite. A **myotome** is that portion of a skeletal muscle innervated by a single spinal cord level or, on one side, by a single spinal nerve.

Myotomes are generally more difficult to test than dermatomes, because each skeletal muscle in the body often develops from more than one somite and is therefore innervated by nerves derived from more than one spinal cord level (Fig. 1.27).

Muscles that abduct the arm are innervated by C5 and C6 spinal levels (spinal nerves) and develop from somites initially associated with C5 and C6 regions of developing spinal cord

Fig. 1.27 Myotomes.

Clinical app

Dermatomes and myotomes

A knowledge of dermatomes and myotomes is absolutely fundamental to carrying out a neurologic examination. A typical dermatome map is shown in Fig. 1.28.

Clinically, a dermatome is that area of skin supplied by a single spinal nerve or spinal cord level. A myotome is that region of skeletal muscle innervated by a single spinal nerve or spinal cord level. Most individual muscles of the body are innervated by more than one spinal cord level, so the evaluation of myotomes is usually accomplished by testing movements of joints or muscle groups.

Fig. 1.28 Dermatomes (anterior view).

Visceral part of the nervous system

The visceral part of the nervous system, as in the somatic part, consists of motor and sensory components:

- Sensory nerves monitor changes in the viscera.
- Motor nerves mainly innervate smooth muscle, cardiac muscle, and glands.

Fig. 1.29 Development of the visceral part of the nervous system.

The visceral motor component is commonly referred to as the **autonomic division of the PNS** and is subdivided into **sympathetic** and **parasympathetic** parts.

Like the somatic part of the nervous system, the visceral part is segmentally arranged and develops in a parallel fashion (Fig. 1.29).

Visceral sensory neurons that arise from neural crest cells send processes medially into the adjacent neural tube and laterally into regions associated with the developing body. Although these sensory neurons and their processes, referred to as **general visceral afferent fibers (GVAs),** are associated primarily with chemoreception, mechanoreception, and stretch reception, they also are associated with visceral pain reception.

Visceral motor neurons that arise from cells in lateral regions of the neural tube send processes out of the anterior aspect of the tube. Unlike in the somatic part, these processes, containing **general visceral efferent fibers (GVEs),** synapse with other cells—usually other visceral motor neurons—that develop outside the CNS from neural crest cells that migrate away from their original positions close to the developing neural tube.

The visceral motor neurons located in the spinal cord are referred to as preganglionic motor neurons, and their axons are called **preganglionic fibers;** the visceral motor neurons located outside the CNS are referred to as *postganglionic motor neurons,* and their axons are called **postganglionic fibers.**

The cell bodies of the visceral motor neurons outside the CNS often associate with each other in a discrete mass called a **ganglion.**

Visceral sensory and motor fibers enter and leave the CNS with their somatic equivalents (Fig. 1.30). Visceral sensory fibers enter the spinal cord together with somatic sensory fibers through posterior roots of spinal nerves. Preganglionic fibers of visceral motor neurons exit the spinal cord in the anterior roots of spinal nerves along with fibers from somatic motor neurons.

Postganglionic fibers traveling to visceral elements in the periphery are found in the posterior and anterior rami (branches) of spinal nerves.

Visceral motor and sensory fibers that travel to and from viscera form named visceral branches that are separate from the somatic branches. These nerves generally form plexuses from which arise branches to the viscera.

Fig. 1.30 Basic anatomy of a thoracic spinal nerve.

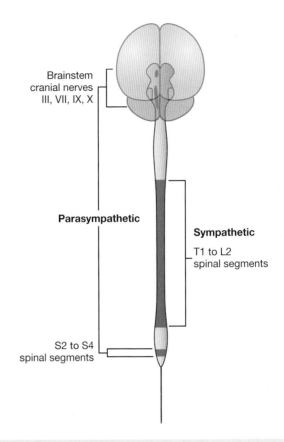

Fig. 1.31 Parts of the central nervous system associated with visceral motor components.

Visceral motor and sensory fibers do not enter and leave the CNS at all levels (Fig. 1.31):

- In the cranial region, visceral components are associated with four of the twelve cranial nerves (visceral efferents with CN III, VII, IX, and X; visceral afferents with IX and X).
- In the spinal cord, visceral components enter and leave the cord at levels T1 to L2 and S2 to S4.

Visceral motor components associated with spinal levels T1 to L2 are termed **sympathetic.** Those visceral motor components in cranial and sacral regions, on either side of the sympathetic region, are termed **parasympathetic:**

- the sympathetic system innervates structures in peripheral regions of the body and viscera; and
- the parasympathetic system is more restricted to innervation of the viscera only.

Sympathetic system

The sympathetic part of the autonomic division of the PNS leaves thoracolumbar regions of the spinal cord with the somatic components of spinal nerves T1 to L2 (Figs. 1.31, 1.32). On each side, a paravertebral sympathetic trunk extends from the base of the skull to the inferior end of the vertebral column where the two trunks converge anteriorly to the coccyx at the ganglion impar. Each trunk is attached

to the anterior rami of spinal nerves and becomes the route by which sympathetics are distributed to the periphery and all viscera.

Visceral motor preganglionic fibers leave the T1 to L2 part of the spinal cord in anterior roots. The fibers then enter the spinal nerves, pass through the anterior rami and into the sympathetic trunks. One trunk is located on each side of the vertebral column (paravertebral) and positioned anterior to the anterior rami. Along the trunk is a series of segmentally arranged ganglia formed from collections of postganglionic neuronal cell bodies where the preganglionic neurons synapse with postganglionic neurons. Anterior rami of T1 to L2 are connected to the sympathetic trunk or to a ganglion by a **white ramus communicans,** which carries preganglionic sympathetic fibers and appears white because the fibers it contains are myelinated (Fig. 1.33).

Preganglionic sympathetic fibers that enter a paravertebral ganglion or the sympathetic trunk through a white ramus communicans may take the following four pathways to target tissues:

1. Peripheral sympathetic innervation at the level of origin of the preganglionic fiber

Preganglionic sympathetic fibers may synapse with postganglionic motor neurons in ganglia associated with the

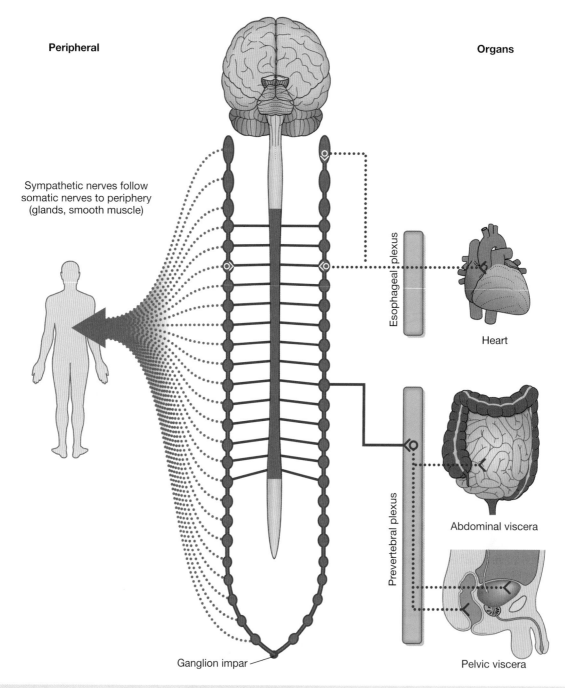

Peripheral

Organs

Sympathetic nerves follow
somatic nerves to periphery
(glands, smooth muscle)

Esophageal plexus

Heart

Prevertebral plexus

Abdominal viscera

Pelvic viscera

Ganglion impar

Fig. 1.32 Sympathetic part of the autonomic division of the PNS.

sympathetic trunk, after which postganglionic fibers enter the same anterior ramus and are distributed with peripheral branches of the posterior and anterior rami of that spinal nerve (Fig. 1.33). The fibers innervate structures at the periphery of the body in regions supplied by the spinal nerve. The **gray ramus communicans** connects the sympathetic trunk or a ganglion to the anterior ramus and contains the postganglionic sympathetic fibers. It appears gray because postganglionic fibers are nonmyelinated. The gray ramus communicans is positioned medial to the white ramus communicans.

2. Peripheral sympathetic innervation above or below the level of origin of the preganglionic fiber

Preganglionic sympathetic fibers may ascend or descend to other vertebral levels where they synapse in ganglia associated with spinal nerves that may or may not have visceral motor input directly from the spinal cord (i.e., those nerves other than T1 to L2) (Fig. 1.34).

The postganglionic fibers leave the distant ganglia via gray rami communicantes and are distributed along the posterior and anterior rami of the spinal nerves.

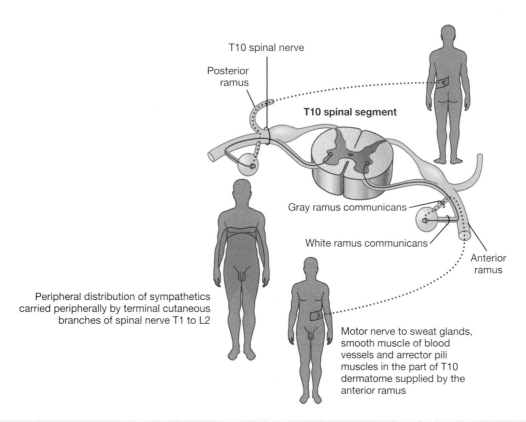

T10 spinal nerve

Posterior ramus

T10 spinal segment

Gray ramus communicans

White ramus communicans

Anterior ramus

Peripheral distribution of sympathetics carried peripherally by terminal cutaneous branches of spinal nerve T1 to L2

Motor nerve to sweat glands, smooth muscle of blood vessels and arrector pili muscles in the part of T10 dermatome supplied by the anterior ramus

Fig. 1.33 Course of sympathetic fibers that travel to the periphery in the same spinal nerves in which they travel out of the spinal cord.

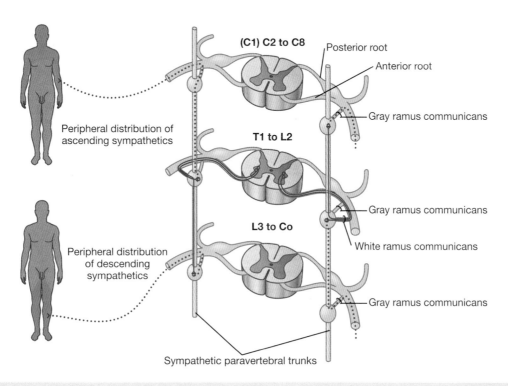

(C1) C2 to C8

Posterior root

Anterior root

Gray ramus communicans

Peripheral distribution of ascending sympathetics

T1 to L2

Gray ramus communicans

L3 to Co

White ramus communicans

Peripheral distribution of descending sympathetics

Gray ramus communicans

Sympathetic paravertebral trunks

Fig. 1.34 Course of sympathetic nerves that travel to the periphery in spinal nerves that are not the ones through which they left the spinal cord.

The ascending and descending fibers, together with all the ganglia, form the **paravertebral sympathetic trunk,** which extends the entire length of the vertebral column (Fig. 1.32). The formation of this trunk, on each side, enables visceral motor fibers of the sympathetic part of the autonomic division of the PNS, which ultimately emerge from only a small region of the spinal cord (T1 to L2) to be distributed to peripheral regions innervated by all spinal nerves.

White rami communicantes only occur in association with spinal nerves T1 to L2, whereas gray rami communicantes are associated with all spinal nerves.

Fibers from spinal cord levels T1 to T5 pass predominantly superiorly, whereas fibers from T5 to L2 pass inferiorly. All sympathetics passing into the head have preganglionic fibers that emerge from spinal cord level T1 and ascend in the sympathetic trunks to the highest ganglion in the neck (the **superior cervical ganglion**) where they synapse. Postganglionic fibers then travel along blood vessels to target tissues in the head, including blood vessels, sweat glands, small smooth muscles associated with the upper eyelids, and the dilator of the pupil.

3. Sympathetic innervation of thoracic and cervical viscera

Preganglionic sympathetic fibers may synapse with postganglionic motor neurons in ganglia and then leave the ganglia medially to innervate thoracic or cervical viscera (Fig. 1.35). They may ascend in the trunk before synapsing; after synapsing, the postganglionic fibers may combine with those from other levels to form named visceral nerves, such as cardiac nerves. Often, these nerves join branches from the parasympathetic system to form plexuses on or near the surface of the target organ (e.g., the cardiac and pulmonary plexuses). Branches of the plexus innervate the organ. Spinal cord levels T1 to T5 mainly innervate cranial, cervical, and thoracic viscera.

4. Sympathetic innervation of the abdomen and pelvic regions and the adrenals

Preganglionic sympathetic fibers may pass through the sympathetic trunk and paravertebral ganglia without synapsing and, together with similar fibers from other levels, form **splanchnic nerves (greater, lesser, least, lumbar,** and **sacral),**

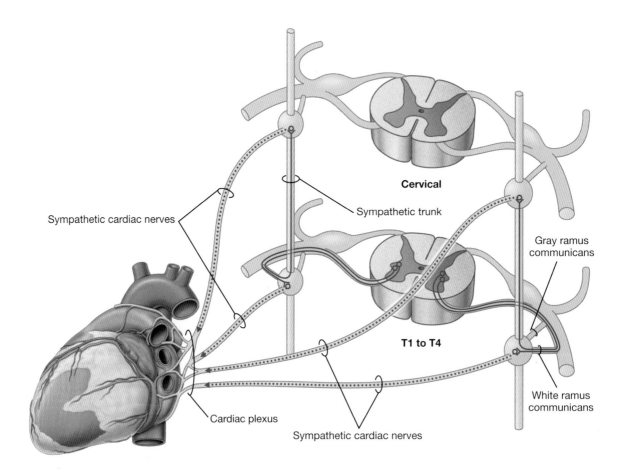

Fig. 1.35 Course of sympathetic nerves traveling to the heart.

which pass into the abdomen and pelvic regions (Fig. 1.36). The preganglionic fibers in these nerves are derived from spinal cord levels T5 to L2.

The splanchnic nerves generally connect with sympathetic ganglia around the roots of major arteries that branch from the abdominal aorta. These ganglia are part of a large prevertebral plexus that also has input from the parasympathetic part of the autonomic division of the PNS. Postganglionic sympathetic fibers are distributed in extensions of this plexus, predominantly along arteries, to viscera in the abdomen and pelvis.

Some of the preganglionic fibers in the prevertebral plexus do not synapse in the sympathetic ganglia of the plexus but pass through the system to the adrenal gland where they synapse directly with cells of the adrenal medulla. These cells are homologues of sympathetic postganglionic neurons and secrete adrenaline and noradrenaline into the vascular system.

Parasympathetic system

The parasympathetic part of the autonomic division of the PNS (Fig. 1.37) leaves cranial and sacral regions of the CNS in association with:

- cranial nerves III, VII, IX, and X: III, VII, and IX carry parasympathetic fibers to structures within the head and neck only, whereas X (the vagus nerve) also innervates thoracic and most abdominal viscera; and
- spinal nerves S2 to S4: sacral parasympathetic fibers innervate inferior abdominal viscera, pelvic viscera, and the arteries associated with erectile tissues of the perineum.

Like the visceral motor nerves of the sympathetic part, the visceral motor nerves of the parasympathetic part generally have two neurons in the pathway. The preganglionic neurons are in the CNS, and fibers leave in the cranial nerves or pelvic splanchnic nerves.

Sacral preganglionic parasympathetic fibers

In the sacral region, the preganglionic parasympathetic fibers form special visceral nerves (the **pelvic splanchnic nerves**), which originate from the anterior rami of S2 to S4 and enter pelvic extensions of the large prevertebral plexus formed around the abdominal aorta. These fibers are distributed to pelvic and abdominal viscera mainly along blood vessels. The

Greater splanchnic nerves

Lesser splanchnic nerves

Least splanchnic nerves

Lumbar splanchnic nerves

T5 to T9

T9 to T10
(T10 to T11)

T12

L1 to L2

Gray ramus communicans

White ramus communicans

Prevertebral plexus and ganglia

Paravertebral sympathetic trunk

Aorta

Abdominal and pelvic viscera

Sacral splanchnic nerves

Fig. 1.36 Course of sympathetic nerves traveling to abdominal and pelvic viscera.

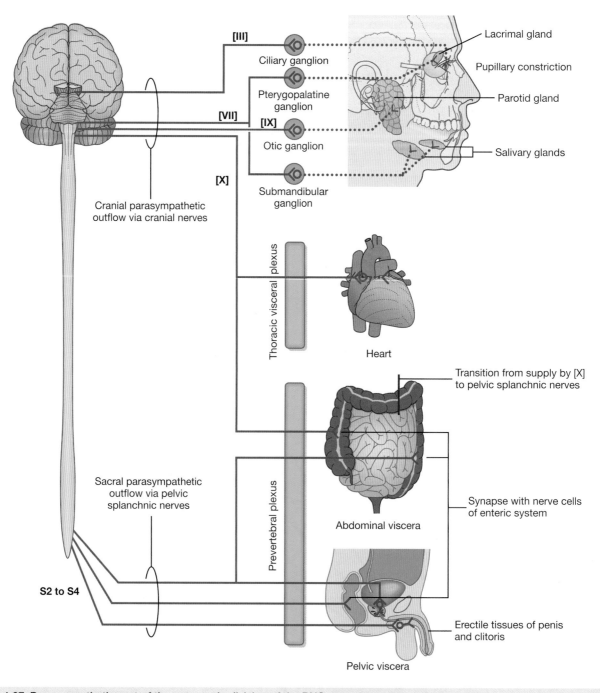

Fig. 1.37 Parasympathetic part of the autonomic division of the PNS.

postganglionic motor neurons are in the walls of the viscera. In organs of the gastrointestinal system, preganglionic fibers do not have a postganglionic parasympathetic motor neuron in the pathway; instead, preganglionic fibers synapse directly on neurons in the ganglia of the enteric system.

Cranial nerve preganglionic parasympathetic fibers

The preganglionic parasympathetic motor fibers in CN III, VII, and IX separate from the nerves and connect with one of four distinct ganglia, which house postganglionic motor neurons. These four ganglia are near major branches of the trigeminal nerve [V]. Postganglionic fibers leave the ganglia, join the branches of the trigeminal nerve [V], and are carried to target tissues (salivary, mucous, and lacrimal glands; constrictor muscle of the pupil; and ciliary muscle in the eye) with these branches.

The vagus nerve [X] gives rise to visceral branches along its course. These branches contribute to plexuses associated with thoracic viscera or to the large prevertebral plexus in the abdomen and pelvis. Many of these plexuses also contain sympathetic fibers.

When present, postganglionic parasympathetic neurons are in the walls of the target viscera.

Visceral sensory innervation (visceral afferents)

Visceral sensory fibers generally accompany visceral motor fibers.

Visceral sensory fibers accompanying sympathetic fibers

Visceral sensory fibers follow the course of sympathetic fibers entering the spinal cord at similar spinal cord levels. However, visceral sensory fibers may also enter the spinal cord at levels other than those associated with motor output. For example, visceral sensory fibers from the heart may enter at levels higher than spinal cord level T1. Visceral sensory fibers that accompany sympathetic fibers are mainly concerned with detecting pain.

Visceral sensory fibers accompanying parasympathetic fibers

Visceral sensory fibers accompanying parasympathetic fibers are carried mainly in the glossopharyngeal nerve [IX] and the vagus nerve [X] and in spinal nerves S2 to S4. These fibers primarily relay information to the CNS about the status of normal physiologic processes and reflex activities.

Visceral sensory fibers in the glossopharyngeal nerve [IX] carry information from chemoreceptors and baroreceptors associated with the walls of major arteries in the neck and from receptors in the pharynx.

Visceral sensory fibers in the vagus nerve [X] include those from cervical viscera and major vessels and viscera in the thorax and abdomen.

Visceral sensory fibers from pelvic viscera and the distal parts of the colon are carried in S2 to S4.

The enteric system

The enteric nervous system consists of motor and sensory neurons and their support cells, which form two interconnected plexuses, the **myenteric** and **submucous nerve plexuses,** within the walls of the gastrointestinal tract (Fig. 1. 38). Each of these plexuses is formed by:

- ganglia, which house the nerve cell bodies and associated cells; and
- bundles of nerve fibers, which pass between ganglia and from the ganglia into surrounding tissues.

Neurons in the enteric system are derived from neural crest cells originally associated with occipitocervical and sacral regions. Interestingly, more neurons are reported to be in the enteric system than in the spinal cord itself.

Sensory and motor neurons within the enteric system control reflex activity within and between parts of the gastrointestinal system. These reflexes regulate peristalsis, secretomotor activity, and vascular tone. These activities can

Legend:
- Preganglionic sympathetic
- Postganglionic sympathetic
- Preganglionic parasympathetic
- Visceral afferent
- Vagal afferent

Prevertebral sympathetic ganglion
Blood vessel
Mesentery
Longitudinal muscle layer
Circular muscle layer
Peritoneum
Myenteric plexus
Submucous plexus
Submucosa muscle
Submucosa
Enteric nervous system

Fig. 1.38 Enteric part of the nervous system.

occur independently of the brain and spinal cord but can also be modified by input from preganglionic parasympathetic and postganglionic sympathetic fibers.

Sensory information from the enteric system is carried back to the CNS by visceral sensory fibers.

Nerve plexuses

Nerve plexuses are either somatic or visceral and combine fibers from different sources or levels to form new nerves with specific targets or destinations (Fig. 1.39). Plexuses of the enteric system also generate reflex activity independent of the CNS.

Somatic plexuses

Major somatic plexuses formed from the anterior rami of spinal nerves are the cervical (C1 to C4), brachial (C5 to T1),

lumbar (L1 to L4), sacral (L4 to S4), and coccygeal (S5 to Co) plexuses (Fig. 1.39). Except for spinal nerve T1, the anterior rami of thoracic spinal nerves remain independent and do not participate in plexuses.

Visceral plexuses

Visceral nerve plexuses are formed in association with viscera and generally contain efferent (sympathetic and parasympathetic) and afferent components (Fig. 1.39). These plexuses include cardiac and pulmonary plexuses in the thorax and a large prevertebral plexus in the abdomen anterior to the aorta, which extends inferiorly onto the lateral walls of the pelvis. The massive prevertebral plexus supplies input to and receives output from all abdominal and pelvic viscera.

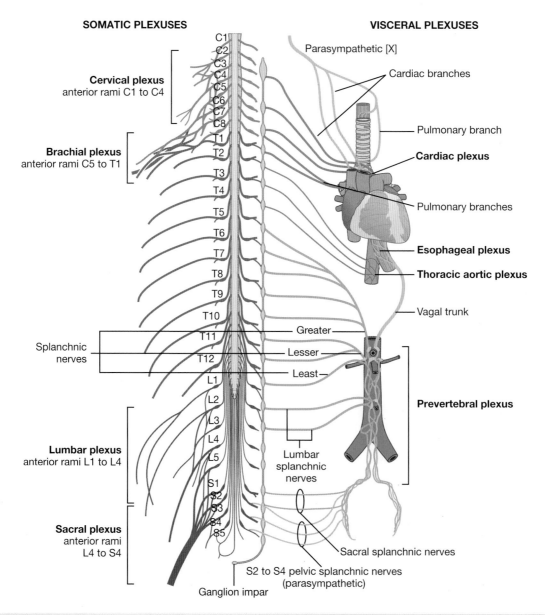

Fig. 1.39 Nerve plexuses.

Referred pain

Referred pain occurs when sensory information comes to the spinal cord from one location but is interpreted by the CNS as coming from another location innervated by the same spinal cord level. Usually, this happens when the pain information comes from a region, such as the gut, which has a low amount of sensory output. These afferents converge on neurons at the same spinal cord level that receive information from the skin, which is an area with a high amount of sensory output. As a result, pain from the normally low output region is interpreted as coming from the normally high output region.

Pain is most often referred from a region innervated by the visceral part of the nervous system to a region innervated, at the same spinal cord level, by the somatic side of the nervous system.

Pain can also be referred from one somatic region to another. For example, irritation of the peritoneum on the inferior surface of the diaphragm, which is innervated by the phrenic nerve, can be referred to the skin on the top of the shoulder, which is innervated by other somatic nerves arising at the same spinal cord level.

OTHER SYSTEMS

Specific information about the organization and components of the respiratory, gastrointestinal, and urogenital systems will be discussed in each of the succeeding chapters of this text.

2

Back

ADDITIONAL LEARNING RESOURCES FOR CHAPTER 2, *BACK,* CAN BE FOUND ON THE ACCOMPANYING EBOOK:

▨ Self-Assessment—National Board style multiple-choice questions, Chapter 2
▨ Short Questions—these are questions requiring short responses, Chapter 2
▨ PT Case Studies
Low back instability
Stenosis
Herniated nucleus pulposus
Atlanto-occipital dysfunction
Atlanto-axial dysfunction
Mid-cervical dysfunction
Cauda equina syndrome
Cervical degenerative joint disease
Cervical radiculopathy
▨ Clinical Cases
Ankylosing spondylitis
Atlas fracture
Cervical facet syndrome
Lumbar puncture
Spinal cord infarction
Sciatica versus lumbago
Cervical spinal cord injury
Psoas abscess
Dissecting thoracic aneurysm
Sacral tumor

Regional anatomy 36
Skeletal framework 36
Vertebrae 36
Intervertebral foramina 40
Posterior spaces between vertebral arches 41
Curvatures of vertebral column 41
Joints 42
Joints between vertebrae in the back 42
Ligaments 46
Anterior and posterior longitudinal ligaments 46
Ligamenta flava 46
Supraspinous ligament and ligamentum nuchae 46
Interspinous ligaments 47
Back musculature 48
Superficial group of back muscles 48
Intermediate group of back muscles 50
Deep group of back muscles 51
Thoracolumbar fascia 53
Spinal cord 55
Vasculature 56
Meninges 57
Arrangement of structures in the vertebral canal 58
Spinal nerves 58

Regional anatomy

The back consists of the posterior aspect of the body and provides the musculoskeletal axis of support for the trunk. The back also contains the spinal cord and proximal parts of the spinal nerves, which send and receive information to and from most of the body.

SKELETAL FRAMEWORK

Skeletal components of the back consist mainly of the vertebrae and associated intervertebral discs. The skull, scapulae, pelvic bones (ileum, ischium, pubis), and ribs also contribute to the bony framework of the back and provide sites for muscle attachment.

Vertebrae

There are approximately 33 vertebrae, which are subdivided into five groups based on morphology and location (Fig. 2.1):

- The seven cervical vertebrae between the thorax and skull are characterized mainly by their small size, bifid spinous processes, and the presence of a foramen in each transverse process (Figs. 2.1, 2.2).
- The 12 thoracic vertebrae are characterized by their articulated ribs (Figs. 2.1, 2.3); ribs are separate bones and articulate via synovial joints with the vertebral bodies and transverse processes of the associated vertebrae; although

all vertebrae have rib elements, these elements are small and are incorporated into the transverse processes in regions other than the thorax.

Imaging app

Typical cervical vertebrae

Fig. 2.2 Radiographs of cervical region of vertebral column. A. Anterior–posterior view. B. Lateral view.

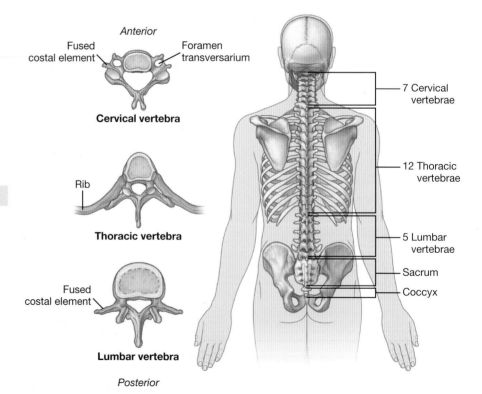

Fig. 2.1 Vertebrae.

Imaging app

Typical thoracic vertebrae

Fig. 2.3 Radiograph of thoracic region of vertebral column. **A.** Anterior–posterior view. **B.** Lateral view.

Imaging app

Typical lumbar vertebrae

Fig. 2.4 Radiograph of lumbar region of vertebral column. **A.** Anterior–posterior view. **B.** Lateral view.

- Inferior to the thoracic vertebrae are five lumbar vertebrae, which form the skeletal support for the posterior abdominal wall and are characterized by their large size (Figs. 2.1, 2.4).
- Next are five sacral vertebrae fused into one single bone called the sacrum, which articulates on each side with a pelvic bone and is a component of the pelvic wall.
- Inferior to the sacrum is a variable number, usually four, of coccygeal vertebrae, which fuse into a single small triangular bone called the *coccyx*.

Typical vertebra

A typical vertebra consists of a vertebral body and a posterior vertebral arch (Fig. 2.5). Extending from the vertebral arch are a number of processes for muscle attachment and articulation with adjacent bones.

The **vertebral body** is the weight-bearing part of the vertebra and is linked to adjacent vertebral bodies by intervertebral discs and ligaments. The size of vertebral bodies increases inferiorly as the amount of weight supported increases.

Fig. 2.5 Typical vertebra.

The **vertebral arch** forms the lateral and posterior parts of the vertebral foramen.

The vertebral foramina of all the vertebrae together form the **vertebral canal,** which contains and protects the spinal cord. Superiorly, the vertebral canal is continuous through the foramen magnum of the skull, with the cranial cavity of the head.

The vertebral arch of each vertebra consists of pedicles and laminae (Fig. 2.5):

- The two **pedicles** are bony pillars that attach the vertebral arch to the vertebral body.
- The two **laminae** are flat sheets of bone that extend from each pedicle to meet in the midline and form the roof of the vertebral arch.

A **spinous process** projects posteriorly and inferiorly from the junction of the two laminae and is a site for muscle and ligament attachment.

A **transverse process** extends posterolaterally from the junction of the pedicle and lamina on each side and is a site for muscle and ligament attachment and articulation with ribs in the thoracic region.

Also projecting from the region where the pedicles join the laminae are **superior** and **inferior articular processes** (Fig. 2.5), which articulate with the inferior and superior articular processes, respectively, of adjacent vertebrae.

Between the vertebral body and the origin of the articular processes, each pedicle is notched on its superior and inferior surfaces. These **superior** and **inferior vertebral notches** participate in forming intervertebral foramina.

Cervical vertebrae

The seven cervical vertebrae are characterized by their small size and by the presence of a foramen in each transverse process. A typical cervical vertebra has the following features (Fig. 2.6A):

- The vertebral body is short in height and square shaped when viewed from above and has a concave superior surface and a convex inferior surface.
- Each transverse process is trough shaped and perforated by a round **foramen transversarium.**
- The spinous process is short and bifid.
- The vertebral foramen is triangular.

The first and second cervical vertebrae—the atlas and axis—are specialized to accommodate movement of the head.

Atlas and axis

Vertebra CI (the **atlas**) articulates with the head (Figs. 2.6B, 2.7). Its major distinguishing feature is that it lacks a vertebral body (Fig. 2.6B). In fact, the vertebral body of CI fuses onto the body of CII during development to become the dens of CII. As a result, there is no intervertebral disc between CI and CII. When viewed from above, the atlas is ring shaped and composed of two **lateral masses** interconnected by an **anterior arch** and a **posterior arch.**

Each lateral mass articulates above with an occipital **condyle** of the skull and below with the superior articular process of vertebra CII (the **axis**). The **superior articular facets** are bean shaped and concave, whereas the **inferior articular facets** are almost circular and flat.

The **atlanto-occipital joint** allows the head to nod up and down on the vertebral column.

The posterior surface of the anterior arch has an articular facet for the **dens,** which projects superiorly from the vertebral body of the axis. The dens is held in position by a strong **transverse ligament of atlas** posterior to it and spanning the distance between the oval attachment facets on the medial surfaces of the lateral masses of the atlas (Fig. 2.6B).

The dens acts as a pivot that allows the atlas and attached head to rotate on the axis, side to side.

The transverse processes of the atlas are large and protrude farther laterally than those of the other cervical vertebrae. They act as levers for muscle action, particularly for muscles that move the head at the **atlanto-axial joints.**

The axis is characterized by the large tooth-like dens, which extends superiorly from the vertebral body (Figs. 2.6B, 2.7). The anterior surface of the dens has an oval facet for articulation with the anterior arch of the atlas.

The two superolateral surfaces of the dens possess circular impressions that serve as attachment sites for strong alar ligaments, one on each side, which connect the dens to the medial surfaces of the occipital condyles. These **alar ligaments** check excessive rotation of the head and atlas relative to the axis (Fig. 2.6B).

Thoracic vertebrae

The twelve thoracic vertebrae are all characterized by their articulation with ribs. A typical thoracic vertebra has two partial facets (superior and inferior costal facets) on each side of the vertebral body for articulation with the head of its own rib and the head of the rib below (Fig. 2.6C). The superior costal facet is much larger than the inferior costal facet.

Each transverse process also has a facet (transverse costal facet) for articulation with the tubercle of its own rib. The vertebral body of the vertebra is somewhat heart-shaped when viewed from above, and the vertebral foramen is circular.

Lumbar vertebrae

The five lumbar vertebrae are distinguished from vertebrae in other regions by their large size (Fig. 2.6D). Also, they lack

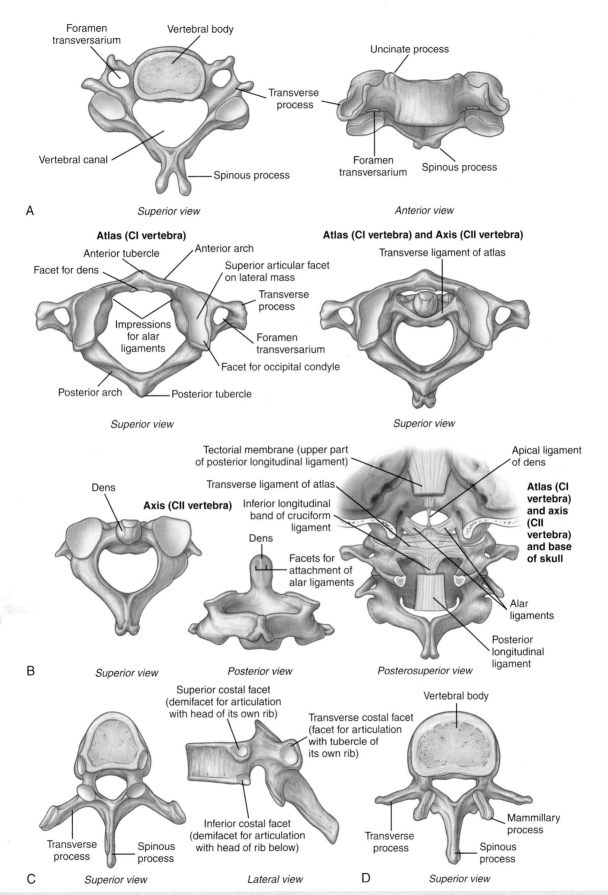

Fig. 2.6 Regional vertebrae. **A.** Typical cervical vertebra. **B.** Atlas and axis. **C.** Typical thoracic vertebra. **D.** Typical lumbar vertebra.

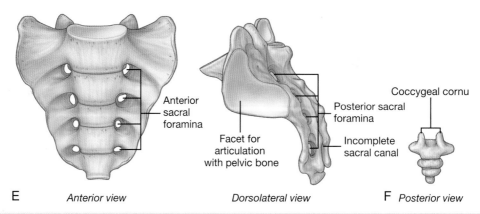

E *Anterior view* Dorsolateral view F *Posterior view*

Fig. 2.6, cont'd Regional vertebrae. E. Sacrum. F. Coccyx.

Imaging app

Articulation between atlas and axis

Superior articular facet of CII Dens Inferior articular facet on lateral mass of CI

Fig. 2.7 Radiograph showing CI (atlas) and CII (axis) vertebrae. Open mouth, anterior–posterior (odontoid peg) view.

facets for articulation with ribs. The transverse processes are generally thin and long, with the exception of those on vertebra LV, which are massive and somewhat cone-shaped for the attachment of **iliolumbar ligaments** to connect the transverse processes to the pelvic bones.

The vertebral body of a typical lumbar vertebra is cylindrical and the vertebral foramen is triangular in shape and larger than in the thoracic vertebrae.

Sacrum

The sacrum is a single bone that represents the five fused sacral vertebrae (Fig. 2.6E). It is triangular in shape with the **apex** pointed inferiorly and is curved so that it has a concave anterior surface and a correspondingly convex posterior surface. It articulates above with vertebra LV and below with the coccyx. It has two large L-shaped facets, one on each lateral surface, for articulation with the pelvic bones.

The posterior surface of the sacrum has four pairs of posterior sacral foramina, and the anterior surface has four pairs of anterior sacral foramina for the passage of the posterior and anterior rami, respectively, of S1 to S4 spinal nerves.

The posterior wall of the vertebral canal may be incomplete near the inferior end of the sacrum.

Coccyx

The coccyx is a small triangular bone that articulates with the inferior end of the sacrum and represents three to four fused coccygeal vertebrae (Fig. 2.6F). It is characterized by its small size and by the absence of vertebral arches and therefore a vertebral canal.

Intervertebral foramina

Intervertebral foramina are formed on each side between adjacent parts of vertebrae and associated intervertebral discs (Fig. 2.9). The foramina allow structures, such as spinal nerves and blood vessels, to pass in and out of the vertebral canal.

An intervertebral foramen is formed by the inferior vertebral notch on the pedicle of the vertebra above and the superior vertebral notch on the pedicle of the vertebra below. The foramen is bordered:

- posteriorly by the zygapophysial joint between the articular processes of the two vertebrae, and
- anteriorly by the intervertebral disc and adjacent vertebral bodies.

Each intervertebral foramen is a confined space surrounded by bone, ligaments, and joints. Pathology in any of these structures, and in the surrounding muscles, can affect structures within the foramen.

Surface anatomy

How to identify specific vertebral spinous processes

Identification of vertebral spinous processes (Fig. 2.8A) can be used to differentiate between regions of the vertebral column and facilitate visualizing the position of deeper structures, such as the inferior ends of the spinal cord and subarachnoid space.

The spinous process of vertebra CII can be identified through deep palpation as the most superior bony protuberance in the midline inferior to the skull.

Most of the other spinous processes, except for that of vertebra CVII, are not readily palpable because they are obscured by soft tissue.

The spinous process of CVII is usually visible as a prominent eminence in the midline at the base of the neck (Fig. 2.8B), particularly when the neck is flexed.

Inferior to the spinous process of CVII is the spinous process of TI, which is also usually visible as a midline protuberance. Often it is more prominent than the spinous process of CVII.

The root of the spine of the scapula is at the same level as the spinous process of vertebra TIII, and the inferior angle of the scapula is level with the spinous process of vertebra TVII.

The spinous process of vertebra TXII is level with the midpoint of a vertical line between the inferior angle of the scapula and the iliac crest.

A horizontal line between the highest point of the iliac crest on each side crosses through the spinous process of vertebra LIV. The LIII and LV vertebral spinous processes can be palpated above and below the LIV spinous process, respectively.

The sacral dimples that mark the position of the posterior superior iliac spine are level with the SII vertebral spinous process.

The tip of the coccyx is palpable at the base of the vertebral column between the gluteal masses.

The tips of the vertebral spinous processes do not always lie in the same horizontal plane as their corresponding vertebral bodies. In thoracic regions, the spinous processes are long and sharply sloped downward so that their tips lie at the level of the vertebral body below. In other words, the tip of the TIII vertebral spinous process lies at vertebral level TIV.

In lumbar and sacral regions, the spinous processes are generally shorter and less sloped than in thoracic regions, and their palpable tips more closely reflect the position of their corresponding vertebral bodies. As a consequence, the palpable end of the spinous process of vertebra LIV lies at approximately the LIV vertebral level.

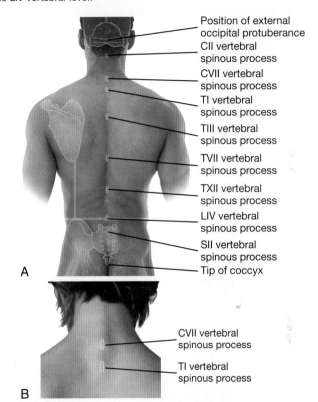

Position of external occipital protuberance
CII vertebral spinous process
CVII vertebral spinous process
TI vertebral spinous process
TIII vertebral spinous process
TVII vertebral spinous process
TXII vertebral spinous process
LIV vertebral spinous process
SII vertebral spinous process
Tip of coccyx

A

CVII vertebral spinous process
TI vertebral spinous process

B

Fig. 2.8 The back with the positions of vertebral spinous processes and associated structures indicated. **A.** In a man. **B.** In a woman with neck flexed. The prominent CVII and TI vertebral spinous processes are labeled.

Posterior spaces between vertebral arches

In most regions of the vertebral column, the laminae and spinous processes of adjacent vertebrae overlap to form a reasonably complete bony posterior (dorsal) wall for the vertebral canal. However, in the lumbar region, large gaps exist between the posterior components of adjacent vertebral arches (Fig. 2.10). These gaps between adjacent laminae and spinous processes become increasingly wide from vertebra LI to vertebra LV. The spaces can be widened further by flexion of the vertebral column. These gaps allow relatively easy access to the vertebral canal for clinical procedures.

Curvatures of vertebral column

The vertebral column has a number of curvatures (Fig. 2.11):

- The primary curvature of the vertebral column is concave anteriorly, reflecting the original shape of the embryo, and is retained in the thoracic and sacral regions in adults.
- Secondary curvatures, which are concave posteriorly, form in the cervical and lumbar regions and bring the center of gravity into a vertical line, which allows the body's weight to be balanced on the vertebral column in a way that expends the least amount of muscular energy to maintain an upright bipedal stance.

Fig. 2.9 Intervertebral foramen.

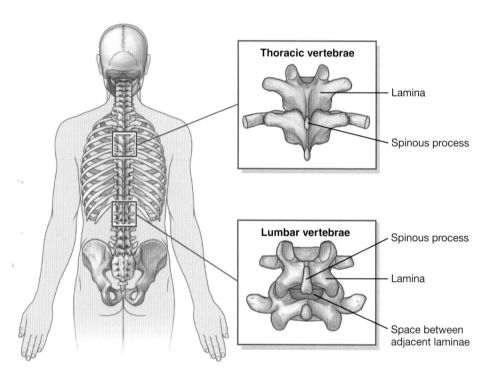

Fig. 2.10 Spaces between adjacent vertebral arches in the lumbar region.

JOINTS

Joints between vertebrae in the back

The two major types of joints between vertebrae are:

- symphyses between vertebral bodies, and
- synovial joints between articular processes.

A typical vertebra has a total of six joints with adjacent vertebrae: four synovial joints (two above and two below) and two symphyses (one above and one below). Each symphysis includes an intervertebral disc.

Although the movement between any two vertebrae is limited, the summation of movement among all vertebrae results in a large range of movement by the vertebral column.

Movements by the vertebral column include flexion, extension, lateral flexion, rotation, and circumduction.

Movements by vertebrae in a specific region (cervical, thoracic, and lumbar) are determined by the shape and orientation of joint surfaces on the articular processes and on the vertebral bodies.

Symphyses between vertebral bodies (intervertebral discs)

The symphysis between adjacent vertebral bodies is formed by a layer of hyaline cartilage on each vertebral body and an intervertebral disc, which lies between the layers.

The **intervertebral disc** consists of an outer anulus fibrosus, which surrounds a central nucleus pulposus (Fig. 2.14).

Early embryo

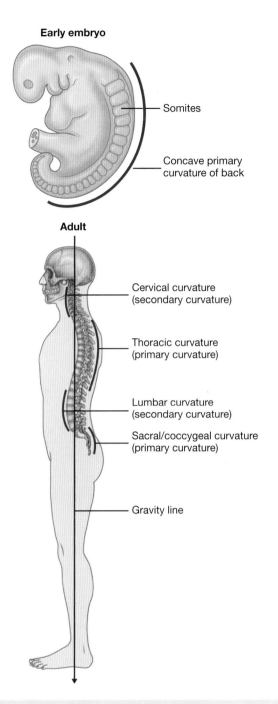

- Somites

- Concave primary curvature of back

Adult

- Cervical curvature (secondary curvature)

- Thoracic curvature (primary curvature)

- Lumbar curvature (secondary curvature)

- Sacral/coccygeal curvature (primary curvature)

- Gravity line

Fig. 2.11 Curvatures of the vertebral column.

- The **anulus fibrosus** consists of an outer ring of collagen surrounding a wider zone of fibrocartilage arranged in a lamellar configuration. This arrangement of fibers limits rotation between vertebrae.
- The **nucleus pulposus** fills the center of the intervertebral disc, is gelatinous, and absorbs compression forces between vertebrae.

Degenerative changes in the anulus fibrosus can lead to herniation of the nucleus pulposus. Posterolateral herniation can impinge on the roots of a spinal nerve in the intervertebral foramen (Fig. 2.17).

Surface anatomy

Primary and secondary curvatures in the sagittal plane

When viewed from the side, the normal vertebral column has primary curvatures in the thoracic and sacral/coccygeal regions and secondary curvatures in the cervical and lumbar regions (Fig. 2.12). The primary curvatures are concave anteriorly. The secondary curvatures are concave posteriorly.

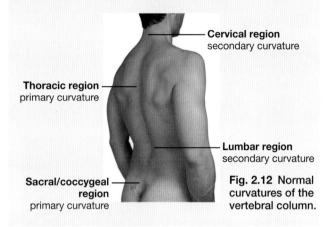

Cervical region secondary curvature

Thoracic region primary curvature

Lumbar region secondary curvature

Sacral/coccygeal region primary curvature

Fig. 2.12 Normal curvatures of the vertebral column.

Clinical app

Spina bifida

Spina bifida is a disorder in which the two sides of vertebral arches, usually in lower vertebrae, fail to fuse during development, resulting in an "open" vertebral canal. There are two types of spina bifida.

- The commonest type is spina bifida occulta in which there is a defect in the vertebral arch of LV or SI. This defect occurs in as many as 10% of individuals and results in failure of the posterior arch to fuse in the midline. Clinically, the patient is asymptomatic, although there may be a tuft of hair over the spinous processes.
- The more severe form of spina bifida involves complete failure of fusion of the posterior arch at the lumbosacral junction with a large outpouching of the meninges. This may contain cerebrospinal fluid (CSF; a **meningocele**) or a portion of the spinal cord (a **myelomeningocele**). These abnormalities may result in a variety of neurologic deficits, including problems with walking and bladder function.

Clinical app

Vertebroplasty

Vertebroplasty is a relatively new technique in which the body of a vertebra can be filled with bone cement (typically methyl methacrylate). The indications for the technique include

Continued

vertebral body collapse and pain from the vertebral body, which may be secondary to tumor infiltration. The procedure is most commonly performed for osteoporotic wedge fractures, which are a considerable cause of morbidity and pain in older patients. These types of fractures typically occur in the thoracolumbar region.

Clinical app

Scoliosis

Scoliosis is an abnormal lateral curvature of the vertebral column (Fig. 2.13).

A true scoliosis involves not only the (right- or left-sided) curvature but also a rotational element of one vertebra on another.

The commonest types of scoliosis are those for which we have little understanding about how or why they occur and are termed *idiopathic scoliosis*. These are never present at birth and tend to occur in either the infantile, juvenile, or adolescent age groups. The vertebral bodies and posterior elements (pedicles and laminae) are normal in these patients.

Fig. 2.13 Volume-rendered CT, anterior view.

Clinical app

Kyphosis

Kyphosis is abnormal curvature (exaggerated anterior concavity) of the vertebral column in the thoracic region, producing a "hunchback" deformity. This condition occurs in certain disease states, the most dramatic of which is usually secondary to tuberculosis infection of a thoracic vertebral body in which the kyphosis becomes angulated at the site of the lesion.

Clinical app

Lordosis

Lordosis is abnormal curvature (exaggerated posterior concavity) of the vertebral column in the lumbar region, producing a swayback deformity.

Clinical app

Variation in vertebral numbers

There are usually seven cervical vertebrae, although in certain diseases these may be fused. Fusion of cervical vertebrae can be associated with other abnormalities in which there is abnormal fusion of vertebrae CI and CII or CV and CVI.

Variations in the number of thoracic vertebrae are well described.

One of the commonest abnormalities in the lumbar vertebrae is a partial fusion of vertebra LV with the sacrum (sacralization of the lumbar vertebra). Partial separation of vertebra SI from the sacrum (lumbarization of first sacral vertebra) may also occur.

A hemivertebra occurs when a vertebra develops only on one side.

Clinical app

The vertebrae and cancer

The vertebrae are common sites for metastatic disease (secondary spread of cancer cells). When cancer cells grow within the vertebral bodies and the posterior elements, they destroy the mechanical properties of the bone. Importantly, vertebrae that contain extensive metastatic disease may extrude fragments of tumor into the vertebral canal, compressing the nerves and spinal cord.

Clinical app

Osteoporosis

Osteoporosis is a pathophysiologic condition in which bone quality is normal, but the quantity of bone is deficient. It is a metabolic bone disorder that commonly occurs in women in their 50s and 60s and in men in their 70s.

Typical complications of osteoporosis include "crush" vertebral body fractures, distal radial fractures, and hip fractures.

Joints between vertebral arches (zygapophysial joints)

The synovial joints between superior and inferior articular processes on adjacent vertebrae are the zygapophysial joints (Fig. 2.15). A thin articular capsule attached to the margins of the articular facets encloses each joint.

In cervical regions, the zygapophysial joints slope inferiorly from anterior to posterior and their shape facilitates

Fig. 2.14 Intervertebral joints.

Fig. 2.16 Uncovertebral joint.

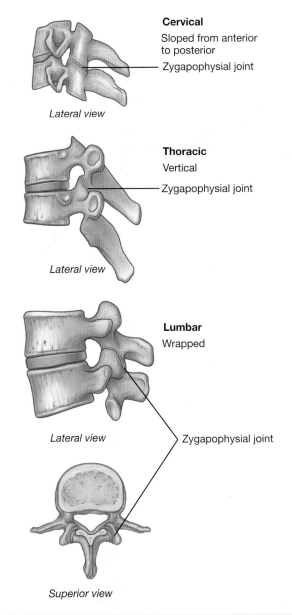

Fig. 2.15 Zygapophysial joints.

flexion and extension. In thoracic regions, the joints are oriented vertically and their shape limits flexion and extension but facilitates rotation. In lumbar regions, the joint surfaces are curved and adjacent processes interlock, thereby limiting range of movement, although flexion and extension are still major movements in the lumbar region.

"Uncovertebral" joints

The lateral margins of the upper surfaces of typical cervical vertebrae are elevated into crests or lips termed *uncinate processes*. These may articulate with the body of the vertebra above to form small "uncovertebral" synovial joints (Fig. 2.16).

Clinical app

Back pain
Back pain is an extremely common disorder. It can be related to mechanical problems or to a disc protrusion impinging on a nerve. In cases involving discs, it may be necessary to operate and remove the disc that is pressing on the nerve.

Clinical app

Herniation of intervertebral discs
The discs between the vertebrae are made up of a central portion (the nucleus pulposus) and a complex series of fibrous rings (anulus fibrosus). A tear can occur within the anulus fibrosus through which the material of the nucleus pulposus can track. After a period of time, this material may track into the vertebral canal or into the intervertebral foramen to impinge on neural structures (Fig. 2.17). This is a common cause of back pain. A disc may protrude posteriorly to directly impinge on the cord or the roots of the lumbar nerves, depending on the level, or may protrude posterolaterally adjacent to the pedicle and impinge on the descending root.

Continued

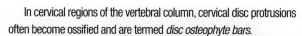

In cervical regions of the vertebral column, cervical disc protrusions often become ossified and are termed *disc osteophyte bars.*

Disc protrusion

Fig. 2.17 Disc protrusion—T2-weighted magnetic resonance images of the lumbar region of the vertebral column. **A.** Sagittal plane. **B.** Axial plane.

Clinical app

Joint diseases

Some diseases have a predilection for synovial joints rather than symphyses. A typical example is rheumatoid arthritis, which primarily affects synovial joints and synovial bursae, resulting in destruction of the joint and its lining. Symphyses are usually preserved.

LIGAMENTS

Joints between vertebrae are reinforced and supported by numerous ligaments, which pass between vertebral bodies and interconnect components of the vertebral arches.

Anterior and posterior longitudinal ligaments

The anterior and posterior longitudinal ligaments are on the anterior and posterior surfaces of the vertebral bodies and extend along most of the vertebral column (Fig. 2.18).

The **anterior longitudinal ligament** is attached superiorly to the base of the skull and extends inferiorly to attach to the anterior surface of the sacrum. Along its length, it is attached to the vertebral bodies and intervertebral discs.

The **posterior longitudinal ligament** is on the posterior surfaces of the vertebral bodies and lines the anterior surface of the vertebral canal. Like the anterior longitudinal ligament, it is attached along its length to the vertebral bodies and intervertebral discs. The upper part of the posterior longitudinal ligament that connects CII to the intracranial aspect of the base of the skull is termed the **tectorial membrane.**

Posterior longitudinal ligament

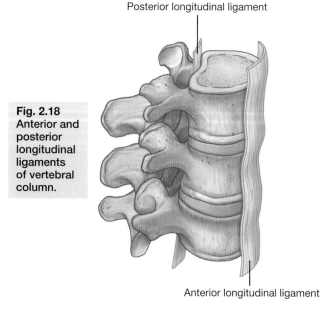

Fig. 2.18 Anterior and posterior longitudinal ligaments of vertebral column.

Anterior longitudinal ligament

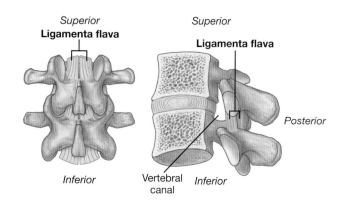

Superior
Ligamenta flava

Superior

Ligamenta flava

Posterior

Inferior

Vertebral canal

Inferior

Fig. 2.19 Ligamenta flava.

Ligamenta flava

The **ligamenta flava**, on each side, pass between the laminae of adjacent vertebrae (Fig. 2.19). These thin, broad ligaments consist predominantly of elastic tissue and form part of the posterior surface of the vertebral canal. Each ligamentum flavum runs between the posterior surface of the lamina on the vertebra below to the anterior surface of the lamina of the vertebra above. The ligamenta flava resist separation of the laminae in flexion and assist in extension back to the anatomical position.

Supraspinous ligament and ligamentum nuchae

The supraspinous ligament connects and passes along the tips of the vertebral spinous processes from vertebra CVII

Fig. 2.20 Supraspinous ligament and ligamentum nuchae.

External occipital protuberance

Ligamentum nuchae

Spinous process of vertebra CVII

Supraspinous ligament

Ligamentum flavum

Supraspinous ligament

Interspinous ligament

Ligamentum flavum

Supraspinous ligament

Fig. 2.21 Interspinous ligaments.

to the sacrum (Fig. 2.20). From vertebra CVII to the skull, the ligament becomes structurally distinct from more caudal parts of the ligament and is called the *ligamentum nuchae*.

The **ligamentum nuchae** is a triangular, sheet-like structure in the median sagittal plane:

- The base of the triangle is attached to the skull, from the external occipital protuberance to the foramen magnum.
- The apex is attached to the tip of the spinous process of vertebra CVII.
- The deep side of the triangle is attached to the posterior tubercle of vertebra CI and the spinous processes of the other cervical vertebrae.

The ligamentum nuchae supports the head. It resists flexion and facilitates returning the head to the anatomical position. The broad lateral surfaces and the posterior edge of the ligament provide attachment for adjacent muscles.

Interspinous ligaments

Interspinous ligaments pass between adjacent vertebral spinous processes (Fig. 2.21). They attach from the base to the apex of each spinous process and blend with the supraspinous ligament posteriorly and the ligamenta flava anteriorly on each side.

Clinical app

Ligamenta flava
In degenerative conditions of the vertebral column, the ligamenta flava may hypertrophy. This is often associated with hypertrophy and arthritic change of the zygapophysial joints. In combination, zygapophysial joint hypertrophy, ligamenta flava hypertrophy, and a mild disc protrusion can reduce the dimensions of the vertebral canal.

Clinical app

Vertebral fractures
Vertebral column stability is divided into three arbitrary clinical "columns:" the **anterior column** consists of the vertebral bodies and the anterior longitudinal ligament; the **middle column** comprises the vertebral body and the posterior longitudinal ligament; and the **posterior column** is made up of the ligamenta flava, interspinous ligaments, supraspinous ligaments, and the ligamentum nuchae in the cervical vertebral column.

Destruction of one of the clinical columns is usually a stable injury requiring little more than rest and appropriate analgesia. Disruption of two columns is likely to be unstable and requires fixation and immobilization. A three-column spinal injury usually results in a significant neurologic event and requires fixation to prevent further extension of the neurologic defect and to create vertebral column stability.

Clinical app

Pars interarticularis fractures

The *pars interarticularis* is a clinical term used to describe the specific region of a vertebra between the superior and inferior facet (zygapophysial) joints. This region is susceptible to trauma, especially in athletes.

If a fracture occurs around the pars interarticularis, the vertebral body may slip anteriorly and compress the vertebral canal. The most common sites for pars interarticularis fractures are the LIV and LV levels. It is possible for a vertebra to slip anteriorly on its inferior counterpart without a pars interarticularis fracture. Usually this is related to abnormal anatomy of the facet joints: facet joint degenerative change. This disorder is termed **spondylolisthesis.**

Clinical app

Surgical procedures on the back
Discectomy

A prolapsed intervertebral disc may impinge on the meningeal (thecal) sac, cord, and most commonly the nerve root, producing symptoms attributable to that level. In some instances the disc protrusion will undergo a degree of involution that may allow symptoms to resolve without intervention. In some instances, pain, loss of function, and failure to resolve may require surgery to remove the disc protrusion.

Spinal fusion

Spinal (vertebral) fusion is performed when it is necessary to fuse one vertebra with the corresponding superior or inferior vertebra, and in some instances multilevel fusion may be necessary. Indications are varied, although they include stabilization after fracture, stabilization related to tumor infiltration, and stabilization when mechanical pain is produced either from the disc or from the posterior elements.

BACK MUSCULATURE

Muscles of the back are organized into superficial, intermediate, and deep groups.

Muscles in the superficial and intermediate groups are extrinsic muscles because they originate embryologically from locations other than the back. They are innervated by anterior rami of spinal nerves:

- The superficial group consists of muscles related to and involved in movements of the upper limb.
- The intermediate group consists of muscles attached to the ribs and may serve a respiratory function.

Muscles of the deep group are intrinsic muscles because they develop in the back. They are innervated by posterior rami of spinal nerves and are directly related to movements of the vertebral column and head.

Superficial group of back muscles

The muscles in the superficial group are immediately deep to the skin and superficial fascia. They attach the superior part of the appendicular skeleton (clavicle, scapula, and humerus) to the axial skeleton (skull, ribs, and vertebral column). Because these muscles are primarily involved with movements of this part of the appendicular skeleton, they are sometimes referred to as the **appendicular group.**

Muscles in the superficial group include the **trapezius, latissimus dorsi, rhomboid major, rhomboid minor,** and **levator scapulae** (Fig. 2.22). Rhomboid major, rhomboid minor, and levator scapulae are located deep to the trapezius in the superior part of the back.

Trapezius

Each **trapezius** muscle is flat and triangular, with the base of the triangle situated along the vertebral column (the muscle's origin) and the apex pointing toward the tip of the

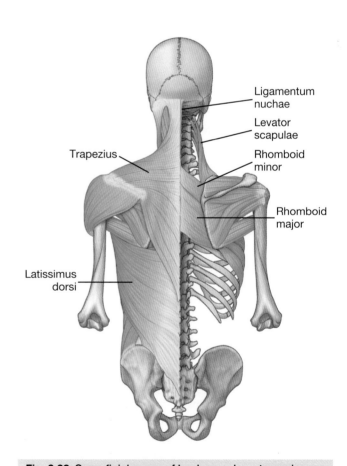

Ligamentum nuchae

Levator scapulae

Rhomboid minor

Trapezius

Rhomboid major

Latissimus dorsi

Fig. 2.22 Superficial group of back muscles—trapezius and latissimus dorsi with rhomboid major, rhomboid minor, and levator scapulae located deep to trapezius in the superior part of the back.

Table 2.1 Superficial (appendicular) group of back muscles

Muscle	Origin	Insertion	Innervation	Function
Trapezius	Superior nuchal line, external occipital protuberance, ligamentum nuchae, spinous processes of CVII to TXII	Lateral one-third of clavicle, acromion, spine of scapula	Motor—accessory nerve [XI]; proprioception—C3 and C4	Assists in rotating the scapula during abduction of humerus above horizontal; upper fibers elevate, middle fibers adduct, and lower fibers depress scapula
Latissimus dorsi	Spinous processes of TVII to LV and sacrum, iliac crest, ribs X to XII	Floor of intertubercular sulcus of humerus	Thoracodorsal nerve (C6 to C8)	Extends, adducts, and medially rotates humerus
Levator scapulae	Transverse processes of CI to CIV	Upper portion medial border of scapula	C3 to C4 and dorsal scapular nerve (C4, C5)	Elevates scapula
Rhomboid major	Spinous processes of TII to TV	Medial border of scapula between spine and inferior angle	Dorsal scapular nerve (C4, C5)	Retracts (adducts) and elevates scapula
Rhomboid minor	Lower portion of ligamentum nuchae, spinous processes of CVII and TI	Medial border of scapula at the spine of scapula	Dorsal scapular nerve (C4, C5)	Retracts (adducts) and elevates scapula

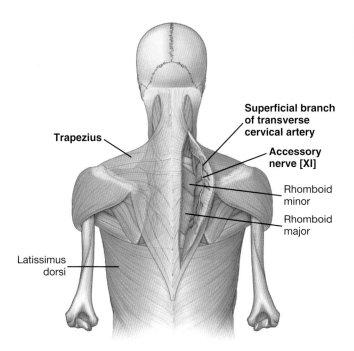

Fig. 2.23 Innervation and blood supply of trapezius.

shoulder (the muscle's insertion) (Table 2.1, Fig. 2.22). The muscles on both sides together form a trapezoid.

Motor innervation of the trapezius is by the accessory nerve [XI], which descends from the neck onto the deep surface of the muscle (Fig. 2.23). Proprioceptive fibers from trapezius pass in the branches of the cervical plexus and enter the spinal cord at spinal cord levels C3 and C4.

The blood supply to trapezius is from the superficial branch of the transverse cervical artery (Fig. 2.23), the acromial branch of the suprascapular artery, and dorsal branches of posterior intercostal arteries.

Latissimus dorsi

Latissimus dorsi is a large, flat triangular muscle that begins in the lower portion of the back and tapers as it ascends to a narrow tendon that attaches to the humerus anteriorly (Table 2.1, Fig. 2.22).

The thoracodorsal nerve of the brachial plexus innervates the latissimus dorsi muscle. Associated with this nerve is the thoracodorsal artery, which is the primary blood supply of the muscle. Additional small arteries come from dorsal branches of posterior intercostal and lumbar arteries.

Levator scapulae

Levator scapulae is a slender muscle that descends from the transverse processes of the upper cervical vertebrae to the upper portion of the scapula on its medial border at the superior angle (Table 2.1, Fig. 2.22). It is innervated by branches from the anterior rami of spinal nerves C3 and C4 and the dorsal scapular nerve, and its arterial supply consists

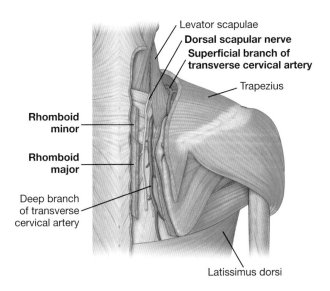

Fig. 2.24 Innervation and blood supply of the rhomboid muscles.

Fig. 2.25 Intermediate group of back muscles—serratus posterior muscles.

of branches primarily from the transverse and ascending cervical arteries.

Rhomboid minor and rhomboid major

The two rhomboid muscles are inferior to levator scapulae (Table 2.1, Fig. 2.22).

The two rhomboid muscles work together to retract or pull the scapula toward the vertebral column. The dorsal scapular nerve, a branch of the brachial plexus, innervates both rhomboid muscles (Fig. 2.24).

An injury to the dorsal scapular nerve, which innervates the rhomboids, may result in a lateral shift in the position of the scapula on the affected side (i.e., the normal position of the scapula is lost because of the affected muscle's inability to prevent antagonistic muscles from pulling the scapula laterally).

Intermediate group of back muscles

The muscles in the intermediate group of back muscles consist of two thin muscular sheets in the superior and inferior regions of the back, immediately deep to the muscles in the superficial group (Table 2.2, Fig. 2.25). Fibers from these two serratus posterior muscles (**serratus posterior superior** and **serratus posterior inferior**) pass obliquely outward from the vertebral column to attach to the ribs. This positioning suggests a respiratory function, and, at times, these muscles have been referred to as the respiratory group.

Serratus posterior superior is deep to the rhomboid muscles, whereas serratus posterior inferior is deep to the latissimus dorsi. They are innervated by segmental branches of the anterior rami of intercostal nerves. Their vascular supply is provided by a similar segmental pattern through the intercostal arteries.

Table 2.2 Intermediate (respiratory) group of back muscles

Muscle	Origin	Insertion	Innervation	Function
Serratus posterior superior	Lower portion of ligamentum nuchae, spinous processes of CVII to TIII and supraspinous ligaments	Upper border of ribs II to V just lateral to their angles	Anterior rami of upper thoracic nerves (T2 to T5)	Elevates ribs II to V
Serratus posterior inferior	Spinous processes of TXI to LIII and supraspinous ligaments	Lower border of ribs IX to XII just lateral to their angles	Anterior rami of lower thoracic nerves (T9 to T12)	Depresses ribs IX to XII and may prevent lower ribs from being elevated when the diaphragm contracts

Table 2.3 Spinotransversales muscles

Muscle	Origin	Insertion	Innervation	Function
Splenius capitis	Lower half of ligamentum nuchae, spinous processes of CVII to TIV	Mastoid process, skull below lateral one-third of superior nuchal line	Posterior rami middle cervical nerves	Together—draw head backward, extending neck; individually—draw and rotate head to one side (turn face to same side)
Splenius cervicis	Spinous processes of TIII to TVI	Transverse processes of CI to CIII	Posterior rami lower cervical nerves	Together—extend neck; individually—draw and rotate head to one side (turn face to same side)

Ligamentum nuchae

Splenius capitis

Levator scapulae

Splenius cervicis

Fig. 2.26 Deep group of back muscles—spinotransversales muscles (splenius capitis and splenius cervicis).

Deep group of back muscles

The deep or intrinsic muscles of the back extend from the pelvis to the skull and are innervated by segmental branches of the posterior rami of spinal nerves. Muscles in this group include the spinotransversales, erector spinae, transversospinales, segmental, and suboccipital muscles.

Spinotransversales muscles

The two spinotransversales muscles run from the spinous processes and ligamentum nuchae upward and laterally (Table 2.3, Fig. 2.26):

- **Splenius capitis** is a broad muscle attached to the occipital bone and mastoid process of the temporal bone.
- **Splenius cervicis** is a narrow muscle attached to the transverse processes of the upper cervical vertebrae.

Erector spinae muscles

The erector spinae is the largest group of intrinsic back muscles. The muscles lie posterolaterally to the vertebral column between the spinous processes medially and the angles of the ribs laterally (Table 2.4, Fig. 2.27). In the upper lumbar region, the erector spinae divides into three vertical columns of muscle, each of which is further subdivided regionally (lumborum, thoracis, cervicis, and capitis), depending on where the muscles attach superiorly.

- The outer or most laterally placed column of the erector spinae muscles is the **iliocostalis.**
- The middle or intermediate column is the **longissimus.**
- The most medial muscle column is the **spinalis.**

The muscles in the erector spinae group are the primary extensors of the vertebral column and head. Acting bilaterally, they straighten the back, returning it to the upright position from a flexed position, and pull the head posteriorly. They also participate in controlling vertebral column flexion by contracting and relaxing in a coordinated fashion. Acting unilaterally, they bend the vertebral column laterally. In addition, unilateral contractions of muscles attached to the head turn the head to the actively contracting side.

Transversospinales muscles

The transversospinales muscles run obliquely upward and medially from transverse processes to spinous processes, filling the groove between these two vertebral projections (Table 2.5, Fig. 2.28). They are deep to the erector spinae and consist of three major subgroups—the semispinalis, multifidus, and rotatores muscles.

- The **semispinalis** muscles are the most superficial collection of muscle fibers in the transversospinales group. They begin in the lower thoracic region and end by attaching to the skull, crossing between four and six vertebrae.
- Deep to the semispinalis is the second group of muscles, the **multifidus.** Muscles in this group span the length

Table 2.4 Erector spinae group of back muscles

Muscle	Origin	Insertion
Iliocostalis lumborum	Sacrum, spinous processes of lumbar and lower two thoracic vertebrae and their supraspinous ligaments, and the iliac crest	Angles of the lower six or seven ribs
Iliocostalis thoracis	Angles of the lower six ribs	Angles of the upper six ribs and the transverse process of CVII
Iliocostalis cervicis	Angles of ribs III to VI	Transverse processes of CIV to CVI
Longissimus thoracis	Blends with iliocostalis in lumbar region and is attached to transverse processes of lumbar vertebrae	Transverse processes of all thoracic vertebrae and just lateral to the tubercles of the lower nine or ten ribs
Longissimus cervicis	Transverse processes of upper four or five thoracic vertebrae	Transverse processes of CII to CVI
Longissimus capitis	Transverse processes of upper four or five thoracic vertebrae and articular processes of lower three or four cervical vertebrae	Posterior margin of the mastoid process
Spinalis thoracis	Spinous processes of TX or TXI to LII	Spinous processes of TI to TVIII (varies)
Spinalis cervicis	Lower part of ligamentum nuchae and spinous process of CVII (sometimes TI to TII)	Spinous process of CII (axis)
Spinalis capitis	Usually blends with semispinalis capitis	With semispinalis capitis

Splenius capitis
Spinous process of CVII
Spinalis
Longissimus
Iliocostalis
Iliac crest
Ligamentum nuchae
Longissimus capitis
Iliocostalis cervicis
Longissimus cervicis
Spinalis thoracis
Longissimus thoracis
Iliocostalis thoracis
Iliocostalis lumborum

Fig. 2.27 Deep group of back muscles—erector spinae muscles.

of the vertebral column spanning between two and four vertebrae.

■ The small **rotatores** muscles are the deepest of the transversospinales group and span the length of the vertebral column, crossing two vertebrae (long rotators) or attaching to adjacent vertebra (short rotators).

When muscles in the transversospinales group contract bilaterally, they extend the vertebral column, an action similar to that of the erector spinae group. However, when muscles on only one side contract, they pull the spinous processes toward the transverse processes on that side, causing the trunk to turn or rotate in the opposite direction.

One muscle in the transversospinales group, the **semispinalis capitis,** has a unique action because it attaches to the skull. Contracting bilaterally, this muscle pulls the head posteriorly, whereas unilateral contraction pulls the head posteriorly and turns it, causing the chin to move superiorly and turn toward the side of the contracting muscle.

Segmental muscles

The two groups of segmental muscles (Table 2.6, Fig. 2.28) are deeply placed in the back and innervated by posterior rami of spinal nerves.

■ The first group of segmental muscles are the **levatores costarum** muscles.
■ The second group of segmental muscles are the true segmental muscles of the back—the **interspinales** and the **intertransversarii.**

Suboccipital muscles

A small group of deep muscles in the upper cervical region at the base of the occipital bone move the head. Because of their location they are sometimes referred to as suboccipital muscles (Table 2.7, Figs. 2.28, 2.29). They include, on each side:

■ **rectus capitis posterior major,**
■ **rectus capitis posterior minor,**
■ **obliquus capitis inferior, and**
■ **obliquus capitis superior.**

Table 2.5 Transversospinales group of back muscles

Muscle	Origin	Insertion
Semispinalis thoracis	Transverse processes of TVI to TX	Spinous processes of upper four thoracic and lower two cervical vertebrae
Semispinalis cervicis	Transverse processes of upper five or six thoracic vertebrae	Spinous processes of CII (axis) to CV
Semispinalis capitis	Transverse processes of TI to TVI (or TVII) and CVII and articular processes of CIV to CVI	Medial area between the superior and inferior nuchal lines of occipital bone
Multifidus	Sacrum, origin of erector spinae, posterior superior iliac spine, mammillary processes of lumbar vertebrae, transverse processes of thoracic vertebrae, and articular processes of lower four cervical vertebrae	Base of spinous processes of all vertebrae from LV to CII (axis)
Rotatores lumborum	Mammillary processes of lumbar vertebrae	Spinous processes of lumbar vertebrae
Rotatores thoracis	Transverse processes of thoracic vertebrae	Spinous processes of thoracic vertebrae
Rotatores cervicis	Articular processes of cervical vertebrae	Spinous processes of cervical vertebrae

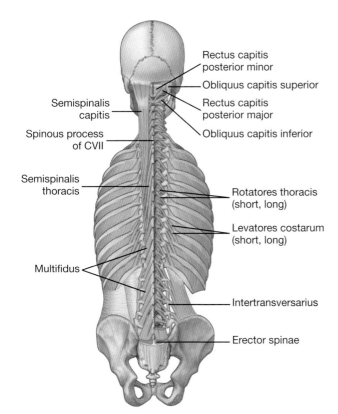

Fig. 2.28 Deep group of back muscles—transversospinales and segmental muscles.

Contraction of the suboccipital muscles extends and rotates the head at the atlanto-occipital and atlanto-axial joints, respectively.

The suboccipital muscles are innervated by the posterior ramus of the first cervical nerve, which enters the area between the vertebral artery and the posterior arch of the atlas (Fig. 2.29). The vascular supply to the muscles in this area is from branches of the vertebral and occipital arteries.

The suboccipital muscles form the boundaries of the **suboccipital triangle** (Fig. 2.29):

- Rectus capitis posterior major forms the medial border of the triangle.
- Obliquus capitis superior muscle forms the lateral border.
- Obliquus capitis inferior muscle forms the inferior border.

The suboccipital triangle contains several important structures:

- Posterior ramus of C1,
- Vertebral artery, and
- Veins

Thoracolumbar fascia

The **thoracolumbar fascia** covers the deep muscles of the back and trunk (Fig. 2.30). This fascial layer is critical to the overall organization and integrity of the region:

- Superiorly, it passes anteriorly to the serratus posterior superior muscle and is continuous with deep fascia in the neck.
- In the thoracic region, it covers the deep muscles and separates them from the muscles in the superficial and intermediate groups.
- Medially, it attaches to the spinous processes of the thoracic vertebrae and, laterally, to the angles of the ribs.

In the lumbar region, the thoracolumbar fascia consists of three layers:

- The posterior layer is thick and is attached to the spinous processes of the lumbar vertebrae, sacral vertebrae, and

Table 2.6 Segmental back muscles

Muscle	Origin	Insertion	Function
Levatores costarum	Short paired muscles arising from transverse processes of CVII to TXI	The rib below vertebra of origin near tubercle	Contraction elevates rib
Interspinales	Short paired muscles attached to the spinous processes of contiguous vertebrae, one on each side of the interspinous ligament		Postural muscles that stabilize adjoining vertebrae during movements of vertebral column
Intertransversarii	Small muscles between the transverse processes of contiguous vertebrae		Postural muscles that stabilize adjoining vertebrae during movements of vertebral column

Table 2.7 Suboccipital group of back muscles

Muscle	Origin	Insertion	Innervation	Function
Rectus capitis posterior major	Spinous process of axis (CII)	Lateral portion of occipital bone below inferior nuchal line	Posterior ramus of C1	Extension of head; rotation of face to same side as muscle
Rectus capitis posterior minor	Posterior tubercle of atlas (CI)	Medial portion of occipital bone below inferior nuchal line	Posterior ramus of C1	Extension of head
Obliquus capitis superior	Transverse process of atlas (CI)	Occipital bone between superior and inferior nuchal lines	Posterior ramus of C1	Extension of head and bends it to same side
Obliquus capitis inferior	Spinous process of axis (CII)	Transverse process of atlas (CI)	Posterior ramus of C1	Rotation of face to same side

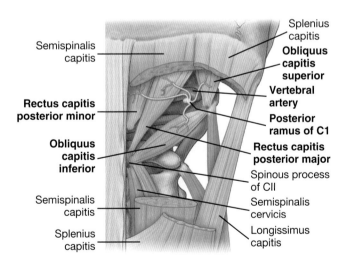

Fig. 2.29 Deep group of back muscles—suboccipital muscles. This also shows the borders of the suboccipital triangle.

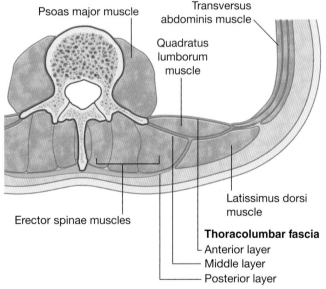

Fig. 2.30 Thoracolumbar fascia and the deep back muscles in the lumbar region (transverse section).

the supraspinous ligament—from these attachments, it extends laterally to cover the erector spinae.

■ The middle layer is attached medially to the tips of the transverse processes of the lumbar vertebrae and intertransverse ligaments—inferiorly it is attached to the iliac crest and superiorly to the lower border of rib XII.

■ The anterior layer covers the anterior surface of the quadratus lumborum muscle (a muscle of the posterior abdominal wall) and is attached medially to the transverse processes of the lumbar vertebrae—inferiorly, it is attached to the iliac crest, and superiorly, it forms the lateral arcuate ligament for attachment of the diaphragm.

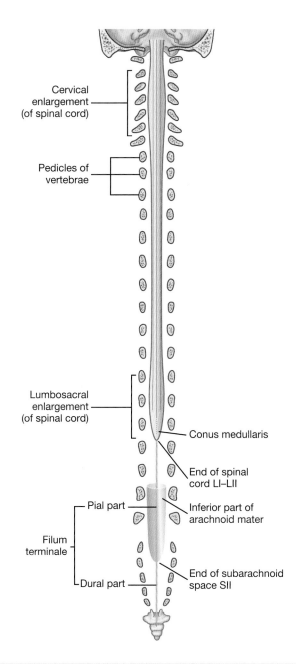

Cervical
enlargement
(of spinal cord)

Pedicles of
vertebrae

Lumbosacral
enlargement
(of spinal cord)

Conus medullaris

End of spinal
cord LI–LII

Pial part

Inferior part of
arachnoid mater

Filum
terminale

Dural part

End of subarachnoid
space SII

Fig. 2.31 Spinal cord.

The posterior and middle layers of the thoracolumbar fascia come together at the lateral margin of the erector spinae (Fig. 2.30). At the lateral border of the quadratus lumborum, the anterior layer joins them and forms the aponeurotic origin for the transversus abdominis muscle of the abdominal wall.

SPINAL CORD

The spinal cord extends from the foramen magnum to approximately the level of the disc between vertebrae LI and LII in adults, although it can end as high as vertebra TXII or

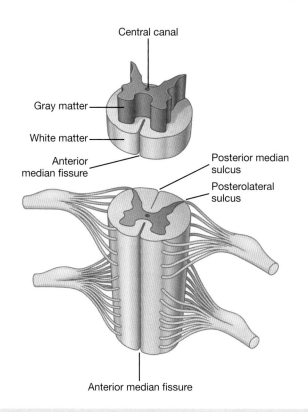

Central canal

Gray matter

White matter

Anterior
median fissure

Posterior median
sulcus

Posterolateral
sulcus

Anterior median fissure

Fig. 2.32 Features of the spinal cord.

as low as the disc between vertebrae LII and LIII (Fig. 2.31). In neonates, the spinal cord extends approximately to vertebra LIII but can reach as low as vertebra LIV. The distal end of the cord (the **conus medullaris**) is cone shaped. A fine filament of connective tissue (the pial part of the **filum terminale**) continues inferiorly from the apex of the **conus medullaris.**

The spinal cord is not uniform in diameter along its length. It has two major swellings or enlargements in regions associated with the origin of spinal nerves that innervate the upper and lower limbs. A **cervical enlargement** occurs in the region associated with the origins of spinal nerves C5 to T1, which innervate the upper limbs. A lumbosacral enlargement occurs in the region associated with the origins of spinal nerves L1 to S3, which innervate the lower limbs (Fig. 2.31).

The external surface of the spinal cord is marked by a number of fissures and sulci (Fig. 2.32):

- The **anterior median fissure** extends the length of the anterior surface.
- The **posterior median sulcus** extends along the posterior surface.
- The **posterolateral sulcus** on each side of the posterior surface marks where the posterior rootlets of spinal nerves enter the cord.

Internally, the cord has a small central canal surrounded by gray and white matter (Fig. 2.32):

- The gray matter is rich in nerve cell bodies, which form longitudinal columns along the cord, and in cross-section, these columns form a characteristic H-shaped appearance in the central regions of the cord.
- The white matter surrounds the gray matter and is rich in nerve cell processes, which form large bundles or tracts that ascend and descend in the cord to other spinal cord levels or carry information to and from the brain.

Vasculature

Arteries

The arterial supply to the spinal cord comes from two sources (Fig. 2.33A). It consists of:

- longitudinally oriented vessels, arising superior to the cervical portion of the cord, that descend on the surface of the cord; and
- feeder arteries that enter the vertebral canal through the intervertebral foramina at every level; these feeder vessels, or **segmental spinal arteries,** arise predominantly from the vertebral and deep cervical arteries in the neck, the posterior intercostal arteries in the thorax, and the lumbar arteries in the abdomen.

After entering an intervertebral foramen, the segmental spinal arteries give rise to **anterior** and **posterior radicular arteries** (Fig. 2.33). This occurs at every vertebral level. The radicular arteries follow and supply the anterior and posterior roots. At various vertebral levels, the **segmental spinal arteries** also give off **segmental medullary arteries** (Fig. 2.33B). These vessels pass directly to the longitudinally oriented vessels, reinforcing these.

The longitudinal vessels consist of:

- a single **anterior spinal artery,** which originates within the cranial cavity as the union of two vessels that arise from the vertebral arteries—the resulting single anterior spinal artery passes inferiorly approximately parallel to the anterior median fissure along the surface of the spinal cord; and
- two **posterior spinal arteries,** which also originate in the cranial cavity, usually arising directly from a terminal branch of each vertebral artery (the posterior inferior cerebellar artery)—the right and left posterior spinal arteries descend along the spinal cord, each as two branches that bracket the posterolateral sulcus and the connection of posterior roots with the spinal cord.

The anterior and posterior spinal arteries are reinforced along their length by 8 to 10 segmental medullary arteries (Fig. 2.33). The largest of these is the **arteria radicularis**

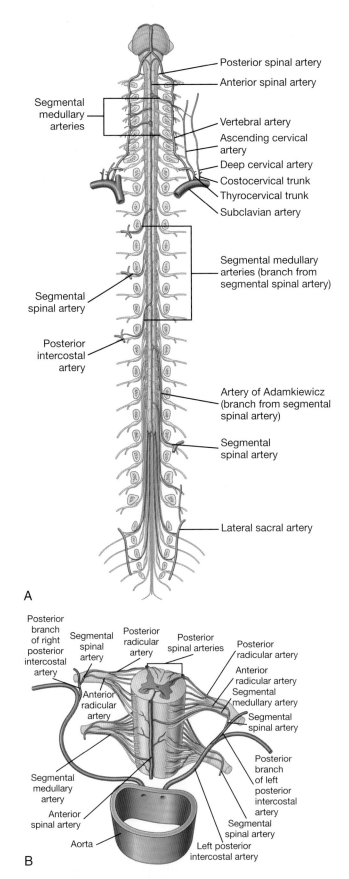

A

B

Fig. 2.33 Arteries that supply the spinal cord. **A.** Anterior view of spinal cord (not all segmental spinal arteries are shown). **B.** Segmental supply of the spinal cord.

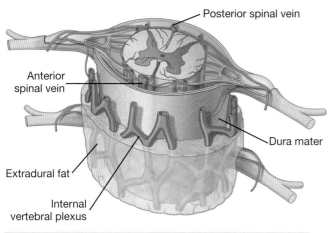

Fig. 2.34 Veins that drain the spinal cord.

Fig. 2.35 Meninges.

magna or the **artery of Adamkiewicz** (Fig. 2.33A). This vessel arises in the lower thoracic or upper lumbar region, usually on the left side, and reinforces the arterial supply to the lower portion of the spinal cord, including the lumbar enlargement.

Veins

Veins that drain the spinal cord form a number of longitudinal channels (Fig. 2.34):

- two pairs of veins on each side bracket the connections of the posterior and anterior roots to the cord;
- one midline channel parallels the anterior median fissure; and
- one midline channel passes along the posterior median sulcus.

These longitudinal channels drain into an extensive internal vertebral plexus in the extradural (epidural) space of the vertebral canal, which then drains into segmentally arranged vessels that connect with major systemic veins, such as the azygos system in the thorax. The internal vertebral venous plexus also communicates with intracranial veins.

Meninges
Spinal dura mater

The **spinal dura mater** (Fig. 2.35) is the outermost meningeal membrane and is separated from the bones forming the vertebral canal by an extradural (epidural) space. Superiorly, it is continuous with the inner meningeal layer of cranial dura mater at the foramen magnum of the skull. Inferiorly, the dural sac dramatically narrows at the level of the lower border of vertebra SII and forms an investing sheath for the pial part of the filum terminale of the spinal cord. This

terminal cord-like extension of dura mater (the dural part of the filum terminale) attaches to the posterior surface of the vertebral bodies of the coccyx.

As spinal nerves and their roots pass laterally, they are surrounded by tubular sleeves of dura mater, which merge with and become part of the outer covering (epineurium) of the nerves.

Arachnoid mater

The **arachnoid mater** is a thin delicate membrane against, but not adherent to, the deep surface of the dura mater (Fig. 2.35). It is separated from the pia mater by the subarachnoid space. The arachnoid mater ends at the level of vertebra SII (see Fig. 2.31).

Subarachnoid space

The subarachnoid space between the arachnoid and pia mater contains CSF (Fig. 2.35). The subarachnoid space around the spinal cord is continuous at the foramen magnum with the subarachnoid space surrounding the brain. Inferiorly, the subarachnoid space terminates at approximately the level of the lower border of vertebra SII (see Fig. 2.31).

Delicate strands of tissue (**arachnoid trabeculae**) are continuous with the arachnoid mater on one side and the pia mater on the other, span the subarachnoid space, and interconnect the two adjacent membranes. Large blood vessels are suspended in the subarachnoid space by similar strands of material, which expand over the vessels to form a continuous external coat.

The subarachnoid space extends further inferiorly than the spinal cord. The spinal cord ends at approximately the disc between vertebrae LI and LII, whereas the subarachnoid space extends to approximately the lower border of vertebra SII (see Fig. 2.31). The subarachnoid space is largest in the region inferior to the terminal end of the spinal cord where it surrounds the cauda equina. As a consequence, CSF can be withdrawn from the subarachnoid space in the lower lumbar region without endangering the spinal cord (Fig. 2.36).

Visualizing the inferior ends of the spinal cord and subarachnoid space

The spinal cord does not occupy the entire length of the vertebral canal. Normally in adults, it terminates at the level of the disc between vertebrae LI and LII; however, it may end as high as TXII or as low as the disc between vertebrae LII and LIII. The subarachnoid space ends at approximately the level of vertebra SII (Fig. 2.36A).

Because the subarachnoid space can be accessed in the lower lumbar region without endangering the spinal cord, it is important to be able to identify the position of the lumbar vertebral spinous processes. The LIV vertebral spinous process is level with a horizontal line between the highest points on the iliac crests. In the lumbar region, the palpable ends of the vertebral spinous processes lie opposite their corresponding vertebral bodies. The subarachnoid space can be accessed between vertebral levels LIII and LIV and between LIV and LV without endangering the spinal cord (Fig. 2.36B). The subarachnoid space ends at vertebral level SII, which is level with the sacral dimples marking the posterior superior iliac spines.

Fig. 2.36 Back with the ends of the spinal cord and subarachnoid space indicated. **A.** In a man. **B.** In a woman lying on her side in a fetal position, which accentuates the lumbar vertebral spinous processes and opens the spaces between adjacent vertebral arches. Cerebrospinal fluid can be withdrawn from the subarachnoid space in lower lumbar regions without endangering the spinal cord.

Pia mater

The spinal pia mater is a vascular membrane that firmly adheres to the surface of the spinal cord (Fig. 2.35). It extends into the anterior median fissure and reflects as sleeve-like coatings onto posterior and anterior rootlets and roots as they cross the subarachnoid space. As the roots exit the space, the sleeve-like coatings reflect onto the arachnoid mater.

On each side of the spinal cord, a longitudinally oriented sheet of pia mater (the **denticulate ligament**) extends laterally from the cord toward the arachnoid and dura mater (Fig. 2.35).

- Medially, each denticulate ligament is attached to the spinal cord in a plane that lies between the origins of the posterior and anterior rootlets.
- Laterally, each denticulate ligament forms a series of triangular extensions along its free border, with the apex of each extension being anchored through the arachnoid mater to the dura mater.

The denticulate ligaments generally occur between the exit points of adjacent posterior and anterior rootlets and position the spinal cord in the center of the subarachnoid space.

Arrangement of structures in the vertebral canal

The vertebral canal is bordered:

- anteriorly by the bodies of the vertebrae, intervertebral discs, and the posterior longitudinal ligament (Fig. 2.37);
- laterally, on each side by the pedicles and intervertebral foramina; and
- posteriorly by the laminae and ligamenta flava and in the median plane the roots of the interspinous ligaments and vertebral spinous processes.

Between the walls of the vertebral canal and the dural sac is an extradural space containing a vertebral plexus of veins embedded in fatty connective tissue.

Spinal nerves

Each spinal nerve is connected to the spinal cord by posterior and anterior roots (Fig. 2.38):

- The **posterior root** contains the processes of sensory neurons carrying information to the central nervous system (CNS). The cell bodies of the sensory neurons,

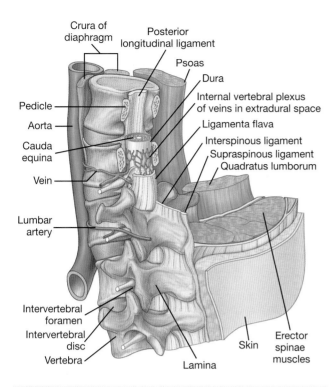

Fig. 2.37 Arrangement of structures in the vertebral canal and the back.

Fig. 2.38 Basic organization of a spinal nerve.

which are derived embryologically from neural crest cells, are clustered in a **spinal ganglion** at the distal end of the posterior root, usually in the intervertebral foramen.

- The **anterior root** contains motor nerve fibers, which carry signals away from the CNS. The cell bodies of the primary motor neurons are in anterior regions of the spinal cord.

Medially, the posterior and anterior roots divide into rootlets, which attach to the spinal cord.

A **spinal segment** is the area of the spinal cord that gives rise to the **posterior** and **anterior rootlets,** which will form a single pair of spinal nerves. Laterally, the posterior and anterior roots on each side join to form a spinal nerve.

Each spinal nerve divides, as it emerges from an intervertebral foramen, into two major branches: a small posterior ramus and a much larger anterior ramus (Fig. 2.38):

- The **posterior rami** innervate only intrinsic back muscles (the epaxial muscles) and an associated narrow strip of skin on the back.
- The **anterior rami** innervate most other skeletal muscles (the hypaxial muscles) of the body, including those of the limbs and trunk, and most remaining areas of the skin, except for certain regions of the head.

Near the point of division into anterior and posterior rami, each spinal nerve gives rise to two to four small recurrent meningeal (sinuvertebral) nerves (see Fig. 2.35). These nerves re-enter the intervertebral foramen to supply dura, ligaments, intervertebral discs, and blood vessels.

All major somatic plexuses (cervical, brachial, lumbar, and sacral) are formed by anterior rami.

Because the spinal cord is much shorter than the vertebral column, the roots of spinal nerves become longer and pass more obliquely from the cervical to coccygeal regions of the vertebral canal (Fig. 2.39).

In adults, the spinal cord terminates at a level approximately between vertebrae LI and LII, but this can range between vertebra TXII and the disc between vertebrae LII and LIII. Consequently, posterior and anterior roots forming spinal nerves emerging between vertebrae in the lower regions of the vertebral column are connected to the spinal cord at higher vertebral levels.

Below the end of the spinal cord, the posterior and anterior roots of lumbar, sacral, and coccygeal nerves pass inferiorly to reach their exit points from the vertebral canal. This terminal cluster of roots is the **cauda equine** (Fig. 2.39).

Clinical app

Lumbar cerebrospinal fluid tap

A lumbar tap (puncture) is carried out to obtain a sample of CSF for examination. In addition, passage of a needle or conduit into the subarachnoid space (CSF space) is used to inject antibiotics, chemotherapeutic agents, and anesthetics. The lumbar region is an ideal site to access the subarachnoid space because the spinal cord terminates around the level of the disc between vertebrae LI and LII in the adult. The subarachnoid space extends to the region of the lower border of the SII vertebra.

Continued

There is therefore a large CSF-filled space containing lumbar and sacral nerve roots but no spinal cord.

Depending on the clinician's preference, the patient is placed in the lateral or prone position. A needle is passed in the midline in between the spinous processes into the extradural space. Further advancement punctures the dura and arachnoid mater to enter the subarachnoid space. Most needles push the roots away from the tip without causing the patient any symptoms. Once the needle is in the subarachnoid space, fluid can be aspirated. In some situations, it is important to measure CSF pressure.

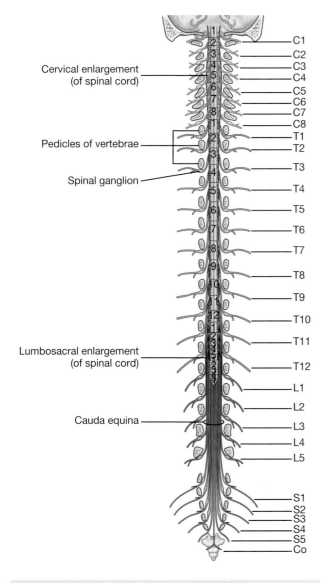

Fig. 2.39 Course of spinal nerves in the vertebral canal.

Nomenclature of spinal nerves

There are approximately 31 pairs of spinal nerves (Fig. 2.39) named according to their position with respect to associated vertebrae:

- eight cervical nerves—C1 to C8,
- twelve thoracic nerves—T1 to T12,
- five lumbar nerves—L1 to L5,
- five sacral nerves—S1 to S5, and
- one coccygeal nerve—Co.

The first cervical nerve (C1) emerges from the vertebral canal between the skull and vertebra CI (Fig. 2.40). Therefore cervical nerves C2 to C7 also emerge from the vertebral canal above their respective vertebrae. Because there are only seven cervical vertebrae, C8 emerges between vertebrae CVII and TI. As a consequence, all remaining spinal nerves, beginning with T1, emerge from the vertebral canal below their respective vertebrae.

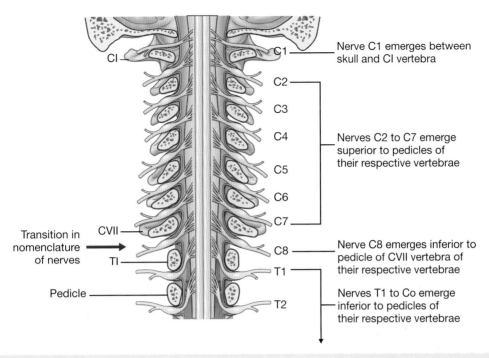

Nerve C1 emerges between skull and CI vertebra

Nerves C2 to C7 emerge superior to pedicles of their respective vertebrae

Nerve C8 emerges inferior to pedicle of CVII vertebra of their respective vertebrae

Nerves T1 to Co emerge inferior to pedicles of their respective vertebrae

Transition in nomenclature of nerves

Pedicle

Fig. 2.40 Nomenclature of the spinal nerves.

3

Thorax

Regional anatomy 64

Pectoral region 64
  Breast 64
  Muscles of the pectoral region 66
Thoracic wall 66
  Superior thoracic aperture 67
  Inferior thoracic aperture 67
  Skeletal framework 68
  Intercostal spaces 75
Diaphragm 81
  Venous drainage 83
  Innervation 83
Movements of the thoracic wall and diaphragm during breathing 84
Pleural cavities 84
  Pleura 84
  Lungs 88
Mediastinum 97
  Anterior mediastinum 102
  Middle mediastinum 102
  Superior mediastinum 126
  Posterior mediastinum 135

Regional anatomy

The **thorax** is an irregularly shaped cylinder with a narrow opening (superior thoracic aperture) superiorly and a relatively large opening (inferior thoracic aperture) inferiorly (Fig. 3.1). The thorax consists of:

- a wall,
- two pleural cavities,
- the lungs, and
- the mediastinum.

The thorax:

- houses and protects the heart, lungs, and great vessels;
- acts as a conduit for structures passing between the neck and the abdomen; and
- plays a principal role in breathing.

The thorax also provides support for the upper limb. Muscles anchored to the anterior thoracic wall provide some of this support and, together with their associated connective tissues, nerves, and vessels and the overlying skin and superficial fascia, define the pectoral region.

PECTORAL REGION

The pectoral region is external to the anterior thoracic wall and helps anchor the upper limb to the trunk. It consists of:

- a superficial compartment containing skin, superficial fascia, and breasts; and
- a deep compartment containing muscles and associated structures.

Breast

The breasts consist of mammary glands, associated skin, and connective tissues. The **mammary glands** are modified sweat glands in the superficial fascia anterior to the pectoral muscles and the anterior thoracic wall (Fig. 3.2).

The mammary glands consist of ducts and associated secretory lobules. These converge, forming 15 to 20 **lactiferous ducts,** which open independently onto the **nipple.** The nipple is surrounded by a circular pigmented area of skin, the **areola** (Fig. 3.2).

A well-developed, connective tissue stroma surrounds the ducts and lobules of the mammary gland. In certain regions, this stroma condenses, forming well-defined

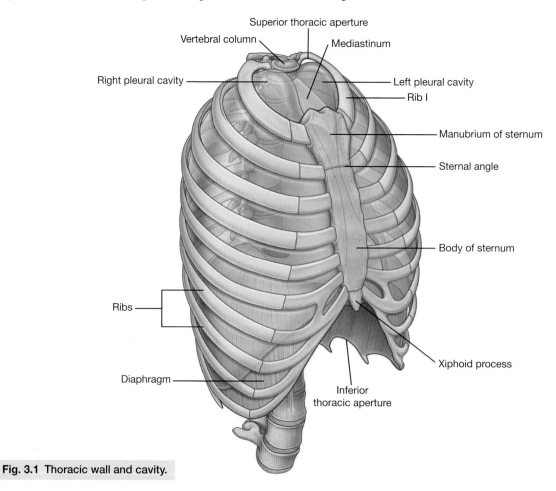

Fig. 3.1 Thoracic wall and cavity.

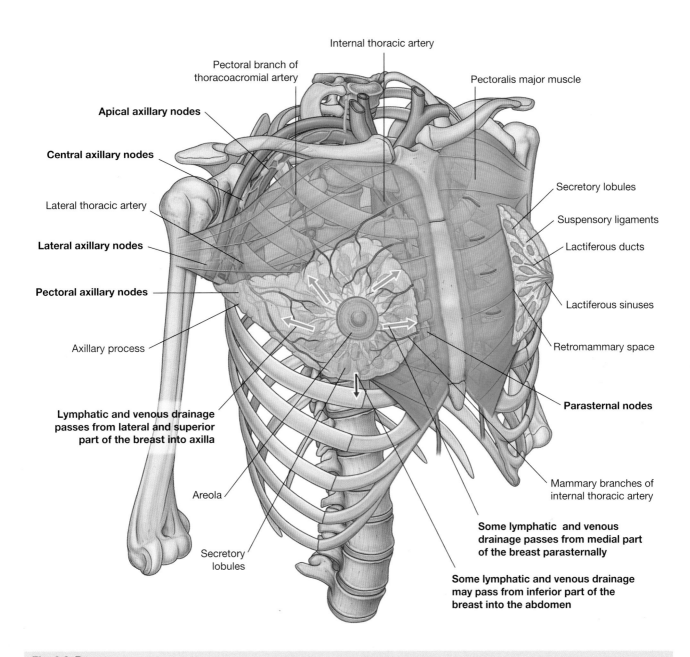

Internal thoracic artery

Pectoral branch of
thoracoacromial artery

Pectoralis major muscle

Apical axillary nodes

Central axillary nodes

Secretory lobules

Lateral thoracic artery

Suspensory ligaments

Lateral axillary nodes

Lactiferous ducts

Pectoral axillary nodes

Lactiferous sinuses

Axillary process

Retromammary space

**Lymphatic and venous drainage
passes from lateral and superior
part of the breast into axilla**

Parasternal nodes

Areola

Mammary branches of
internal thoracic artery

Secretory
lobules

**Some lymphatic and venous
drainage passes from medial part
of the breast parasternally**

**Some lymphatic and venous drainage
may pass from inferior part of the
breast into the abdomen**

Fig. 3.2 Breasts.

ligaments, the **suspensory ligaments of breast,** which are continuous with the dermis of the skin and support the breast.

In nonlactating women, the predominant component of the breasts is fat, whereas glandular tissue is more abundant in lactating women.

The breast lies on the deep fascia of the pectoralis major muscle and other surrounding muscles. A layer of loose connective tissue (the **retromammary space**) separates the breast from the deep fascia and provides some degree of movement over underlying structures.

The base, or attached surface, of each breast extends vertically from ribs II to VI and transversely from the sternum to as far laterally as the midaxillary line.

Clinical app

Axillary process of breast

It is important for clinicians to remember, when evaluating the breast for pathology, that the upper lateral region of the mammary gland and supporting tissues can project around the lateral margin of the pectoralis major muscle and into the axilla. This axillary process (axillary tail) may perforate deep fascia and extend as far superiorly as the apex of the axilla (Fig. 3.2).

Arterial supply

The breast is related to the thoracic wall and to structures associated with the upper limb; therefore vascular supply and drainage can occur by multiple routes (Fig. 3.2):

laterally, vessels from the axillary artery—superior thoracic, thoracoacromial, lateral thoracic, and subscapular arteries;
- medially, branches from the internal thoracic artery; and
- from the second to fourth intercostal arteries via branches that perforate the thoracic wall and overlying muscle.

Venous drainage

Veins draining the breast parallel the arteries and ultimately drain into the axillary, internal thoracic, and intercostal veins.

Innervation

Innervation of the breast is via anterior and lateral cutaneous branches of the second to sixth intercostal nerves. The nipple is innervated by the fourth intercostal nerve.

Lymphatic drainage

Lymphatic drainage of the breast is as follows:

- Approximately 75% is via lymphatic vessels that drain laterally and superiorly into **axillary nodes** (see Fig. 3.2).
- Most of the remaining drainage is into parasternal nodes deep to the anterior thoracic wall and associated with the internal thoracic artery.
- Some drainage may occur via lymphatic vessels that follow the lateral branches of posterior intercostal arteries and connect with intercostal nodes situated near the heads and necks of ribs.

Axillary nodes drain into the subclavian trunks, parasternal nodes drain into the bronchomediastinal trunks, and intercostal nodes drain either into the thoracic duct or into the bronchomediastinal trunks.

Breast in men

The breast in men is rudimentary. The mammary gland consists only of small ducts, often composed of cords of cells, which normally do not extend beyond the areola. Breast cancer can occur in men.

Clinical app

Breast cancer
Breast cancer is one of the most common malignancies in women. Breast cancer develops in the cells of the acini, lactiferous ducts, and lobules of the breast. Tumor growth and spread depend on the exact cellular site of origin of the cancer. Breast tumors spread via the lymphatics and veins or by direct invasion.

Subcutaneous lymphatic obstruction and tumor growth pull on connective tissue ligaments, the suspensory ligaments, in the breast resulting in the appearance of an orange peel texture **(peau d'orange)** on the surface of the breast. Further subcutaneous spread can induce a rare manifestation of breast cancer that produces a hard, woody texture to the skin **(cancer en cuirasse).**

Patients who have undergone chest masculinization surgery (e.g., some transgender men) may not have had all breast tissue removed. If an irregularity is palpated over the chest wall, clinical suspicion for breast pathology should remain and needs to be investigated. Ultrasound is the favored imaging modality rather than mammography because of the technical difficulties of mammography with a masculinized chest. Because the lymphatics remain intact, malignancies in the breast can still spread into the thorax via the axilla. In patients on feminizing hormones (e.g., some transgender women), estrogen and progesterone stimulates the growth of breast tissue. Extended lengths of time on feminizing hormones may increase the risk of breast cancer to those levels seen in cisgender women.

Muscles of the pectoral region

Each pectoral region contains the **pectoralis major, pectoralis minor,** and **subclavius muscles** (Table 3.1, Fig. 3.4). All originate from the anterior thoracic wall and insert into bones of the upper limb.

A continuous layer of deep fascia, **clavipectoral fascia,** encloses the subclavius and pectoralis minor and attaches to the clavicle above and to the floor of the axilla below.

The muscles of the pectoral region form the anterior wall of the axilla, a region between the upper limb and the neck through which all major structures pass.

THORACIC WALL

The **thoracic wall** consists of skeletal elements and muscles (see Fig. 3.1):

- Posteriorly, it is made up of 12 thoracic vertebrae and their intervening intervertebral discs.
- Laterally, the wall is formed by **ribs** (12 on each side) and three layers of flat muscles, which span the intercostal spaces between adjacent ribs, move the ribs, and provide support for the intercostal spaces.
- Anteriorly, the wall is made up of the **sternum,** which consists of the manubrium of sternum, body of sternum, and xiphoid process.

The thoracic wall extends between:

- the superior thoracic aperture bordered by vertebra TI, rib I, and the manubrium of sternum; and
- the inferior thoracic aperture bordered by vertebra TXII, rib XII, the end of rib XI, the costal margin, and the xiphoid process of the sternum.

Surface anatomy

The breast in women
Although breasts vary in size, they are normally positioned on the thoracic wall between ribs II and VI and overlie the pectoralis major muscles. Each mammary gland extends superolaterally around the lower margin of the pectoralis major muscle and enters the axilla (Fig. 3.3). This portion of the gland is the axillary tail or axillary process. The positions of the nipple and areola vary relative to the chest wall depending on breast size.

Areola   Nipple

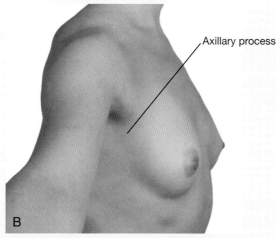

Axillary process

Fig. 3.3 A. Close-up view of the nipple and surrounding areola of the breast. **B.** Lateral view of the chest wall of a woman showing the axillary process of the breast.

Superior thoracic aperture

The **superior thoracic aperture** (Fig. 3.5; also see Fig. 3.1) consists of:

- the body of vertebra TI posteriorly,
- the medial margin of rib I on each side, and
- the manubrium anteriorly.

The superior margin of the manubrium is in approximately the same horizontal plane as the intervertebral disc between vertebrae TII and TIII.

The first ribs slope inferiorly from their posterior articulation with vertebra TI to their anterior attachment to the manubrium. Consequently, the plane of the superior thoracic aperture is at an oblique angle, facing somewhat anteriorly (Fig. 3.5).

At the superior thoracic aperture, the superior aspects of the pleural cavities, which surround the lungs, lie on either side of the entrance to the mediastinum (Fig. 3.6).

Structures that pass between the upper limb and thorax pass over rib I and the superior part of the pleural cavity as they enter and leave the mediastinum (Fig. 3.6). Structures that pass between the neck and head and the thorax pass more vertically through the superior thoracic aperture (Fig. 3.5).

Inferior thoracic aperture

The **inferior thoracic aperture** is large and expandable, and bone, cartilage, and ligaments form its margin (Fig. 3.7). It is closed by the diaphragm (Fig. 3.7B), and structures passing between the abdomen and thorax pierce or pass posteriorly to this structure. Skeletal elements of the inferior thoracic aperture are:

- the body of vertebra TXII posteriorly,
- rib XII and the distal end of rib XI posterolaterally,
- the distal cartilaginous ends of ribs VII to X, which unite to form the costal margin anterolaterally, and
- the xiphoid process anteriorly.

Clinical app

Thoracic outlet syndrome
Clinically, thoracic outlet syndrome is used to describe symptoms resulting from abnormal compression of the brachial plexus of nerves as it passes over the first rib and through the axillary inlet into the upper limb. The anterior ramus of T1 passes superiorly out of the superior thoracic aperture to join and become part of the brachial plexus. A connective tissue band that can extend from the tip of a cervical rib to rib I is one cause of thoracic outlet syndrome by putting upward stresses on the lower parts of the brachial plexus as they pass over the first rib.

Joints between the costal margin and sternum lie roughly in the same horizontal plane as the intervertebral disc between vertebrae TIX and TX. Thus the posterior margin of the inferior thoracic aperture is inferior to the anterior margin.

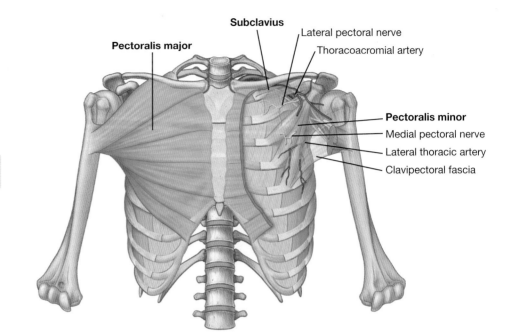

Fig. 3.4 Muscles and fascia of the pectoral region.

Labels: Pectoralis major, Subclavius, Lateral pectoral nerve, Thoracoacromial artery, Pectoralis minor, Medial pectoral nerve, Lateral thoracic artery, Clavipectoral fascia

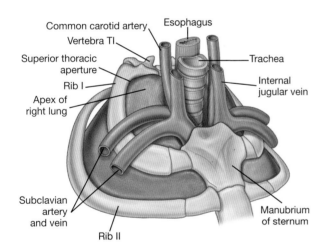

Fig. 3.5 Superior thoracic aperture.

Labels: Common carotid artery, Esophagus, Vertebra TI, Superior thoracic aperture, Trachea, Rib I, Internal jugular vein, Apex of right lung, Subclavian artery and vein, Rib II, Manubrium of sternum

Skeletal framework

The skeletal elements of the thoracic wall consist of thoracic vertebrae, intervertebral discs, ribs, and sternum.

Thoracic vertebrae

There are 12 **thoracic vertebrae,** each of which is characterized by articulations with the ribs.

A typical thoracic vertebra

A typical thoracic vertebra has a heart-shaped **vertebral body,** with roughly equal dimensions in the transverse and anteroposterior directions and a long spinous process (Fig. 3.8). The **vertebral foramen** is generally circular,

and the **laminae** are broad and overlap with those of the vertebra below. The **superior articular processes** are flat, with their articular surfaces facing almost directly posteriorly, whereas the **inferior articular processes** project from the laminae and their articular facets face anteriorly. The **transverse processes** are club shaped and project posterolaterally.

Articulation with ribs

A typical thoracic vertebra has three sites for articulations with ribs on each side (Fig. 3.8).

- Two demifacets (i.e., partial facets) located on the superior and inferior aspects of the body for articulation with corresponding sites on the heads of adjacent ribs. The **superior costal facet** articulates with part of the head of its own rib, and the **inferior costal facet** articulates with part of the head of the rib below.
- An oval facet **(transverse costal facet)** at the end of the transverse process articulates with the tubercle of its own rib.

Not all vertebrae articulate with ribs in the same fashion (Fig. 3.9):

- The superior costal facets on the body of vertebra TI are complete and articulate with a single facet on the head of its own rib—in other words, the head of rib I does not articulate with vertebra CVII.
- Similarly, vertebra TX (and often TIX) articulates only with its own ribs and therefore lacks inferior demifacets on the body.

Table 3.1 Muscles of the pectoral region

Muscle	Origin	Insertion	Innervation	Function
Pectoralis major	Medial half of clavicle and anterior surface of sternum, first seven costal cartilages, aponeurosis of external oblique	Lateral lip of intertubercular sulcus of humerus	Medial and lateral pectoral nerves	Adduction, medial rotation, and flexion of the humerus at the shoulder joint
Subclavius	Rib I at junction between rib and costal cartilage	Groove on inferior surface of middle third of clavicle	Nerve to subclavius	Pulls clavicle medially to stabilize sternoclavicular joint; depresses tip of shoulder
Pectoralis minor	Anterior surfaces of the third, fourth, and fifth ribs and deep fascia overlying the related intercostal spaces	Coracoid process of scapula	Medial pectoral nerves	Depresses tip of shoulder; protracts scapula

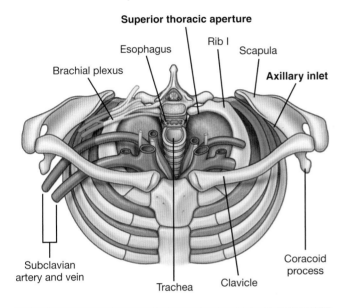

Superior thoracic aperture

Esophagus
Rib I
Scapula
Brachial plexus
Axillary inlet

Subclavian artery and vein
Trachea
Clavicle
Coracoid process

Fig. 3.6 Superior thoracic aperture and axillary inlet.

- Vertebrae TXI and TXII articulate only with the heads of their own ribs—they lack transverse costal facets and have only a single complete facet on each side of their bodies.

Ribs

There are 12 pairs of ribs, each terminating anteriorly in a costal cartilage (Fig. 3.10). The anterior end is continuous

Although all ribs articulate with the vertebral column, only the costal cartilages of the upper seven ribs, known as **true ribs**, articulate directly with the sternum. The remaining five pairs of ribs are **false ribs**:

- The costal cartilages of ribs VIII to X articulate anteriorly with the costal cartilages of the ribs above.
- Ribs XI and XII have no anterior connection with other ribs or with the sternum and are often called **floating ribs.**

A typical rib consists of a curved shaft with anterior and posterior ends (Fig. 3.11). The anterior end is continuous

with its costal cartilage. The posterior end articulates with the vertebral column and is characterized by a head, neck, and tubercle.

The **head** is somewhat expanded and typically presents two articular surfaces separated by a **crest.** The smaller superior surface articulates with the inferior costal facet on the body of the vertebra above, whereas the larger inferior facet articulates with the superior costal facet of its own vertebra.

The **neck** is a short flat region of bone that separates the head from the tubercle.

The **tubercle** projects posteriorly from the junction of the neck with the shaft and consists of two regions, an articular part and a nonarticular part:

- The articular part is medial and has an oval facet for articulation with a corresponding facet on the transverse process of the associated vertebra.
- The raised nonarticular part is roughened by ligament attachments.

The shaft is generally thin and flat with internal and external surfaces.

The superior margin is smooth and rounded, whereas the inferior margin is sharp. The shaft bends forward just laterally to the tubercle at a site termed the **angle.** It also has a gentle twist around its longitudinal axis so that the external surface of the anterior part of the shaft faces somewhat superiorly relative to the posterior part. The inferior margin of the internal surface is marked by a distinct **costal groove.**

Distinct features of upper and lower ribs

The upper and lower ribs have distinct features (Fig. 3.12).

Rib I

Rib I is flat in the horizontal plane and has broad superior and inferior surfaces. From its articulation with vertebra TI, it slopes inferiorly to its attachment to the manubrium of sternum. The head articulates with the

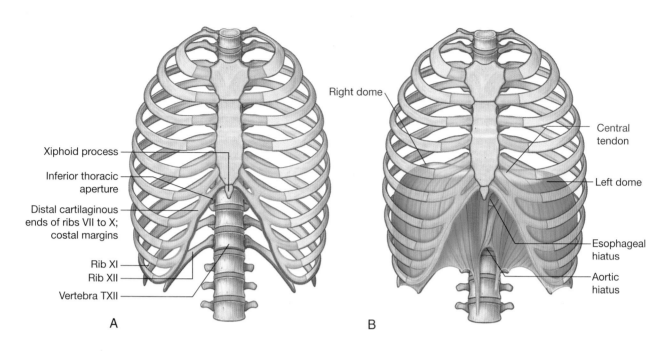

Fig. 3.7 A. Inferior thoracic aperture. **B.** Diaphragm.

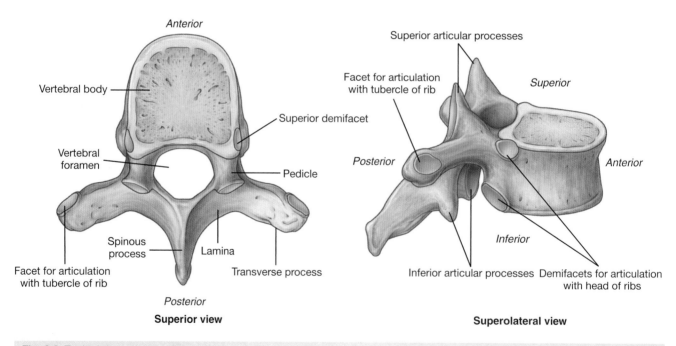

Fig. 3.8 Typical thoracic vertebra.

body of vertebra TI and has only one articular surface. The tubercle has a facet for articulation with the transverse process. The superior surface of the rib is characterized by a distinct tubercle, the **scalene tubercle,** which separates two smooth grooves that cross the rib approximately midway along the shaft. The anterior groove is caused by the subclavian vein, and the posterior groove is caused by the subclavian artery. Anterior and posterior to these grooves, the shaft is roughened by muscle and ligament attachments.

Rib II

Rib II, like rib I, is flat but twice as long. It articulates with the vertebral column in a way typical of most ribs.

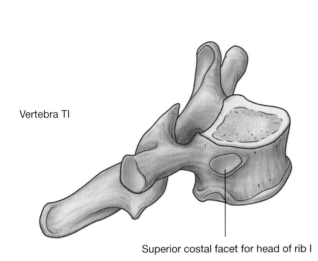

Vertebra TI

Superior costal facet for head of rib I

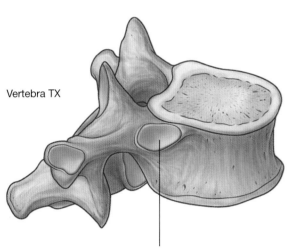

Vertebra TX

Single complete costal facet for head of rib X

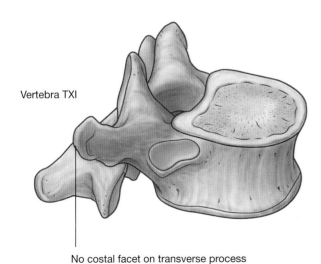

Vertebra TXI

No costal facet on transverse process

Fig. 3.9 Thoracic vertebrae.

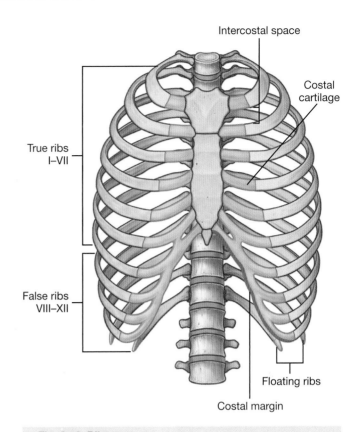

Intercostal space

Costal cartilage

True ribs I–VII

False ribs VIII–XII

Floating ribs

Costal margin

Fig. 3.10 Ribs.

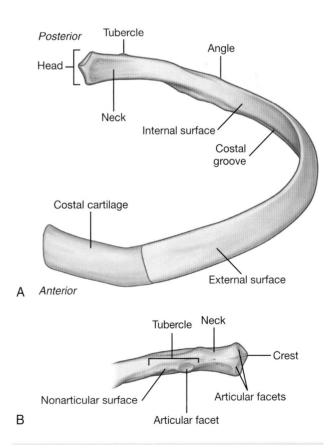

Posterior   Tubercle

Head   Angle

Neck

Internal surface

Costal groove

Costal cartilage

External surface

A   *Anterior*

Tubercle   Neck

Crest

Articular facets

Nonarticular surface

B   Articular facet

Fig. 3.11 A typical rib. **A.** Anterior view. **B.** Posterior view of proximal end of rib.

Rib X

The head of **rib X** has a single facet for articulation with its own vertebra.

Ribs XI and XII

Ribs XI and **XII** articulate only with the bodies of their own vertebrae and have no tubercles or necks. Both ribs are short, have little curve, and are pointed anteriorly.

Clinical apps

Cervical ribs

Cervical ribs are present in approximately 1% of the population.

A cervical rib is an accessory rib articulating with vertebra CVII; the anterior end attaches to the superior border of the anterior aspect of rib I.

Plain radiographs may demonstrate cervical ribs as small horn-like structures.

It is often not appreciated by clinicians that a fibrous band commonly extends from the anterior tip of the small cervical ribs to rib I, producing a "cervical band" that is not visualized on radiography. In patients with cervical ribs and cervical bands, structures that normally pass over rib I are elevated by, and pass over, the cervical rib and band.

Clinical apps

Rib fractures

Single rib fractures are of little consequence, though extremely painful.

After severe trauma, ribs may be broken in two or more places. If enough ribs are broken, a loose segment of chest wall, a flail segment **(flail chest),** is produced. When the patient takes a deep inspiration, the flail segment moves in the opposite direction to the chest wall, preventing full lung expansion and creating a paradoxically moving segment. If a large enough segment of chest wall is affected, ventilation may be impaired and assisted ventilation may be required until the ribs have healed.

Sternum

The adult **sternum** consists of three major elements: the broad and superiorly positioned manubrium of sternum, the narrow and longitudinally oriented body of sternum, and the small and inferiorly positioned xiphoid process (Fig. 3.13).

Manubrium of sternum

The **manubrium of sternum** forms part of the bony framework of the neck and the thorax.

The superior surface of the manubrium is expanded laterally and bears a distinct and palpable notch, the **jugular notch (suprasternal notch),** in the midline (Fig. 3.13). On either side of this notch is a large oval fossa for articulation with the clavicle. Immediately inferior to this fossa, on each lateral surface of the manubrium, is a facet for the attachment of the first costal cartilage. At the lower end of the lateral border is a demifacet for articulation with the upper half of the anterior end of the second costal cartilage.

Body of the sternum

The **body of the sternum** is flat (Fig. 3.13).

The anterior surface of the body of the sternum is often marked by transverse ridges that represent lines of fusion between the segmental elements called *sternbrae* from which this part of the sternum arises embryologically.

The lateral margins of the body of the sternum have articular facets for costal cartilages. Superiorly, each lateral margin has a demifacet for articulation with the inferior aspect of the second costal cartilage. Inferior to this demifacet are four facets for articulation with the costal cartilages of ribs III to VI.

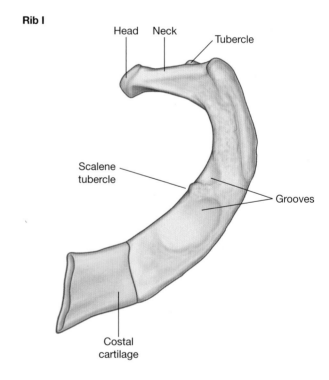

Rib I

Head · Neck · Tubercle

Scalene tubercle · Grooves

Costal cartilage

Rib XII

Fig. 3.12 Atypical ribs.

At the inferior end of the body of the sternum is a demifacet for articulation with the upper demifacet on the seventh costal cartilage. The inferior end of the body of the sternum is attached to the xiphoid process.

Xiphoid process

The **xiphoid process** is the smallest part of the sternum (Fig. 3.13). Its shape is variable: it may be wide, thin, pointed, bifid, curved, or perforated. It begins as a cartilaginous structure, which becomes ossified in the adult. On each side of its upper lateral margin is a demifacet for articulation with the inferior end of the seventh costal cartilage.

Clinical app

Collection of sternal bone marrow
The subcutaneous position of the sternum makes it possible to place a needle through the hard outer cortex into the internal (or medullary) cavity containing bone marrow. Once the needle is in this position, bone marrow can be aspirated. Evaluation of this material under the microscope helps clinicians diagnose certain blood diseases such as leukemia.

Joints

Costovertebral joints

A typical rib articulates with:

- the bodies of adjacent vertebrae, forming a joint with the head of the rib, and
- the transverse process of its related vertebra, forming a **costotransverse joint** (Fig. 3.14).

Together, the costovertebral joints and related ligaments allow the necks of the ribs either to rotate around their longitudinal axes, which occurs mainly in the upper ribs, or to ascend and descend relative to the vertebral column, which occurs mainly in the lower ribs. The combined movements of all of the ribs on the vertebral column are essential for altering the volume of the thoracic cavity during breathing.

Joint with head of rib

The two facets on the head of the rib articulate with the superior facet on the body of its own vertebra and with the inferior facet on the body of the vertebra above (Fig. 3.14). This joint is divided into two synovial compartments by an intra-articular ligament, which attaches the crest to the adjacent intervertebral disc and separates the two articular surfaces

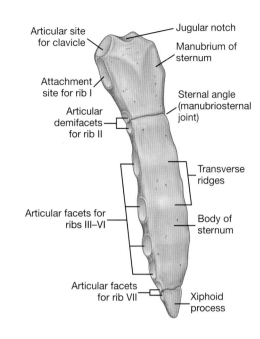

Fig. 3.13 Sternum.

on the head of the rib. The two synovial compartments and the intervening ligament are surrounded by a single joint capsule attached to the outer margins of the combined articular surfaces of the head and vertebral column.

Costotransverse joints

Costotransverse joints are synovial joints between the tubercle of a rib and the transverse process of the related vertebra (Fig. 3.14). The joint is stabilized by two strong extracapsular ligaments that span the space between the transverse process and the rib on the medial and lateral sides of the joint:

- The **costotransverse ligament** is medial to the joint and attaches the neck of the rib to the transverse process.
- The **lateral costotransverse ligament** is lateral to the joint and attaches the tip of the transverse process to the roughened nonarticular part of the tubercle of the rib.

A third ligament, the **superior costotransverse ligament,** attaches the superior surface of the neck of the rib to the transverse process of the vertebra above.

Slight gliding movements occur at the costotransverse joints.

Sternocostal joints

The sternocostal joints are joints between the upper seven costal cartilages and the sternum (Fig. 3.15).

The joint between rib I and the manubrium is not synovial and consists of a fibrocartilaginous connection between

Fig. 3.14 Costovertebral joints.

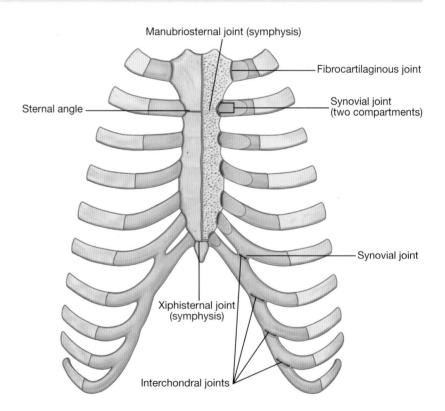

Fig. 3.15 Sternocostal joints.

the manubrium and the costal cartilage. The joints between rib II through VII and the sternum are synovial and have thin capsules reinforced by surrounding sternocostal ligaments.

The joint between the second costal cartilage and the sternum is divided into two compartments by an intra-articular ligament. This ligament attaches the second costal cartilage to the junction of the manubrium and the body of the sternum.

Interchondral joints

Interchondral joints occur between the costal cartilages of adjacent ribs (Fig. 3.15), mainly between the costal cartilages of ribs VII to X but may also involve the costal cartilages of ribs V and VI.

Interchondral joints provide indirect anchorage to the sternum and contribute to the formation of a smooth inferior costal margin. They are usually synovial, and the thin fibrous capsules are reinforced by interchondral ligaments.

Manubriosternal and xiphisternal joints

The joints between the manubrium and body of sternum and between the body of sternum and the xiphoid process are usually symphyses (Fig. 3.15). Only slight angular movements occur between the manubrium and body of sternum during respiration. The joint between the body of sternum and the xiphoid process often becomes ossified with age.

Additionally, the sternal angle is on a horizontal plane that passes through the intervertebral disc between vertebrae TIV and TV (Fig. 3.16). This plane separates the superior mediastinum from the inferior mediastinum and marks the superior border of the pericardium. It also separates the end of the ascending aorta from the beginning of the arch of the aorta, the end of the arch of the aorta from the beginning of the thoracic aorta, and passes through the bifurcation of the trachea just superior to the pulmonary trunk.

Clinical app

The manubriosternal joint as reference
A clinically useful feature of the manubriosternal joint is that it can be palpated easily. This is because the manubrium normally angles posteriorly on the body of sternum, forming a raised feature referred to as the *sternal angle.* This elevation marks the site of articulation of rib II with the sternum. Rib I is not palpable because it lies inferior to the clavicle and is embedded in tissues at the base of the neck. Therefore rib II is used as a reference for counting ribs and can be felt immediately lateral to the sternal angle.

Intercostal spaces

Intercostal spaces lie between adjacent ribs and are filled by intercostal muscles (Fig. 3.19).

Intercostal nerves and associated major arteries and veins lie in the costal groove along the inferior margin of the superior rib and pass in the plane between the inner two layers of muscles (Fig. 3.19). In each space, the vein is the most superior structure and is therefore highest in the costal groove. The artery is inferior to the vein, and the nerve is inferior to the artery and often not protected by the groove. Therefore the nerve is the structure most at risk

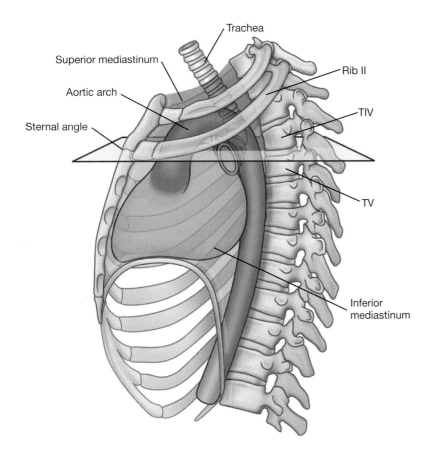

Fig. 3.16 Vertebral level TIV/V.

Surface anatomy

How to count ribs

Knowing how to count ribs is important because different ribs provide palpable landmarks for the positions of deeper structures. To determine the location of specific ribs, palpate the **jugular notch** at the superior extent of the manubrium of the sternum. Move down the sternum until a ridge is felt. This ridge is the **sternal angle,** which identifies the articulation between the manubrium of sternum and the body of sternum. The costal cartilage of rib II articulates with the sternum at this location. Identify rib II. Then continue counting the ribs, moving in a downward and lateral direction (Fig. 3.17).

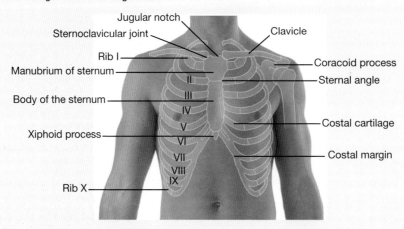

Fig. 3.17 Anterior view of chest wall with the locations of skeletal structures shown. In women, the location of the nipple relative to a specific intercostal space varies depending on the size of the breasts, which may not be symmetric. In men, the location of the nipple is in the fourth intercostal space.

Surface anatomy

Visualizing structures at the TIV/V vertebral level

The TIV/V vertebral level is a transverse plane that passes through the sternal angle on the anterior chest wall and the intervertebral disc between TIV and TV vertebrae posteriorly. This plane can be easily located, because the joint between the manubrium of sternum and the body of sternum forms a distinct bony protuberance that can be palpated. At the TIV/V level (Fig. 3.18):

- The costal cartilage of rib II articulates with the sternum.
- The superior mediastinum is separated from the inferior mediastinum.
- The ascending aorta ends and the arch of aorta begins.
- The arch of aorta ends and the thoracic aorta begins.
- The trachea bifurcates.

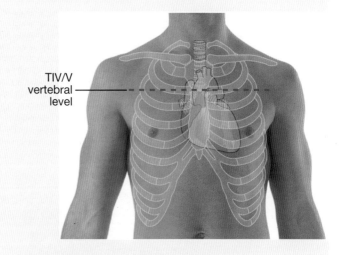

Fig. 3.18 Anterior view of the chest wall of a man showing the locations of various structures related to the TIV/V level.

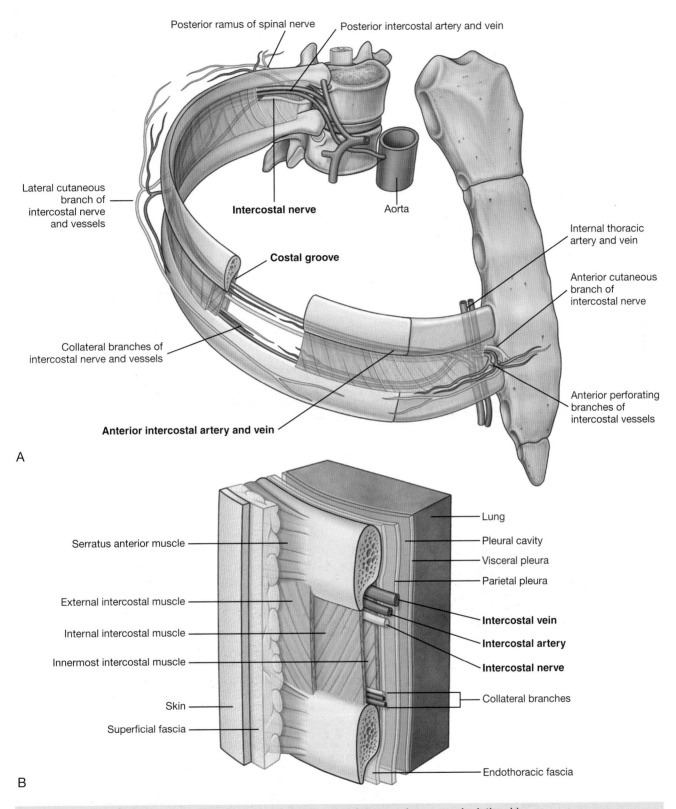

Posterior ramus of spinal nerve

Posterior intercostal artery and vein

Lateral cutaneous branch of intercostal nerve and vessels

Intercostal nerve

Aorta

Costal groove

Internal thoracic artery and vein

Anterior cutaneous branch of intercostal nerve

Collateral branches of intercostal nerve and vessels

Anterior intercostal artery and vein

Anterior perforating branches of intercostal vessels

A

Serratus anterior muscle

Lung

Pleural cavity

Visceral pleura

Parietal pleura

External intercostal muscle

Internal intercostal muscle

Intercostal vein

Intercostal artery

Innermost intercostal muscle

Intercostal nerve

Skin

Collateral branches

Superficial fascia

Endothoracic fascia

B

Fig. 3.19 Intercostal space. **A.** Anterolateral view. **B.** Details of an intercostal space and relationships.

when objects perforate the upper aspect of an intercostal space.

Deep to the intercostal spaces and ribs and separating these structures from the underlying pleura is a layer of loose connective tissue called **endothoracic fascia,** which contains variable amounts of fat (Fig. 3.19B).

Muscles

Muscles of the thoracic wall include those that fill and support the intercostal spaces (**external, internal,** and **innermost intercostal muscles** [Table 3.2, Figs. 3.19, 3.20]); those that cross several ribs between the costal attachments (**subcostal muscles** [Table 3.2, Fig. 3.21A]); and those that pass between the sternum and the ribs (**transversus thoracis muscles** [Table 3.2, Fig. 3.21B]).

The muscles of the thoracic wall, together with muscles between the vertebrae and ribs posteriorly (i.e., the **levatores costarum** and **serratus posterior superior** and **serratus posterior inferior muscles**), alter the position of the ribs and sternum, changing the thoracic volume during breathing. They also reinforce the thoracic wall.

Intercostal muscles

The **intercostal muscles** are three flat muscles found in each intercostal space that pass between adjacent ribs (Figs. 3.19B, 3.20). Individual muscles in this group are named according to their positions:

- The external intercostal muscles are the most superficial and their fibers pass from the rib above anteroinferiorly to the rib below (these muscles extend around the thoracic wall from the regions of the tubercles of the ribs to the costal cartilages where each muscle continues as a thin connective tissue aponeurosis termed the *external intercostal membrane*).

- The internal intercostal muscles are sandwiched between the external and innermost muscles, and their fibers run in the opposite direction to those of the external intercostal muscles (the internal intercostal muscles extend around the thoracic wall from the sternum to the angles of the ribs where each muscle continues as a thin connective tissue aponeurosis termed the *internal intercostal membrane*).

- The innermost intercostal muscles are the deepest of the three muscles and their fibers course in a similar direction as the internal intercostal muscles.

The intercostal muscles are innervated by the related intercostal nerves. As a group, the intercostal muscles provide structural support for the intercostal spaces during breathing. They can also move the ribs.

Arterial supply

Vessels that supply the thoracic wall consist mainly of posterior and anterior intercostal arteries, which pass around the wall between adjacent ribs in intercostal spaces (Fig. 3.19A). These arteries originate from the aorta and internal thoracic arteries, which in turn arise from the subclavian arteries in the root of the neck. Together, the intercostal arteries form a basket-like pattern of vascular supply around the thoracic wall.

Posterior intercostal arteries

Posterior intercostal arteries originate from vessels associated with the posterior thoracic wall. The upper two posterior intercostal arteries on each side come from the **supreme intercostal artery,** which descends into the thorax as a branch of the costocervical trunk in the neck. The **costocervical trunk** is a posterior branch of the subclavian artery (Fig. 3.22).

Table 3.2 Muscles of the thoracic wall

Muscle	Superior attachment	Inferior attachment	Innervation	Function
External intercostal	Inferior margin of rib above	Superior margin of rib below	Intercostal nerves; T1-T11	Most active during inspiration; supports intercostal space; moves ribs superiorly
Internal intercostal	Lateral edge of costal groove of rib above	Superior margin of rib below deep to the attachment of the related external intercostal	Intercostal nerves; T1-T11	Most active during expiration; supports intercostal space; moves ribs inferiorly
Innermost intercostal	Medial edge of costal groove of rib above	Internal aspect of superior margin of rib below	Intercostal nerves; T1-T11	Acts with internal intercostal muscles
Subcostals	Internal surface (near angle) of lower ribs	Internal surface of second or third rib below	Related intercostal nerves	May depress ribs
Transversus thoracis	Inferior margins and internal surfaces of costal cartilages of second to sixth ribs	Inferior aspect of deep surface of body of sternum, xiphoid process, and costal cartilages ribs IV-VII	Related intercostal nerves	Depresses costal cartilages

Fig. 3.20 Intercostal muscles.

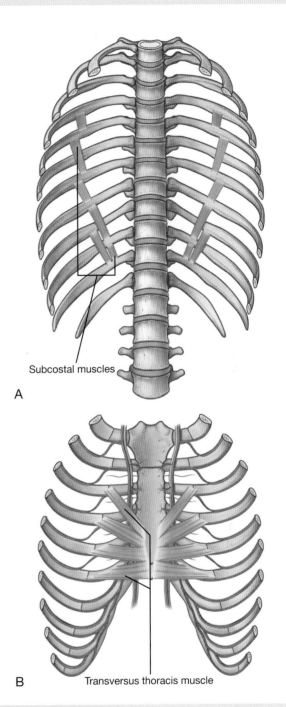

A

B Transversus thoracis muscle

Fig. 3.21 A. Subcostal muscles. B. Transversus thoracis muscles.

The remaining nine pairs of posterior intercostal arteries arise from the posterior surface of the thoracic aorta. Because the aorta is on the left side of the vertebral column, those posterior intercostal vessels passing to the right side of the thoracic wall cross the midline anterior to the bodies of the vertebrae and therefore are longer than the corresponding vessels on the left.

In addition to having numerous branches that supply various components of the wall, the posterior intercostal arteries have branches that accompany lateral cutaneous branches of the intercostal nerves to the superficial regions.

Anterior intercostal arteries

The **anterior intercostal arteries** originate directly or indirectly as lateral branches from the internal thoracic arteries (Fig. 3.22).

Each **internal thoracic artery** arises as a major branch of the subclavian artery in the neck. It passes anteriorly over the cervical dome of pleura and descends vertically through the superior thoracic aperture and along the deep aspect of the anterior thoracic wall. On each side, the internal thoracic artery lies posterior to the costal cartilages of the upper six ribs and about 1 cm lateral to the sternum. At approximately the level of the sixth intercostal space, it divides into two terminal branches (Fig. 3.22):

■ the **superior epigastric artery,** which continues inferiorly into the anterior abdominal wall, and

■ the **musculophrenic artery,** which passes along the costal margin, goes through the diaphragm, and ends near the last intercostal space.

Anterior intercostal arteries that supply the upper six intercostal spaces arise as lateral branches from the internal thoracic artery, whereas those supplying the lower spaces arise from the musculophrenic artery.

In each intercostal space, the anterior intercostal arteries usually have two branches:

- One passes below the margin of the upper rib.
- The other passes above the margin of the lower rib and meets a collateral branch of the posterior intercostal artery.

The distributions of the anterior and posterior intercostal vessels overlap and can develop anastomotic connections. The anterior intercostal arteries are generally smaller than the posterior vessels.

In addition to anterior intercostal arteries and a number of other branches, the internal thoracic arteries give rise to perforating branches that pass directly forward between the costal cartilages to supply structures external to the thoracic wall. These vessels travel with the anterior cutaneous branches of the intercostal nerves.

Venous drainage

Venous drainage from the thoracic wall generally parallels the pattern of arterial supply (Fig. 3.23).

Centrally, the intercostal veins ultimately drain into the azygos system of veins or into **internal thoracic veins,** which connect with the **brachiocephalic veins** in the neck.

Often the upper posterior intercostal veins on the left side come together and form the **left superior intercostal vein,** which empties into the left brachiocephalic vein.

Similarly, the upper posterior intercostal veins on the right side may come together and form the **right superior intercostal vein,** which empties into the **azygos vein.**

Lymphatic drainage

Lymphatic vessels of the thoracic wall drain mainly into lymph nodes associated with the internal thoracic arteries **(parasternal nodes),** with the heads and necks of ribs **(intercostal nodes)** and with the diaphragm **(diaphragmatic nodes)** (Fig. 3.24). Diaphragmatic nodes are posterior to the xiphoid and at sites where the phrenic nerves penetrate the diaphragm. They also occur in regions where the diaphragm is attached to the vertebral column.

Parasternal nodes drain into **bronchomediastinal trunks.** Intercostal nodes in the upper thorax also drain into bronchomediastinal trunks, whereas intercostal nodes in the lower thorax drain into the **thoracic duct.**

Nodes associated with the diaphragm interconnect with parasternal, prevertebral, juxta-esophageal nodes, **brachiocephalic nodes** (anterior to the brachiocephalic veins in the superior mediastinum), and **lateral aortic/lumbar nodes** (in the abdomen).

Superficial regions of the thoracic wall drain mainly into **axillary lymph nodes** in the axilla or parasternal nodes.

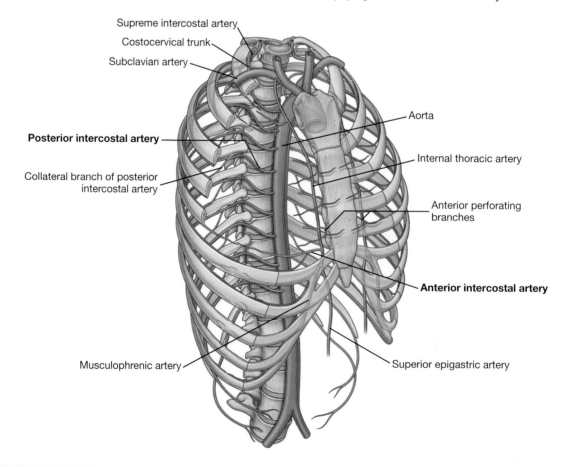

Fig. 3.22 Arteries of the thoracic wall.

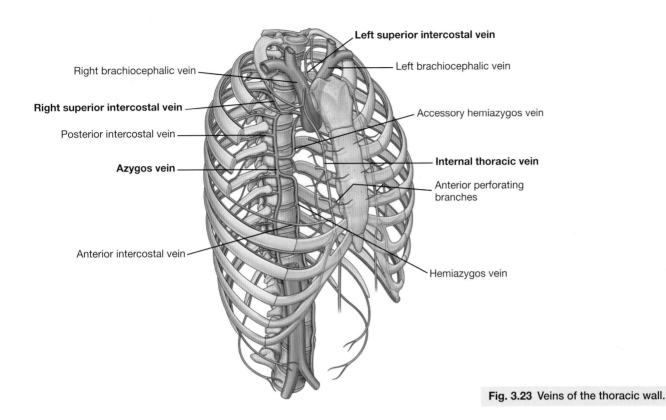

Left superior intercostal vein

Right brachiocephalic vein

Left brachiocephalic vein

Right superior intercostal vein

Accessory hemiazygos vein

Posterior intercostal vein

Internal thoracic vein

Azygos vein

Anterior perforating branches

Anterior intercostal vein

Hemiazygos vein

Fig. 3.23 Veins of the thoracic wall.

Innervation

Intercostal nerves

Innervation of the thoracic wall is mainly by the **intercostal nerves,** which are the anterior rami of spinal nerves T1 to T11 and lie in the intercostal spaces between adjacent ribs (Fig. 3.25). The anterior ramus of spinal nerve T12 (the **subcostal nerve**) is inferior to rib XII.

A typical intercostal nerve passes laterally around the thoracic wall in an intercostal space. The largest of the branches is the **lateral cutaneous branch,** which pierces the lateral thoracic wall and divides into an anterior branch and a posterior branch that innervate the overlying skin.

The intercostal nerves end as **anterior cutaneous branches,** which emerge either parasternally between adjacent costal cartilages or laterally to the midline on the anterior abdominal wall to supply the skin.

In addition to these major branches, small collateral branches can be found in the intercostal space running along the superior border of the lower rib.

In the thorax, the intercostal nerves carry:

- somatic motor innervation to the muscles of the thoracic wall (intercostal, subcostal, and transversus thoracis muscles),

- somatic sensory innervation from the skin and parietal pleura, and
- postganglionic sympathetic fibers to the periphery.

Sensory innervation from the skin overlying the upper thoracic wall is supplied by cutaneous branches (supraclavicular nerves), which descend from the cervical plexus in the neck.

In addition to innervating the thoracic wall, intercostal nerves innervate other regions:

- The anterior ramus of T1 contributes to the brachial plexus.
- The lateral cutaneous branch of the second intercostal nerve (the **intercostobrachial nerve**) contributes to cutaneous innervation of the medial surface of the upper arm.
- The lower intercostal nerves supply muscles, skin, and parietal peritoneum of the abdominal wall.

DIAPHRAGM

The **diaphragm** is a thin musculotendinous structure that fills the inferior thoracic aperture and separates the thoracic cavity from the abdominal cavity (Figs. 3.26, 3.27, and see Chapter 4). It is attached peripherally to the:

- xiphoid process of the sternum,
- costal margin of the thoracic wall,
- ends of ribs XI and XII,
- ligaments that span across structures of the posterior abdominal wall, and
- vertebrae of the lumbar region.

From these peripheral attachments, muscle fibers converge to join the central tendon. The pericardium is attached to the middle part of the central tendon.

In the median sagittal plane, the diaphragm slopes inferiorly from its anterior attachment to the xiphoid, approximately at vertebral level TVIII/IX, to its posterior

Clinical app

Surgical access to the chest

Surgical access is challenging in the chest given the rigid nature of the thoracic cage. Moreover, the access site is also dependent on the organ that is operated upon and its relationships to subdiaphragmatic structures and structures in the neck.

Minimally invasive thoracic surgery (video-assisted thoracic surgery [VATS]) involves making small (1-cm) incisions in the intercostal spaces, inserting a small camera, and manipulating other instruments through additional small incisions. A number of procedures can be performed in this manner, including lobectomy, lung biopsy, and esophagectomy. A standard incision site would include a median sternotomy to obtain access to the heart, including the coronary arteries and the cardiac valves.

A left lateral thoracotomy or a right lateral thoracotomy is an incision through an intercostal space to access the lungs and the more lateral mediastinal structures.

Clinical app

Thoracostomy (chest) tube insertion

Insertion of a chest tube is a commonly performed procedure and is indicated to relieve air or fluid trapped in the thorax between the lung and the chest wall (pleural cavity). This procedure is done for pneumothorax, hemothorax, hemopneumothorax, malignant pleural effusion empyema, hydrothorax, chylothorax, and after thoracic surgery.

The position of the thoracostomy tube should be between the anterior axillary and midaxillary anatomical lines from anterior to posterior and either the fourth or fifth intercostal space from cephalad to caudad. The position of the ribs in this region should be clearly marked. Anesthetic should be applied to the superior border of the rib and the inferior aspect of the intercostal space, including one rib and space above and one rib and space below. The neurovascular bundle runs in the neurovascular plane, which lies in the superior aspect of the intercostal space (just below the rib), hence the reason for positioning the tube on the superior border of a rib (i.e., at the lowest position in the intercostal space).

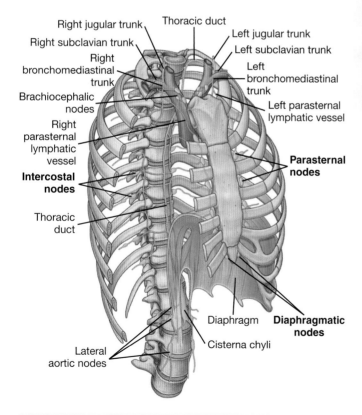

Fig. 3.24 Major lymphatic vessels and nodes of the thoracic wall.

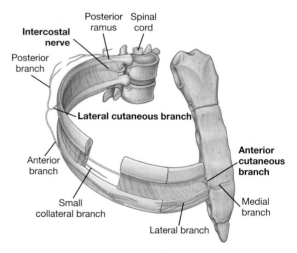

Fig. 3.25 Intercostal nerves.

Clinical app

Intercostal nerve block

Local anesthesia of intercostal nerves produces excellent analgesia in patients with chest trauma and those patients requiring anesthesia for a thoracotomy, mastectomy, and upper abdominal surgical procedures.

The intercostal nerves are situated inferior to the rib borders in the neurovascular bundle. Each neurovascular bundle is situated deep to the external and internal intercostal muscle groups.

The nerve block may be undertaken using a "blind" technique or under direct imaging guidance.

The patient is placed in the appropriate position to access the rib. Typically, under ultrasound guidance, a needle may be advanced into the region of the subcostal groove followed by an injection with local anesthesia. Depending on the type of local anesthetic, analgesia may be short- or long-acting.

Given the position of the neurovascular bundle and the subcostal groove, complications may include puncture of the parietal pleura and an ensuing pneumothorax. Bleeding may also occur if the artery or vein is damaged during the procedure.

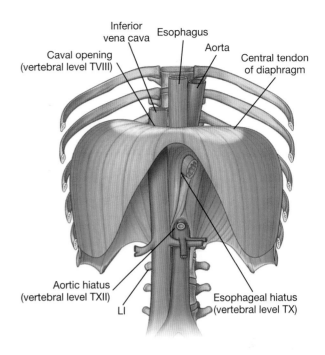

Fig. 3.26 Major structures passing between abdomen and thorax.

attachment to the **median arcuate ligament,** crossing anteriorly to the aorta at approximately vertebral level TXII.

Structures traveling between the thorax and abdomen pass through the diaphragm or between the diaphragm and its peripheral attachments (Figs. 3.26, 3.27):

- The inferior vena cava passes through the central tendon at approximately vertebral level TVIII.
- The esophagus passes through the muscular part of the diaphragm, just to the left of midline, approximately at vertebral level TX.
- The vagus nerves pass through the diaphragm with the esophagus.
- The aorta passes behind the posterior attachment of the diaphragm at vertebral level TXII.
- The thoracic duct passes behind the diaphragm with the aorta.
- The azygos and hemiazygos veins may also pass through the aortic hiatus or through the crura of the diaphragm.

Other structures outside the posterior attachments of the diaphragm lateral to the aortic hiatus include the sympathetic trunks. The greater, lesser, and least splanchnic nerves penetrate the crura.

Arterial supply

The arterial supply to the diaphragm is from vessels that arise superiorly and inferiorly to it (see Fig. 3.27). From above, pericardiacophrenic and musculophrenic arteries supply the diaphragm. These vessels are branches of the internal thoracic arteries. **Superior phrenic arteries,** which arise directly from lower parts of the thoracic aorta, and small branches from intercostal arteries contribute to the supply. The largest arteries supplying the diaphragm arise from below it. These arteries are the **inferior phrenic arteries,** which branch directly from the abdominal aorta.

Venous drainage

Venous drainage of the diaphragm is by veins that generally parallel the arteries. The veins drain into:

- the brachiocephalic veins in the neck,
- the **azygos system of veins,** or
- the abdominal veins (left suprarenal vein and inferior vena cava).

Innervation

The diaphragm is innervated by the **phrenic nerves** (C3, C4, and C5), which penetrate the diaphragm and innervate it from its abdominal surface (Fig. 3.27).

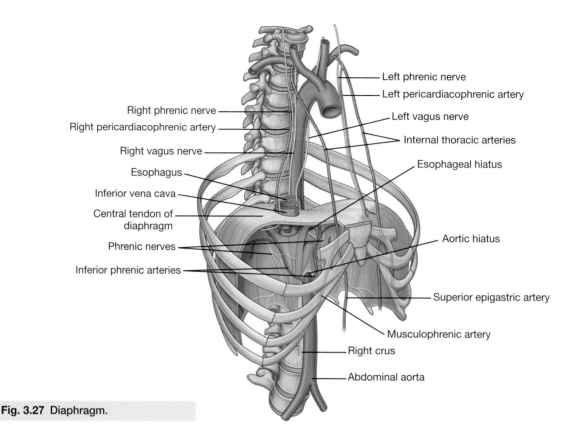

Fig. 3.27 Diaphragm.

Contraction of the domes of the diaphragm flattens the diaphragm, increasing thoracic volume. Movements of the diaphragm are essential for normal breathing.

MOVEMENTS OF THE THORACIC WALL AND DIAPHRAGM DURING BREATHING

During breathing, the dimensions of the thorax change in the vertical, lateral, and anteroposterior directions. Elevation and depression of the diaphragm significantly alter the vertical dimensions of the thorax. Depression results when the muscle fibers of the diaphragm contract. Elevation occurs when the diaphragm relaxes.

Changes in the anteroposterior and lateral dimensions result from elevation and depression of the ribs (Fig. 3.28). The posterior ends of the ribs articulate with the vertebral column, whereas the anterior ends of most ribs articulate with the sternum or adjacent ribs.

Because the anterior ends of the ribs are inferior to the posterior ends, when the ribs are elevated, they move the sternum upward and forward. Also, the angle between the body of the sternum and the manubrium may become slightly less acute. When the ribs are depressed, the sternum moves downward and backward. This "pump handle" movement changes the dimensions of the thorax in the anteroposterior direction (Fig. 3.28A).

As well as the anterior ends of the ribs being lower than the posterior ends, the middle of the shafts tend to be lower than the two ends. When the shafts are elevated, the middle of the shafts move laterally. This "bucket handle" movement increases the lateral dimensions of the thorax (Fig. 3.28B).

PLEURAL CAVITIES

Two **pleural cavities,** one on either side of the mediastinum, surround the lungs (Figs. 3.29, 3.30):

- superiorly, they extend above rib I into the root of the neck;
- inferiorly, they extend to a level just above the costal margin; and
- the medial wall of each pleural cavity is the mediastinum (Fig. 3.31).

Pleura

Each pleural cavity is lined by a single layer of flat cells, mesothelium, and an associated layer of supporting connective tissue; together, they form the pleura.

The **pleura** is divided into two major types based on location:

Clinical app

The arrangement of pleural cavities is clinically significant

The pleural cavities are completely separated from each other by the mediastinum. Therefore abnormal events in one pleural cavity do not necessarily affect the other cavity. This also means that the mediastinum can be entered surgically without opening the pleural cavities.

Another important feature of the pleural cavities is that they extend above the level of rib I. The apex of each lung actually extends into the root of the neck. As a consequence, abnormal events in the root of the neck can involve the adjacent pleura and lung, and events in the adjacent pleura and lung can involve the root of the neck.

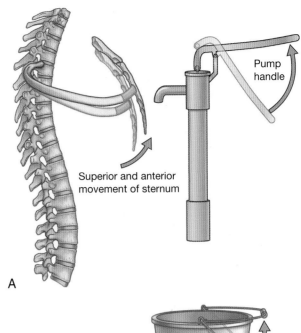

A

- pleura associated with the walls of a pleural cavity is **parietal pleura (Fig. 3.30)**, and
- pleura that reflects from the medial wall and onto the surface of the lung is **visceral pleura** (Fig. 3.30), which adheres to and covers the lung.

Each pleural cavity is the potential space enclosed between the visceral and parietal pleurae. They normally contain only a very thin layer of serous fluid. As a result, the surface of the lung, which is covered by visceral pleura, directly opposes and freely slides over the parietal pleura attached to the wall.

Parietal pleura

The names given to the parietal pleura correspond to the parts of the wall with which they are associated (Fig. 3.32):

- Pleura related to the ribs and intercostal spaces is termed the **costal part.**
- Pleura covering the diaphragm is the **diaphragmatic part.**
- Pleura covering the mediastinum is the **mediastinal part.**
- The dome-shaped layer of parietal pleura lining the cervical extension of the pleural cavity is **cervical pleura (dome of pleura** or **pleural cupola).**

Covering the superior surface of the cervical pleura is a distinct dome-like layer of fascia, the **suprapleural membrane** (Fig. 3.32). This connective tissue membrane is attached laterally to the medial margin of the first rib and behind to the transverse process of vertebra CVII. Superiorly, the membrane receives muscle fibers from some of the deep muscles in the neck (scalene muscles) that function to keep the membrane taught. The suprapleural membrane provides apical support for the pleural cavity in the root of the neck.

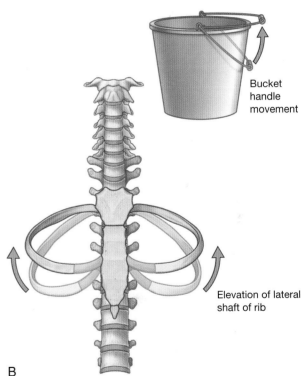

B

Fig. 3.28 Movement of thoracic wall during breathing. **A.** Pump handle movement of ribs and sternum. **B.** Bucket handle movement of ribs.

In the region of vertebrae TV to TVII, the mediastinal pleura reflects off the mediastinum as a tubular, sleeve-like covering for structures (i.e., airway, vessels, nerves, lymphatics) that pass between the lung and mediastinum. This sleeve-like covering and the structures it contains form the **root of the lung.** The root joins the medial surface of the lung at an area referred to as the **hilum of lung.** Here, the mediastinal pleura is continuous with the visceral pleura.

Fig. 3.29 Pleural cavities.

Fig. 3.30 Pleural cavities.

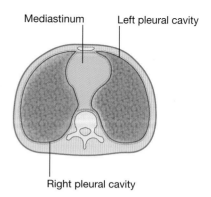

Fig. 3.31 Cross-section of the thorax showing the position of the mediastinum.

Clinical app

Innervation of parietal and visceral pleura

The parietal pleural is innervated by somatic afferent fibers. The costal pleura is innervated by branches from the intercostal nerves, and pain would be felt in relation to the thoracic wall. The diaphragmatic pleura and the mediastinal pleura are innervated mainly by the phrenic nerves (originating at spinal cord levels C3, C4, and C5). Pain from these areas would refer to the C3, C4, and C5 dermatomes (lateral neck and the supraclavicular region of the shoulder).

The visceral pleural is innervated by visceral afferent fibers that accompany bronchial vessels, and pain is generally not elicited from this tissue.

Peripheral reflections

The peripheral reflections of parietal pleura mark the extent of the pleural cavities (Fig. 3.33).

Superiorly, the pleural cavity can project as much as 3 to 4 cm above the first costal cartilage but does not extend above the neck of rib I. This limitation is caused by the inferior slope of rib I to its articulation with the manubrium.

Anteriorly, the pleural cavities approach each other posterior to the upper part of the sternum. However, posterior to the lower part of the sternum, the parietal pleura does not come as close to the midline on the left side as it does on the right because the middle mediastinum, containing the pericardium and heart, bulges to the left.

Inferiorly, the costal pleura reflects onto the diaphragm above the costal margin. In the midclavicular line, the pleural cavity extends inferiorly to approximately rib VIII (Fig. 3.34). In the midaxillary line, it extends to rib X. From this point, the inferior margin courses somewhat horizontally, crossing ribs XI and XII to reach vertebra TXII. From the midclavicular line to the vertebral column, the inferior boundary of the pleura can be approximated by a line that runs between rib VIII, rib X, and vertebra TXII.

Visceral pleura

The visceral pleura is continuous with the parietal pleura at the hilum of each lung where structures enter and leave the organ. The visceral pleura is firmly attached to the surface of the lung, including both opposed surfaces of the fissures that divide the lungs into lobes.

Costomediastinal recesses

Anteriorly, a **costomediastinal recess** occurs on each side where the costal pleura is opposed to the mediastinal pleura. The largest is on the left side in the region overlying the heart (Fig. 3.34).

Costodiaphragmatic recesses

The largest and clinically most important recesses are the **costodiaphragmatic recesses,** which occur in each pleural cavity between the costal pleura and diaphragmatic pleura (Fig. 3.34). The costodiaphragmatic recesses are the regions between the inferior margin of the lungs and inferior margin of the pleural cavities. They are deepest after forced expiration and shallowest after forced inspiration.

During quiet respiration, the inferior margin of the lung crosses rib VI in the midclavicular line, rib VIII in the midaxillary line, and then courses somewhat horizontally to reach the vertebral column at vertebral level TX. From the midclavicular line and around the thoracic wall to the vertebral column, the inferior margin of the lung can be approximated by a line running between rib VI, rib VIII, and vertebra TX. The inferior margin of the pleural cavity at the same points is rib VIII, rib X, and vertebra TXII. The costodiaphragmatic recess is the region between the two margins.

During expiration, the inferior margin of the lung rises and the costodiaphragmatic recess becomes larger.

Fig. 3.32 Parietal pleura.

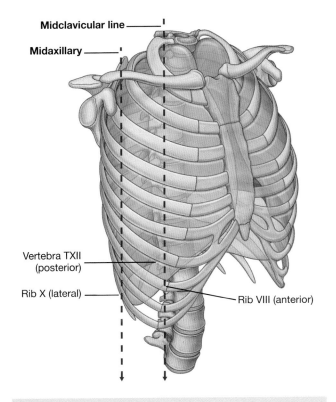

Fig. 3.33 Pleural reflections.

Clinical app

Pleural recesses

The lungs do not completely fill the anterior or posterior inferior regions of the pleural cavities (Fig. 3.34). This results in recesses in which two layers of parietal pleura become opposed. Expansion of the lungs into these spaces usually occurs only during forced inspiration; the recesses also provide potential spaces in which fluids can collect and from which fluids can be aspirated.

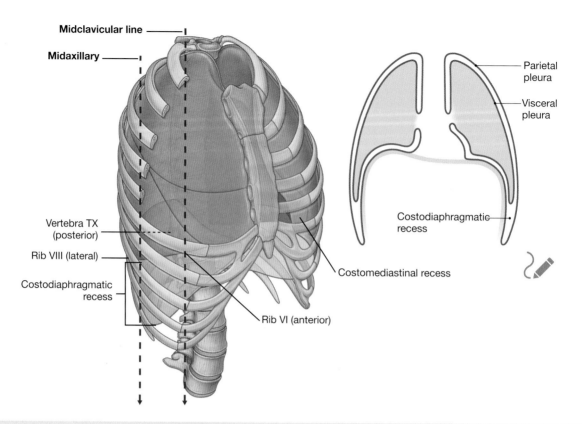

Fig. 3.34 Parietal pleural reflections and recesses.

Clinical app

Pleural effusion

A pleural effusion occurs when excess fluid accumulates within the pleural space. As the fluid accumulates within the pleural space, the underlying lung is compromised and may collapse as the volume of fluid increases. Once a pleural effusion has been diagnosed, fluid often will be aspirated to determine the cause, which can include infection, malignancy, cardiac failure, hepatic disease, and pulmonary embolism.

Lungs

The two lungs are organs of respiration and lie on either side of the mediastinum surrounded by the right and left pleural cavities. Air enters and leaves the lungs via the main bronchi, which are branches of the trachea.

The pulmonary arteries deliver deoxygenated blood to the lungs from the right ventricle of the heart. Oxygenated blood returns to the left atrium via the pulmonary veins.

The right lung is normally a little larger than the left lung because the middle mediastinum, containing the heart, bulges more to the left than to the right.

Each lung has a half-cone shape with a base, apex, two surfaces, and three borders (Fig. 3.35).

Clinical app

Pneumothorax

A pneumothorax is a collection of gas or air within the pleural cavity. When air enters the pleural cavity the tissue elasticity of the parenchyma causes the lung to collapse within the chest, impairing lung function. Occasionally, the gas within the pleural cavity may accumulate to such an extent that the mediastinum is "pushed" to the opposite side, compromising the other lung. This is termed a *tension pneumothorax* and requires urgent treatment.

Most pneumothoraces are spontaneous (i.e., they occur in the absence of pathology and lung disease.) Secondly, pneumothoraces may occur as a result of trauma, inflammation, smoking, and other underlying pulmonary diseases.

The symptoms of pneumothorax are often determined by the degree of air leak and the rate at which the accumulation of gas occurs and the ensuing lung collapse. They include pain, shortness of breath, and cardiorespiratory collapse if severe.

■ The **base** sits on the diaphragm.
■ The **apex** projects above rib I and into the root of the neck.
■ The two surfaces—the **costal surface** lies immediately adjacent to the ribs and intercostal spaces of the thoracic wall. The **mediastinal surface** lies against the mediastinum

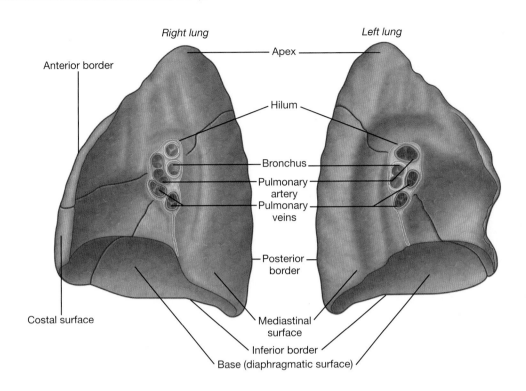

Right lung — Apex — *Left lung*

Anterior border

Hilum

Bronchus

Pulmonary artery

Pulmonary veins

Posterior border

Costal surface

Mediastinal surface

Inferior border

Base (diaphragmatic surface)

Fig. 3.35 Lungs.

anteriorly and the vertebral column posteriorly and contains the comma-shaped hilum of the lung through which structures enter and leave.

- The three borders—the **inferior border** of the lung is sharp and separates the base from the costal surface. The **anterior** and **posterior borders** separate the costal surface from the medial surface. Unlike the anterior and inferior borders, which are sharp, the posterior border is smooth and rounded.

The lungs lie directly adjacent to and are indented by structures contained in the overlying area. The heart and major vessels form bulges in the mediastinum that indent the medial surfaces of the lung; the ribs indent the costal surfaces. Pathology, such as tumors, or abnormalities in one structure can affect the related structure.

Root and hilum

The **root** of each lung is a short tubular collection of structures that together attach the lung to structures in the mediastinum (Fig. 3.36). It is covered by a sleeve of mediastinal pleura that reflects onto the surface of the lung as visceral pleura. The region outlined by this pleural reflection on the medial surface of the lung is the **hilum** where structures enter and leave.

A thin blade-like fold of pleura projects inferiorly from the root of the lung and extends from the hilum to the mediastinum. This structure is the **pulmonary ligament** (Fig. 3.36). It may stabilize the position of the inferior lobe and may also accommodate the down-and-up translocation of structures in the root during breathing.

In the mediastinum, the vagus nerves pass immediately posterior to the roots of the lungs, while the phrenic nerves pass immediately anterior to them.

Within each root and located in the hilum are:

- a pulmonary artery,
- two pulmonary veins,
- a main bronchus,
- bronchial vessels,
- nerves, and
- lymphatics.

Generally, the pulmonary artery is superior at the hilum, the pulmonary veins are inferior, and the bronchi are somewhat posterior in position.

On the right side, the lobar bronchus to the superior lobe branches from the main bronchus in the root, unlike on the left where it branches within the lung itself and is superior to the pulmonary artery.

Right lung

The **right lung** has three lobes and two fissures (Fig. 3.37A). Normally, the lobes are freely movable against each other because they are separated almost to the hilum by invaginations of visceral pleura. These invaginations form the fissures:

- the **oblique fissure** separates the **inferior lobe (lower lobe)** from the **superior lobe (upper lobe)** and the **middle lobe of the right lung,**

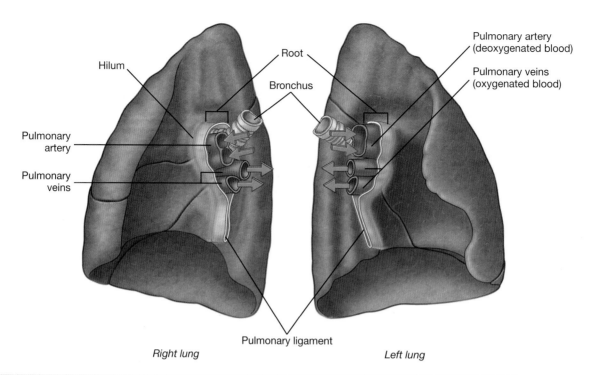

Hilum

Root

Bronchus

Pulmonary artery
(deoxygenated blood)

Pulmonary veins
(oxygenated blood)

Pulmonary
artery

Pulmonary
veins

Pulmonary ligament

Right lung

Left lung

Fig. 3.36 Roots and hila of the lungs.

the **horizontal fissure** separates the superior lobe (upper lobe) from the middle lobe.

The horizontal fissure follows the fourth intercostal space from the sternum until it meets the oblique fissure as it crosses rib V.

The largest surface of the superior lobe is in contact with the upper part of the anterolateral wall and the apex of this lobe projects into the root of the neck. The surface of the middle lobe lies mainly adjacent to the lower anterior and lateral walls. The costal surface of the inferior lobe is in contact with the posterior and inferior walls.

The medial surface of the right lung lies adjacent to a number of important structures in the mediastinum and the root of the neck (Fig. 3.37B). These include the:

- heart,
- inferior vena cava,
- superior vena cava,
- azygos vein, and
- esophagus.

The right subclavian artery and vein arch over and are related to the superior lobe of the right lung as they pass over the dome of cervical pleura and into the axilla.

Left lung

The **left lung** is smaller than the right lung and has two lobes separated by an oblique fissure (Fig. 3.38A). The **oblique** fissure of the left lung is slightly more oblique than the corresponding fissure of the right lung.

The largest surface of the **superior lobe** is in contact with the upper part of the anterolateral wall, and the apex of this lobe projects into the root of the neck. The costal surface of the **inferior lobe** is in contact with the posterior and inferior walls.

The inferior portion of the medial surface of the left lung, unlike the right lung, is notched because of the heart's projection into the left pleural cavity from the middle mediastinum.

From the anterior border of the lower part of the superior lobe, a tongue-like extension (the **lingula of left lung**) projects over the heart bulge (Fig. 3.38A).

The medial surface of the left lung lies adjacent to a number of important structures in the mediastinum and root of the neck (Fig. 3.38B). These include the:

- heart,
- aortic arch,
- thoracic aorta, and
- esophagus.

The left subclavian artery and vein arch over and are related to the superior lobe of the left lung as they pass over the dome of the cervical pleura and into the axilla.

Bronchial tree

The **trachea** is a flexible tube that extends from vertebral level CVI in the lower neck to vertebral level TIV/V in the

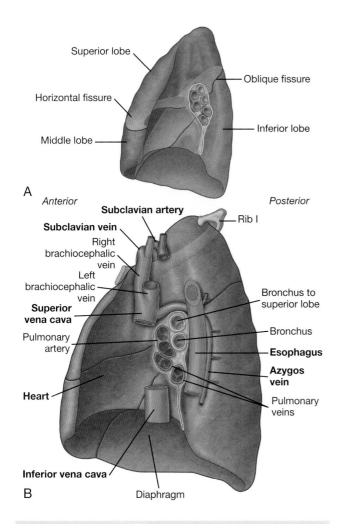

Fig. 3.37 A. Right lung. B. Major structures related to the right lung.

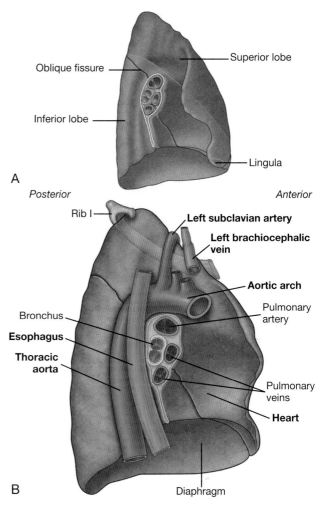

Fig. 3.38 A. Left lung. B. Major structures related to the left lung.

Surface anatomy

Visualizing the pleural cavities and lungs, pleural recesses, and lung lobes and fissures

Palpable surface landmarks can be used to visualize the normal outlines of the pleural cavities and the lungs and to determine the positions of the lobes and fissures of each lung.

Superiorly, the parietal pleura projects above the first costal cartilage. Anteriorly, the costal pleura approaches the midline posterior to the upper portion of the sternum. Posterior to the lower portion of the sternum, the left parietal pleura does not come as close to the midline as it does on the right side. This is because the heart bulges onto the left side (Fig. 3.39A).

Inferiorly, the pleura reflects onto the diaphragm above the costal margin and courses around the thoracic wall following an VIII, X, XII contour (i.e., rib VIII in the midclavicular line, rib X in the midaxillary line, and vertebra TXII posteriorly).

The lungs do not completely fill the area surrounded by the pleural cavities, particularly anteriorly and inferiorly.

Continued

Surface anatomy—cont'd

- Costomediastinal recesses occur anteriorly, particularly on the left side in relationship to the heart bulge (Fig. 3.39A).
- Costodiaphragmatic recesses occur inferiorly between the lower lung margin and the lower margin of the pleural cavity (Fig. 3.39A,B).

In quiet respiration, the inferior margin of the lungs travel around the thoracic wall following a VI, VIII, X contour (i.e., rib VI in the midclavicular line, rib VIII in the midaxillary line, and vertebra TX posteriorly).

In the posterior view, the oblique fissure on both sides is located in the midline near the spine of vertebra TIV (Figs. 3.39B and 3.40A). It moves laterally in a downward direction, crossing the fourth and fifth intercostal spaces and reaches rib VI laterally.

In the anterior view, the horizontal fissure on the right side follows the contour of rib IV and its costal cartilage and the oblique fissures on both sides follow the contour of rib VI and its costal cartilage (Fig. 3.40B).

Fig. 3.39 Views of the chest wall showing the surface projections of the lobes and the fissures of the lungs. **A.** Anterior view in a woman. On the right side, the superior, middle, and inferior lobes are illustrated. On the left side, the superior and inferior lobes are illustrated. **B.** Posterior view in a woman. On both sides, the superior and inferior lobes are illustrated. The middle lobe on the right side is not visible in this view.

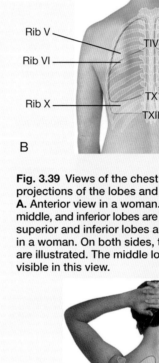

Fig. 3.40 Views of the chest wall. **A.** Posterior view in a woman with arms abducted and hands positioned behind her head. On both sides, the superior and inferior lobes of the lungs are illustrated. When the scapula is rotated into this position, the medial border of the scapula parallels the position of the oblique fissure and can be used as a guide for determining the surface projection of the superior and inferior lobes of the lungs. **B.** Lateral view in a man with his right arm abducted. The superior, middle, and inferior lobes of the right lung are illustrated. The oblique fissure begins posteriorly at the level of the spine of vertebra TIV and passes inferiorly, crossing rib IV, the fourth intercostal space, and rib V. It crosses the fifth intercostal space at the midaxillary line and continues anteriorly along the contour of rib VI. The horizontal fissure crosses rib V in the midaxillary space and continues anteriorly, crossing the fourth intercostal space and following the contour of rib IV and its costal cartilage to the sternum.

Surface anatomy

Where to listen for lung sounds

The stethoscope placements for listening for lung sounds are shown in Fig. 3.41.

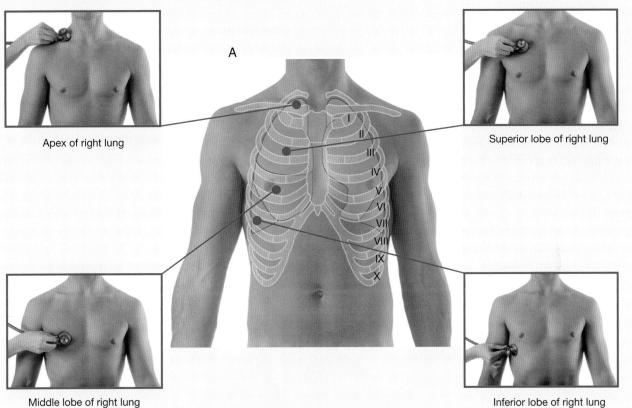

A

Apex of right lung

Superior lobe of right lung

Middle lobe of right lung

Inferior lobe of right lung

B

Apex of left lung

Superior lobe of left lung

Inferior lobe of left lung

Fig. 3.41 Views of the chest wall of a man with stethoscope placements for listening to the lobes of the lungs. **A.** Anterior views. **B.** Posterior views.

mediastinum where it bifurcates into a right and a left main bronchus (Fig. 3.42). The trachea is held open by C-shaped transverse cartilage rings embedded in its wall—the open part of the C facing posteriorly. The lowest tracheal ring has a hook-shaped structure, the carina, that projects backward in the midline between the origins of the two main bronchi. The posterior wall of the trachea is composed mainly of smooth muscle.

Each main bronchus enters the root of a lung and passes through the hilum into the lung itself.

The main bronchus divides within the lung into **lobar bronchi** (secondary bronchi), each of which supplies a lobe. On the right side, the lobar bronchus to the superior lobe originates within the root of the lung.

The lobar bronchi further divide into **segmental bronchi** (tertiary bronchi), which supply bronchopulmonary segments (Fig. 3.42B).

Within each bronchopulmonary segment, the segmental bronchi give rise to multiple generations of divisions and, ultimately, to bronchioles, which further subdivide and supply the respiratory surfaces. The walls of the bronchi are

held open by discontinuous elongated plates of cartilage, but these are not present in bronchioles.

Clinical app

Inhaled objects

The right main bronchus is wider and takes a more vertical course through the root and hilum than the left main bronchus (Fig. 3.42A). Therefore inhaled foreign bodies tend to lodge more frequently on the right side than on the left.

Bronchopulmonary segments

A **bronchopulmonary segment** is the area of lung supplied by a segmental (tertiary) bronchus and its accompanying pulmonary artery branch.

Tributaries of the pulmonary vein tend to pass intersegmentally between and around the margins of segments.

Each bronchopulmonary segment is shaped like an irregular cone with the apex at the origin of the segmental (tertiary)

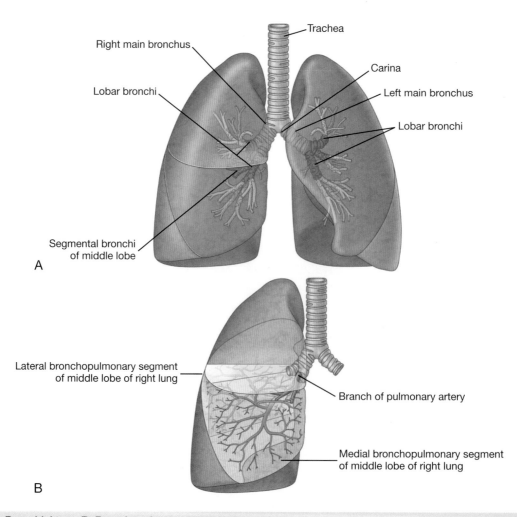

Fig. 3.42 A. Bronchial tree. **B.** Bronchopulmonary segments.

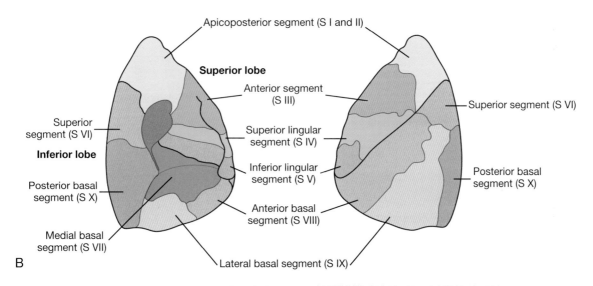

Fig. 3.43 Bronchopulmonary segments. **A.** Right lung. **B.** Left lung. (Bronchopulmonary segments are numbered and named.)

bronchus and the base projected peripherally onto the surface of the lung.

A bronchopulmonary segment is the smallest, functionally independent region of a lung and the smallest area of lung that can be isolated and removed without affecting adjacent regions.

There are 10 bronchopulmonary segments in each lung (Fig. 3.43); some of them fuse in the left lung.

Pulmonary arteries

The right and left pulmonary arteries originate from the **pulmonary trunk** and carry deoxygenated blood to the lungs from the right ventricle of the heart (Fig. 3.44).

The bifurcation of the pulmonary trunk occurs to the left of the midline just inferior to vertebral level TIV/V and anteroinferiorly to the left of the bifurcation of the trachea.

Right pulmonary artery

The **right pulmonary artery** is longer than the left and passes horizontally across the mediastinum (Fig. 3.44). It passes:

- anteriorly and slightly inferiorly to the tracheal bifurcation and anteriorly to the right main bronchus and
- posteriorly to the ascending aorta, superior vena cava, and upper right pulmonary vein.

The right pulmonary artery enters the root of the lung and gives off a large branch to the superior lobe of the lung. The main vessel continues through the hilum of the lung, gives off a second (recurrent) branch to the superior lobe, and then divides to supply the middle and inferior lobes.

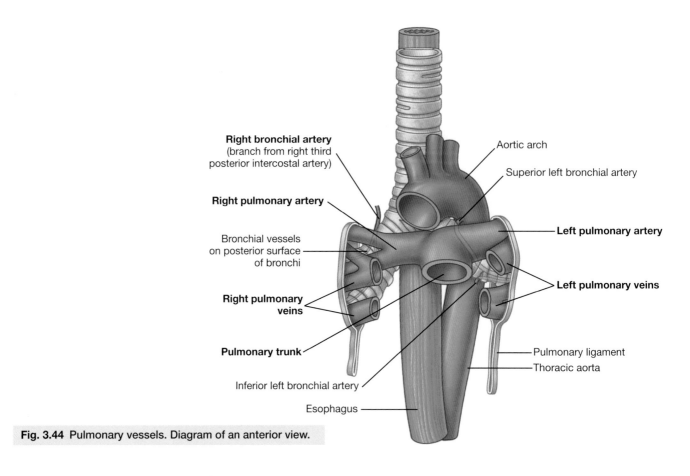

Right bronchial artery
(branch from right third posterior intercostal artery)

Aortic arch

Right pulmonary artery

Superior left bronchial artery

Bronchial vessels on posterior surface of bronchi

Left pulmonary artery

Right pulmonary veins

Left pulmonary veins

Pulmonary trunk

Pulmonary ligament

Thoracic aorta

Inferior left bronchial artery

Esophagus

Fig. 3.44 Pulmonary vessels. Diagram of an anterior view.

Imaging app

Visualizing the pulmonary trunk by computed tomography

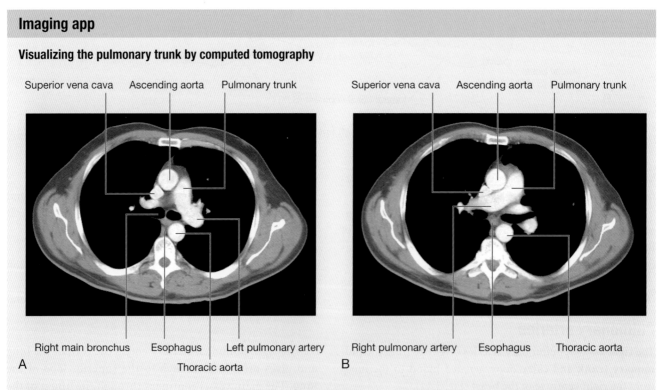

Superior vena cava   Ascending aorta   Pulmonary trunk

Superior vena cava   Ascending aorta   Pulmonary trunk

Right main bronchus   Esophagus   Left pulmonary artery

Thoracic aorta

A

Right pulmonary artery   Esophagus   Thoracic aorta

B

Fig. 3.45 Pulmonary vessels. **A.** Axial computed tomography image showing the left pulmonary artery branching from the pulmonary trunk. **B.** Axial computed tomography image (just inferior to the image in **A**) showing the right pulmonary artery branching from the pulmonary trunk.

Fig. 3.46 Pulmonary innervation.

Right vagus nerve

Anterior pulmonary plexus

Posterior pulmonary plexus

Esophageal plexus

Cervical cardiac nerves

Left recurrent laryngeal nerve

Left vagus nerve

Ligamentum arteriosum

Sympathetic trunk

Left pulmonary artery

The **left pulmonary artery** is shorter than the right and lies anterior to the descending aorta and posterior to the superior pulmonary vein (Fig. 3.44). It passes through the root and hilum and branches within the lung.

Pulmonary veins

On each side a **superior pulmonary vein** and an **inferior pulmonary vein** carry oxygenated blood from the lungs back to the heart (Fig. 3.44). The veins begin at the hilum of the lung, pass through the root of the lung, and immediately drain into the left atrium.

Bronchial arteries and veins

The bronchial arteries (Fig. 3.44) and veins constitute the "nutritive" vascular system of the pulmonary tissues (bronchial walls and glands, walls of large vessels, and visceral pleura). They interconnect within the lung with branches of the pulmonary arteries and veins.

The bronchial arteries originate from the thoracic aorta or one of its branches:

■ A single **right bronchial artery** normally arises from the third posterior intercostal artery, but occasionally it originates from the **upper left bronchial artery.**

■ Two **left bronchial arteries** arise directly from the anterior surface of the thoracic aorta—the **superior left bronchial artery** arises at vertebral level TV and the inferior one inferior to the left bronchus.

The bronchial arteries run on the posterior surfaces of the bronchi and ramify in the lungs to supply pulmonary tissues.
The **bronchial veins** drain into:

■ either the pulmonary veins or the left atrium and
■ into the azygos vein on the right or into the superior intercostal vein or hemiazygos vein on the left.

Innervation

Structures of the lung and the visceral pleura are supplied by visceral afferents and efferents distributed through the anterior pulmonary plexus and posterior pulmonary plexus (Fig. 3.46). These interconnected plexuses lie anteriorly and posteriorly to the tracheal bifurcation and main bronchi. The anterior plexus is much smaller than the posterior plexus.

Branches of these plexuses, which ultimately originate from the sympathetic trunks and vagus nerves, are distributed along branches of the airway and vessels.
Visceral efferents from:

■ the vagus nerves constrict the bronchioles;
■ the sympathetic system dilates the bronchioles.

Lymphatic drainage

Superficial, or subpleural, and deep lymphatics of the lung drain into lymph nodes called **tracheobronchial nodes** around the roots of lobar and main bronchi and along the sides of the trachea (Fig. 3.47). As a group, these lymph nodes extend from within the lung, through the hilum and root, and into the posterior mediastinum.

Efferent vessels from these nodes pass superiorly along the trachea to unite with similar vessels from parasternal nodes and brachiocephalic nodes, which are anterior to brachiocephalic veins in the superior mediastinum, to form the **right** and **left bronchomediastinal trunks.** These trunks drain directly into deep veins at the base of the neck or may drain into the right lymphatic trunk or thoracic duct.

MEDIASTINUM

The **mediastinum** is a broad central partition that separates the two laterally placed pleural cavities (Fig. 3.52). It extends:

■ from the sternum to the bodies of the vertebrae and
■ from the superior thoracic aperture to the diaphragm.

The mediastinum contains the thymus gland, the pericardial sac, the heart, the trachea, and the major arteries and

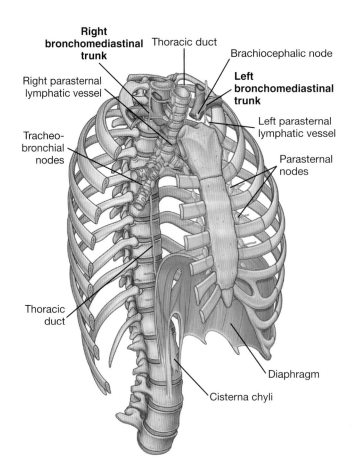

Fig. 3.47 Lymphatic drainage of lungs.

Imaging app

Visualizing the lungs

Medical imaging of the lungs is important because they are one of the commonest sites for disease in the body. While the body is at rest, the lungs exchange up to 5 L of air per minute, and this may contain pathogens and other potentially harmful elements (e.g., allergens).

Techniques to visualize the lung range from bronchoscopy, to high-resolution computed tomography (HRCT), to plain chest radiographs.

Bronchoscopy

Patients who have an endobronchial lesion (i.e., a lesion within a bronchus) may undergo bronchoscopic evaluation of the trachea and its main branches (Fig. 3.48). The bronchoscope is passed

Fig. 3.48 Bronchoscopic evaluation. **A.** Of the lower end of the normal trachea and its main branches. **B.** Of tracheal bifurcation showing a tumor at the carina.

through the nose into the pharynx and is then directed by a control system into the larynx and then past the vocal cords into the trachea. The bronchi are inspected and, if necessary, small biopsies are obtained.

High-resolution lung computed tomography

HRCT is a diagnostic method for assessing the lungs but more specifically the interstitium of the lungs (Fig. 3.49). The technique involves obtaining narrow cross-sectional slices of 1 to 2 mm. These scans enable the physician and radiologist to view the patterns of disease and their distribution. Diseases that may be easily demonstrated using this procedure include emphysema, pneumoconiosis (coal worker's pneumoconiosis), and asbestosis.

Fig. 3.49 CT images, with contrast, in axial plane: **A.** Right lung and left lung demonstrating superior and inferior lobes. The oblique fissures are visible. **B.** Right lung demonstrating superior, middle, and inferior lobes and the left lung demonstrating superior and inferior lobes. The oblique fissure associated with the left lung is visible. **C.** Right lung demonstrating middle and inferior lobes and the left lung demonstrating superior and inferior lobes. The oblique fissures are visible.

Imaging app

Plain chest radiograph

Plain chest radiographs are the most common method of visualizing the lungs (Fig. 3.50).

Fig. 3.50 Chest radiograph, anteroposterior view.

Clinical app

Lung cancer

It is important to stage lung cancer because the treatment depends on its stage.

If a small malignant nodule is found within the lung, it can sometimes be excised and the prognosis is excellent. Unfortunately, many patients present with a tumor mass that has invaded structures in the mediastinum or the pleurae or has metastasized. The tumor may then be inoperable and is treated with radiotherapy and chemotherapy.

Spread of the tumor is by lymphatics to lymph nodes within the hila, mediastinum, and root of the neck.

Imaging methods to assess spread include plain radiography, computed tomography (CT) (Fig. 3.51), and magnetic resonance imaging (MRI). Increasingly, radionuclide studies using fluorodeoxyglucose positron emission tomography (FDG-PET) are being used.

In FDG-PET, a gamma radiation emitter is attached to a glucose molecule. In areas of excessive metabolic activity (i.e., the tumor), excessive uptake occurs and is recorded by a gamma camera.

Fig. 3.51 Axial CT image of lungs showing tumor *(arrow)* in right lung.

Clinical app

Pneumonia

Chest infection is a common disease. In most patients the infection affects the large airways and bronchi. If the infection continues, exudates and transudates are produced, filling the alveoli and the secondary pulmonary lobules. The diffuse, patchy nature of this type of infection is termed *bronchial pneumonia.*

veins. It also serves as a passageway for structures such as the esophagus, thoracic duct, and various components of the nervous system as they traverse the thorax on their way to the abdomen.

For organizational purposes, the mediastinum is subdivided into several smaller regions. A transverse plane extending from the sternal angle (the junction between the manubrium and the body of the sternum) to the intervertebral disc between vertebrae TIV and TV separates the mediastinum into the (Fig. 3.53):

- **superior mediastinum** and
- **inferior mediastinum,** which is further partitioned into the **anterior, middle,** and **posterior mediastinum** by the pericardial sac.

The area anterior to the pericardial sac and posterior to the body of the sternum is the anterior mediastinum. The region

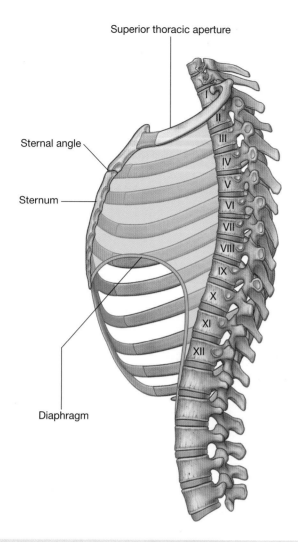

Fig. 3.52 Lateral view of the mediastinum.

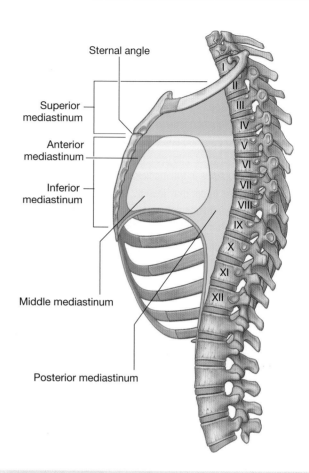

Fig. 3.53 Subdivisions of the mediastinum.

posterior to the pericardial sac and the diaphragm and anterior to the bodies of the vertebrae is the posterior mediastinum. The area in the middle, which includes the pericardial sac and its contents, is the middle mediastinum (Fig. 3.53).

Anterior mediastinum

The **anterior mediastinum** is posterior to the body of the sternum and anterior to the pericardial sac (see Fig. 3.53).

- Its superior boundary is a transverse plane passing from the sternal angle to the intervertebral disc between vertebrae TIV and TV, separating it from the superior mediastinum.
- Its inferior boundary is the diaphragm.
- Laterally, it is bordered by the mediastinal part of parietal pleura on either side.

The major structure in the anterior mediastinum is a portion of thymus, described later (see Fig. 3.85). Also present are fat, connective tissue, lymph nodes, mediastinal branches of the internal thoracic vessels, and sternopericardial ligaments, which pass from the posterior surface of the body of the sternum to the fibrous pericardium.

Middle mediastinum

The **middle mediastinum** is centrally located in the thoracic cavity. It contains the pericardium, heart, origins of the great vessels, various nerves, and smaller vessels.

Pericardium

The **pericardium** is a fibroserous sac surrounding the heart and the roots of the great vessels. It consists of two components, the fibrous pericardium and the serous pericardium (Fig. 3.54).

The **fibrous pericardium** is a tough connective tissue outer layer that defines the boundaries of the middle mediastinum. The **serous pericardium** is thin and consists of two parts:

- The **parietal layer** lines the inner surface of the fibrous.
- The **visceral layer (epicardium)** of serous pericardium adheres to the heart and forms its outer covering.

The parietal and visceral layers of serous pericardium are continuous at the roots of the great vessels. The narrow space created between the two layers of serous pericardium, containing a small amount of fluid, is the **pericardial cavity.**

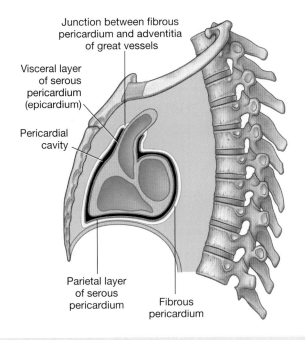

Junction between fibrous pericardium and adventitia of great vessels

Visceral layer of serous pericardium (epicardium)

Pericardial cavity

Parietal layer of serous pericardium

Fibrous pericardium

Fig. 3.54 Sagittal section of the pericardium.

This potential space allows for the relatively uninhibited movement of the heart.

Fibrous pericardium

The **fibrous pericardium** is a cone-shaped bag with its base attached to the **central tendon of the diaphragm** and a small muscular area on the left side of the diaphragm and its apex continuous with the **adventitia** of the great vessels (Fig. 3.54). Anteriorly, it is attached to the posterior surface of the sternum by **sternopericardial ligaments.** These attachments help to retain the heart in its position in the thoracic cavity. The sac also limits cardiac distention.

The phrenic nerves, which innervate the diaphragm and originate from spinal cord levels C3 to C5, pass through the fibrous pericardium and innervate this structure as they travel from their point of origin to their final destination (Fig. 3.55). Their location within the fibrous pericardium is directly related to the embryological origin of the diaphragm and the formation of the pericardial cavity. Similarly, the **pericardiacophrenic vessels** are also located within and supply the fibrous pericardium as they pass through the thoracic cavity.

Serous pericardium

The parietal layer of serous pericardium is continuous with the visceral layers of serous pericardium around the roots

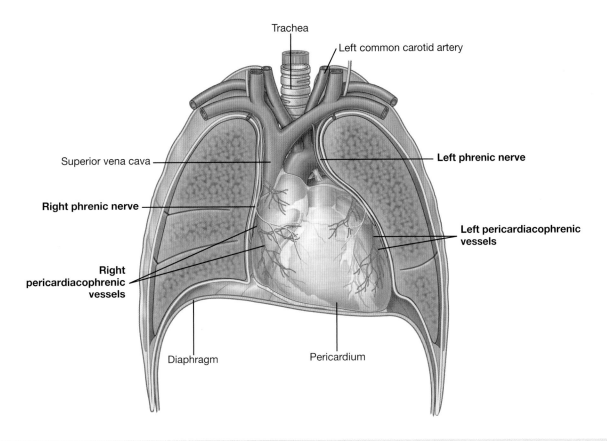

Trachea

Left common carotid artery

Superior vena cava

Left phrenic nerve

Right phrenic nerve

Left pericardiacophrenic vessels

Right pericardiacophrenic vessels

Diaphragm

Pericardium

Fig. 3.55 Phrenic nerves and pericardiacophrenic vessels.

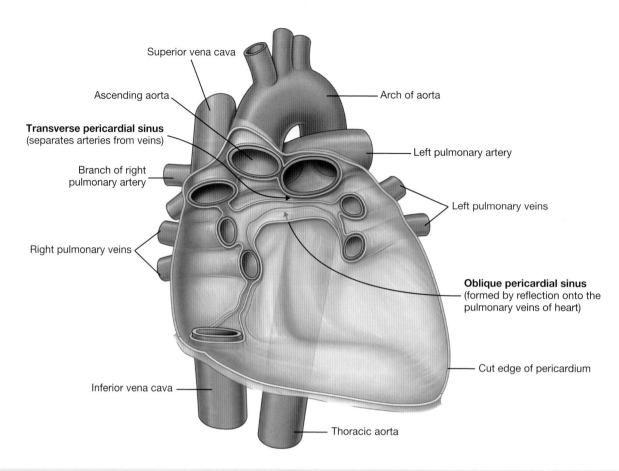

Fig. 3.56 Posterior portion of pericardial sac showing reflections of serous pericardium.

of the great vessels. These reflections of serous pericardium (Fig. 3.56) occur in two locations:

- one superiorly, surrounding the arteries—the aorta and the pulmonary trunk; and
- the second more posteriorly, surrounding the veins—the superior and inferior vena cava and the pulmonary veins.

The zone of reflection surrounding the veins is J-shaped, and the cul-de-sac formed within the J, posterior to the left atrium, is the **oblique pericardial sinus.**

A passage between the two sites of reflected serous pericardium is the **transverse pericardial sinus.** This sinus lies posteriorly to the ascending aorta and the pulmonary trunk, anteriorly to the superior vena cava, and superiorly to the left atrium.

When the pericardium is opened anteriorly during surgery, a finger placed in the transverse sinus separates arteries from veins. A hand placed under the apex of the heart and moved superiorly slips into the oblique sinus.

Vessels and nerves

Arteries supplying the pericardium are branches from the internal thoracic, pericardiacophrenic, musculophrenic, and inferior phrenic arteries and the thoracic aorta.

Veins from the pericardium enter the azygos system of veins and the internal thoracic and superior phrenic veins.

Nerves supplying the pericardium arise from the vagus nerve [X], the sympathetic trunks, and the phrenic nerves.

Clinical app

Pericardial innervation
It is important to note that the source of somatic sensation (pain) from the parietal pericardium is carried by somatic afferent fibers in the phrenic nerves. For this reason, "pain" related to a pericardial problem may be referred to the supraclavicular region of the shoulder or lateral neck area, dermatomes for spinal cord segments C3, C4, and C5.

Clinical app

Pericarditis
Pericarditis is an inflammatory condition of the pericardium. Common causes are viral and bacterial infections, systemic illnesses (e.g., chronic renal failure), and postmyocardial infarction.

Pericardial effusion

Normally, only a tiny amount of fluid is present between the visceral and parietal layers of the serous pericardium. In certain situations, this space can be filled with excess fluid (pericardial effusion).

Because the fibrous pericardium is a "relatively fixed" structure that cannot expand easily, a rapid accumulation of excess fluid within the pericardial sac compresses the heart (cardiac tamponade), resulting in biventricular failure. Removing the fluid with a needle inserted into the pericardial sac can relieve the symptoms.

Constrictive pericarditis

Abnormal thickening of the pericardial sac (constrictive pericarditis) can compress the heart, impairing heart function and resulting in heart failure.

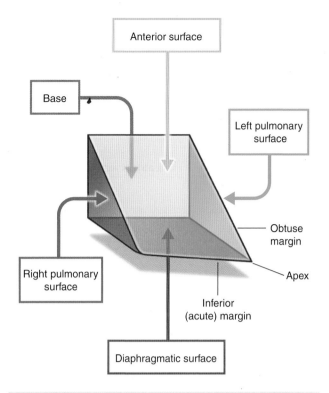

Fig. 3.57 Schematic illustration of the heart showing orientation, surfaces, and margins.

Heart

Cardiac orientation

The shape and orientation of the heart is that of a pyramid that has fallen over and is resting on one of its sides. Placed in the thoracic cavity, the apex of this pyramid projects forward, downward, and to the left, whereas the base is opposite the apex and faces in a posterior direction (Fig. 3.57). The sides of the pyramid consist of:

- a diaphragmatic (inferior) surface on which the pyramid rests,
- an anterior (sternocostal) surface oriented anteriorly,
- a right pulmonary surface, and
- a left pulmonary surface.

Base (posterior surface) and apex

The **base of the heart** is quadrilateral and directed posteriorly (Fig. 3.58). It consists of:

- the left atrium,
- a small portion of the right atrium, and
- the proximal parts of the great veins (superior and inferior venae cavae and the pulmonary veins).

Because the great veins enter the base of the heart with the pulmonary veins entering the right and left sides of the left atrium and the superior and inferior venae cavae at the upper and lower ends of the right atrium, the base

of the heart is fixed posteriorly to the pericardial wall, opposite the bodies of vertebrae TV to TVIII (TVI to TIX when standing). The esophagus lies immediately posterior to the base.

From the base the heart projects forward, downward, and to the left, ending in the apex. The **apex of the heart** is formed by the inferolateral part of the left ventricle (Fig. 3.59) and is posterior to the left fifth intercostal space, 8 to 9 cm from the midsternal line.

Surfaces of the heart

The **anterior surface** faces anteriorly and consists mostly of the right ventricle, with some of the right atrium on the right and some of the left ventricle on the left (Fig. 3.59).

The heart in the anatomical position rests on the **diaphragmatic surface,** which consists of the left ventricle and a small portion of the right ventricle separated by the posterior interventricular groove (Fig. 3.60). This surface faces inferiorly, rests on the diaphragm, is separated from the base of the heart by the coronary sinus, and extends from the base to the apex of the heart.

The **left pulmonary surface** faces the left lung, is broad and convex, and consists of the left ventricle and a portion of the left atrium.

The **right pulmonary surface** faces the right lung, is broad and convex, and consists of the right atrium.

Fig. 3.58 Base of the heart.

Margins and borders

Some general descriptions of cardiac orientation refer to right, left, inferior (acute), and obtuse margins:

- The **right** and **left margins** are the same as the right and left pulmonary surfaces of the heart.
- The **inferior margin** is defined as the sharp edge between the anterior and diaphragmatic surfaces of the heart (Figs. 3.57, 3.59)—it is formed mostly by the right ventricle and a small portion of the left ventricle near the apex.
- The **obtuse margin** separates the anterior and left pulmonary surfaces (Fig. 3.57)—it is round and extends from the left auricle to the cardiac apex (Fig. 3.59) and is formed mostly by the left ventricle and superiorly by a small portion of the left auricle.

External sulci

Internal partitions divide the heart into four chambers (i.e., two atria and two ventricles) and produce surface or external grooves referred to as *sulci*.

- The **coronary sulcus** circles the heart, separating the atria from the ventricles (Fig. 3.62). It contains the right coronary artery, the small cardiac vein, the coronary sinus, and the circumflex branch of the left coronary artery.
- The **anterior** and **posterior interventricular sulci** separate the two ventricles—the anterior interventricular

sulcus on the anterior surface of the heart containing the anterior interventricular artery and the great cardiac vein and the posterior interventricular sulcus on the diaphragmatic surface of the heart containing the posterior interventricular artery and the middle cardiac vein.

These sulci are continuous inferiorly just to the right of the apex of the heart.

Cardiac chambers

Functionally, the heart consists of two pumps separated by a partition (Fig. 3.63).

- The right pump receives deoxygenated blood from the body and sends it to the lungs.
- The left pump receives oxygenated blood from the lungs and sends it to the body.

Each pump consists of an atrium and a ventricle separated by a valve.

The thin-walled atria receive blood coming into the heart, whereas the relatively thick-walled ventricles pump blood out of the heart. More force is required to pump blood through the body than through the lungs, so the muscular wall of the left ventricle is thicker than the right.

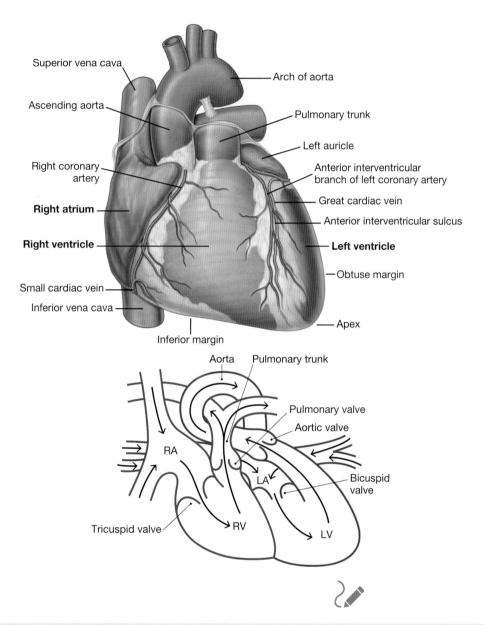

Superior vena cava

Ascending aorta

Right coronary artery

Right atrium

Right ventricle

Small cardiac vein

Inferior vena cava

Inferior margin

Arch of aorta

Pulmonary trunk

Left auricle

Anterior interventricular branch of left coronary artery

Great cardiac vein

Anterior interventricular sulcus

Left ventricle

Obtuse margin

Apex

Aorta   Pulmonary trunk

Pulmonary valve

Aortic valve

RA

LA

Bicuspid valve

Tricuspid valve   RV   LV

Fig. 3.59 Anterior surface of the heart.

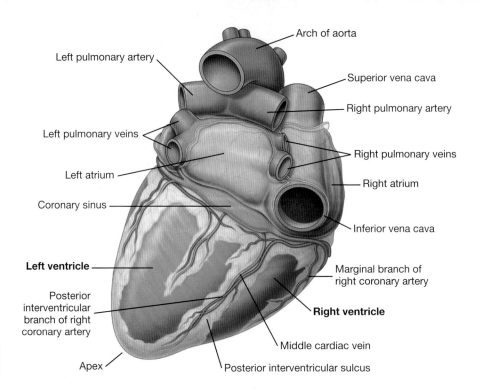

Imaging app

Visualizing the heart

For radiological evaluations, a thorough understanding of the structures defining the cardiac borders is critical. The right border in a standard posterior–anterior view consists of the superior vena cava, the right atrium, and the inferior vena cava (Fig. 3.61A). The left border in a similar view consists of the arch of the aorta, the pulmonary trunk, the left auricle, and the left ventricle. The inferior border in this radiological study consists of the right ventricle and the left ventricle at the apex. In lateral views, the right ventricle is seen anteriorly, and the left atrium is visualized posteriorly (Fig. 3.61B).

Fig. 3.61 Chest radiographs. **A.** Standard posterior–anterior view of the chest. **B.** Standard lateral view of the heart.

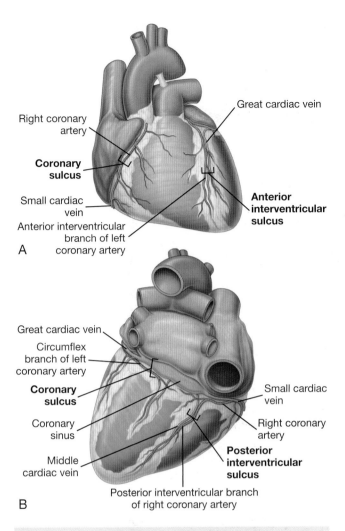

A

B

Fig. 3.62 Sulci of the heart. **A.** Anterior surface of the heart. **B.** Diaphragmatic surface and base of the heart.

Interatrial, interventricular, and atrioventricular septa separate the four chambers of the heart (Fig. 3.64). The internal anatomy of each chamber is critical to its function.

Right atrium

In the anatomical position, the **right atrium** forms the right border of the heart and contributes to the right portion of the heart's anterior surface (Fig. 3.66).

Blood returning to the right atrium enters through one of three vessels. These are:

- the superior and inferior venae cavae, which together deliver blood to the heart from the body, and
- the coronary sinus, which returns blood from the walls of the heart itself.

The superior vena cava enters the upper posterior portion of the right atrium, and the inferior vena cava and coronary sinus enter the lower posterior portion of the right atrium (Fig. 3.66).

From the right atrium, blood passes into the right ventricle through the **right atrioventricular orifice.** This opening faces forward and medially and is closed during ventricular contraction by the tricuspid valve.

The interior of the right atrium is divided into two continuous spaces. Externally, this separation is indicated by a shallow, vertical groove (the **sulcus terminalis cordis**), which extends from the right side of the opening of the superior vena cava to the right side of the opening of the inferior vena cava. Internally, this division is indicated by the **crista terminalis** (Fig. 3.66), which is a smooth, muscular ridge that begins on the roof of the atrium just in front of

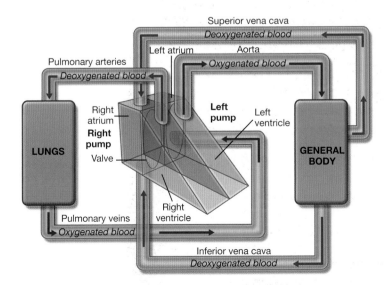

Fig. 3.63 The heart has two pumps.

Imaging app

Visualizing the chambers of the heart

Right ventricle

Right atrium

Thoracic aorta

Left ventricle

Interventricular septum

Left atrium

Fig. 3.64 Magnetic resonance image of midthorax showing all four chambers and septa.

Surface anatomy

Visualizing the margins of the heart

Surface landmarks can be palpated to visualize the outline of the heart (Fig. 3.65).

- The upper limit of the heart reaches as high as the third costal cartilage on the right side of the sternum and the second intercostal space on the left side of the sternum.
- The right margin of the heart extends from the right third costal cartilage to near the right sixth costal cartilage.
- The left margin of the heart descends laterally from the second intercostal space to the apex located near the midclavicular line in the fifth intercostal space.
- The lower margin of the heart extends from the sternal end of the right sixth costal cartilage to the apex in the fifth intercostal space near the midclavicular line.

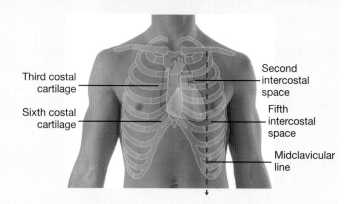

Third costal cartilage

Sixth costal cartilage

Second intercostal space

Fifth intercostal space

Midclavicular line

Fig. 3.65 Anterior view of the chest wall of a man showing skeletal structures and the surface projection of the heart.

the opening of the superior vena cava and extends down the lateral wall to the anterior lip of the inferior vena cava.

The space posterior to the crista is the **sinus of venae cavae** and is derived embryologically from the right horn of the sinus venosus. This component of the right atrium has smooth, thin walls, and both venae cavae empty into this space.

The space anterior to the crista, including the **right auricle,** is sometimes referred to as the **atrium proper.** This terminology is based on its origin from the embryonic primitive atrium. Its walls are covered by ridges called the **musculi pectinati (pectinate muscles),** which fan out from the crista like the "teeth of a comb." These ridges are also found in the right auricle, which is an ear-like, conical, muscular pouch that externally overlaps the ascending aorta.

An additional structure in the right atrium is the **opening of coronary sinus,** which receives blood from most of the cardiac veins and opens medially to the **opening of inferior vena cava.** Associated with these openings are small folds of tissue derived from the valve of the embryonic sinus venosus (the **valve of coronary sinus** and the **valve of inferior vena cava,** respectively). During development, the valve of inferior vena cava helps direct incoming oxygenated blood through the foramen ovale and into the left atrium.

Separating the right atrium from the left atrium is the **interatrial septum,** which faces forward and to the right because the left atrium lies posteriorly and to the left of the right atrium. A depression is clearly visible in the septum just above the orifice of the inferior vena cava. This is the

Arch of aorta

Superior vena cava

Right auricle

Limbus of fossa ovalis

Crista terminalis

Right ventricle

Musculi pectinati

Fossa ovalis

Inferior vena cava

Valve of inferior vena cava

Opening of coronary sinus

Valve of coronary sinus

Fig. 3.66 Internal view of right atrium.

fossa ovalis (oval fossa) with its prominent margin, the **limbus fossa ovalis (border of oval fossa)** (Fig. 3.66).

The fossa ovalis marks the location of the embryonic **foramen ovale,** which is an important part of fetal circulation. The foramen ovale allows oxygenated blood entering the right atrium through the inferior vena cava to pass directly to the left atrium and so bypass the lungs, which are nonfunctional before birth.

Finally, numerous small openings—the **openings of the smallest cardiac veins (the foramina of the venae cordis minimae)**—are scattered along the walls of the right atrium. These are small veins that drain the myocardium directly into the right atrium.

Right ventricle

In the anatomical position, the right ventricle forms most of the anterior surface of the heart and a portion of the diaphragmatic surface (Fig. 3.67). It is to the right of the right atrium and located in front of and to the left of the right atrioventricular orifice. Blood entering the right ventricle from the right atrium therefore moves in a horizontal and forward direction.

The outflow tract of the right ventricle, which leads to the pulmonary trunk, is the **conus arteriosus (infundibulum)** (Fig. 3.67). This area has smooth walls and derives from the embryonic bulbus cordis.

The walls of the inflow portion of the right ventricle have numerous muscular, irregular structures called **trabeculae carneae** (Fig. 3.67). Most of these are either attached to the ventricular walls throughout their length, forming ridges, or attached at both ends, forming bridges.

A few trabeculae carneae **(papillary muscles)** have only one end attached to the ventricular surface, whereas the other end serves as the point of attachment for tendon-like fibrous cords (the **chordae tendineae**), which connect to the free edges of the cusps of the tricuspid valve.

There are three papillary muscles in the right ventricle. Named relative to their point of origin on the ventricular surface, they are the anterior, posterior, and septal papillary muscles (Fig. 3.67).

■ The **anterior papillary muscle** is the largest and most constant papillary muscle and arises from the anterior wall of the ventricle.

111

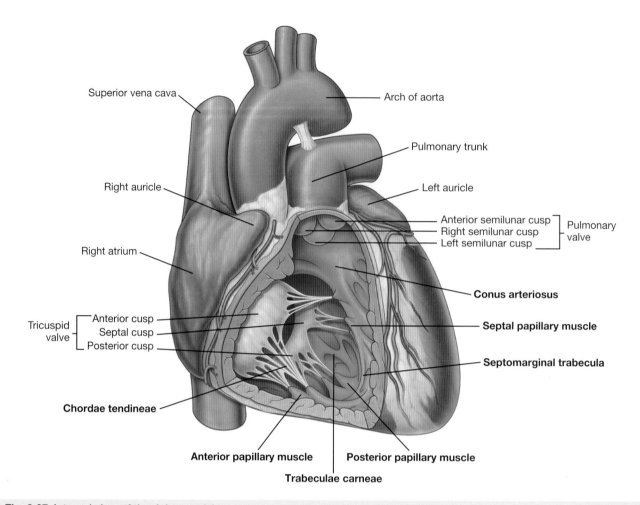

Superior vena cava

Arch of aorta

Pulmonary trunk

Right auricle

Left auricle

Anterior semilunar cusp
Right semilunar cusp ⎤ Pulmonary
Left semilunar cusp ⎦ valve

Right atrium

Conus arteriosus

Tricuspid valve ⎡ Anterior cusp
Septal cusp
Posterior cusp ⎦

Septal papillary muscle

Septomarginal trabecula

Chordae tendineae

Anterior papillary muscle

Posterior papillary muscle

Trabeculae carneae

Fig. 3.67 Internal view of the right ventricle.

- The **posterior papillary muscle** may consist of one, two, or three structures with some chordae tendineae arising directly from the ventricular wall.
- The **septal papillary muscle** is the most inconsistent papillary muscle, being either small or absent with chordae tendineae emerging directly from the septal wall.

A single specialized trabeculum, the **septomarginal trabecula (moderator band),** forms a bridge between the lower portion of the **interventricular septum** and the base of the anterior papillary muscle. The septomarginal trabecula carries a portion of the cardiac conduction system, the right bundle of the atrioventricular bundle, to the anterior wall of the right ventricle.

Tricuspid valve

The right atrioventricular orifice is closed during ventricular contraction by the **tricuspid valve (right atrioventricular valve),** so named because it usually consists of three cusps or leaflets (Fig. 3.67). The base of each cusp is secured to a fibrous ring surrounding the atrioventricular orifice. This fibrous ring helps maintain the shape of the opening. The

cusps are continuous with each other near their bases at sites termed **commissures.**

The naming of the three cusps, the **anterior, septal,** and **posterior cusps,** is based on their relative position in the right ventricle (Fig. 3.67). The free margins of the cusps are attached to the chordae tendineae, which arise from the tips of the papillary muscles.

During filling of the right ventricle, the tricuspid valve is open, and the three cusps project into the right ventricle.

Without the presence of a compensating mechanism, when the ventricular musculature contracts, the valve cusps would be forced upward with the flow of blood and blood would move back into the right atrium. However, contraction of the papillary muscles attached to the cusps by chordae tendineae prevent the cusps from being everted into the right atrium.

Simply put, the papillary muscles and associated chordae tendineae keep the valves closed during the dramatic changes in ventricular size that occur during contraction.

In addition, chordae tendineae from two papillary muscles attach to each cusp. This helps prevent separation of the cusps during ventricular contraction. Proper closing of the

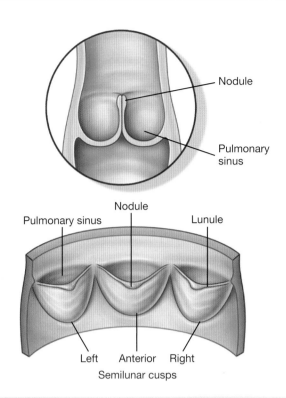

Fig. 3.68 Posterior view of the pulmonary valve.

Visualizing the left atrium and pulmonary veins

Fig. 3.69 Axial computed tomography image showing the pulmonary veins entering the left atrium.

tricuspid valve causes blood to exit the right ventricle and move into the pulmonary trunk.

Necrosis of a papillary muscle following a myocardial infarction (heart attack) may result in prolapse of the related valve.

Pulmonary valve

At the apex of the infundibulum, the outflow tract of the right ventricle, the opening into the pulmonary trunk is closed by the **pulmonary valve** (Fig. 3.68), which consists of three **semilunar cusps** with free edges projecting upward into the lumen of the pulmonary trunk. The free superior edge of each cusp has a middle, thickened portion, the **nodule of the semilunar cusp;** and a thin lateral portion, the **lunula of the semilunar cusp** (Fig. 3.68).

The cusps are named the **left, right,** and **anterior semilunar cusps** (see Fig. 3.75). Each cusp forms a pocket-like sinus (Fig. 3.68)—a dilation in the wall of the initial portion of the pulmonary trunk. After ventricular contraction, the recoil of blood fills these **pulmonary sinuses** and forces the cusps closed. This prevents blood in the pulmonary trunk from refilling the right ventricle.

Left atrium

The **left atrium** forms most of the base or posterior surface of the heart.

As with the right atrium, the left atrium is derived embryologically from two structures.

- The posterior half, or inflow portion, receives the four pulmonary veins (Fig. 3.70). It has smooth walls and derives from the proximal parts of the pulmonary veins that are incorporated into the left atrium during development.
- The anterior half is continuous with the left auricle. It contains musculi pectinati and derives from the embryonic primitive atrium. Unlike the crista terminalis in the right atrium, no distinct structure separates the two components of the left atrium.

The interatrial septum is part of the anterior wall of the left atrium. The thin area or depression in the septum is the valve of the foramen ovale and is opposite the floor of the fossa ovalis in the right atrium.

During development, the **valve of foramen ovale** prevents blood from passing from the left atrium to the right atrium. This valve may not be completely fused in some adults, leaving a "probe patent" passage between the right atrium and the left atrium.

Left ventricle

The left ventricle lies anterior to the left atrium. It contributes to the anterior, diaphragmatic, and left pulmonary surfaces of the heart and forms the apex.

Blood enters the ventricle through the **left atrioventricular orifice** and flows in a forward direction to the apex (Fig. 3.71). The chamber itself is conical, is longer than the right ventricle, and has the thickest layer of **myocardium.** The outflow tract (the **aortic vestibule**) is posterior to the infundibulum of the right ventricle, has smooth walls, and is derived from the embryonic bulbus cordis.

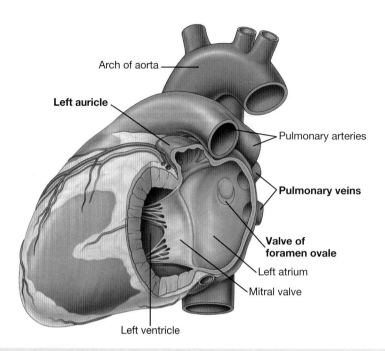

Arch of aorta

Left auricle

Pulmonary arteries

Pulmonary veins

**Valve of
foramen ovale**

Left atrium

Mitral valve

Left ventricle

Fig. 3.70 Internal view of left atrium

The **trabeculae carneae** in the left ventricle are fine and delicate in contrast to those in the right ventricle. The general appearance of the trabeculae with muscular ridges and bridges is similar to that of the right ventricle (Fig. 3.71).

Papillary muscles, together with chordae tendineae, are also observed and their structure is as described above for the right ventricle. Two papillary muscles, the **anterior** and **posterior papillary muscles,** are usually found in the left ventricle and are larger than those of the right ventricle (Fig. 3.71).

In the anatomical position, the left ventricle is somewhat posterior to the right ventricle. The interventricular septum therefore forms the anterior wall and some of the wall on the right side of the left ventricle. The septum is described as having two parts:

- a **muscular part,** and
- a **membranous part.**

The muscular part is thick and forms the major part of the septum, whereas the membranous part is the thin, upper part of the septum. A third part of the septum may be considered an atrioventricular part because of its position above the septal cusp of the tricuspid valve. This superior location places this part of the septum between the left ventricle and right atrium.

Mitral valve

The left atrioventricular orifice opens into the posterior right side of the superior part of the left ventricle. It is closed during ventricular contraction by the **mitral valve (left atrioventricular valve),** which is also referred to as the bicuspid valve because it has two cusps, the **anterior** and **posterior cusps** (Fig. 3.71). At their base, the cusps are secured to a fibrous ring surrounding the opening and are continuous with each other at the commissures. The coordinated action of the papillary muscles and chordae tendineae is as described for the right ventricle.

Aortic valve

The aortic vestibule, or outflow tract of the left ventricle, is continuous superiorly with the ascending aorta. The opening from the left ventricle into the aorta is closed by the **aortic valve.** This valve is similar in structure to the pulmonary valve. It consists of three **semilunar cusps** with the free edge of each projecting upward into the lumen of the ascending aorta (Fig. 3.72).

Between the semilunar cusps and the wall of the ascending aorta are pocket-like sinuses—the **right, left,** and **posterior aortic sinuses.** The right and left coronary arteries originate from the right and left aortic sinuses. Because of this, the posterior aortic sinus and cusp are sometimes referred to as the **noncoronary sinus and cusp.**

The functioning of the aortic valve is similar to that of the pulmonary valve with one important additional process: as blood recoils after ventricular contraction and fills the aortic sinuses, it is automatically forced into the coronary arteries because these vessels originate from the right and left aortic sinuses.

Arch of aorta

Mitral valve anterior cusp

Chordae tendineae

Anterior papillary muscle

Trabeculae carneae

Posterior papillary muscle

Mitral valve posterior cusp

Pulmonary arteries

Pulmonary veins

Left atrium

Coronary sinus

Fig. 3.71 Internal view of the left ventricle.

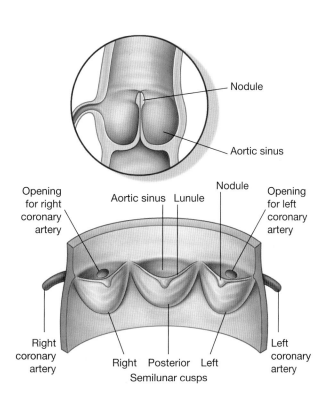

Nodule

Aortic sinus

Opening for right coronary artery

Aortic sinus

Lunule

Nodule

Opening for left coronary artery

Right coronary artery

Right

Posterior

Left

Semilunar cusps

Left coronary artery

Fig. 3.72 Anterior view of the aortic valve.

Surface anatomy

Where to listen for heart sounds

To listen for valve sounds, position the stethoscope downstream from the flow of blood through the valves (Fig. 3.73).

- The tricuspid valve is heard just to the left of the lower part of the sternum near the fifth intercostal space.

- The mitral valve is heard over the apex of the heart in the left fifth intercostal space at the midclavicular line.
- The pulmonary valve is heard over the medial end of the left second intercostal space.
- The aortic valve is heard over the medial end of the right second intercostal space.

Auscultation position for aortic valve

Auscultation position for pulmonary valve

Pulmonary valve

Aortic valve

Mitral valve

Tricuspid valve

Auscultation position for tricuspid valve

Auscultation position for mitral valve

Fig. 3.73 Anterior view of the chest wall of a man showing skeletal structures, heart, location of the heart valves, and auscultation points.

Clinical app

Valve disease

Valve problems consist of two basic types:

- incompetence (insufficiency), which results from poorly functioning valves, and
- stenosis, a narrowing of the orifice caused by the valve's inability to open fully.

Mitral valve disease is usually a mixed pattern of stenosis and incompetence, one of which usually predominates. Both stenosis and incompetence lead to a poorly functioning valve and subsequent heart changes, which include:

- left ventricular hypertrophy (this is appreciably less marked in patients with mitral stenosis),
- increased pulmonary venous pressure,
- pulmonary edema, and
- enlargement (dilation) and hypertrophy of the left atrium.

Aortic valve disease, both aortic stenosis and aortic regurgitation (backflow), can produce heart failure.

Valve disease in the right side of the heart (affecting the tricuspid or pulmonary valve) is most likely caused by infection. The resulting valve dysfunction produces abnormal pressure changes in the right atrium and right ventricle, and these can induce cardiac failure.

Common congenital heart defects

The most common abnormalities that occur during development are those produced by a defect in the interatrial and interventricular septa.

A **defect in the interatrial septum** allows blood to pass from one side of the heart to the other from the chamber with the higher pressure; this is clinically referred to as a shunt. An **atrial septal defect (ASD)** allows oxygenated blood to flow from the left atrium (higher pressure) across the ASD into the right atrium (lower pressure). Many patients with ASD are asymptomatic, but in some cases the ASD may need to be closed surgically or by endovascular devices. The most common of all congenital heart defects are those that occur in the interventricular septum—**ventricular septal defect (VSD).** These lesions are most frequent in the membranous portion of the septum and they allow blood to move from the left ventricle (higher pressure) to the right ventricle (lower pressure); this leads to right ventricular hypertrophy and pulmonary arterial hypertension. If large enough and left untreated, VSDs can produce marked clinical problems that might require surgery.

Occasionally, the **ductus arteriosus,** which connects the left branch of the pulmonary artery to the inferior aspect of the aortic arch, fails to close at birth. When this occurs, the oxygenated blood in the aortic arch (higher pressure) passes into the left branch of the pulmonary artery (lower pressure) and produces pulmonary hypertension. This is termed a **patent** or **persistent ductus arteriosus (PDA).**

Cardiac skeleton

The cardiac skeleton consists of dense, fibrous connective tissue in the form of four rings with interconnecting areas between the atria and the ventricles (Fig. 3.75). The four rings surround the two atrioventricular orifices, the aortic orifice, and the opening of the pulmonary trunk. They are the **anulus fibrosus.** The interconnecting areas include:

- the **right fibrous trigone**—a thickened area of connective tissue between the aortic ring and right atrioventricular ring (Fig. 3.75); and
- the **left fibrous trigone**—a thickened area of connective tissue between the aortic ring and the left atrioventricular ring (Fig. 3.75).

The cardiac skeleton helps maintain the integrity of the openings it surrounds and provides points of attachment for the cusps. It also separates the atrial musculature from the ventricular musculature. The atrial myocardium originates from the upper border of the rings, whereas the ventricular myocardium originates from the lower border of the rings.

The cardiac skeleton also serves as a dense connective tissue partition that electrically isolates the atria from the ventricles. The atrioventricular bundle, which passes through

Cardiac auscultation

Auscultation of the heart reveals the normal audible cardiac cycle, which allows the clinician to assess heart rate, rhythm, and regularity. Furthermore, cardiac murmurs that have characteristic sounds within the phases of the cardiac cycle can be demonstrated (Fig. 3.74).

Fig. 3.74 Heart sounds and how they relate to valve closure, the electrocardiogram, and ventricular pressure.

the anulus, is the single connection between these two groups of myocardium.

Coronary vasculature

Two coronary arteries arise from the aortic sinuses in the initial portion of the ascending aorta and supply the muscle and other tissues of the heart. They circle the heart in the coronary sulcus, with marginal and interventricular branches, in the interventricular sulci, converging toward the apex of the heart.

The returning venous blood passes through cardiac veins, most of which empty into the coronary sinus. This large venous structure is located in the coronary sulcus on the posterior surface of the heart between the left atrium and left ventricle. The coronary sinus empties into the right atrium between the opening of the inferior vena cava and the right atrioventricular orifice.

Coronary arteries

The right coronary artery branches from the right aortic sinus of the ascending aorta, passing anterior and to the right between the right auricle and the pulmonary trunk. It then

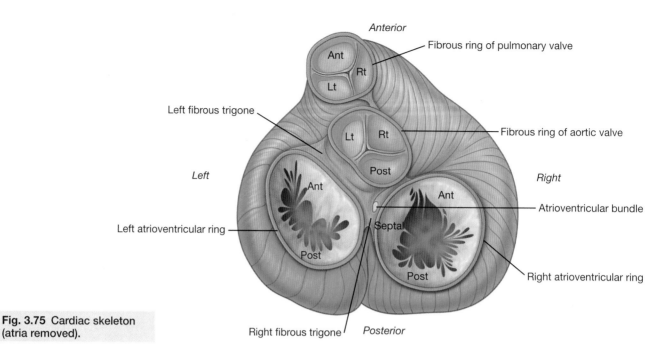

Fig. 3.75 Cardiac skeleton (atria removed).

descends vertically between the right atrium and right ventricle in the coronary sulcus (Fig. 3.76). Reaching the inferior margin of the heart, it turns posteriorly and continues in the sulcus onto the diaphragmatic surface and base of the heart. During this course, the following branches arise:

- an early **atrial branch,** passing between the right auricle and ascending aorta, gives off the **sinu-atrial nodal branch,** which passes posteriorly around the superior vena cava to supply the sinu-atrial node;
- a **right marginal branch** arising as the right coronary artery approaches the inferior (acute) margin of the heart. This branch continues along this border toward the apex of the heart;
- a small branch to the atrioventricular node as the right coronary artery continues on the base/diaphragmatic surface of the heart; and
- the **posterior interventricular branch,** its final branch, which lies in the posterior interventricular sulcus.

The right coronary artery supplies the right atrium and right ventricle, the sinu-atrial and atrioventricular nodes, the interatrial septum, a portion of the left atrium, the posteroinferior one-third of the interventricular septum, and a portion of the posterior part of the left ventricle.

The **left coronary artery** branches from the left aortic sinus of the ascending aorta passing between the pulmonary trunk and the left auricle before entering the coronary sulcus. Posterior to the pulmonary trunk, the artery divides into its two terminal branches, the anterior interventricular and the circumflex (Fig. 3.76).

- The **anterior interventricular branch (left anterior descending artery—LAD)** continues around the left side

of the pulmonary trunk and descends obliquely toward the apex of the heart in the anterior interventricular sulcus. During its course, one or two large **diagonal branches** may arise and descend diagonally across the anterior surface of the left ventricle.

- The **circumflex branch** continues to the left in the coronary sulcus and onto the base/diaphragmatic surface of the heart. It usually ends before reaching the posterior interventricular sulcus. A large branch, the **left marginal artery,** usually arises from it and continues across the rounded obtuse margin of the heart.

The left coronary artery supplies most of the left atrium and left ventricle and most of the interventricular septum, including the atrioventricular bundle and its branches.

Variations in the distribution patterns of coronary arteries. Several major variations in the basic distribution patterns of the coronary arteries occur.

- The distribution pattern described above for both right and left coronary arteries is the most common and consists of a right dominant coronary artery. This means that the posterior interventricular branch arises from the right coronary artery. The right coronary artery therefore supplies a large portion of the posterior wall of the left ventricle, and the circumflex branch of the left coronary artery is relatively small.
- In contrast, in hearts with a left dominant coronary artery, the posterior interventricular branch arises from an enlarged circumflex branch and supplies most of the posterior wall of the left ventricle (Fig. 3.77).
- Another point of variation relates to the arterial supply to the sinu-atrial and atrioventricular nodes. In most

Atrial branch

Left coronary artery

Left auricle

**Circumflex branch
of left coronary artery**

**Left marginal branch
of circumflex branch**

**Anterior interventricular
branch of left
coronary artery**

Left ventricle

**Diagonal branch of
anterior interventricular branch**

**Sinu-atrial nodal branch
of right coronary artery**

Right coronary artery

Right atrium

Right ventricle

**Right marginal branch
of right coronary artery**

**Posterior interventricular
branch of right coronary artery**

Fig. 3.76 Anterior view of coronary arterial system. Right dominant coronary artery.

Left coronary artery

Circumflex branch
of left coronary artery

Left marginal branch
of circumflex branch

Anterior interventricular
branch of left coronary artery

Diagonal branch of
anterior interventricular branch

**Sinu-atrial nodal branch
of left coronary artery**

Right coronary artery

Marginal branch
of right coronary artery

**Posterior interventricular branch of
circumflex branch of left coronary artery**

Fig. 3.77 Left dominant coronary artery.

cases, these two structures are supplied by the right coronary artery. However, vessels from the circumflex branch of the left coronary artery occasionally supply these structures.

Clinical app

Clinical terminology for coronary arteries
In practice, physicians use alternative names for the coronary vessels. The short left coronary artery is referred to as the **left main stem vessel.** One of its primary branches, the anterior interventricular artery, is termed the **left anterior descending artery (LAD).** Similarly, the terminal branch of the right coronary artery, the posterior interventricular artery, is termed the **posterior descending artery (PDA).**

Cardiac veins

The **coronary sinus** receives four major tributaries: the great, middle, small, and posterior cardiac veins.

The **great cardiac vein** begins at the apex of the heart (Fig. 3.78A) and ascends in the anterior interventricular sulcus where it travels with the anterior interventricular artery. In this location it may be referred to as the **anterior interventricular vein.** At the coronary sulcus, it turns to the left and continues onto the base/diaphragmatic surface of the heart and is associated with the circumflex branch of the left coronary artery. Continuing along its path in the coronary sulcus, the great cardiac vein gradually enlarges becoming the coronary sinus, which enters the right atrium (Fig. 3.78B).

The **middle cardiac vein (posterior interventricular vein)** begins near the apex of the heart and ascends in the posterior interventricular sulcus toward the coronary sinus (Fig. 3.78B). It is associated with the posterior interventricular branch of the right or left coronary artery throughout its course.

The **small cardiac vein** begins in the lower anterior section of the coronary sulcus between the right atrium and right ventricle (Fig. 3.78A). It continues in this groove onto the base/diaphragmatic surface of the heart and enters the coronary sinus at its atrial end. It is a companion of the right coronary artery throughout its course and may receive the **right marginal vein** (Fig. 3.78A). This small vein accompanies the marginal branch of the right coronary artery along the acute margin of the heart. If the right marginal vein does not join the small cardiac vein, it enters the right atrium directly.

The **posterior cardiac vein** lies on the posterior surface of the left ventricle just to the left of the middle cardiac vein (Fig. 3.78B). It either enters the coronary sinus directly or joins the great cardiac vein.

Other cardiac veins. Two additional groups of cardiac veins are also involved in the venous drainage of the heart.

- The **anterior veins of right ventricle (anterior cardiac veins)** are small veins that arise on the anterior surface of the right ventricle (Fig. 3.78A). They cross the coronary sulcus and enter the anterior wall of the right atrium. They drain the anterior portion of the right ventricle. The right marginal vein may be part of this group if it does not enter the small cardiac vein.
- A group of the smallest cardiac veins (**venae cordis minimae** or **veins of Thebesius**) have also been described. Draining directly into the cardiac chambers, they are numerous in the right atrium and right ventricle, are occasionally associated with the left atrium, and are rarely associated with the left ventricle.

Coronary lymphatics

The lymphatic vessels of the heart follow the coronary arteries and drain mainly into:

- brachiocephalic nodes, anterior to the brachiocephalic veins; and
- tracheobronchial nodes, at the inferior end of the trachea.

Cardiac conduction system

The cardiac conduction system initiates and coordinates contraction of the musculature of the atria and ventricles (Fig. 3.79). It consists of nodes and networks of specialized cardiac muscle cells organized into four basic components:

- the sinu-atrial node,
- the atrioventricular node,
- the atrioventricular bundle with its right and left bundle branches, and
- the subendocardial plexus of conduction cells (the Purkinje fibers).

The unique distribution pattern of the cardiac conduction system is an important unidirectional pathway of excitation/contraction. Throughout its course, large branches of the conduction system are insulated from the surrounding myocardium by connective tissue. This tends to decrease inappropriate stimulation and contraction of cardiac muscle fibers.

Thus a unidirectional wave of excitation and contraction is established, which moves from the papillary muscles and apex of the ventricles to the arterial outflow tracts.

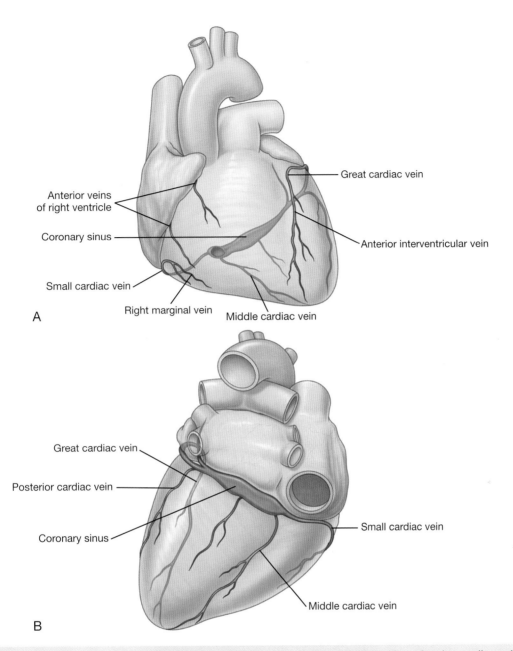

Great cardiac vein

Anterior veins
of right ventricle

Coronary sinus

Small cardiac vein

Right marginal vein

Middle cardiac vein

Anterior interventricular vein

A

Great cardiac vein

Posterior cardiac vein

Coronary sinus

Small cardiac vein

Middle cardiac vein

B

Fig. 3.78 Major cardiac veins. **A.** Anterior view of major cardiac veins. **B.** Posteroinferior view of major cardiac veins.

Clinical app

Cardiac conduction system

The cardiac conduction system can be affected by coronary artery disease. The normal rhythm may be disturbed if the blood supply to the coronary conduction system is disrupted. If a dysrhythmia affects the heart rate or the order in which the chambers contract, heart failure and death may ensue.

Sinu-atrial node

Impulses begin at the **sinu-atrial node,** the cardiac pacemaker. This collection of cells is located at the superior end of the crista terminalis at the junction of the superior vena cava and the right atrium (Fig. 3.79A). This is also the junction between the parts of the right atrium derived from the embryonic sinus venosus and the atrium proper.

The excitation signals generated by the sinu-atrial node spread across the atria, causing the muscle to contract.

Atrioventricular node

Concurrently, the wave of excitation in the atria stimulates the **atrioventricular node,** which is located near the opening of the coronary sinus, close to the attachment of the septal cusp of the tricuspid valve, and within the atrioventricular septum (Fig. 3.79A).

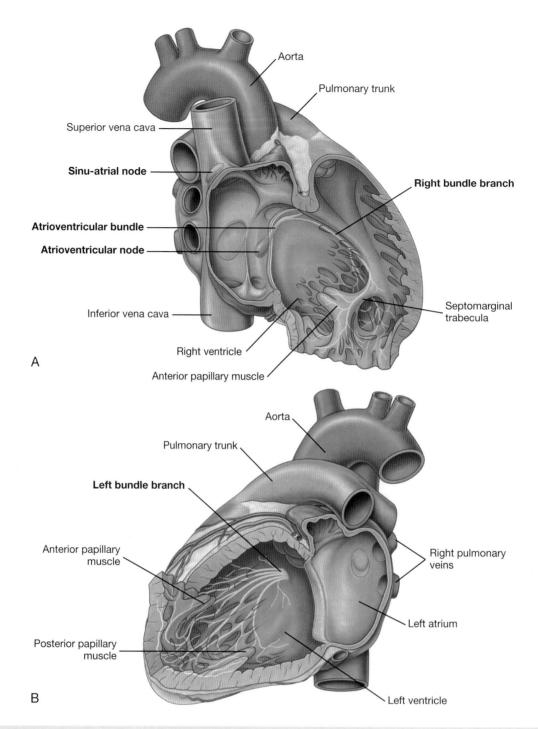

Fig. 3.79 Conduction system of the heart. **A.** Right chambers. **B.** Left chambers.

The atrioventricular node is a collection of specialized cells that form the beginning of an elaborate system of conducting tissue, the atrioventricular bundle, which extends the excitatory impulse to all ventricular musculature.

Atrioventricular bundle

The **atrioventricular bundle** is a direct continuation of the atrioventricular node (Fig. 3.79A). It follows the lower border

of the membranous part of the interventricular septum before splitting into right and left bundles.

The **right bundle branch** continues on the right side of the interventricular septum toward the apex of the right ventricle. From the septum it enters the septomarginal trabecula to reach the base of the anterior papillary muscle. At this point, it divides and is continuous with the final component of the cardiac conduction system, the **subendocardial plexus of ventricular conduction cells (Purkinje fibers).**

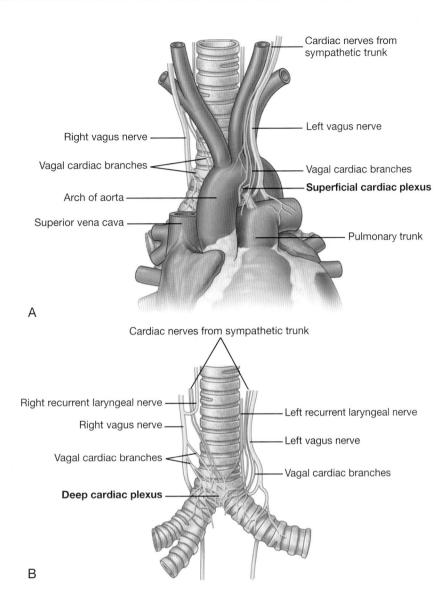

Cardiac nerves from sympathetic trunk

Right vagus nerve

Vagal cardiac branches

Arch of aorta

Superior vena cava

Left vagus nerve

Vagal cardiac branches

Superficial cardiac plexus

Pulmonary trunk

A

Cardiac nerves from sympathetic trunk

Right recurrent laryngeal nerve

Right vagus nerve

Vagal cardiac branches

Deep cardiac plexus

Left recurrent laryngeal nerve

Left vagus nerve

Vagal cardiac branches

B

Fig. 3.80 Cardiac plexus. A. Superficial. B. Deep.

This network of specialized cells spreads throughout the ventricle to supply ventricular musculature including the papillary muscles.

The **left bundle branch** passes to the left side of the muscular interventricular septum and descends to the apex of the left ventricle (Fig. 3.79B). Along its course it gives off branches that eventually become continuous with the **subendocardial plexus of conduction cells (Purkinje fibers).** As with the right side, this network of specialized cells spreads the excitation impulses throughout the left ventricle.

Cardiac innervation

The autonomic division of the peripheral nervous system is directly responsible for regulating:

- heart rate,
- force of each contraction, and
- cardiac output.

Branches from both the parasympathetic and sympathetic systems contribute to the formation of the **cardiac plexus.** This plexus consists of a **superficial part,** inferior to the aortic arch and between it and the pulmonary trunk (Fig. 3.80A), and a **deep part,** between the aortic arch and the tracheal bifurcation (Fig. 3.80B).

From the cardiac plexus, small branches that are mixed nerves containing both sympathetic and parasympathetic fibers supply the heart. These branches affect nodal tissue and other components of the conduction system, coronary blood vessels, and atrial and ventricular musculature.

Parasympathetic innervation

Stimulation of the parasympathetic system:

- decreases heart rate,
- reduces force of contraction, and
- constricts the coronary arteries.

The preganglionic parasympathetic fibers reach the heart as cardiac branches from the right and left vagus nerves (Fig. 3.80). They enter the cardiac plexus and synapse in ganglia located either within the plexus or in the walls of the atria.

Sympathetic innervation

Stimulation of the sympathetic system:

- increases heart rate and
- increases the force of contraction.

Sympathetic fibers reach the cardiac plexus through the cardiac nerves from the sympathetic trunk (Fig. 3.80). Preganglionic sympathetic fibers from the upper four or five segments of the thoracic spinal cord enter and move through the sympathetic trunk. They synapse in cervical and upper thoracic sympathetic ganglia, and postganglionic fibers proceed as bilateral branches from the sympathetic trunk to the cardiac plexus.

Visceral afferents

Visceral afferents from the heart are also a component of the cardiac plexus. These fibers pass through the cardiac plexus and return to the central nervous system in the cardiac nerves from the sympathetic trunk and in the vagal cardiac branches.

The afferents associated with the vagal cardiac nerves return to the vagus nerve [X]. They sense alterations in blood pressure and blood chemistry and are therefore primarily concerned with cardiac reflexes.

The afferents associated with the cardiac nerves from the sympathetic trunks return to either the cervical or the thoracic portions of the sympathetic trunk. If they are in the cervical portion of the trunk, they normally descend to the thoracic region where they re-enter the upper four or five thoracic spinal cord segments along with the afferents from the thoracic region of the sympathetic trunk.

Pulmonary trunk

The **pulmonary trunk** is within the pericardial sac (Fig. 3.82A), covered by the visceral layer of serous pericardium

Clinical app

Referred pain

When cardiac cells die during an MI, pain fibers (visceral afferents) are stimulated. They detect events at the cellular level as tissue-damaging events (i.e., cardiac ischemia). These visceral sensory fibers follow the course of sympathetic fibers that innervate the heart and enter the spinal cord between T1 and T4 spinal levels. At this level, somatic sensory fibers from spinal nerves T1 to T4 also enter the spinal cord via the posterior roots. Both types of fibers (visceral and somatic) synapse with interneurons, which then synapse with second neurons whose fibers pass across the cord and then ascend to the somatosensory areas of the brain that represent the T1 to T4

Clinical app—cont'd

levels. The brain is unable to distinguish clearly between the visceral sensory distribution and the somatic sensory distribution, and therefore the pain is interpreted as arising from the somatic regions rather than the visceral organ (i.e., the heart; Fig. 3.81).

Clinical app

Are heart attack symptoms the same in men and women?

Although men and women can experience the typical symptoms of severe chest pain, cold sweats, and pain in the left arm, women are more likely than men to have subtler, less recognizable symptoms. These may include abdominal pain, achiness in the jaw or back, nausea, shortness of breath and/or simply fatigue. The mechanism of this difference is not understood, but it is important to consider cardiac ischemia for a wide range of symptoms.

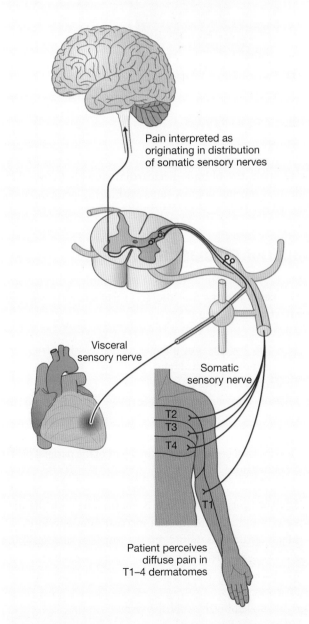

Pain interpreted as originating in distribution of somatic sensory nerves

Visceral sensory nerve

Somatic sensory nerve

T2
T3
T4

T1

Patient perceives diffuse pain in T1–4 dermatomes

Fig. 3.81 Mechanism for perceiving heart pain in T1–T4 dermatomes.

and enclosed in a common sheath with the ascending aorta. Arising from the conus arteriosus of the right ventricle, it is slightly anterior to the aortic orifice and ascends, moving posteriorly and to the left, lying initially anterior and then to the left of the ascending aorta. At approximately the level of the intervertebral disc between vertebrae TV and TVI opposite the left border of the sternum and posterior to the third left costal cartilage, the pulmonary trunk divides into:

- the right pulmonary artery, which passes to the right, posterior to the ascending aorta and the superior vena cava, to enter the right lung (Fig. 3.82B); and
- the left pulmonary artery, which passes inferiorly to the arch of the aorta and anteriorly to the descending aorta to enter the left lung (Fig. 3.82A,B).

Ascending aorta

The **ascending aorta** is within the pericardial sac and covered by a visceral layer of serous pericardium, which also surrounds the pulmonary trunk in a common sheath (Fig. 3.82A).

The origin of the ascending aorta is the aortic orifice at the base of the left ventricle, which is level with the lower edge of the third left costal cartilage and posterior to the left half of the sternum. Moving superiorly, slightly forward, and to the right, the ascending aorta continues to the level of the second right costal cartilage. At this point, it enters the superior mediastinum and is then referred to as the **arch of the aorta.**

Ascending aorta

Pulmonary trunk

Arch of aorta

Superior vena cava

Superior vena cava

Left pulmonary artery

Right pulmonary artery

Left pulmonary veins

Right pulmonary veins

Right atrium

Inferior vena cava

A

B   Oblique pericardial sinus

Fig. 3.82 Major vessels within the middle mediastinum. **A.** Anterior view. **B.** Posterior view.

Immediately superior to the point where the ascending aorta arises from the left ventricle are three small outward bulges opposite the semilunar cusps of the aortic valve. These are the posterior, right, and left aortic sinuses. The right and left coronary arteries originate from the right and left aortic sinuses, respectively.

Other vasculature

Passing through the fibrous pericardium at approximately the level of the second costal cartilage, the inferior half of the **superior vena cava** is within the pericardial sac (Fig. 3.82B). It enters the right atrium at the lower level of the third costal cartilage. The portion within the pericardial sac is covered with serous pericardium except for a small area on its posterior surface.

After passing through the diaphragm at approximately the level of vertebra TVIII, the **inferior vena cava** enters the fibrous pericardium. A short portion of this vessel is within the pericardial sac before entering the right atrium. While within the pericardial sac, it is covered by serous pericardium except for a small portion of its posterior surface (Fig. 3.82B).

A very short segment of each of the pulmonary veins is also within the pericardial sac. These veins, usually two from each lung, pass through the fibrous pericardium and enter the superior region of the left atrium on its posterior surface. In the pericardial sac, all but a portion of the posterior surface of these veins is covered by serous pericardium.

In addition, the **oblique pericardial sinus** is between the right and left pulmonary veins within the pericardial sac (Fig. 3.82B).

Superior mediastinum

Posterior to the manubrium of the sternum and anterior to the bodies of the first four thoracic vertebrae is the **superior mediastinum** (see Fig. 3.53).

- Superior border—an oblique plane passing from the jugular notch upward and posteriorly to the superior border of vertebra TI.
- Inferior border—a transverse plane passing from the sternal angle to the intervertebral disc between vertebra TIV/V separates it from the inferior mediastinum.
- Lateral borders—the mediastinal part of the parietal pleura on either side.

The superior mediastinum is continuous with the neck superiorly and with the inferior mediastinum inferiorly.

Major structures found in the superior mediastinum (Figs. 3.83, 3.84) include the:

- thymus,
- right and left brachiocephalic veins,
- left superior intercostal vein,
- superior vena cava,

- arch of the aorta with its three large branches,
- trachea,
- esophagus,
- phrenic nerves,
- vagus nerves,
- left recurrent laryngeal branch of the left vagus nerve,
- thoracic duct, and
- other small nerves, blood vessels, and lymphatics.

Thymus

Lying immediately posterior to the manubrium of the sternum, the thymus, asymmetric and bilobed, is the most anterior component of the superior mediastinum (Fig. 3.85).

The upper extent of the thymus can reach into the neck as high as the thyroid gland, and a lower portion typically extends into the anterior mediastinum over the pericardial sac.

Involved in the early development of the immune system, the thymus is a large structure in the child that begins to atrophy after puberty and shows considerable size variation in the adult. In the elderly adult, it is barely identifiable as an organ, consisting mostly of fatty tissue that is sometimes arranged as two lobulated fatty structures.

Arteries to the thymus are small branches from the internal thoracic arteries. Venous drainage is usually into the left brachiocephalic vein and possibly into the internal thoracic veins.

Lymphatic drainage returns to multiple groups of nodes at one or more of the following locations:

- along the internal thoracic arteries (parasternal),
- at the tracheal bifurcation (tracheobronchial), and
- in the root of the neck.

Clinical app

Ectopic parathyroid glands in the thymus

The parathyroid glands develop from the third pharyngeal pouch, which also forms the thymus. The thymus is therefore a common site for ectopic parathyroid glands and, potentially, ectopic parathyroid hormone production.

Right and left brachiocephalic veins

The **left and right brachiocephalic veins** are located immediately posterior to the thymus and form on each side at the junction between the internal jugular and subclavian veins (see Fig. 3.83). The left brachiocephalic vein crosses the midline and joins with the right brachiocephalic vein to form the superior vena cava (Fig. 3.86).

- The **right brachiocephalic vein** begins posterior to the medial end of the right clavicle and passes vertically downward, forming the superior vena cava when it is joined by the left brachiocephalic vein (Fig. 3.83). Venous tributaries include the vertebral, first posterior intercostal, and internal thoracic veins. The inferior thyroid and thymic veins may also drain into it.
- The **left brachiocephalic vein** begins posterior to the medial end of the left clavicle (Fig. 3.83). It crosses to the right, moving in a slightly inferior direction, and joins with the right brachiocephalic vein to form the superior vena cava posterior to the lower edge of the right first costal cartilage close to the right sternal border. Venous tributaries include the vertebral, first posterior intercostal, left superior intercostal, inferior thyroid, and internal thoracic veins. It may also receive thymic and pericardial veins.

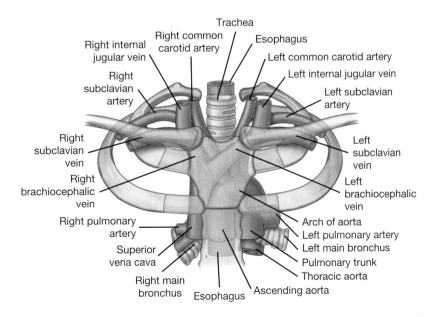

Fig. 3.83 Structures in the superior mediastinum.

Imaging app

Visualizing structures in the superior mediastinum

A

Brachiocephalic trunk

Thymus — Manubrium of sternum

Right brachiocephalic vein — Left brachiocephalic vein

Right phrenic nerve — Left phrenic nerve

Left common carotid artery

Trachea

Left vagus nerve

Left subclavian artery

Left recurrent laryngeal nerve

TIII

Right vagus nerve

Esophagus — Thoracic duct

B

Brachiocephalic trunk

Right brachiocephalic vein — Left brachiocephalic vein

Trachea

Esophagus

Left subclavian artery

Left common carotid artery

Fig. 3.84 Cross-section through the superior mediastinum at the level of vertebra TIII. **A.** Diagram. **B.** Axial computed tomography image.

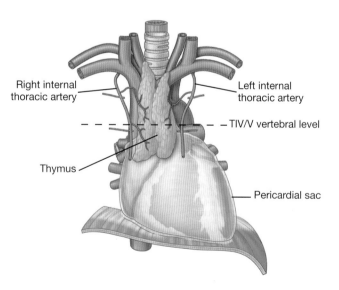

Right internal thoracic artery

Left internal thoracic artery

TIV/V vertebral level

Thymus

Pericardial sac

Fig. 3.85 Thymus.

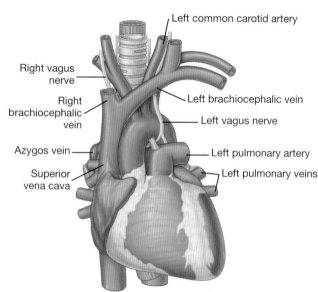

Left common carotid artery

Right vagus nerve

Right brachiocephalic vein

Left brachiocephalic vein

Left vagus nerve

Azygos vein

Superior vena cava

Left pulmonary artery

Left pulmonary veins

Fig. 3.86 Superior mediastinum with thymus removed.

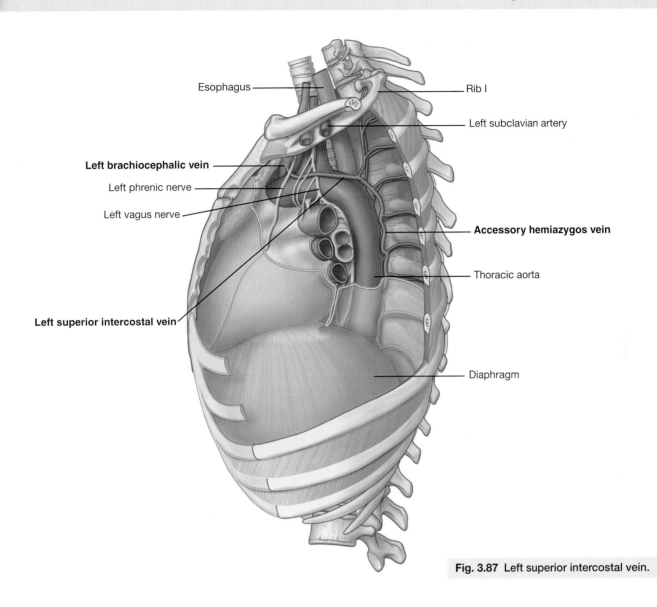

Esophagus — — Rib I

— Left subclavian artery

Left brachiocephalic vein —

Left phrenic nerve —

Left vagus nerve —

— **Accessory hemiazygos vein**

— Thoracic aorta

Left superior intercostal vein —

— Diaphragm

Fig. 3.87 Left superior intercostal vein.

Clinical app

Left brachiocephalic vein

The left brachiocephalic vein crosses the midline posterior to the manubrium in the adult. In infants and children, the left brachiocephalic vein rises above the superior border of the manubrium and therefore is less protected.

Left superior intercostal vein

The **left superior intercostal vein** receives the second, third, and sometimes the left fourth posterior intercostal veins, usually the left bronchial veins, and sometimes the left pericardiacophrenic vein. It passes over the left side of the aortic arch, lateral to the left vagus nerve and medial to the left phrenic nerve, before entering the left brachiocephalic vein (Fig. 3.87). Inferiorly, it may connect with the **accessory hemiazygos vein (superior hemiazygos vein)**. The left first intercostal vein drains directly into the left brachiocephalic vein or into the left vertebral vein.

Superior vena cava

The vertically oriented **superior vena** cava begins posterior to the lower edge of the right first costal cartilage where the right and left brachiocephalic veins join and terminates at the lower edge of the right third costal cartilage where it joins the right atrium (see Fig. 3.83).

The lower half of the superior vena cava is within the pericardial sac and contained in the middle mediastinum.

The superior vena cava receives the azygos vein immediately before entering the pericardial sac and may also receive pericardial and mediastinal veins.

Arch of aorta and its branches

The thoracic portion of the aorta can be divided into **ascending aorta, arch of aorta,** and **thoracic (descending) aorta.** Only the arch of the aorta is in the superior mediastinum. It begins when the ascending aorta emerges from the pericardial sac and courses upward, backward, and to the left as it passes through the superior mediastinum, ending on the left side at vertebral level TIV/V. Extending as high as the midlevel of the manubrium of sternum, the arch is initially anterior and finally lateral to the trachea (Figs. 3.88, 3.89).

Clinical app

Venous access for central and dialysis lines
Large systemic veins are used to establish central venous access for administering large amounts of fluid, drugs, and blood. Most of these lines (small bore tubes) are introduced through venous puncture into the axillary, subclavian, or internal jugular veins. The lines are then passed through the main veins of the superior mediastinum, with the tips of the lines usually residing in the distal portion of the superior vena cava or in the right atrium.

Similar devices, such as dialysis lines, are inserted into patients who have renal failure, so that a large volume of blood can be aspirated through one channel and re-infused through a second channel.

Clinical app

Using the superior vena cava to access the inferior vena cava
Because the superior and inferior vena cava are oriented along the same vertical axis, a guide-wire, catheter, or line can be passed from the superior vena cava through the right atrium and into the inferior vena cava. This is a common route of access for such procedures as:

- transjugular liver biopsy,
- transjugular intrahepatic portosystemic shunts (TIPS), and
- insertion of an inferior vena cava filter to catch emboli dislodged from veins in the lower limb and pelvis (i.e., patients with deep vein thrombosis [DVT]).

Fig. 3.88 Superior mediastinum with thymus and venous channels removed.

Three branches arise from the superior border of the arch of the aorta and, at their origins, all three are crossed anteriorly by the left brachiocephalic vein.

The first branch

Beginning on the right, the first branch of the arch of aorta is the **brachiocephalic trunk** (Fig. 3.88). It is the largest of the three branches and, at its point of origin behind the manubrium of sternum, is slightly anterior to the other two branches. It ascends slightly posteriorly and to the right. At the level of the upper edge of the right sternoclavicular joint, the brachiocephalic trunk divides into:

- the **right common carotid artery** and
- the **right subclavian artery.**

The arteries mainly supply the right side of the head and neck and the right upper limb, respectively.

Occasionally, the brachiocephalic trunk has a small branch, the **thyroid ima artery,** which contributes to the vascular supply of the thyroid gland.

The second branch

The second branch of the arch of aorta is the **left common carotid artery** (Fig. 3.88). It arises from the arch immediately to the left and slightly posterior to the brachiocephalic trunk and ascends through the superior mediastinum along the left side of the trachea.

The left common carotid artery supplies the left side of the head and neck.

The third branch

The third branch of the arch of the aorta is the **left subclavian artery** (Fig. 3.88). It arises from the arch of aorta immediately to the left of, and slightly posterior to, the left common carotid artery and ascends through the superior mediastinum along the left side of the trachea.

The left subclavian artery is the major blood supply to the left upper limb.

Ligamentum arteriosum

The **ligamentum arteriosum** is also in the superior mediastinum and is important in embryonic circulation, when it is a patent vessel (the **ductus arteriosus**). It connects the pulmonary trunk with the arch of aorta and allows blood to bypass the lungs during development (Fig. 3.88). The vessel closes soon after birth and forms the ligamentous connection observed in the adult.

Trachea and esophagus

The **trachea** is a midline structure that is palpable in the jugular notch as it enters the superior mediastinum.

Clinical app

Coarctation of the aorta
Coarctation of the aorta is a congenital abnormality in which the aortic lumen is constricted just distal to the origin of the left subclavian artery. At this point, the aorta becomes significantly narrowed and the blood supply to the lower limbs and abdomen is diminished. Over time, collateral vessels develop around the chest wall and abdomen to supply the lower body. The coarctation also affects the heart, which has to pump the blood at higher pressure to maintain peripheral perfusion. This in turn may produce cardiac failure.

Clinical app

Traumatic injury to the aorta
The aorta has three fixed points of attachment:
- the aortic valve,
- the ligamentum arteriosum, and
- the point of entry behind the crura of the diaphragm.

A serious deceleration injury (e.g., in a traffic accident) is most likely to cause aortic trauma at these fixed points. The rest of the aorta is relatively free from attachment to other structures of the mediastinum and is less likely to be injured.

Posterior to it is the **esophagus,** which is immediately anterior to the vertebral column (Fig. 3.89; also see Fig. 3.83). Significant mobility exists in the vertical positioning of these structures as they pass through the superior mediastinum.

As the trachea and esophagus pass through the superior mediastinum, they are crossed laterally by the azygos vein on the right side and the arch of aorta on the left side.

The trachea divides into the right and left main bronchi at, or just inferior to, the transverse plane between the sternal angle and vertebral level TIV/V (Fig. 3.90), whereas the esophagus continues into the posterior mediastinum.

Nerves of the superior mediastinum
Vagus nerves

The **vagus nerves** [X] pass through the superior and posterior divisions of the mediastinum on their way to the abdominal cavity. As they pass through the thorax, they provide parasympathetic innervation to the thoracic viscera and carry visceral afferents from the thoracic viscera.

Visceral afferents in the vagus nerves relay information to the central nervous system about normal physiological processes and reflex activities. They do not transmit pain sensation.

Imaging app

Visualizing structures at the TIV vertebral level

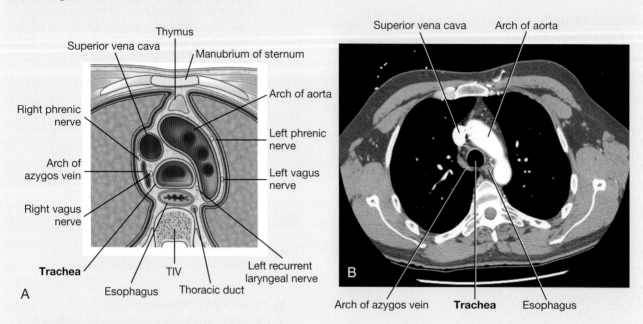

Fig. 3.89 Cross-section through the superior mediastinum at the level of vertebra TIV. **A.** Diagram. **B.** Axial computed tomography image.

Fig. 3.90 Trachea in the superior mediastinum.

Right vagus nerve

The **right vagus nerve** enters the superior mediastinum between the right brachiocephalic vein and the brachiocephalic trunk. It descends in a posterior direction toward the trachea (Fig. 3.91), crosses the lateral surface of the trachea, and passes posteriorly to the root of the right lung to reach the esophagus. Just before the esophagus, it is crossed by the arch of the azygos vein.

Clinical app

Aortic dissection

In certain conditions, such as in severe arteriovascular disease, the wall of the aorta can split longitudinally, creating a false channel, which may or may not rejoin into the true lumen distally. This aortic dissection occurs between the intima and media anywhere along its length. If it occurs in the ascending aorta or arch of the aorta, blood flow in the coronary and cerebral arteries may be disrupted, resulting in MI or stroke. In the abdomen the visceral vessels may be disrupted, producing ischemia to the gut or kidneys.

Clinical app

Aortic arch and its anomalies

A right-sided arch of aorta occasionally occurs and may be asymptomatic. It can be associated with **dextrocardia** (right-sided heart) and, in some instances, with complete **situs inversus** (left-to-right inversion of the body's organs). It can also be associated with abnormal branching of the great vessels.

Clinical app

Abnormal origin of great vessels

Great vessels occasionally have an abnormal origin, including:

- a common origin of the brachiocephalic trunk and the left common carotid artery,
- the left vertebral artery originating from the aortic arch, and
- the right subclavian artery originating from the distal portion of the aortic arch and passing behind the esophagus to supply the right arm—as a result, the great vessels form a vascular ring around the trachea and the esophagus, which can potentially produce difficulty swallowing.

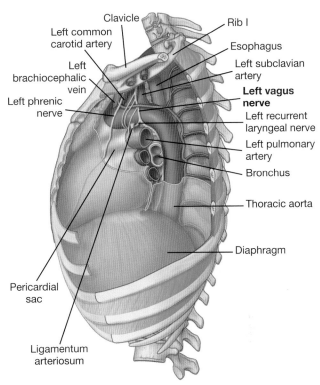

Fig. 3.92 Left vagus nerve passing through the superior mediastinum.

As the left vagus nerve passes through the superior mediastinum, branches go to the esophagus, cardiac plexus, and pulmonary plexus.

The left vagus nerve also gives rise to the **left recurrent laryngeal nerve,** which arises at the inferior margin of the arch of aorta just lateral to the ligamentum arteriosum (Fig. 3.92). The left recurrent laryngeal nerve passes inferior to the arch of aorta before ascending on its medial surface. Entering a groove between the trachea and esophagus, the left recurrent laryngeal nerve continues superiorly to enter the neck and terminate in the larynx (Fig. 3.93).

Phrenic nerves

The phrenic nerves arise in the cervical region from the third, fourth, and fifth cervical spinal cord segments. They descend through the thorax to supply motor and sensory innervation to the diaphragm and its associated membranes. As they pass through the thorax, they provide innervation through somatic afferent fibers to the mediastinal pleura, fibrous pericardium, and parietal layer of the serous pericardium.

Right phrenic nerve

The **right phrenic nerve** enters the superior mediastinum lateral to the right vagus nerve and lateral and slightly posterior to the beginning of the right brachiocephalic vein (see

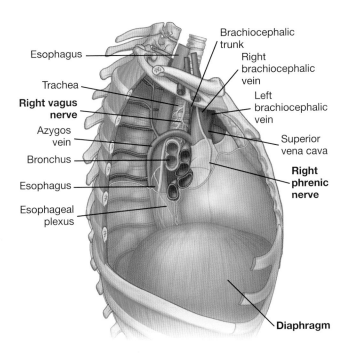

Fig. 3.91 Right vagus nerve passing through the superior mediastinum.

As it passes through the superior mediastinum, branches are given off to the esophagus, cardiac plexus, and pulmonary plexus.

Left vagus nerve

The **left vagus nerve** enters the superior mediastinum posterior to the left brachiocephalic vein between the left common carotid and left subclavian arteries (Fig. 3.92). It passes into the superior mediastinum just deep to the mediastinal part of the parietal pleura and crosses the left side of the arch of aorta. It descends in a posterior direction and passes posterior to the root of the left lung to reach the esophagus in the posterior mediastinum.

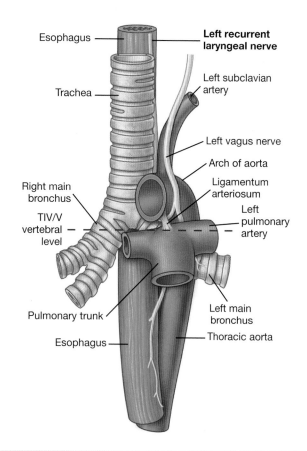

Fig. 3.93 Left recurrent laryngeal nerve passing through the superior mediastinum.

Fig. 3.91). It continues inferiorly along the right side of this vein and the superior vena cava.

On entering the middle mediastinum, the right phrenic nerve descends along the right side of the pericardial sac within the fibrous pericardium, anterior to the root of the right lung. The pericardiacophrenic vessels accompany it through most of its course in the thorax (see Fig. 3.55). It leaves the thorax by passing through the diaphragm with the inferior vena cava.

Left phrenic nerve

The **left phrenic nerve** enters the superior mediastinum in a position similar to the path taken by the right phrenic nerve. It lies lateral to the left vagus nerve and lateral and slightly posterior to the beginning of the left brachiocephalic vein (Fig. 3.92) and continues to descend across the left lateral surface of the arch of aorta, passing superficially to the left vagus nerve and the left superior intercostal vein.

On entering the middle mediastinum, the left phrenic nerve follows the left side of the pericardial sac within the fibrous pericardium, anterior to the root of the left lung, and is accompanied by the pericardiacophrenic vessels (see Fig. 3.55). It leaves the thorax by piercing the diaphragm near the apex of the heart.

Surface anatomy

Visualizing structures in the superior mediastinum
A number of structures in the superior mediastinum in adults can be visualized based on their positions relative to skeletal landmarks that can be palpated through the skin (Fig. 3.94).

- On each side, the internal jugular and subclavian veins join to form the brachiocephalic veins behind the sternal ends of the clavicles near the sternoclavicular joints.
- The left brachiocephalic vein crosses from left to right behind the manubrium of sternum.
- The brachiocephalic veins unite to form the superior vena cava behind the lower border of the costal cartilage of the right first rib.
- The arch of aorta begins and ends at the transverse plane between the sternal angle anteriorly and vertebral level TIV/V posteriorly. The arch may reach as high as the midlevel of the manubrium of sternum.

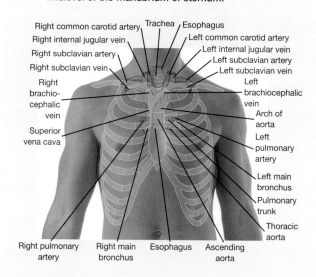

Fig. 3.94 Anterior view of the chest wall of a man showing the locations of different structures in the superior mediastinum as they relate to the skeleton.

Clinical app

The vagus nerves, recurrent laryngeal nerves, and hoarseness
The left recurrent laryngeal nerve is a branch of the left vagus nerve. It passes between the pulmonary artery and the aorta, a region known clinically as the **aortopulmonary window,** and may be compressed in any patient with a pathological mass in this region. This compression results in left vocal cord paralysis and hoarseness of the voice. Lymph node enlargement, often

Clinical app—cont'd

associated with the spread of lung cancer, is a common condition that may produce compression. Chest radiography is therefore usually carried out for all patients whose symptoms include a hoarse voice.

More superiorly, the right vagus nerve gives off the right recurrent laryngeal nerve, which "hooks" around the right subclavian artery at the superior sulcus of the right lung. If a patient has a hoarse voice and a right vocal cord palsy is demonstrated with a laryngoscopy, a chest CT should be obtained to assess for cancer in the right lung apex **(Pancoast's tumor)**.

Thoracic duct in the superior mediastinum

The **thoracic duct,** the major lymphatic vessel in the body, passes through the posterior portion of the superior mediastinum (see Figs. 3.84A, 3.89A). It:

- enters the superior mediastinum inferiorly, slightly to the left of the midline, having moved to this position just before leaving the posterior mediastinum opposite vertebral level TIV/V; and
- continues through the superior mediastinum, posterior to the arch of aorta, and the initial portion of the left subclavian artery between the esophagus and the left mediastinal part of the parietal pleura.

Posterior mediastinum

The **posterior mediastinum** is posterior to the pericardial sac and diaphragm and anterior to the bodies of the mid and lower thoracic vertebrae (see Fig. 3.53).

- Its superior boundary is a transverse plane from the sternal angle to the TIV and TV intervertebral disc.
- Its inferior boundary is the diaphragm.
- Laterally, it is bordered by the mediastinal part of parietal pleura on either side.
- Superiorly, it is continuous with the superior mediastinum.

Major structures in the posterior mediastinum include the:

- esophagus and its associated nerve plexus,
- thoracic aorta and its branches,
- azygos system of veins,
- thoracic duct and associated lymph nodes,
- sympathetic trunks, and
- thoracic splanchnic nerves.

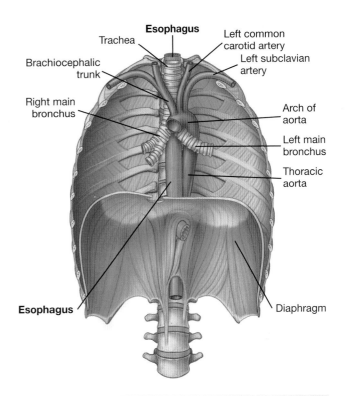

Fig. 3.95 Esophagus.

Esophagus

The **esophagus** is a muscular tube passing between the pharynx in the neck and the stomach in the abdomen. It begins at the inferior border of the cricoid cartilage opposite vertebra CVI and ends at the cardiac opening of the stomach opposite vertebra TXI.

The esophagus descends on the anterior aspect of the bodies of the vertebrae generally in a midline position as it moves through the thorax (Fig. 3.95). As it approaches the diaphragm, it moves anteriorly and to the left, crossing from the right side of the thoracic aorta to a position anterior to it. It passes through the esophageal hiatus, an opening in the muscular part of the diaphragm, at vertebral level TX.

The esophagus has a slight anterior-to-posterior curvature that parallels the thoracic portion of the vertebral column and is secured superiorly in the neck by its attachment to the pharynx and inferiorly in the thorax by its attachment to the diaphragm.

Relationships to important structures in the posterior mediastinum

In the posterior mediastinum, the right side of the esophagus is covered by the mediastinal part of the parietal pleura.

Posterior to the esophagus, the thoracic duct is on the right side inferiorly but crosses to the left more superiorly. Also on the left side of the esophagus is the thoracic aorta.

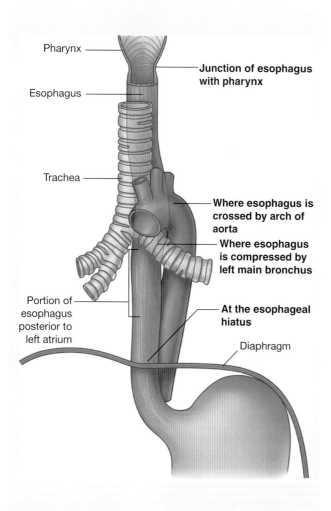

Fig. 3.96 Sites of normal esophageal constrictions.

Anterior to the esophagus, below the level of the tracheal bifurcation, are the right pulmonary artery and the left main bronchus. The esophagus then passes immediately posteriorly to the left atrium, separated from it only by pericardium. Inferior to the left atrium, the esophagus is related to the diaphragm.

Structures other than the thoracic duct posterior to the esophagus include portions of the hemiazygos veins, the right posterior intercostal vessels, and, near the diaphragm, the thoracic aorta.

Arterial supply and venous and lymphatic drainage

The arterial supply and venous drainage of the esophagus in the posterior mediastinum involve many vessels. Esophageal arteries arise from the thoracic aorta, bronchial arteries, and ascending branches of the left gastric artery in the abdomen.

Venous drainage involves small vessels returning to the azygos vein, hemiazygos vein, and esophageal branches to the left gastric vein in the abdomen.

Lymphatic drainage of the esophagus in the posterior mediastinum returns to posterior mediastinal and left gastric nodes.

Innervation

Innervation of the esophagus, in general, is complex. Esophageal branches arise from the vagus nerves and sympathetic trunks.

Striated muscle fibers in the superior portion of the esophagus originate from the branchial arches and are innervated by branchial efferents from the vagus nerves.

Smooth muscle fibers are innervated by cranial components of the parasympathetic part of the autonomic division of the peripheral nervous system, visceral efferents from the vagus nerves. These are preganglionic fibers that synapse in the myenteric and submucosal plexuses of the enteric nervous system in the esophageal wall.

Sensory innervation of the esophagus involves visceral afferent fibers originating in the vagus nerves, sympathetic trunks, and splanchnic nerves.

The visceral afferents from the vagus nerves are involved in relaying information back to the central nervous system about normal physiological processes and reflex activities. They are not involved in the relay of pain recognition.

The visceral afferents that pass through the sympathetic trunks and the splanchnic nerves are the primary participants in detection of esophageal pain and transmission of this information to various levels of the central nervous system.

Esophageal plexus

After passing posteriorly to the root of the lungs, the right and left vagus nerves approach the esophagus. As they reach the esophagus, each nerve divides into several branches that spread over this structure, forming the **esophageal plexus** (Fig. 3.97). There is some mixing of fibers from the two vagus nerves as the plexus continues inferiorly on the esophagus toward the diaphragm. Just above the diaphragm, fibers of the plexus converge to form two trunks:

- the **anterior vagal trunk** on the anterior surface of the esophagus, mainly from fibers originally in the left vagus nerve, and
- the **posterior vagal trunk** on the posterior surface of the esophagus, mainly from fibers originally in the right vagus nerve.

The vagal trunks continue on the surface of the esophagus as it passes through the diaphragm into the abdomen.

Fig. 3.97 Esophageal plexus.

Clinical app

Esophageal cancer

When patients present with esophageal cancer, it is important to note which portion of the esophagus contains the tumor, because tumor location determines the sites to which the disease will spread.

Esophageal cancer spreads quickly to lymphatics, draining to lymph nodes in the neck and around the celiac artery in the abdomen. Endoscopy or barium swallow is used to assess the site. CT and MRI may be necessary to stage the disease.

Once the extent of the disease has been assessed, treatment can be planned.

Clinical app

Esophageal rupture

The first case of esophageal rupture was described by Herman Boerhaave in 1724. This case was fatal, but early diagnosis has increased the survival rate up to 65%. If the disease is left untreated, mortality is 100%.

Typically, the rupture occurs in the lower third of the esophagus with a sudden rise in intraluminal esophageal pressure produced by vomiting together with failure of the cricopharyngeus muscle in the lower neck to relax. Because the tears typically occur on the left, they are often associated with a large left pleural effusion that contains the gastric contents.

Thoracic aorta

The thoracic portion of the descending aorta (**thoracic aorta**) begins at the lower edge of vertebra TIV where it is continuous with the arch of aorta. It ends anterior to the lower edge of vertebrae TXII where it passes through the aortic hiatus posterior to the diaphragm. Situated to the left of the vertebral column superiorly, it approaches the midline inferiorly, lying directly anterior to the lower thoracic vertebral bodies (Fig. 3.98). Throughout its course, it gives off a number of branches, which are summarized in Table 3.3.

Azygos system of veins

The azygos system of veins consists of a series of longitudinal vessels on each side of the body that drain blood from the body wall and move it superiorly to the superior vena cava. Blood from some of the thoracic viscera may also enter the system, and there are anastomotic connections with abdominal veins.

The longitudinal vessels may or may not be continuous and are connected to each other from side to side at various points throughout their course (Fig. 3.99).

The azygos system of veins serves as an important anastomotic pathway capable of returning venous blood from the lower part of the body to the heart if the inferior vena cava is blocked.

The major veins in the system are:

- the azygos vein on the right and
- the hemiazygos vein and the accessory hemiazygos vein on the left.

There is significant variation in the origin, course, tributaries, anastomoses, and termination of these vessels.

Azygos vein

The **azygos vein** arises opposite vertebra LI or LII at the junction of the **right ascending lumbar vein** and the **right subcostal vein** (Fig. 3.99). It may also arise as a direct branch of the inferior vena cava, which is joined by a common trunk from the junction of the right ascending lumbar vein and the right subcostal vein.

The azygos vein enters the thorax through the aortic hiatus of the diaphragm or through or posterior to the right crus of the diaphragm. It ascends through the posterior mediastinum, usually to the right of the thoracic duct. At approximately vertebral level TIV, it arches anteriorly over the root of the right lung to join the superior vena cava before the superior vena cava enters the pericardial sac.

Tributaries of the azygos vein include:

- the **right superior intercostal vein** (a single vessel formed by the second, third, and fourth intercostal veins; the first right intercostal vein drains directly into the right brachiocephalic vein or into the vertebral vein),
- fifth to eleventh right posterior intercostal veins,
- the hemiazygos vein,
- the accessory hemiazygos vein,
- esophageal veins,
- mediastinal veins,
- pericardial veins, and
- right bronchial veins.

Hemiazygos vein

The **hemiazygos vein (inferior hemiazygos vein)** usually arises at the junction between the **left ascending lumbar vein** and the **left subcostal vein** (Fig. 3.99). It may also arise

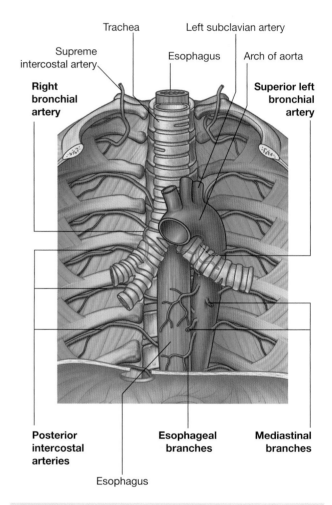

Fig. 3.98 Thoracic aorta and branches.

Branches	Origin and course
Pericardial branches	A few small vessels to the posterior surface of the pericardial sac
Bronchial branches	Vary in number, size, and origin—usually two left bronchial arteries from the thoracic aorta and one right bronchial artery from the third posterior intercostal artery or the superior left bronchial artery
Esophageal branches	Four or five vessels from the anterior aspect of the thoracic aorta, which form a continuous anastomotic chain—anastomotic connections include esophageal branches of the inferior thyroid artery superiorly and esophageal branches of the left inferior phrenic and the left gastric arteries inferiorly
Mediastinal branches	Several small branches supplying lymph nodes, vessels, nerves, and areolar tissue in the posterior mediastinum
Posterior intercostal arteries	Usually nine pairs of vessels branching from the posterior surface of the thoracic aorta—usually supply the lower nine intercostal spaces (first two spaces are supplied by the supreme intercostal artery—a branch of the costocervical trunk)
Superior phrenic arteries	Small vessels from the lower part of the thoracic aorta supplying the posterior part of the superior surface of the diaphragm—they anastomose with the musculophrenic and pericardiacophrenic arteries
Subcostal artery	The lowest pair of branches from the thoracic aorta located inferior to rib XII

Table 3.3 Branches of the thoracic aorta

from either of these veins alone and often has a connection to the left renal vein.

The hemiazygos vein usually enters the thorax through the left crus of the diaphragm but may enter through the aortic hiatus. It ascends through the posterior mediastinum on the left side to approximately vertebral level TIX. At this point, it crosses the vertebral column posterior to the thoracic aorta, esophagus, and thoracic duct to enter the azygos vein.

Tributaries joining the hemiazygos vein include:

- the lowest four or five left posterior intercostal veins,
- esophageal veins, and
- mediastinal veins.

Accessory hemiazygos vein

The **accessory hemiazygos vein (superior hemiazygos vein)** descends on the left side from the superior portion of the posterior mediastinum to approximately vertebral level TVIII (Fig. 3.99). At this point, it crosses the vertebral column to join the azygos vein, ends in the hemiazygos vein, or has a connection to both veins. Usually, it also has a connection superiorly to the **left superior intercostal vein.**

Vessels that drain into the accessory hemiazygos vein include:

- the fourth to eighth left posterior intercostal veins and
- sometimes, the left bronchial veins.

Thoracic duct in the posterior mediastinum

The thoracic duct is the principal channel through which lymph from most of the body is returned to the venous system. It begins as a confluence of lymph trunks in the abdomen, sometimes forming a saccular dilation referred to as the **cisterna chyli (chyle cistern),** which drains the abdominal viscera and walls, pelvis, perineum, and lower limbs.

The thoracic duct extends from vertebra LII to the root of the neck.

Entering the thorax posterior to the aorta through the aortic hiatus of the diaphragm, the thoracic duct ascends through the posterior mediastinum to the right of midline between the thoracic aorta on the left and the azygos vein on the right (Fig. 3.100). It lies posterior to the diaphragm and the esophagus and anterior to the bodies of the vertebrae.

At vertebral level TV, the thoracic duct moves to the left of midline and enters the superior mediastinum. It continues through the superior mediastinum and into the neck.

After being joined, in most cases, by the **left jugular trunk,** which drains the left side of the head and neck, and the **left subclavian trunk,** which drains the left upper limb, the thoracic duct empties into the junction of the left subclavian and left internal jugular veins.

The thoracic duct usually receives the contents from:

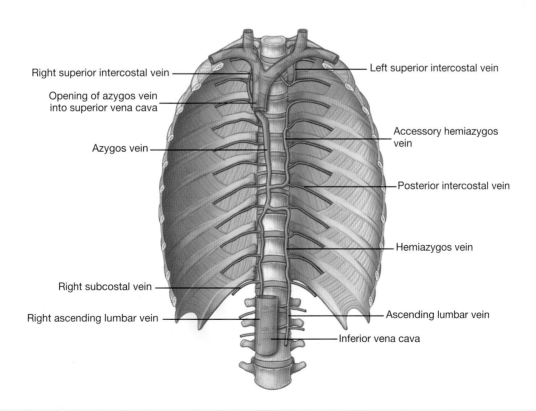

Right superior intercostal vein

Opening of azygos vein into superior vena cava

Azygos vein

Right subcostal vein

Right ascending lumbar vein

Left superior intercostal vein

Accessory hemiazygos vein

Posterior intercostal vein

Hemiazygos vein

Ascending lumbar vein

Inferior vena cava

Fig. 3.99 Azygos system of veins.

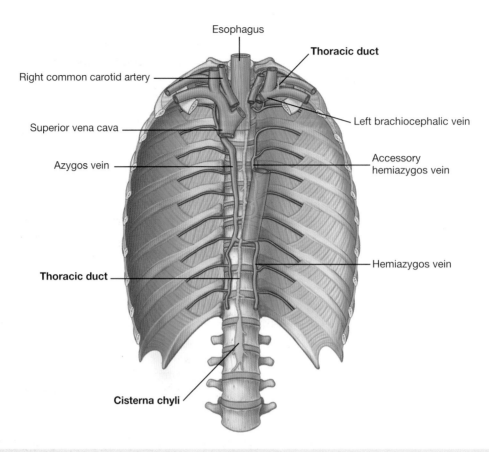

Esophagus

Thoracic duct

Right common carotid artery

Superior vena cava

Left brachiocephalic vein

Azygos vein

Accessory
hemiazygos vein

Hemiazygos vein

Thoracic duct

Cisterna chyli

Fig. 3.100 Thoracic duct.

- the confluence of lymph trunks in the abdomen,
- descending thoracic lymph trunks draining the lower six or seven intercostal spaces on both sides,
- upper intercostal lymph trunks draining the upper left five or six intercostal spaces,
- ducts from posterior mediastinal nodes, and
- ducts from posterior diaphragmatic nodes.

Sympathetic trunks

The **sympathetic trunks** are an important component of the sympathetic part of the autonomic division of the peripheral nervous system and are usually considered a component of the posterior mediastinum as they pass through the thorax (also see Chapter 1, pp. 23–26).

This portion of the sympathetic trunks consists of two parallel cords punctuated by 11 or 12 **ganglia** (Fig. 3.101). The ganglia are connected to adjacent thoracic spinal nerves by **white** and **gray rami communicantes** and are numbered according to the thoracic spinal nerve with which they are associated.

In the superior portion of the posterior mediastinum, the trunks are anterior to the neck of the ribs. Inferiorly, they

become more medial in position until they lie on the lateral aspect of the vertebral bodies. The sympathetic trunks leave the thorax by passing posterior to the diaphragm under the medial arcuate ligament or through the crura of the diaphragm. Throughout their course the trunks are covered by parietal pleura.

Branches from the ganglia

Two types of medial branches are given off by the ganglia:

- The first type includes branches from the upper five ganglia.
- The second type includes branches from the lower seven ganglia.

The first type includes branches from the upper five ganglia and is mainly postganglionic sympathetic fibers, which supply the various thoracic viscera. These branches are relatively small and contain visceral afferent fibers.

The second type includes branches from the lower seven ganglia and is mainly preganglionic sympathetic fibers, which supply the various abdominal and pelvic viscera. These

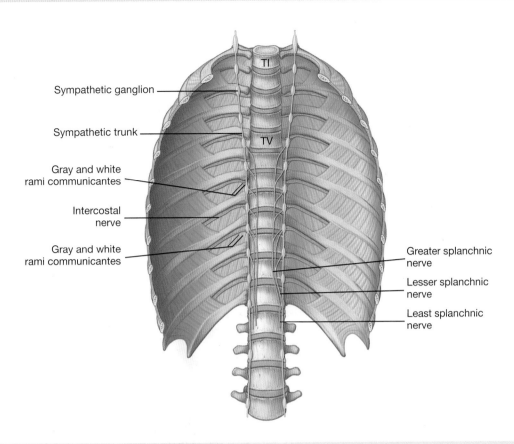

Fig. 3.101 Thoracic portion of sympathetic trunks.

branches are large, carry visceral afferent fibers, and form the three thoracic splanchnic nerves referred to as the greater, lesser, and least splanchnic nerves (Fig. 3.101).

- The **greater splanchnic nerve** on each side usually arises from the fifth to ninth or tenth thoracic ganglia. It descends across the vertebral bodies moving in a medial direction, passes into the abdomen through the crus of the diaphragm, and ends in the celiac ganglion.

- The **lesser splanchnic nerve** usually arises from the ninth and tenth or tenth and eleventh thoracic ganglia. It descends across the vertebral bodies moving in a medial direction and passes into the abdomen through the crus of the diaphragm to end in the aorticorenal ganglion.

- The **least splanchnic nerve (lowest splanchnic nerve),** when present, usually arises from the twelfth thoracic ganglion. It descends and passes into the abdomen through the crus of the diaphragm to end in the renal plexus.

Imaging app

Visualizing the mediastinum in the axial plane
Fig. 3.102A through I
This is a series of images that pass through the thorax from superior to inferior showing the various mediastinal structures and their relationships with each other. CT images, with contrast, in axial plane.

Continued

Imaging app—cont'd

Right common carotid artery

Right brachiocephalic vein

Right subclavian artery

Trachea

Left brachiocephalic vein

Left common carotid artery

Left subclavian artery

Esophagus

A

Right brachiocephalic vein

Trachea

Left brachiocephalic vein

Brachiocephalic trunk

Left common carotid artery

Left subclavian artery

Esophagus

TIII

B

Superior vena cava

Trachea

Brachiocephalic trunk

Left common carotid artery

Left subclavian artery

Esophagus

C

Fig. 3.102

Imaging app—cont'd

Superior vena cava
Trachea
Azygos vein
Arch of aorta
Esophagus
TIV
D

Ascending aorta
Superior vena cava
Right pulmonary artery
Right main bronchus
Carina
Pulmonary trunk
Left pulmonary artery
Left main bronchus
Esophagus
Thoracic aorta
E

Ascending aorta
Superior vena cava
Right pulmonary artery
Right main bronchus
Esophagus
Pulmonary trunk
Left pulmonary artery
Left main bronchus
Thoracic aorta
TV
F

Fig. 3.102, cont'd

Continued

Imaging app—cont'd

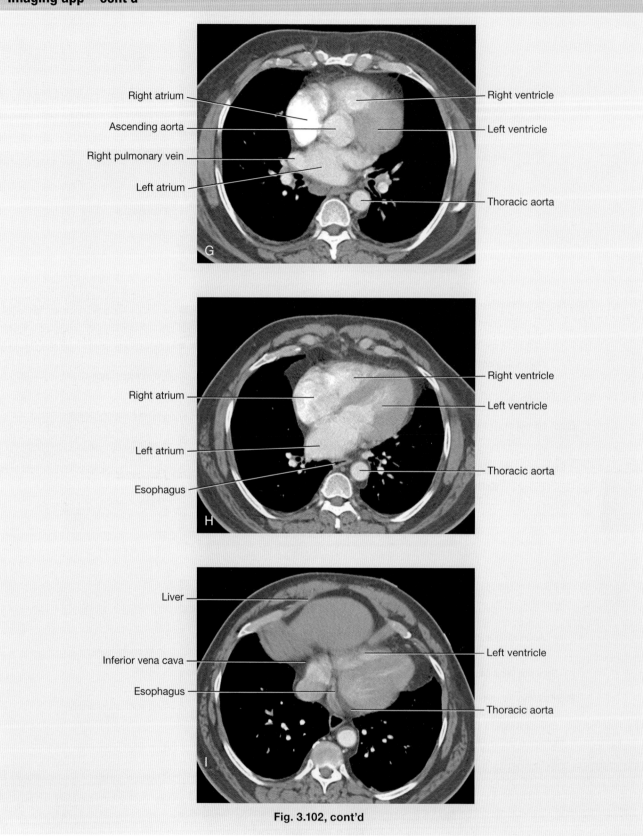

Fig. 3.102, cont'd

4

Abdomen

Regional anatomy   146

Surface topography   146
   Four-quadrant pattern   146
   Nine-region pattern   146
Abdominal wall   147
   Superficial fascia   148
   Anterolateral muscles   149
   Extraperitoneal fascia   152
   Peritoneum   153
   Innervation   153
   Arterial supply and venous drainage   155
   Lymphatic drainage   155
Groin   156
   Inguinal canal   157
Abdominal viscera   163
   Peritoneum   163
   Peritoneal cavity   164
   Organs   167
   Arterial supply to the gastrointestinal tract   187
   Venous drainage   193
   Lymphatics   196
   Innervation   196
Posterior abdominal region   201
   Posterior abdominal wall   201
   Viscera   206
   Vasculature   212
   Lymphatic system   216
   Nervous system in the posterior abdominal
      region   217
   Sympathetic trunks and splanchnic nerves   217

Regional anatomy

The abdomen is the part of the trunk inferior to the thorax (Fig. 4.1). Its musculomembranous walls surround a large cavity (the **abdominal cavity**), which is bounded superiorly by the diaphragm and inferiorly by the pelvic inlet.

The abdominal cavity may extend superiorly as high as the fourth intercostal space and is continuous inferiorly with the pelvic cavity. It contains the **peritoneal cavity** and the abdominal viscera.

SURFACE TOPOGRAPHY

Topographical divisions of the abdomen are used to describe the location of abdominal organs and the pain associated with abdominal problems. The two schemes most often used are:

- a four-quadrant pattern and
- a nine-region pattern.

Four-quadrant pattern

A horizontal transumbilical plane passing through the umbilicus and the intervertebral disc between vertebrae LIII and LIV and intersecting with the vertical median plane divides the abdomen into four quadrants—the right upper, left upper, right lower, and left lower quadrants (Fig. 4.2).

Nine-region pattern

The nine-region pattern is based on two horizontal and two vertical planes (Fig. 4.3).

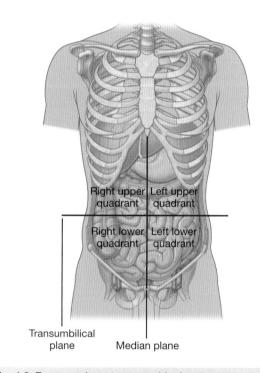

Fig. 4.2 Four-quadrant topographical pattern.

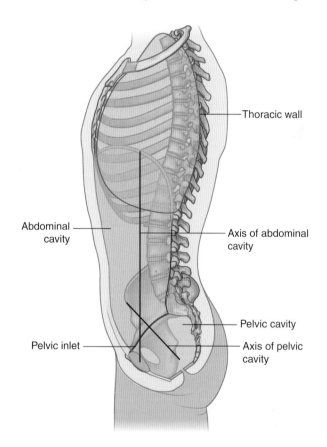

Fig. 4.1 Boundaries of the abdominal cavity.

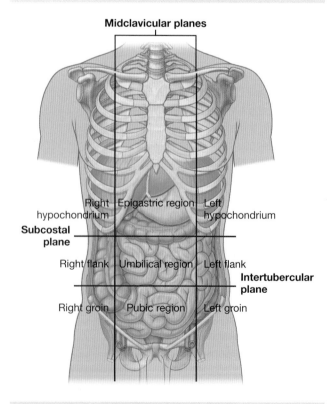

Fig. 4.3 Nine-region organizational pattern.

The superior horizontal plane (the **subcostal plane**) is immediately inferior to the costal margins, which places it at the lower border of the costal cartilage of rib X and passes posteriorly through the body of vertebra LIII. (Note, however, that sometimes the **transpyloric plane,** halfway between the jugular notch and the symphysis pubis or halfway between the umbilicus and the inferior end of the body of the sternum, passing posteriorly through the lower border of vertebrae LI and intersecting with the costal margin at the ends of the ninth costal cartilages, is used instead.)

The inferior horizontal plane (the **intertubercular plane**) connects the tubercles of the iliac crests, which are palpable structures 5 cm posterior to the anterior superior iliac spines, and passes through the upper part of the body of vertebra LV.

The vertical planes pass from the midpoint of the clavicles inferiorly to a point midway between the anterior superior iliac spine and pubic symphysis.

These four planes establish the topographical divisions in the nine-region organization. The following designations are used for each region: superiorly the right hypochondrium, the epigastric region, and the left hypochondrium; inferiorly the right groin (inguinal region), pubic region, and left groin (inguinal region); and in the middle the right flank (lateral region), the umbilical region, and the left flank (lateral region) (Fig. 4.3).

Surface anatomy

Using abdominal quadrants to locate major viscera

The abdomen can be divided into quadrants by a vertical median plane and a horizontal transumbilical plane (Fig. 4.4):

- The liver and gallbladder are in the right upper quadrant.

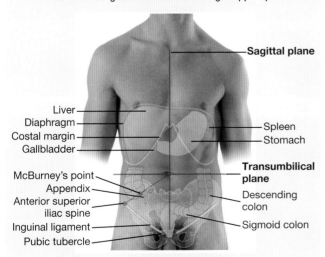

Fig. 4.4 Abdominal quadrants and the positions of major viscera. Anterior view of a man.

- The stomach and spleen are in the left upper quadrant.
- The cecum and appendix are in the right lower quadrant.
- The end of the descending colon and sigmoid colon are in the left lower quadrant.

Most of the liver is under the right dome of the diaphragm and is deep to the lower thoracic wall. The inferior margin of the liver can be palpated descending below the right costal margin when a patient is asked to inhale deeply. On deep inspiration, the edge of the liver can be felt "slipping" under the palpating fingers placed under the costal margin.

A common surface projection of the appendix is McBurney's point, which is one-third of the way up a line from the right anterior superior iliac spine to the umbilicus.

Surface anatomy

Defining surface regions to which pain from the gut is referred

The abdomen can be divided into nine regions by a midclavicular sagittal plane on each side and by the subcostal and intertubercular planes, which pass through the body transversely (Fig. 4.5).

Pain from the abdominal part of the foregut is referred to the epigastric region, pain from the midgut is referred to the umbilical region, and pain from the hindgut is referred to the pubic region.

Fig. 4.5 The nine regions of the abdomen. Anterior view of a woman.

ABDOMINAL WALL

The abdominal wall covers a large area. It is bounded superiorly by the xiphoid process and costal margins, posteriorly by the vertebral column, and inferiorly by the upper parts of the pelvic bones.

Its layers consist of skin, superficial fascia (subcutaneous tissue), muscles and their associated deep fascias, extraperitoneal fascia, and parietal peritoneum (Fig. 4.6).

Superficial fascia

The superficial fascia of the abdominal wall (subcutaneous tissue of abdomen) is a layer of fatty connective tissue. It is usually a single layer similar to, and continuous with, the superficial fascia throughout other regions of the body.

However, in the lower region of the anterior part of the abdominal wall, below the umbilicus, it forms two layers: a superficial fatty layer and a deeper membranous layer.

Superficial layer

The superficial fatty layer of superficial fascia (**Camper's fascia**) contains fat and varies in thickness (Figs. 4.7, 4.8). It is continuous over the inguinal ligament with the superficial fascia of the thigh and with a similar layer in the perineum.

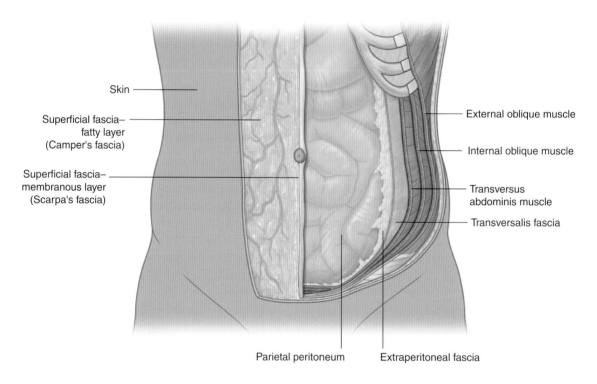

Fig. 4.6 Layers of the abdominal wall.

Fig. 4.7 Superficial fascia.

External oblique muscle and aponeurosis

Continuity with superficial penile fascia

Attachment to ischiopubic rami

Continuity with dartos fascia

Membranous layer of superficial fascia (Scarpa's fascia)

Attachment to fascia lata

Superficial perineal fascia (Colles' fascia)

Fig. 4.8 Continuity of membranous layer of superficial fascia into other areas.

In men, this superficial layer continues over the penis and, after losing its fat and fusing with the deeper layer of superficial fascia, continues into the scrotum where it forms a specialized fascial layer containing smooth muscle fibers (the **dartos fascia**). In women, this superficial layer retains some fat and is a component of the labia majora.

Deeper layer

The deeper membranous layer of superficial fascia (**Scarpa's fascia**) is thin and membranous and contains little or no fat (Fig. 4.7). Inferiorly, it continues into the thigh, but just below the inguinal ligament, it fuses with the deep fascia of the thigh (the **fascia lata;** Fig. 4.8). In the midline, it is firmly attached to the linea alba and the pubic symphysis. It continues into the anterior part of the perineum where it is firmly attached to the ischiopubic rami and to the posterior margin of the perineal membrane. Here, it is referred to as the **superficial perineal fascia (Colles' fascia).**

In men, the deeper membranous layer of superficial fascia blends with the superficial layer as they both pass over the penis, forming the superficial fascia of the penis before they continue into the scrotum where they form the dartos fascia (Figs. 4.7, 4.8). Also in men, extensions of the deeper membranous layer of superficial fascia attached to the pubic symphysis pass inferiorly onto the dorsum and sides of the penis to form the **fundiform ligament of the penis.** In women, the membranous layer of the superficial fascia continues into the labia majora and the anterior part of the perineum.

Anterolateral muscles

There are five muscles in the anterolateral group of abdominal wall muscles (Table 4.1):

- three flat muscles whose fibers begin posterolaterally, pass anteriorly and are replaced by an aponeurosis as the muscle continues toward the midline—the external oblique, internal oblique, and transversus abdominis muscles and
- two vertical muscles near the midline, which are enclosed within a tendinous sheath formed by the aponeuroses of the flat muscles—the rectus abdominis and pyramidalis muscles.

Each of these five muscles has specific actions, but together the muscles are critical:

- for the maintenance of many normal physiological functions,
- to keep the abdominal viscera within the abdominal cavity,
- to protect the viscera from injury, and
- to help maintain the position of the viscera in the erect posture against the action of gravity.

Contraction of these muscles assists in both quiet and forced expiration by pushing the viscera upward (which helps push the relaxed diaphragm farther into the thoracic cavity) and in coughing and vomiting.

All these muscles are also involved in any action that increases intra-abdominal pressure, including parturition (childbirth), micturition (urination), and defecation (expulsion of feces from the rectum).

Flat muscles
External oblique

The most superficial of the three flat muscles in the anterolateral group of abdominal wall muscles is the **external oblique,** which is immediately deep to the superficial fascia (Table 4.1, Fig. 4.9). Its laterally placed muscle fibers pass in an inferomedial direction, while its large aponeurotic component covers the anterior part of the abdominal wall to the midline. Approaching the midline, the aponeuroses are entwined, forming the linea alba, which extends from the xiphoid process to the pubic symphysis.

Table 4.1 Abdominal wall muscles

Muscle	Origin	Insertion	Innervation	Function
External oblique	Muscular slips from the outer surfaces of the lower eight ribs (ribs V to XII)	Lateral lip of iliac crest; aponeurosis ending in midline raphe (linea alba)	Anterior rami of lower six thoracic spinal nerves (T7 to T12)	Compress abdominal contents; both muscles flex trunk; each muscle bends trunk to same side, turning anterior part of abdomen to opposite side
Internal oblique	Thoracolumbar fascia; iliac crest between origins of external and transversus; lateral two-thirds of inguinal ligament	Inferior border of the lower three or four ribs; aponeurosis ending in linea alba; pubic crest and pectineal line	Anterior rami of lower six thoracic spinal nerves (T7 to T12) and L1	Compress abdominal contents; both muscles flex trunk; each muscle bends trunk and turns anterior part of abdomen to same side
Transversus abdominis	Thoracolumbar fascia; medial lip of iliac crest; lateral one-third of inguinal ligament; costal cartilages lower six ribs (ribs VII to XII)	Aponeurosis ending in linea alba; pubic crest and pectineal line	Anterior rami of lower six thoracic spinal nerves (T7 to T12) and L1	Compress abdominal contents
Rectus abdominis	Pubic crest, pubic tubercle, and pubic symphysis	Costal cartilages of ribs V to VII; xiphoid process	Anterior rami of lower seven thoracic spinal nerves (T7 to T12)	Compress abdominal contents; flex vertebral column; tense abdominal wall
Pyramidalis	Front of pubis and pubic symphysis	Into linea alba	Anterior ramus of T12	Tenses the linea alba

Fig. 4.9 External oblique muscle and its aponeurosis.

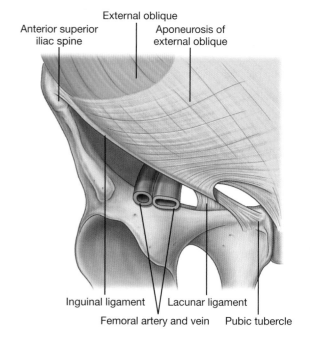

Fig. 4.10 Ligaments formed from the external oblique aponeurosis.

Associated ligaments

The lower border of the external oblique aponeurosis forms the **inguinal ligament** on each side (Fig. 4.9). This thickened reinforced free edge of the external oblique aponeurosis passes between the anterior superior iliac spine laterally and the pubic tubercle medially (Fig. 4.10). It folds under itself forming a trough, which plays an important role in the formation of the inguinal canal.

Several other ligaments are also formed from extensions of the fibers at the medial end of the inguinal ligament:

- The **lacunar ligament** is a crescent-shaped extension of fibers at the medial end of the inguinal ligament that pass backward to attach to the **pecten pubis** on the superior ramus of the pubic bone (Figs. 4.10, 4.11).

- Additional fibers extend from the lacunar ligament along the pecten pubis of the pelvic brim to form the **pectineal (Cooper's) ligament.**

Internal oblique

Deep to the external oblique muscle is the **internal oblique** muscle, which is the second of the three flat muscles (Table 4.1, Fig. 4.12). This muscle is smaller and thinner than the external oblique, with most of its muscle fibers passing in a superomedial direction. Its lateral muscular components end anteriorly as an aponeurosis that blends into the linea alba at the midline.

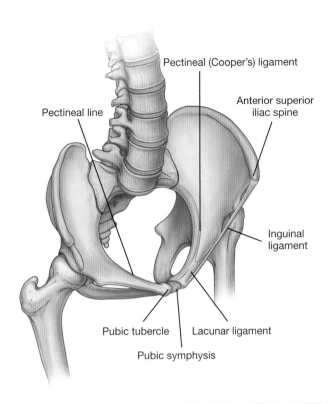

Fig. 4.11 Ligaments of the inguinal region.

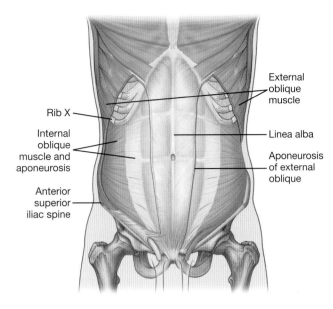

Fig. 4.12 Internal oblique muscle and its aponeurosis.

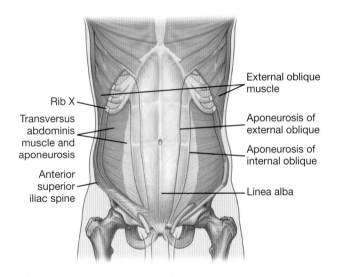

Fig. 4.13 Transversus abdominis muscle and its aponeurosis.

Transversus abdominis

Deep to the internal oblique muscle is the **transversus abdominis** muscle (Table 4.1, Fig. 4.13), so named because of the direction of most of its muscle fibers. It ends in an anterior aponeurosis, which blends with the linea alba at the midline.

Transversalis fascia

Each of the three flat muscles is covered on its anterior and posterior surfaces by a layer of deep (or investing) fascia. In general, these layers are unremarkable except for the layer deep to the transversus abdominis muscle (the **transversalis fascia**), which is better developed.

The transversalis fascia is a continuous layer of deep fascia that lines the abdominal cavity and continues into the pelvic cavity. It crosses the midline anteriorly, associating with the transversalis fascia of the opposite side, and is continuous with the fascia on the inferior surface of the diaphragm. It is continuous posteriorly with the deep fascia covering the muscles of the posterior abdominal wall and attaches to the thoracolumbar fascia.

After attaching to the crest of the ilium, the transversalis fascia blends with the fascia covering the muscles associated with the upper regions of the pelvic bones and with similar fascia covering the muscles of the pelvic cavity. At this point, it is referred to as the **parietal pelvic** (or **endopelvic**) **fascia.**

There is therefore a continuous layer of deep fascia surrounding the abdominal cavity that is thick in some areas, thin in others, attached or free, and participates in the formation of specialized structures.

Vertical muscles

The two vertical muscles in the anterolateral group of abdominal wall muscles are the large rectus abdominis and the small pyramidalis (Table 4.1, Fig. 4.14).

Rectus abdominis

The **rectus abdominis** is a long, flat muscle that extends the length of the anterior abdominal wall. It is a paired muscle, separated in the midline by the linea alba, and it widens and thins as it ascends from the pubic symphysis to the costal margin. Along its course, it is intersected by three or four transverse fibrous bands or **tendinous intersections**

Abdomen

(Fig. 4.14). These are easily visible on individuals with a well-developed rectus abdominis muscle.

Pyramidalis

The second vertical muscle is the **pyramidalis.** This small, triangular muscle, which may be absent, is anterior to the rectus abdominis, has its base on the pubis, and its apex is attached superiorly and medially to the linea alba (Fig. 4.14).

Rectus sheath

The rectus abdominis and pyramidalis muscles are enclosed in an aponeurotic tendinous sheath (the **rectus sheath**) formed by a unique layering of the aponeuroses of the external and internal oblique and transversus abdominis muscles (Fig. 4.15).

The rectus sheath completely encloses the upper three-quarters of the rectus abdominis and covers the anterior

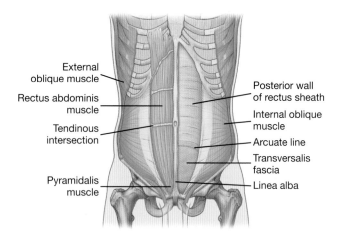

Fig. 4.14 Rectus abdominis and pyramidalis muscles.

surface of the lower one-quarter of the muscle. As no sheath covers the posterior surface of the lower quarter of the rectus abdominis muscle, the muscle at this point is in direct contact with the transversalis fascia.

The formation of the rectus sheath surrounding the upper three-quarters of the rectus abdominis muscle has the following pattern:

- The anterior wall consists of the aponeurosis of the external oblique and half of the aponeurosis of the internal oblique, which splits at the lateral margin of the rectus abdominis.
- The posterior wall of the rectus sheath consists of the other half of the aponeurosis of the internal oblique and the aponeurosis of the transversus abdominis.

At a point midway between the umbilicus and the pubic symphysis, corresponding to the beginning of the lower one-fourth of the rectus abdominis muscle, all of the aponeuroses move anterior to the rectus muscle. There is no posterior wall of the rectus sheath and the anterior wall of the sheath consists of the aponeuroses of the external oblique, the internal oblique, and the transversus abdominis muscles. From this point inferiorly, the rectus abdominis muscle is in direct contact with the transversalis fascia. Marking this point of transition is an arch of fibers (the **arcuate line;** see Fig. 4.14).

Extraperitoneal fascia

Deep to the transversalis fascia is a layer of connective tissue, the **extraperitoneal fascia,** that separates the transversalis fascia from the peritoneum (Fig. 4.16). Containing varying amounts of fat, this layer not only lines the abdominal cavity but is also continuous with a similar layer lining the pelvic

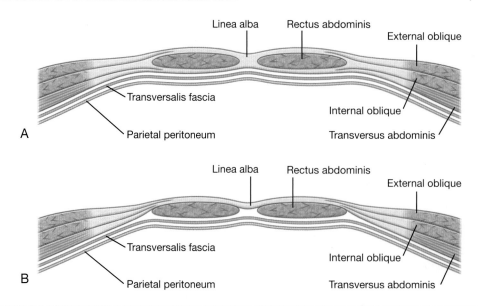

Fig. 4.15 Organization of the rectus sheath. A. Transverse section through the upper three-quarters of the rectus sheath. **B.** Transverse section through the lower one-quarter of the rectus sheath.

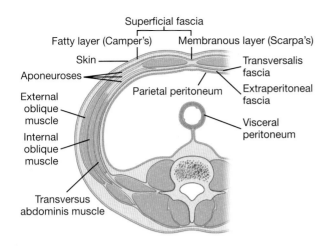

Fig. 4.16 Transverse section showing the layers of the abdominal wall.

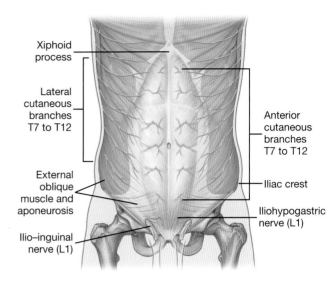

Fig. 4.18 Innervation of the anterolateral abdominal wall.

cavity. It is abundant on the posterior abdominal wall, especially around the kidneys, continues over organs covered by peritoneal reflections, and, as the vasculature is located in this layer, extends into mesenteries with the blood vessels. Viscera in the extraperitoneal fascia are referred to as **retroperitoneal.**

Clinical app

Preperitoneal vs. retroperitoneal

In the description of specific surgical procedures, the terminology used to describe the extraperitoneal fascia is further modified. The fascia toward the anterior side of the body is described as preperitoneal (or, less commonly, properitoneal), and the fascia toward the posterior side of the body has been described as retroperitoneal (Fig. 4.17). Examples of the use of these terms would be the continuity of fat in the inguinal canal with the preperitoneal fat and a transabdominal preperitoneal laparoscopic repair of an inguinal hernia.

Fig. 4.17 Subdivisions of the extraperitoneal fascia.

Peritoneum

Deep to the extraperitoneal fascia is the peritoneum (Fig. 4.16). This thin serous membrane lines the walls of the abdominal cavity and, at various points, reflects onto the abdominal viscera, providing either a complete or a partial covering. The peritoneum lining the walls is the parietal peritoneum; the peritoneum covering the viscera is the visceral peritoneum.

The continuous lining of the abdominal walls by the parietal peritoneum forms a sac. This sac is closed in men but has two openings in women where the uterine tubes provide a passage to the outside. The closed sac in men and the semi-closed sac in women is called the *peritoneal cavity.*

Innervation

The skin, muscles, and parietal peritoneum of the anterolateral abdominal wall are supplied by T7 to T12 and L1 spinal nerves. The anterior rami of these spinal nerves pass around the body, from posterior to anterior, in an inferomedial direction (Fig. 4.18). As they proceed, they give off a lateral cutaneous branch and end as an anterior cutaneous branch.

The intercostal nerves (T7 to T11) leave their intercostal spaces, passing deep to the costal cartilages, and continue onto the anterolateral abdominal wall between the internal oblique and transversus abdominis muscles (Fig. 4.19). Reaching the lateral edge of the rectus sheath, they enter the rectus sheath and pass posterior to the lateral aspect of the rectus abdominis muscle. Approaching the midline, an anterior cutaneous branch passes through the rectus abdominis muscle and the anterior wall of the rectus sheath to supply the skin.

Spinal nerve T12 (the **subcostal nerve**) follows a similar course as the intercostals. Branches of L1 (the **iliohypogastric nerve** and **ilio-inguinal nerve**), which originate from

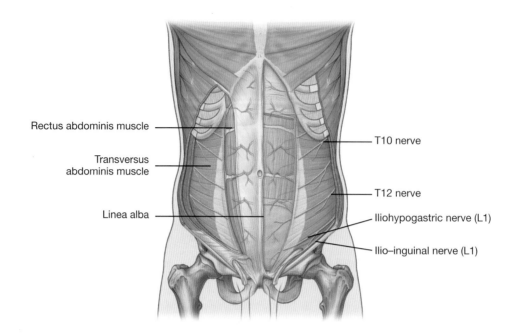

Fig. 4.19 Path taken by the nerves innervating the anterolateral abdominal wall.

Rectus abdominis muscle

Transversus abdominis muscle

Linea alba

T10 nerve

T12 nerve

Iliohypogastric nerve (L1)

Ilio–inguinal nerve (L1)

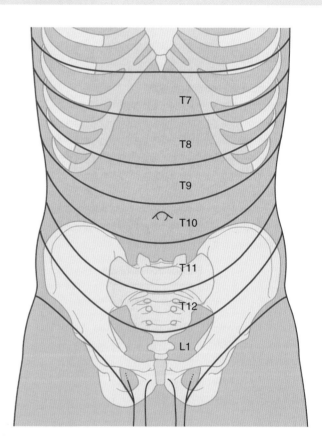

T7

T8

T9

T10

T11

T12

L1

Fig. 4.20 Dermatomes of the anterolateral abdominal wall.

the lumbar plexus, follow similar courses initially but deviate from this pattern near their final destination.

Along their course, nerves T7 to T12 and L1 supply branches to the anterolateral abdominal wall muscles and the underlying parietal peritoneum. All terminate by supplying skin (Fig. 4.20):

- Nerves T7 to T9 supply the skin from the xiphoid process to just above the umbilicus.
- T10 supplies the skin around the umbilicus.
- T11, T12, and L1 supply the skin from just below the umbilicus to, and including, the pubic region.

Intercostal arteries

Musculophrenic artery

Superficial circumflex iliac artery

Superficial epigastric artery

Internal thoracic artery

Superior epigastric artery

Deep circumflex iliac artery

Inferior epigastric artery

Fig. 4.21 Arterial supply to the anterolateral abdominal wall.

- Additionally, the ilio-inguinal nerve (a branch of L1) supplies the anterior surface of the scrotum or labia majora and sends a small cutaneous branch to the thigh.

Arterial supply and venous drainage

Numerous blood vessels supply the anterolateral abdominal wall (Fig. 4.21). Superficially:

- The superior part of the wall is supplied by branches from the **musculophrenic artery,** a terminal branch of the **internal thoracic artery.**
- The inferior part of the wall is supplied by the medially placed **superficial epigastric artery** and the laterally placed **superficial circumflex iliac artery,** both branches of the **femoral artery.**

At a deeper level:

- The superior part of the wall is supplied by the **superior epigastric artery,** a terminal branch of the internal thoracic artery.
- The lateral part of the wall is supplied by branches of the **tenth** and **eleventh intercostal arteries** and the **subcostal artery.**

- The inferior part of the wall is supplied by the medially placed **inferior epigastric artery** and the laterally placed **deep circumflex iliac artery,** both branches of the **external iliac artery.**

The superior and inferior epigastric arteries both enter the rectus sheath. They are posterior to the rectus abdominis muscle throughout their course and anastomose with each other (Fig. 4.22).

Veins of similar names follow the arteries and are responsible for venous drainage.

Lymphatic drainage

Lymphatic drainage of the anterolateral abdominal wall follows the basic principles of lymphatic drainage:

- Superficial lymphatics above the umbilicus pass in a superior direction to the **axillary nodes,** while drainage below the umbilicus passes in an inferior direction to the **superficial inguinal nodes.**
- Deep lymphatic drainage follows the deep arteries back to **parasternal nodes** along the internal thoracic artery, lumbar nodes along the abdominal aorta, and external iliac nodes along the external iliac artery.

155

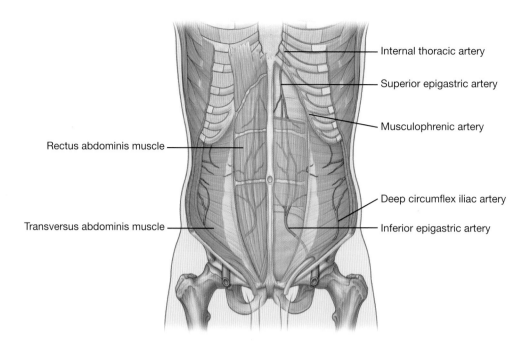

Rectus abdominis muscle

Transversus abdominis muscle

Internal thoracic artery

Superior epigastric artery

Musculophrenic artery

Deep circumflex iliac artery

Inferior epigastric artery

Fig. 4.22 Superior and inferior epigastric arteries.

GROIN

The groin (**inguinal region**) is the area of junction between the anterior abdominal wall and the thigh. In this area, the abdominal wall is weakened from changes that occur during development, and a peritoneal sac or diverticulum, with or without abdominal contents, can therefore protrude through it, creating an inguinal hernia. This type of hernia can occur in both sexes, but it is more common in males.

The inherent weakness in the anterior abdominal wall in the groin is caused by changes that occur during the development of the gonads. Before the descent of the testis and ovaries from their initial position high in the posterior abdominal wall, a peritoneal outpouching (the processus vaginalis) forms (Fig. 4.23), protruding through the various layers of the anterior abdominal wall and acquiring coverings from each:

- The transversalis fascia forms its deepest covering.
- The second covering is formed by the musculature of the internal oblique (a covering from the transversus abdominis muscle is not acquired because the processus vaginalis passes under the arching fibers of this abdominal wall muscle).
- Its most superficial covering is the aponeurosis of the external oblique.

As a result, the processus vaginalis is transformed into a tubular structure with multiple coverings from the layers of the anterior abdominal wall. This forms the basic structure of the **inguinal canal.**

The final event in this development is the descent of the testes into the scrotum or of the ovaries into the pelvic cavity. This

Parietal peritoneum

Extraperitoneal fascia

Transversalis fascia

Internal oblique muscle

Transversus abdominis muscle

External oblique muscle

Testis

Gubernaculum

Processus vaginalis

Fig. 4.23 Descent of the testes from week 7 (postfertilization) to birth.

process depends on the development of the **gubernaculum** (Fig. 4.23), which extends from the inferior border of the developing gonad to labioscrotal swellings in the developing perineum.

The processus vaginalis is immediately anterior to the gubernaculum within the inguinal canal.

In men, as the testes descend, the testes and their accompanying vessels, ducts, and nerves pass through the inguinal canal and are therefore surrounded by the same fascial layers of the abdominal wall. Testicular descent completes the formation of the spermatic cord in men.

In women, the ovaries descend into the pelvic cavity and become associated with the developing uterus. Therefore the

Fig. 4.24 Inguinal canal.

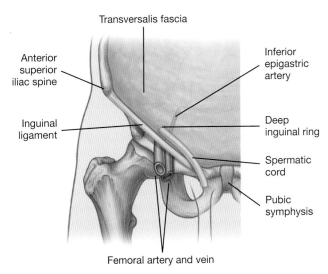

Fig. 4.25 Deep inguinal ring and the transversalis fascia.

only remaining structure passing through the inguinal canal is the round ligament of the uterus, which is a remnant of the gubernaculum.

The development sequence is concluded in both sexes when the processus vaginalis obliterates. If this does not occur or is incomplete, a potential weakness exists in the anterior abdominal wall and an inguinal hernia may develop. In males, only proximal regions of the processus vaginalis obliterate. The distal end expands to enclose most of the testes in the scrotum. In other words, the cavity of the tunica vaginalis in men forms as an extension of the developing peritoneal cavity that becomes separated off during development.

Inguinal canal

The inguinal canal is a slit-like passage that extends in a downward and medial direction just above and parallel to the lower half of the inguinal ligament. It begins at the deep inguinal ring and continues for approximately 4 cm, ending at the superficial inguinal ring (Fig. 4.24). The contents of the canal are the genital branch of the genitofemoral nerve, the **spermatic cord** in men, and the **round ligament of the uterus** in women. Additionally, in both sexes, the ilio-inguinal nerve passes through part of the canal, exiting through the superficial inguinal ring with the other contents.

Deep inguinal ring

The deep (internal) inguinal ring is the beginning of the inguinal canal and is at a point midway between the anterior superior iliac spine and the pubic symphysis (Fig. 4.25). It is just above the inguinal ligament and immediately lateral to the inferior epigastric vessels. Although sometimes referred to as a defect or opening in the transversalis fascia, it is actually the beginning of the tubular evagination of transversalis fascia that forms one of the coverings (the **internal spermatic fascia**) of the spermatic cord in men or the round ligament of the uterus in women.

Superficial inguinal ring

The superficial (external) inguinal ring is the end of the inguinal canal and is superior to the pubic tubercle (Fig. 4.26). It is a triangular opening in the aponeurosis of the external oblique, with its apex pointing superolaterally and its base formed by the pubic crest. The two remaining sides of the triangle (the **medial crus** and the **lateral crus**) are attached to the pubic symphysis and the pubic tubercle, respectively. At the apex of the triangle the two crura are held together by crossing (intercrural) fibers, which prevent further widening of the superficial ring.

As with the deep inguinal ring, the superficial inguinal ring is actually the beginning of the tubular evagination of the aponeurosis of the external oblique onto the structures traversing the inguinal canal and emerging from the superficial inguinal ring. This continuation of tissue over the spermatic cord is the **external spermatic fascia.**

Anterior wall

The anterior wall of the inguinal canal is formed along its entire length by the aponeurosis of the external oblique muscle (Fig. 4.26). It is also reinforced laterally by the lower fibers of the internal oblique that originate from the lateral two-thirds of the inguinal ligament (Fig. 4.27). This adds an additional covering over the deep inguinal ring, which is a potential point of weakness in the anterior abdominal wall. Furthermore, as the internal oblique muscle covers the deep inguinal ring, it also contributes a layer (the **cremasteric fascia** containing the **cremasteric muscle**) to the coverings of the structures traversing the inguinal canal.

Posterior wall

The posterior wall of the inguinal canal is formed along its entire length by the transversalis fascia (see Fig. 4.25). It is reinforced along its medial one-third by the **conjoint tendon** (**inguinal falx;** Fig. 4.27). This tendon is the combined insertion of the transversus abdominis and internal oblique muscles into the pubic crest and pectineal line.

As with the internal oblique muscle's reinforcement of the area of the deep inguinal ring, the position of the conjoint tendon posterior to the superficial inguinal ring provides additional support to a potential point of weakness in the anterior abdominal wall.

Roof

The roof (superior wall) of the inguinal canal is formed by the arching fibers of the transversus abdominis and internal oblique muscles (Figs. 4.27, 4.28). They pass from their lateral points of origin from the inguinal ligament to their common medial attachment as the conjoint tendon.

Floor

The floor (inferior wall) of the inguinal canal is formed by the medial one-half of the inguinal ligament. This rolled-under, free margin of the lowest part of the aponeurosis of the external oblique forms a gutter or trough on which the contents of the inguinal canal are positioned. The lacunar ligament reinforces most of the medial part of the gutter.

Contents

The contents of the inguinal canal are:

- the spermatic cord in men,
- the round ligament of the uterus in women, and
- the genital branch of the genitofemoral nerve in both men and women.

These structures enter the inguinal canal through the deep inguinal ring and exit it through the superficial inguinal ring.

Additionally, the ilio-inguinal nerve (L1) passes through part of the inguinal canal. This nerve is a branch of the lumbar plexus and enters the abdominal wall posteriorly by piercing the internal surface of the transversus abdominis muscle and continues through the layers of the anterior abdominal wall by piercing the internal oblique muscle. As it continues to pass inferomedially, it enters the inguinal canal. It continues down the canal to exit through the superficial inguinal ring.

Spermatic cord

The spermatic cord begins to form proximally at the deep inguinal ring and consists of structures passing between the

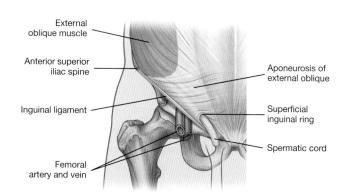

Fig. 4.26 Superficial inguinal ring and the aponeurosis of the external oblique.

Fig. 4.27 Internal oblique muscle and the inguinal canal.

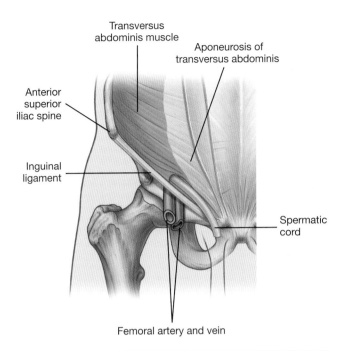

Fig. 4.28 Transversus abdominis muscle and the inguinal canal.

abdominopelvic cavities and the testes and the three fascial coverings that enclose these structures (Fig. 4.29A).

The structures in the spermatic cord include:

- the ductus deferens,
- the artery to ductus deferens (from the inferior vesical artery),
- the testicular artery (from the abdominal aorta),
- the pampiniform plexus of veins (testicular veins),
- the cremasteric artery and vein (small vessels associated with the cremasteric fascia),
- the genital branch of the genitofemoral nerve (innervation to the cremasteric muscle),
- sympathetic and visceral afferent nerve fibers,
- lymphatics, and
- remnants of the processus vaginalis.

These structures enter the deep inguinal ring, proceed down the inguinal canal, and exit from the superficial inguinal ring, having acquired the three fascial coverings during their journey. This collection of structures and fascias

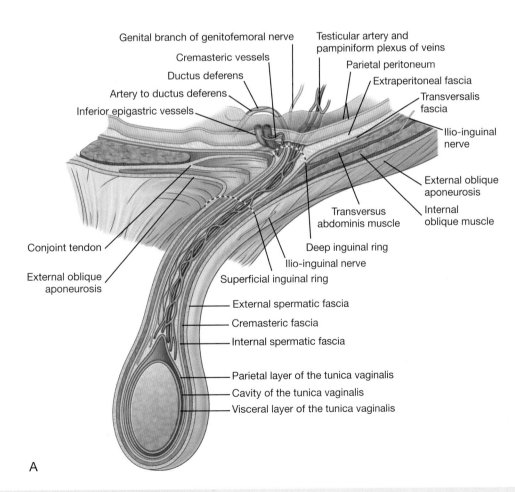

Fig. 4.29 A. Spermatic cord (men).

Continued

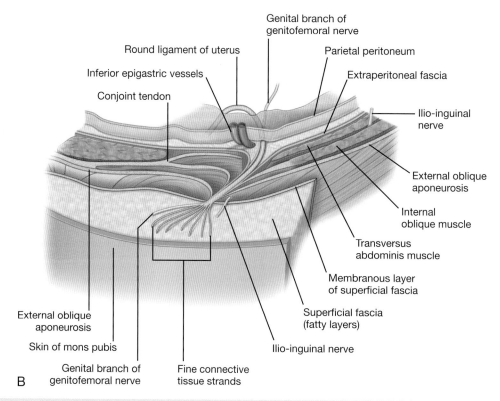

Genital branch of
genitofemoral nerve

Round ligament of uterus

Parietal peritoneum

Inferior epigastric vessels

Extraperitoneal fascia

Conjoint tendon

Ilio-inguinal
nerve

External oblique
aponeurosis

Internal
oblique muscle

Transversus
abdominis muscle

Membranous layer
of superficial fascia

External oblique
aponeurosis

Superficial fascia
(fatty layers)

Skin of mons pubis

Ilio-inguinal nerve

B

Genital branch of
genitofemoral nerve

Fine connective
tissue strands

Fig. 4.29, cont'd B. Round ligament of uterus (women).

continues into the scrotum where the structures connect with the testes and the fascias surround the testes.

The fascias enclosing the contents of the spermatic cord include (Fig. 4.29):

- the internal spermatic fascia, which is the deepest layer, arises from the transversalis fascia and is attached to the margins of the deep inguinal ring;
- the cremasteric fascia with the associated cremasteric muscle, which is the middle fascial layer and arises from the internal oblique muscle; and
- the external spermatic fascia, which is the most superficial covering of the spermatic cord, arises from the aponeurosis of the external oblique muscle, and is attached to the margins of the superficial inguinal ring (Fig. 4.29A).

Round ligament of the uterus

The round ligament of the uterus is a cord-like structure that passes from the uterus to the deep inguinal ring where it enters the inguinal canal (Fig. 4.29B). It passes down the inguinal canal and exits through the superficial inguinal ring. At this point, it has changed from a cord-like structure to a few strands of tissue that attach to the connective tissue associated with the labia majora. As it traverses the inguinal canal, it acquires the same coverings as the spermatic cord in men.

The round ligament of the uterus is the long distal part of the original gubernaculum in the fetus that extends

from the ovary to the labioscrotal swellings. From its attachment to the uterus, the round ligament of the uterus continues to the ovary as the ligament of the ovary that develops from the short proximal end of the gubernaculum.

Clinical app

Surgical incisions

Traditionally, incisions have been placed at and around the region of surgical interest. The size of these incisions was usually large to allow good access and optimal visualization of the abdominal cavity.

Currently, the most commonly used large abdominal incision is a central craniocaudad incision from the xiphoid process to the pubic symphysis, which provides wide access to the whole of the abdominal contents and allows an exploratory procedure to be performed (laparotomy).

With the advent of small cameras and the development of minimal access surgery, tiny incisions can be made in the anterior abdominal wall and cameras inserted. The peritoneal cavity is "inflated" with carbon dioxide to increase the space in which the procedure is performed. Further instruments may be inserted through small portholes, and procedures such as cholecystectomy (removal of the gallbladder) and appendectomy (removal of the appendix) can be carried out, allowing the patient to return home sooner.

Surface anatomy

How to find the superficial inguinal ring

The superficial inguinal ring is superior to the pubic crest and tubercle and to the medial end of the inguinal ligament (Fig. 4.30):

- In men, the superficial inguinal ring can be easily located by following the spermatic cord superiorly to the lower abdominal wall—the external spermatic fascia of the spermatic cord is continuous with the margins of the superficial inguinal ring.
- In women, the pubic tubercle can be palpated and the ring is superior and lateral to it.
- The deep inguinal ring, which is the internal opening to the inguinal canal, lies superior to the inguinal ligament midway between the anterior superior iliac spine and pubic symphysis. The pulse of the femoral artery can be felt in the same position but below the inguinal ligament.

Because the superficial inguinal ring is the site where inguinal hernias appear, particularly in men, the ring and related parts of the inguinal canal are often evaluated during physical examination.

Fig. 4.30 Groin. **A.** In a man. **B.** In a woman.
C. Examination of the superficial inguinal ring and related regions of the inguinal canal in a man.

Clinical app

Cremasteric reflex

In men, the cremaster muscle and cremasteric fascia form the middle or second covering of the spermatic cord. This muscle and its associated fascia are supplied by the genital branch of the genitofemoral nerve (L1/L2). Contraction of this muscle can be stimulated by a reflex arc. Gentle touch at and around the skin of the medial aspect of the superior part of the thigh stimulates the sensory fibers in the ilio-inguinal nerve. These sensory fibers enter the spinal cord at level L1. At this level, the sensory fibers stimulate the motor fibers carried in the genital branch of the genitofemoral nerve and the testis elevates on the stimulated side.

Clinical app

Masses around the groin

The most common masses in the groin are hernias. A hernia is the protrusion of a viscus, in part or in whole, through a normal or abnormal opening. The viscus usually carries a covering of parietal peritoneum, which forms the lining of the hernial sac.

The key to groin examination is determining the position of the inguinal ligament. The inguinal ligament passes between the anterior superior iliac spine laterally and the pubic tubercle medially. Inguinal hernias are above the inguinal ligament and are usually more apparent on standing. A visual assessment of the lump is necessary, bearing in mind the anatomical landmarks of the inguinal ligament.

In men, it is wise to examine the scrotum to check for a lump. If an abnormal mass is present, an inability to feel its upper edge suggests that it may originate from the inguinal canal and might be a hernia. By placing the hand over the lump and asking the patient to cough, the lump bulges outward.

An attempt should be made to reduce the swelling by applying gentle, firm pressure over the lump. If the lump is reducible, the hand should be withdrawn and careful observation will reveal recurrence of the mass.

The position of an abnormal mass in the groin relative to the pubic tubercle is very important as are the presence of increased temperature and pain, which may represent early signs of strangulation or infection.

As a general rule:

- An inguinal hernia appears through the superficial inguinal ring above the pubic tubercle and crest.
- A femoral hernia appears through the femoral canal below and lateral to the pubic tubercle.

Abdomen

Clinical app

Inguinal hernias

An inguinal hernia is the protrusion or passage of a peritoneal sac, with or without abdominal contents, through a weakened part of the abdominal wall in the groin. It occurs because the peritoneal sac enters the inguinal canal either:

- indirectly through the deep inguinal ring or
- directly through the posterior wall of the inguinal canal.
- Inguinal hernias are therefore classified as either indirect or direct and occur more commonly in men than in women possibly because men have a much larger inguinal canal than women.

Clinical app

Indirect inguinal hernias

The indirect inguinal hernia is the most common of the two types of inguinal hernias and is much more common in men than in women (Fig. 4.31). It usually occurs because some part or all of the embryonic processus vaginalis remains open or patent. It is therefore referred to as being congenital in origin.

The protruding peritoneal sac enters the inguinal canal by passing through the deep inguinal ring just lateral to the inferior epigastric vessels. The extent of its excursion down the inguinal canal depends on the amount of processus vaginalis that remains patent. If the entire processus vaginalis remains patent, the peritoneal sac may traverse the length of the canal, exit the superficial inguinal ring, and continue into the scrotum in men or the labia majus in women. In this case, the protruding peritoneal sac acquires the same coverings as those associated with the spermatic cord in men or the round ligament of the uterus in women.

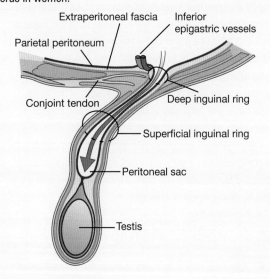

Fig. 4.31 Indirect inguinal hernia.

Clinical app

Direct inguinal hernias

A peritoneal sac that enters the medial end of the inguinal canal directly through a weakened posterior wall is a direct inguinal hernia (Fig. 4.32). It is usually described as acquired because it develops when abdominal musculature has been weakened and is commonly seen in mature men.

This type of inguinal hernia does not traverse the entire length of the inguinal canal but may exit through the superficial inguinal ring. When this occurs, the peritoneal sac acquires a layer of external spermatic fascia and can extend, like an indirect hernia, into the scrotum. Also, unlike indirect inguinal hernias that originate lateral to the inferior epigastric artery, direct inguinal hernias originate medial to the artery (Fig. 4.32).

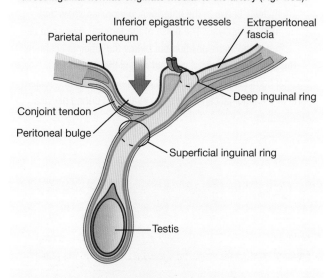

Fig. 4.32 Direct inguinal hernia.

Clinical app

Femoral hernias

A femoral hernia passes through the femoral canal and into the medial aspect of the anterior thigh. The femoral canal lies at the medial edge of the femoral sheath, which contains the femoral artery, femoral vein, and lymphatics. The neck of the femoral canal is extremely narrow and is prone to trapping bowel within the sac, making this type of hernia irreducible and susceptible to bowel strangulation. Femoral hernias are usually acquired, and most commonly occur in middle-aged and elderly populations. In addition, because women generally have wider pelvises than men, they tend to occur more commonly in women.

Clinical app

Umbilical hernias

Umbilical hernias are rare. Occasionally, they are congenital and result from failure of the small bowel to return to the abdominal cavity from the umbilical cord during development. After birth, umbilical hernias may result from incomplete closure of the umbilicus (navel). Overall, most of these hernias close in the first year of life, and surgical repair is not generally attempted until later.

Para-umbilical hernias may occur in adults at and around the umbilicus and often have small necks, so requiring surgical treatment.

Clinical app

Incisional hernias

Incisional hernias occur through a defect in a scar of a previous abdominal operation. Usually, the necks of these hernias are wide and do not therefore strangulate the viscera they contain.

Clinical app

Sportsmen's groin/sportsmen's hernia

The groin can loosely be defined as the area where the leg meets the trunk near the midline. Here the abdominal muscles of the trunk blend in with the adductor muscles of the thigh, the medial end of the inguinal ligament attaches to the pubic tubercle, the pubic symphysis attaches the two pubic bones together, and the superficial (external) inguinal ring occurs. It also is in and around this region where there is considerable translation of force during most athletic and sporting activities. Pain in the groin or pubic region can be due to numerous causes, which include inflammatory changes at the pubic symphysis, insertional problems of the rectus abdominus/adductor longus, and hernias.

Clinical app

Other hernias

A spigelian hernia passes upward through the arcuate line into the lateral border at the lower part of the posterior rectus sheath. It may appear as a tender mass on one side of the lower anterior abdominal wall.

Abdominopelvic cavity hernias can also develop in association with the pelvic walls, and sites include the obturator canal, the greater sciatic foramen, and above and below the piriformis muscle.

Clinical app

Potential problem of hernias

One of the potential problems with hernias is that bowel and fat may become stuck within the hernial sac. This can cause appreciable pain and bowel obstruction, necessitating urgent surgery. Another potential risk is **strangulation** of the hernia in which the blood supply to the bowel is cut off at the neck of the hernial sac, rendering the bowel ischemic and susceptible to perforation.

ABDOMINAL VISCERA

Peritoneum

A thin membrane (the **peritoneum**) lines the walls of the abdominal cavity and covers much of the viscera. The **parietal peritoneum** lines the walls of the cavity, and the **visceral peritoneum** covers the viscera. Between the parietal and visceral layers of peritoneum is a potential space (the **peritoneal cavity**). Abdominal viscera either are suspended in the peritoneal cavity by folds of peritoneum (**mesenteries**) or are outside the peritoneal cavity. Organs suspended in the cavity are referred to as **intraperitoneal** (Fig. 4.33); organs outside

Fig. 4.33 A. Intraperitoneal. **B.** Retroperitoneal.

the peritoneal cavity, with only one surface or part of one surface covered by peritoneum, are *retroperitoneal.*

Peritoneal cavity

The peritoneal cavity is subdivided into the **greater sac** and the **omental bursa (lesser sac;** Fig. 4.34).

- The greater sac accounts for most of the space in the peritoneal cavity, beginning superiorly at the diaphragm and continuing inferiorly into the pelvic cavity. It is entered once the parietal peritoneum has been penetrated.
- The omental bursa is a smaller subdivision of the peritoneal cavity posterior to the stomach and liver and is continuous with the greater sac through an opening, the omental (epiploic) foramen (Fig. 4.35).

Surrounding the **omental (epiploic) foramen** are numerous structures covered with peritoneum (Fig. 4.35). They include:

- the portal vein, hepatic artery proper, and bile duct anteriorly;
- the inferior vena cava posteriorly;
- the caudate lobe of the liver superiorly; and
- the first part of the duodenum inferiorly.

Clinical app

The peritoneum
The peritoneum has a large surface area, which facilitates the spread of disease through the peritoneal cavity and over the bowel and visceral surfaces. Conversely, this large surface area can be used for administering certain types of treatment and a number of procedures.

Clinical app

Innervation of peritoneum
The parietal peritoneum associated with the abdominal wall is innervated by somatic afferents carried in branches of the associated spinal nerves and is therefore sensitive to well-localized pain. The visceral peritoneum is innervated by visceral afferents that accompany autonomic nerves (sympathetic and parasympathetic) back to the central nervous system. Activation of these fibers can lead to referred pain and poorly localized sensations of discomfort and to reflex visceral motor activity.

Clinical app

Ventriculoperitoneal shunts
Patients with obstructive hydrocephalus (an excessive accumulation of cerebrospinal fluid within the cerebral ventricular system) require continuous drainage of this fluid. This is achieved by placing a catheter through the skull into the cerebral ventricles and placing the extracranial part of the tube beneath the scalp and skin of the chest wall and then passing it through the abdominal wall into the peritoneal cavity. Cerebrospinal fluid drains through the tube into the peritoneal cavity where it is absorbed.

Clinical app

Hemodialysis and peritoneal dialysis
People who develop renal failure require dialysis to live. There are two methods.

In the first method **(hemodialysis),** blood is taken from the circulation, dialyzed through a complex artificial membrane, and returned to the body. A high rate of blood flow is required to remove excess body fluid, exchange electrolytes, and remove noxious metabolites. To accomplish this, either an arteriovenous fistula is established surgically and is cannulated each time the patient returns for dialysis, or a large-bore cannula is placed into the right atrium through which blood can be aspirated and returned.

In the second method (peritoneal dialysis), the peritoneum is used as the dialysis membrane. The large surface area of the peritoneal cavity is an ideal dialysis membrane for fluid and electrolyte exchange. To accomplish dialysis, a small tube is inserted through the abdominal wall and dialysis fluid is injected into the peritoneal cavity. Electrolytes and molecules are exchanged across the peritoneum between the fluid and blood. Once dialysis is completed, the fluid is drained.

Clinical app

Peritoneal spread of disease
The large surface area of the peritoneal cavity allows infection and malignant disease to spread easily throughout the abdomen. If malignant cells enter the peritoneal cavity by direct invasion (e.g., from colon or ovarian cancer), spread may be rapid. Similarly, a surgeon excising a malignant tumor and releasing malignant cells into the peritoneal cavity may cause an appreciable worsening of the patient's prognosis.

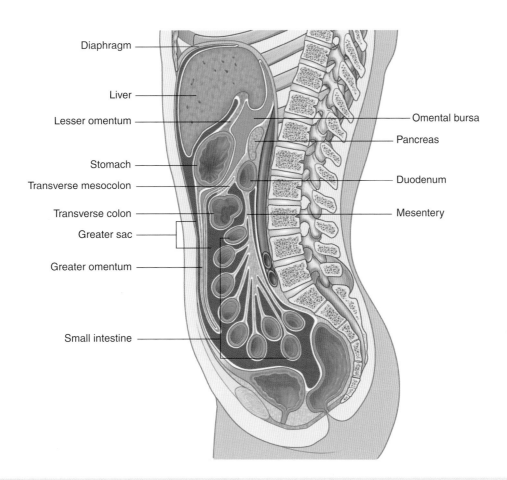

Fig. 4.34 Greater and lesser sacs of the peritoneal cavity.

Clinical app

Perforated bowel

A perforated bowel (e.g., caused by a perforated duodenal ulcer) often leads to the release of gas into the peritoneal cavity. This peritoneal gas can be easily visualized on a chest radiograph with the patient standing, where gas can be demonstrated in extremely small amounts beneath the diaphragm. A patient with severe abdominal pain and subdiaphragmatic gas needs a laparotomy.

Omenta, mesenteries, and ligaments

Throughout the peritoneal cavity, numerous peritoneal folds connect organs to each other or to the abdominal wall. These folds (omenta, mesenteries, and ligaments) develop from the original dorsal and ventral mesenteries, which suspend the developing gastrointestinal tract in the embryonic coelomic cavity. Some contain vessels and nerves supplying the viscera, whereas others help maintain the proper positioning of the viscera.

Omenta

The omenta consist of two layers of peritoneum, which pass from the stomach and the first part of the duodenum to other viscera. There are two:

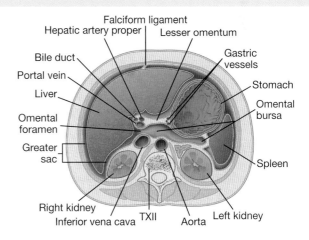

Fig. 4.35 Transverse section illustrating the continuity between the greater and lesser sacs through the omental (epiploic) foramen.

■ the greater omentum derived from the dorsal mesentery and

■ the lesser omentum derived from the ventral mesentery.

Greater omentum

The **greater omentum** is a large, apron-like, peritoneal fold that attaches to the greater curvature of the stomach and the first part of the duodenum (Fig. 4.36). It drapes inferiorly over the

Abdomen

Liver   Xiphoid process   Stomach

Greater omentum

Fig. 4.36 Greater omentum.

The hepatoduodenal ligament ends laterally as a free margin and serves as the anterior border of the omental foramen (see Fig. 4.35). Enclosed in this free edge are the hepatic artery proper, the bile duct, and the portal vein. Additionally, the right and left gastric vessels are between the layers of the lesser omentum near the lesser curvature of the stomach.

Clinical app

The greater omentum

When a laparotomy is performed and the peritoneal cavity is opened, the first structure usually encountered is the greater omentum. This fatty double-layered vascular membrane hangs like an apron from the greater curvature of the stomach, drapes over the transverse colon, and lies freely suspended within the abdominal cavity. It is often referred to as the *policeman of the abdomen* because of its apparent ability to migrate to any inflamed area and wrap itself around the organ to wall off inflammation.

The greater omentum is also an important site for metastatic tumor spread. Direct omental spread by a transcoelomic route is common for carcinoma of the ovary.

transverse colon and the coils of the jejunum and ileum (see Fig. 4.34). Turning posteriorly, it ascends to associate with, and become adherent to, the peritoneum on the superior surface of the transverse colon and the anterior layer of the transverse mesocolon before arriving at the posterior abdominal wall.

Usually a thin membrane, the greater omentum always contains an accumulation of fat, which may become substantial in some individuals. Additionally, there are two arteries and accompanying veins, the **right** and **left gastro-omental vessels,** between this double-layered peritoneal apron just inferior to the greater curvature of the stomach.

Lesser omentum

The other two-layered peritoneal omentum is the **lesser omentum** (Fig. 4.37). It extends from the lesser curvature of the stomach and the first part of the duodenum to the inferior surface of the liver (Fig. 4.37; also see Fig. 4.34).

A thin membrane continuous with the peritoneal coverings of the anterior and posterior surfaces of the stomach and the first part of the duodenum, the lesser omentum is divided into:

- a medial **hepatogastric ligament,** which passes between the stomach and liver, and
- a lateral **hepatoduodenal ligament,** which passes between the duodenum and liver.

Mesenteries

Mesenteries are peritoneal folds that attach viscera to the posterior abdominal wall. They allow some movement and provide a conduit for vessels, nerves, and lymphatics to reach the viscera and include:

- the mesentery—associated with parts of the small intestine,
- the transverse mesocolon—associated with the transverse colon, and
- the sigmoid mesocolon—associated with the sigmoid colon.

All of these are derivatives of the dorsal mesentery.

Mesentery

The **mesentery** is a large, fan-shaped, double-layered fold of peritoneum that connects the jejunum and ileum to the posterior abdominal wall (Fig. 4.38). Its superior attachment is at the duodenojejunal junction just to the left of the upper lumbar part of the vertebral column. It passes obliquely downward and to the right, ending at the ileocecal junction near the upper border of the right sacro-iliac joint. In the fat between the two peritoneal layers of the mesentery are the arteries, veins, nerves, and lymphatics that supply the jejunum and ileum.

Fig. 4.37 Lesser omentum.

Fig. 4.38 Peritoneal reflections, forming mesenteries, outlined on the posterior abdominal wall.

Transverse mesocolon

The **transverse mesocolon** is a fold of peritoneum that connects the transverse colon to the posterior abdominal wall (Fig. 4.38, also see Fig. 4.34). Its two layers of peritoneum leave the posterior abdominal wall across the anterior surface of the head and body of the pancreas and pass outward to surround the transverse colon. Between its layers are the arteries, veins, nerves, and lymphatics related to the transverse colon. The anterior layer of the transverse mesocolon is adherent to the posterior layer of the greater omentum.

Sigmoid mesocolon

The **sigmoid mesocolon** is an inverted, V-shaped peritoneal fold that attaches the sigmoid colon to the abdominal wall (Fig. 4.38). The apex of the V is near the division of the left common iliac artery into its internal and external branches, with the left limb of the descending V along the medial border of the left psoas major muscle and the right limb descending into the pelvis to end at the level of vertebra SIII. The sigmoid and superior rectal vessels, along with the nerves and lymphatics associated with the sigmoid colon, pass through this peritoneal fold.

Ligaments

Peritoneal ligaments consist of two layers of peritoneum that connect two organs to each other or attach an organ to the body wall and may form part of an omentum. They are usually named after the structures being connected. For example, the splenorenal ligament connects the left kidney to the spleen and the gastrophrenic ligament connects the stomach to the diaphragm.

Organs
Abdominal esophagus

The abdominal esophagus represents the short distal part of the esophagus located in the abdominal cavity. Emerging through the right crus of the diaphragm usually at the level of vertebra TX, it passes from the esophageal hiatus to the cardial orifice of the stomach just left of the midline (Fig. 4.39).

Associated with the esophagus as it enters the abdominal cavity are the anterior and posterior vagal trunks:

- The **anterior vagal trunk** consists of several smaller trunks whose fibers mostly come from the left vagus nerve; rotation of the gut during development moves these trunks to the anterior surface of the esophagus.
- Similarly, the **posterior vagal trunk** consists of a single trunk whose fibers mostly come from the right vagus nerve, and rotational changes during development move this trunk to the posterior surface of the esophagus.

Fig. 4.39 Abdominal esophagus.

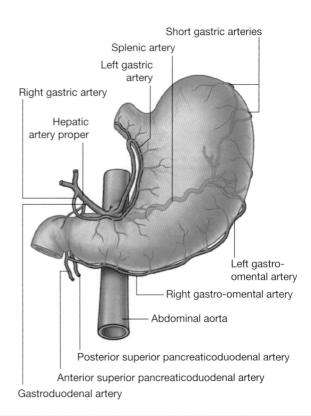

Fig. 4.40 Arterial supply to the abdominal esophagus and stomach.

The arterial supply to the abdominal esophagus (Fig. 4.40) includes:

- esophageal branches from the left gastric artery (from the celiac trunk) and
- esophageal branches from the left inferior phrenic artery (from the abdominal aorta).

Stomach

The stomach is the most dilated part of the gastrointestinal tract and has a J-like shape (Figs. 4.41, 4.42). Positioned between the abdominal esophagus and the small intestine, the stomach is in the epigastric, umbilical, and left hypochondrium regions of the abdomen.

The stomach is divided into four regions (Fig. 4.41):

- the **cardia,** which surrounds the opening of the esophagus into the stomach,
- the **fundus of stomach,** which is the area above the level of the cardial orifice,
- the **body of stomach,** which is the largest region of the stomach; and

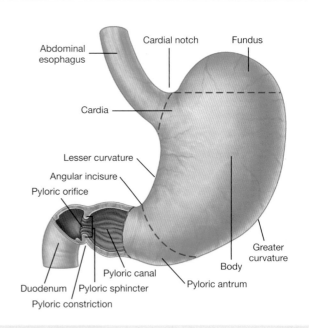

Fig. 4.41 Stomach.

- the **pyloric part,** which is divided into the **pyloric antrum** and **pyloric canal** and is the distal end of the stomach (Fig. 4.41).

The most distal portion of the pyloric part of the stomach is the **pylorus** (Fig. 4.41). It is marked on the surface of the organ by the **pyloric constriction** and contains a thickened ring of gastric circular muscle, the **pyloric sphincter,** which surrounds the distal opening of the stomach, the **pyloric orifice.** The pyloric orifice is just to the right of midline in a plane that passes through the lower border of vertebra LI (the **transpyloric plane**).

Other features of the stomach include:

- the **greater curvature,** which is a point of attachment for the gastrosplenic ligament and the greater omentum;
- the **lesser curvature,** which is a point of attachment for the lesser omentum;
- the **cardial notch,** which is the superior angle created when the esophagus enters the stomach; and
- the **angular incisure,** which is a bend on the lesser curvature.

The arterial supply to the stomach (Fig. 4.40) includes:

- the left gastric artery from the celiac trunk,
- the right gastric artery often from the hepatic artery proper,
- the right gastro-omental artery from the gastroduodenal artery,
- the left gastro-omental artery from the splenic artery, and
- the posterior gastric artery from the splenic artery (variant and not always present).

Imaging app

Visualizing the stomach

Superior part of duodenum   Esophagus
Pyloric antrum   Fundus of stomach

Descending part of duodenum   Body of stomach
Duodenal jejunal flexure

Fig. 4.42 Double-contrast radiograph of the stomach and duodenum.

Small intestine

The small intestine is the longest part of the gastrointestinal tract and extends from the pyloric orifice of the stomach to the ileocecal fold. This hollow tube, which is approximately 6 to 7 m long with a narrowing diameter from beginning to end, consists of the duodenum, the jejunum, and the ileum.

Duodenum

The first part of the small intestine is the duodenum. This C-shaped structure adjacent to the head of the pancreas is 20 to 25 cm long and is above the level of the umbilicus; its lumen is the widest of the small intestine (Fig. 4.43). It is retroperitoneal except for its beginning, which is connected to the liver by the hepatoduodenal ligament, a part of the lesser omentum.

The duodenum is divided into four parts (Fig. 4.43).

- The **superior part** (first part) extends from the pyloric orifice of the stomach to the neck of the gallbladder, is just to the right of the body of vertebra LI, and passes anteriorly to the bile duct, gastroduodenal artery, portal vein, and inferior vena cava. Clinically, the beginning of this part of the duodenum is referred to as the *ampulla* or *duodenal cap,* and most duodenal ulcers occur in this part of the duodenum.
- The **descending part** (second part) of the duodenum is just to the right of midline and extends from the neck of the gallbladder to the lower border of vertebra LIII. Its anterior surface is crossed by the transverse colon, posterior to it is the right kidney, and medial to it is the head of the pancreas. This part of the duodenum contains the **major duodenal papilla,** which is the common entrance for the bile and pancreatic ducts, and the **minor duodenal papilla,** which is the entrance for the accessory pancreatic duct. The junction of the foregut and the midgut occurs just below the major duodenal papilla.
- The **inferior part** (third part) of the duodenum is the longest section crossing the inferior vena cava, the aorta, and the vertebral column (Figs. 4.42, 4.43). It is crossed anteriorly by the superior mesenteric artery and vein.
- The **ascending part** (fourth part) of the duodenum passes upward on, or to the left of, the aorta to approximately the upper border of vertebra LII and terminates at the **duodenojejunal flexure.**

This duodenojejunal flexure is surrounded by a fold of peritoneum containing muscle fibers called the **suspensory muscle (ligament) of duodenum (ligament of Treitz).**

169

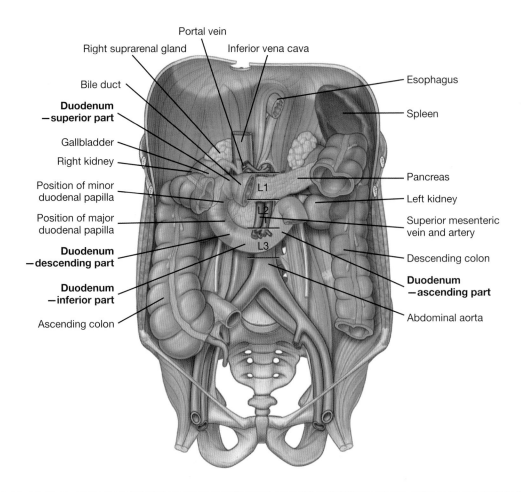

Fig. 4.43 Duodenum.

The arterial supply to the duodenum (Fig. 4.44) includes:

- branches from the gastroduodenal artery,
- the supraduodenal artery from the gastroduodenal artery,
- duodenal branches from the anterior superior pancreatico-duodenal artery (from the gastroduodenal artery),
- duodenal branches from the posterior superior pancreaticoduodenal artery (from the gastroduodenal artery),
- duodenal branches from the anterior inferior pancreaticoduodenal artery (from the inferior pancreaticoduodenal artery—a branch of the superior mesenteric artery),
- duodenal branches from the posterior inferior pancreaticoduodenal artery (from the inferior pancreaticoduodenal artery—a branch of the superior mesenteric artery), and
- the first jejunal branch from the superior mesenteric artery.

Jejunum

The jejunum and ileum make up the last two sections of the small intestine (Fig. 4.45). The jejunum represents the proximal two-fifths. It is mostly in the left upper quadrant of the abdomen and is larger in diameter and has a thicker wall than the ileum. Additionally, the inner mucosal lining of the jejunum is characterized by numerous prominent folds that circle the lumen (plicae circulares). The less prominent arterial arcades and longer vasa recta (straight arteries) compared with those of the ileum are a unique characteristic of the jejunum (Fig. 4.46).

The arterial supply to the jejunum includes jejunal arteries from the superior mesenteric artery (Fig. 4.47).

Ileum

The ileum makes up the distal three-fifths of the small intestine and is mostly in the right lower quadrant. Compared with the jejunum, the ileum has thinner walls, fewer and less prominent mucosal folds (plicae circulares), shorter vasa recta, more mesenteric fat, and more arterial arcades (Fig. 4.46).

The ileum opens into the large intestine where the cecum and ascending colon join together. Two flaps

Posterior superior
pancreaticoduodenal artery

Left gastric artery

Hepatic artery proper

Gastroduodenal
artery

Right gastro-
omental artery

Supraduodenal
artery

Anterior superior
pancreaticoduodenal
artery

Superior mesenteric
artery

Posterior inferior
pancreaticoduodenal
artery

Abdominal aorta

Anterior inferior
pancreaticoduodenal artery

Fig. 4.44 Arterial supply to the duodenum.

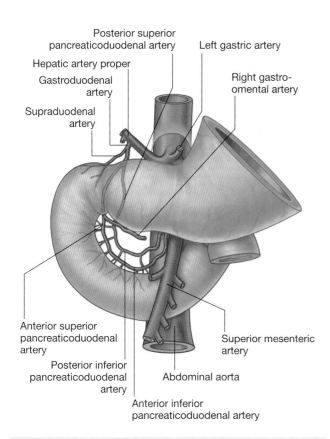

Vasa recta

Arterial arcades

A

Vasa recta

Arterial arcades

B

Fig. 4.46 Differences in the arterial supply to the small intestine. **A.** Jejunum. **B.** Ileum.

Imaging app

Visualizing the jejunum and ileum

Jejunum

Ileum

Stomach

Fig. 4.45 Radiograph of the jejunum and ileum.

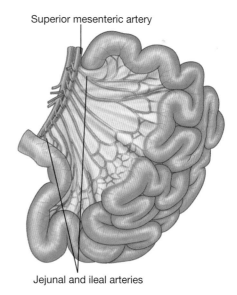

Superior mesenteric artery

Jejunal and ileal arteries

Fig. 4.47 Arterial supply to the ileum and jejunum.

Clinical app

Epithelial transition between the abdominal esophagus and stomach

The gastroesophageal junction is demarcated by a transition from one epithelial type (nonkeratinized stratified squamous

Continued 171

Clinical app—cont'd

epithelium) to another epithelial type (columnar epithelium). In some people, the histological junction does not lie at the anatomical gastroesophageal junction but occurs more proximally in the lower one-third of the esophagus. This may predispose these people to esophageal ulceration and is also associated with an increased risk of adenocarcinoma.

Clinical app

Surgery for obesity
Surgical procedures for obesity are divided into malabsorption and restrictive procedures.

Malabsorption procedures
In these procedures, the stomach is surgically anastomosed to the distal jejunum/ileum so that the stomach contents bypass most of the small intestine. There are certain complications of malabsorption procedures, which include anemia, osteoporosis, and diarrhea.

Restrictive procedures
These procedures involve placing bands around the stomach to reduce the amount of food that can be ingested and also produce an earlier feeling of satiety.

Clinical app

Duodenal ulceration
Duodenal ulcers usually occur in the superior part of the duodenum:

- Posterior duodenal ulcers erode either directly onto the gastroduodenal artery or, more commonly, onto the posterior superior pancreaticoduodenal artery, which can produce torrential hemorrhage and may be fatal in some patients. Treatment may involve extensive upper abdominal surgery with ligation of the vessels or by endovascular means, whereby the radiologist may place a very fine catheter retrograde from the femoral artery into the celiac artery. The common hepatic artery and the gastroduodenal artery are cannulated, and the bleeding area may be blocked using small coils, which stem the flow of blood.
- Anterior duodenal ulcers erode into the peritoneal cavity, causing peritonitis. This intense inflammatory reaction and the local ileus promote adhesion of the greater omentum, which attempts to seal off the perforation. The stomach and duodenum usually contain considerable amounts of gas, which enters the peritoneal cavity and can be observed on a chest radiograph of an erect patient as subdiaphragmatic gas.

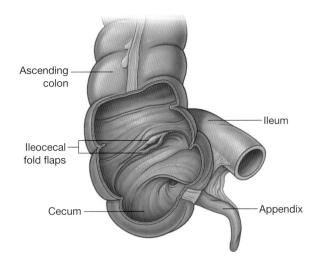

Fig. 4.48 Illustration showing ileocecal junction and the ileocecal fold.

Clinical app

Examination of the bowel lumen
Barium sulfate solutions may be swallowed by the patient and can be visualized using an X-ray fluoroscopy unit. The lumen can be examined for masses (e.g., polyps and tumors), and peristaltic waves can be assessed. Patients may also be given carbon dioxide–releasing granules to fill the stomach so that the barium thinly coats the mucosa, resulting in images displaying fine mucosal detail.

Clinical app

Meckel's diverticulum
A Meckel's diverticulum is the remnant of the proximal part of the yolk stalk (vitelline duct), which extends into the umbilical cord in the embryo and lies on the antimesenteric border of the ileum. Although it is an uncommon finding (occurring in approximately 2% of the population), it is always important to consider the diagnosis of Meckel's diverticulum because it does produce symptoms in a small number of patients.

Clinical app

Carcinoma of the stomach
Carcinoma of the stomach is a common gastrointestinal malignancy. Chronic gastric inflammation (gastritis), pernicious anemia, and polyps predispose to the development of this aggressive cancer, which is usually not diagnosed until late in the course of the disease.

Clinical app—cont'd

The diagnosis may be made using barium and conventional radiology or endoscopy, which allows a biopsy to be obtained at the same time. Ultrasound scanning is used to check the liver for metastatic spread, and, if negative, computed tomography is carried out to assess for surgical resectability. If carcinoma of the stomach is diagnosed early, a curative surgical resection is possible.

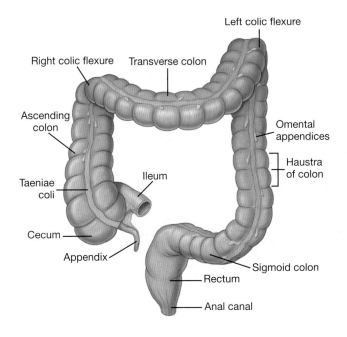

Fig. 4.49 Large intestine.

Imaging app

Visualizing the large intestine

Fig. 4.50 Radiograph, using barium, showing the large intestine.

projecting into the lumen of the large intestine (the **ileocecal fold**) surround the opening (Fig. 4.48). The flaps of the ileocecal fold come together at their end, forming ridges. Musculature from the ileum continues into each flap, forming a sphincter. Possible functions of the ileocecal fold include preventing reflux from the cecum to the ileum and regulating the passage of contents from the ileum to the cecum.

The arterial supply to the ileum (Fig. 4.47) includes:

- ileal arteries from the superior mesenteric artery and
- an ileal branch from the ileocolic artery (from the superior mesenteric artery).

Large intestine

The large intestine extends from the distal end of the ileum to the anus, a distance of approximately 1.5 m in adults. It absorbs fluids and salts from the gut contents, thus forming feces, and consists of the cecum, appendix, colon, rectum, and anal canal (Figs. 4.49, 4.50).

Beginning in the right groin as the cecum with its associated appendix, the large intestine continues upward as the **ascending colon** through the right flank and into the right hypochondrium (Fig. 4.51). Just below the liver it bends to the left, forming the **right colic flexure (hepatic flexure),** and crosses the abdomen as the **transverse colon** to the left hypochondrium. At this position just below the spleen, the large intestine bends downward, forming the **left colic flexure (splenic flexure),** and continues as the **descending colon** through the left flank and into the left groin.

It enters the upper part of the pelvic cavity as the sigmoid colon, continues on the posterior wall of the pelvic cavity as the rectum, and terminates as the anal canal.

The general characteristics of most of the large intestine (Fig. 4.49) are:

- its large internal diameter compared to that of the small intestine;
- peritoneal-covered accumulations of fat (the **omental appendices**) are associated with the colon;

Abdomen

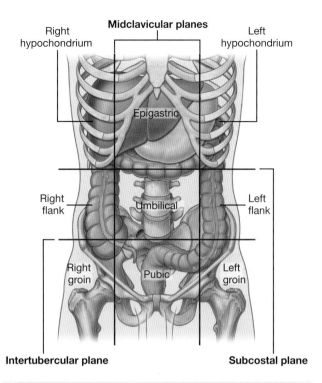

Fig. 4.51 Position of the large intestine in the nine-region organizational pattern.

Fig. 4.52 Cecum and appendix.

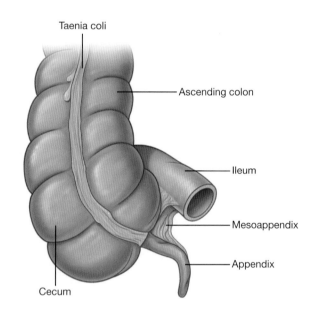

Fig. 4.53 Mesoappendix.

- the segregation of longitudinal muscle in its walls into three narrow bands (the **taenia coli**), which are primarily observed in the cecum and colon and less visible in the rectum; and
- the sacculations of the colon (the **haustra of colon**).

Cecum and appendix

The **cecum** is the first part of the large intestine (Fig. 4.52). It is inferior to the ileocecal opening and in the right iliac fossa. It is generally considered to be an intraperitoneal structure because of its mobility, even though it normally is not suspended in the peritoneal cavity by a mesentery.

The cecum is continuous with the ascending colon at the entrance of the ileum and is usually in contact with the anterior abdominal wall. It may cross the pelvic brim to lie in the true pelvis. The appendix is attached to the posteromedial wall of the cecum just inferior to the end of the ileum (Fig. 4.52).

The **appendix** is a narrow, hollow, blind-ended tube connected to the cecum. It has large aggregations of lymphoid tissue in its walls and is suspended from the terminal ileum by the **mesoappendix** (Fig. 4.53), which contains the **appendicular vessels**. Its point of attachment to the cecum is consistent with the highly visible free taenia leading directly to the base of the appendix, but the location of the rest of the appendix varies considerably (Fig. 4.54). It may be:

- posterior to the cecum or the lower ascending colon, or both, in a retrocecal or retrocolic position;
- suspended over the pelvic brim in a pelvic or descending position;
- below the cecum in a subcecal location; or
- anterior to the terminal ileum, possibly contacting the body wall in a preileal position or posterior to the terminal ileum in a postileal position.

The surface projection of the base of the appendix is at the junction of the lateral and middle one-third of a line from the anterior superior iliac spine to the umbilicus (McBurney's point). People with appendicular problems may describe pain near this location.

174

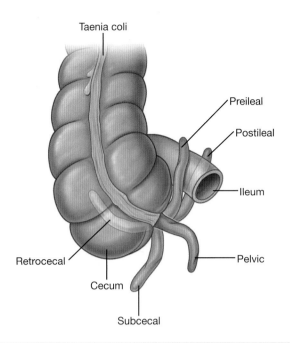

Fig. 4.54 Positions of the appendix.

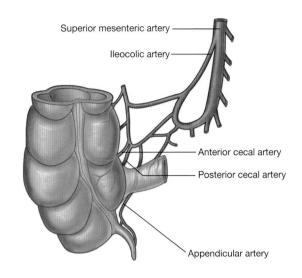

Fig. 4.55 Arterial supply to the cecum and appendix.

The arterial supply to the cecum and appendix (Fig. 4.55) includes:

■ the anterior cecal artery from the ileocolic artery (from the superior mesenteric artery),

■ the posterior cecal artery from the ileocolic artery (from the superior mesenteric artery), and

■ the appendicular artery from the ileocolic artery (from the superior mesenteric artery).

Clinical app

Appendicitis

Acute appendicitis is an abdominal emergency. It usually occurs when the appendix is obstructed by either a fecalith or enlargement of the lymphoid nodules. Within the obstructed appendix, bacteria proliferate and invade the appendix wall, which becomes damaged by pressure necrosis. In some instances, this may resolve spontaneously; in other cases, inflammatory change continues and perforation ensues, which may lead to localized or generalized peritonitis.

Most patients with acute appendicitis have localized tenderness in the right groin. Initially, the pain begins as a central/periumbilical, which tends to come and go. As the disease progresses, the pain shifts to the lower right groin and is focal.

When the appendix first becomes inflamed, the visceral sensory fibers are stimulated (Fig. 4.56). These fibers enter the spinal cord at spinal cord level T10. The pain is referred to the dermatome of T10 in the periumbilical region. The pain is diffuse, not focal; every time a peristaltic wave passes through

the ileocecal region, the pain recurs. This intermittent type of pain is referred to as *colic*.

In later stages of the disease, the appendix contacts and irritates the parietal peritoneum in the right iliac fossa, which is innervated by somatic sensory nerves. This produces a constant focal pain, which predominates over the colicky pain that the patient felt some hours previously, and the patient no longer perceives the referred pain.

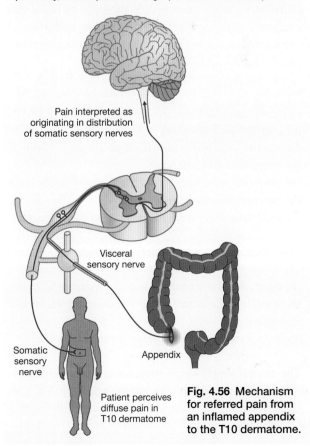

Fig. 4.56 Mechanism for referred pain from an inflamed appendix to the T10 dermatome.

Colon

The colon extends superiorly from the cecum and consists of the ascending, transverse, descending, and sigmoid colon (Fig. 4.57). Its ascending and descending segments are (secondarily) retroperitoneal, and its transverse and sigmoid segments are intraperitoneal.

At the junction of the ascending and transverse colon is the right colic flexure, which is just inferior to the right lobe of the liver (Fig. 4.58). A similar but more acute bend (the left colic flexure) occurs at the junction of the transverse and descending colon (Fig. 4.58). This bend is just inferior to the spleen, higher and more posterior than the right colic flexure, and is attached to the diaphragm by the phrenicocolic ligament.

Immediately lateral to the ascending and descending colons are the **right** and **left paracolic gutters** (Fig. 4.57). These depressions are formed between the lateral margins of the ascending and descending colon and the posterolateral abdominal wall and are gutters through which material can pass from one region of the peritoneal cavity to another. Because major vessels and lymphatics are on the medial or posteromedial sides of the ascending and descending colon, a relatively blood-free mobilization of the ascending and descending colon is possible by cutting the peritoneum along these lateral paracolic gutters.

The final segment of the colon (the sigmoid colon) begins above the pelvic inlet and extends to the level of vertebra SIII where it is continuous with the rectum (Fig. 4.57). This S-shaped structure is quite mobile except at its beginning, where it continues from the descending colon, and at its end, where it continues as the rectum. Between these points, it is suspended by the sigmoid mesocolon.

The arterial supply to the ascending colon includes (Fig. 4.59):

- the colic branch from the ileocolic artery (from the superior mesenteric artery),
- the anterior cecal artery from the ileocolic artery (from the superior mesenteric artery),
- the posterior cecal artery from the ileocolic artery (from the superior mesenteric artery), and
- the right colic artery from the superior mesenteric artery.

The arterial supply to the transverse colon includes (Fig. 4.59):

- the right colic artery from the superior mesenteric artery,
- the middle colic artery from the superior mesenteric artery, and
- the left colic artery from the inferior mesenteric artery.

The arterial supply to the descending colon includes the left colic artery from the inferior mesenteric artery (Fig. 4.59).

The arterial supply to the sigmoid colon includes sigmoidal arteries from the inferior mesenteric artery (Fig. 4.59).

Anastomotic connections between arteries supplying the colon can result in a marginal artery that courses along the ascending, transverse, and descending parts of the large bowel (Fig. 4.59).

Rectum and anal canal

Extending from the sigmoid colon is the rectum (Fig. 4.60). The rectosigmoid junction is usually described as being at the level of vertebra SIII or at the end of the sigmoid mesocolon because the rectum is a retroperitoneal structure.

The anal canal is the continuation of the large intestine inferior to the rectum.

The arterial supply to the rectum and anal canal includes (Fig. 4.61):

- the superior rectal artery from the inferior mesenteric artery,
- the middle rectal artery from the internal iliac artery, and
- the inferior rectal artery from the internal pudendal artery (from the internal iliac artery).

Fig. 4.57 Colon.

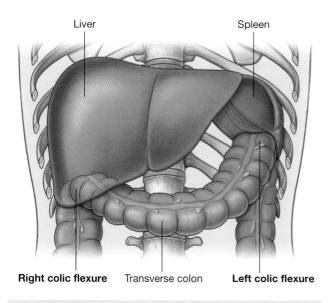

Liver Spleen

Right colic flexure Transverse colon **Left colic flexure**

Fig. 4.58 Right and left colic flexures.

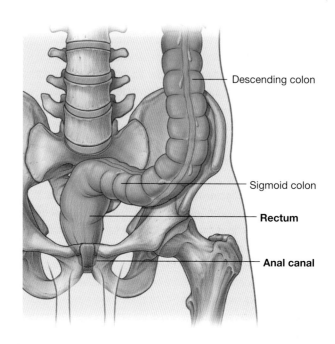

Descending colon

Sigmoid colon

Rectum

Anal canal

Fig. 4.60 Rectum and anal canal.

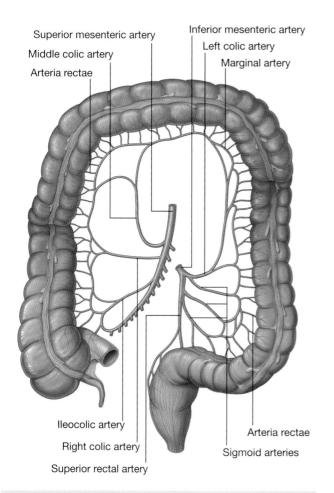

Superior mesenteric artery Inferior mesenteric artery
Middle colic artery Left colic artery
Arteria rectae Marginal artery

Ileocolic artery

Right colic artery

Superior rectal artery Arteria rectae Sigmoid arteries

Fig. 4.59 Arterial supply to the colon.

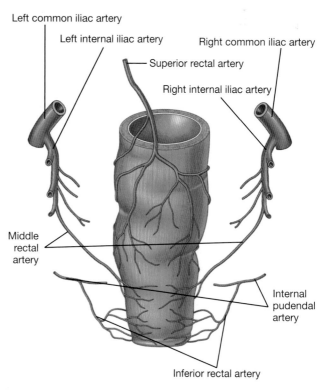

Left common iliac artery

Left internal iliac artery Right common iliac artery

Superior rectal artery

Right internal iliac artery

Middle rectal artery

Internal pudendal artery

Inferior rectal artery

Fig. 4.61 Arterial supply to the rectum and anal canal. Posterior view.

Abdomen

Clinical app

Congenital disorders of the gastrointestinal tract

The normal positions of the abdominal viscera result from a complex series of rotations that the gut tube undergoes and from the growth of the abdominal cavity to accommodate changes in the size of the developing organs.

Malrotation is incomplete rotation and fixation of the midgut after it has passed from the umbilical sac and returned to the abdominal cavity. The proximal attachment of the small bowel mesentery begins at the **suspensory muscle of duodenum (ligament of Treitz)**, which determines the position of the duodenojejunal junction. The mesentery of the small bowel ends at the level of the ileocecal junction in the right lower quadrant. This long line of fixation of the mesentery prevents accidental twists of the gut.

If the duodenojejunal flexure or the cecum does not end up in its usual site, the origin of the small bowel mesentery shortens, which permits twisting of the small bowel around the axis of the superior mesenteric artery. Twisting of the bowel, in general, is termed **volvulus**. Volvulus of the small bowel may lead to a reduction of blood flow and infarction.

Clinical app

Bowel obstruction

A bowel obstruction can be either mechanical or functional:

- Mechanical obstruction is caused by an intraluminal, mural, or extrinsic mass that can be secondary to a foreign body, obstructing tumor in the wall extrinsic compression from an adhesion, or an embryological band.
- A functional obstruction is usually due to an inability of the bowel to peristalse, which, again, has a number of causes and most frequently is a postsurgical state due to excessive intraoperative bowel handling. Small bowel obstruction is typically caused by adhesions following previous surgery, and history should always be sought for any operations or abdominal interventions (e.g., previous appendectomy). Other causes include bowel passing into hernias (e.g., inguinal) and bowel twisting on its own mesentery (volvulus). Large bowel obstruction is commonly caused by a tumor. Other potential causes include hernias and inflammatory diverticular disease of the sigmoid colon.

Clinical app

Diverticular disease

Diverticular disease is the development of multiple colonic diverticula, predominantly throughout the sigmoid colon, though the whole colon may be affected (Fig. 4.62). The sigmoid colon has the smallest diameter of any portion of the colon and is therefore the site where intraluminal pressure is potentially the highest.

Patients tend to develop symptoms and signs when the neck of the diverticulum becomes obstructed by feces and becomes infected. Inflammation may spread along the wall, causing abdominal pain.

Because of the anatomical position of the sigmoid colon, there are a number of complications that may occur. The diverticula can perforate to form an abscess in the pelvis. The inflammation may produce an inflammatory mass, obstructing the left ureter. Inflammation may also spread to the bladder, producing a fistula between the sigmoid colon and the bladder.

Descending colon

Diverticula

Fig. 4.62 This double-contrast barium enema demonstrates numerous small outpouchings throughout the distal large bowel, predominantly within the descending colon and the sigmoid colon. These small outpouchings are diverticula and in most instances remain quiescent.

Imaging app

Endoscopic examination of the abdominal gastrointestinal tract

Endoscopy is a minimally invasive diagnostic medical procedure that can be used to assess the interior surfaces of an organ by inserting a tube into the body. The instrument is typically made of a flexible plastic material through which a light source and eye piece are attached at one end.

In gastrointestinal and abdominal medicine, an endoscope is used to assess the esophagus, stomach, duodenum, and proximal small bowel (Fig. 4.63A-E). The tube is swallowed by the patient under light sedation and is extremely well tolerated.

Assessment of the colon is performed by passage of the tube through the anus and into the rectum. The whole of the colon can be readily assessed (Fig. 4.63F-J).

Fig. 4.63 Endoscopy and colonoscopy showing different parts of the gastrointestinal tract. **A.** Gastroesophageal junction. **B.** Cardiac orifice and fundus of stomach—retroflexed view. **C.** Body of stomach. **D.** Pylorus of stomach and pyloric sphincter. **E.** Duodenum. **F.** Cecum showing appendiceal opening. **G.** Transverse colon. **H.** Sigmoid colon. **I.** Rectum—retroflexed view. **J.** Pectinate line.

Liver

The liver is the largest visceral organ in the body and is primarily in the right hypochondrium and epigastric region, extending into the left hypochondrium (or in the right upper quadrant, extending into the left upper quadrant) (see Fig. 4.4).

Surfaces of the liver include:

- a **diaphragmatic surface** in the anterior, superior, and posterior directions and
- a **visceral surface** in the inferior direction (Fig. 4.64).

Diaphragmatic surface

The diaphragmatic surface of the liver, which is smooth and domed, lies against the inferior surface of the diaphragm (Fig. 4.65). Associated with it are the subphrenic and hepatorenal recesses (Fig. 4.64):

- The **subphrenic recess** separates the diaphragmatic surface of the liver from the diaphragm and is divided into right and left areas by the **falciform ligament,** a structure derived from the ventral mesentery in the embryo.
- The **hepatorenal recess** is a part of the peritoneal cavity on the right side between the liver and the right kidney and right suprarenal gland.

The subphrenic and hepatorenal recesses are continuous anteriorly.

Visceral surface

The visceral surface of the liver is covered with visceral peritoneum except in the **fossa for the gallbladder** and at the **porta hepatis** (gateway to the liver; Fig. 4.66). Structures related to it include the following (Fig. 4.66):

- esophagus,
- right anterior part of the stomach,
- superior part of the duodenum,
- lesser omentum,
- gallbladder,
- right colic flexure,
- right transverse colon,
- right kidney, and
- right suprarenal gland.

The **porta hepatis** serves as the point of entry into the liver for the hepatic arteries and the portal vein and the exit point for the hepatic ducts (Fig. 4.66).

Associated ligaments

The liver is attached to the anterior abdominal wall by the **falciform ligament** and, except for a small area of the liver against the diaphragm (the **bare area**), the liver is almost completely surrounded by visceral peritoneum (Fig. 4.66). Additional folds of peritoneum connect the liver to the stomach (**hepatogastric ligament),** the duodenum (**hepatoduodenal ligament),** and the diaphragm (**right** and **left triangular ligaments** and **anterior** and **posterior coronary ligaments**).

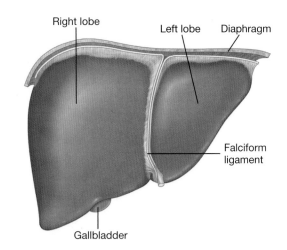

Fig. 4.65 Diaphragmatic surface of the liver.

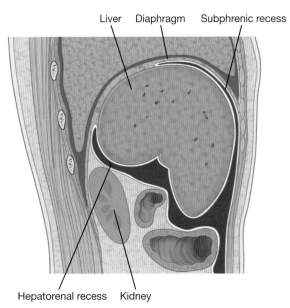

Fig. 4.64 Surfaces of the liver and recesses associated with the liver.

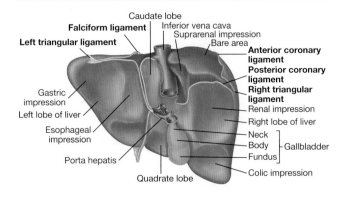

Fig. 4.66 Posterior view of the bare area of the liver and associated ligaments.

The bare area of the liver is a part of the liver on the diaphragmatic surface where there is no intervening peritoneum between the liver and the diaphragm (Fig. 4.66):

- The anterior boundary of the bare area is indicated by a reflection of peritoneum—the anterior coronary ligament.
- The posterior boundary of the bare area is indicated by a reflection of peritoneum—the posterior coronary ligament.
- Where the coronary ligaments come together laterally, they form the right and left triangular ligaments.

Lobes

The liver is divided into right and left lobes by the falciform ligament anterosuperiorly and the fissure for the ligametum venosum and ligamentum teres on the visceral surface (Figs. 4.66, 4.67, 4.68). The **right lobe of liver** is the largest lobe, whereas the **left lobe of liver** is smaller. The quadrate and caudate lobes are described as arising from the right lobe of the liver but functionally are distinct.

- The **quadrate lobe** is visible on the anterior part of the visceral surface of the liver and is bounded on the left by the fissure for ligamentum teres and on the right by the fossa for the gallbladder. Functionally it is related to the left lobe of the liver.
- The **caudate lobe** is visible on the posterior part of the visceral surface of the liver. It is bounded on the left by the fissure for the ligamentum venosum and on the right by the groove for the inferior vena cava. Functionally, it is separate from the right and the left lobes of the liver.

Fig. 4.67 Visceral surface of the liver.

Imaging app

Visualizing the liver

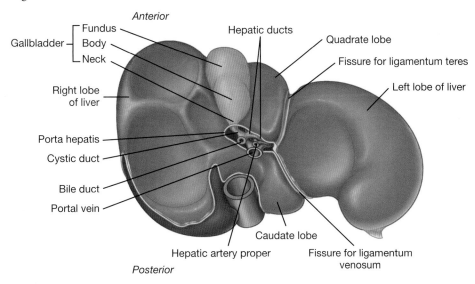

Fig. 4.68 Abdominal computed tomogram with contrast in the axial plane, showing the visceral surface of the liver.

The arterial supply to the liver includes (Fig. 4.69):

- the right hepatic artery from the hepatic artery proper (a branch of the common hepatic artery from the celiac trunk), and
- the left hepatic artery from the hepatic artery proper (a branch of the common hepatic artery from the celiac trunk).

Clinical app

Ostomies

It is occasionally necessary to surgically externalize bowel to the anterior abdominal wall. Externalization of bowel plays an important role in patient management.

Gastrostomy is performed when the stomach is attached to the anterior abdominal wall and a tube is placed through the skin into the stomach. Typically this is performed to feed the patient when it is impossible to take food and fluid orally (e.g., complex head and neck cancer).

In **jejunostomy,** the jejunum is brought to the anterior abdominal wall and fixed. The jejunostomy is used as a site where a feeding tube is placed through the anterior abdominal wall into the proximal efferent small bowel.

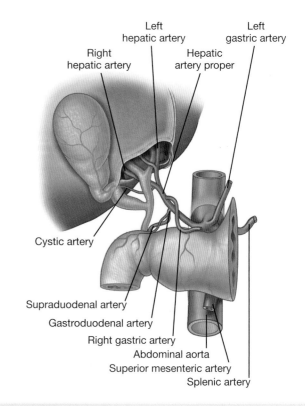

Fig. 4.69 Arterial supply to the liver and gallbladder.

Clinical app

Segmental anatomy of the liver

For many years the segmental anatomy of the liver was of little importance. However, since the development of liver resection surgery, the size, shape, and segmental anatomy of the liver has become clinically important, especially with regard to liver resection for metastatic disease.

The liver is divided by the principal plane, which divides the organ into halves of approximately equal size. This imaginary line is defined by a parasagittal line that passes through the gallbladder fossa to the inferior vena cava. It is in this plane that the middle hepatic vein is found. Importantly, the principal plane divides the left half of the liver from the right half. The lobes of the liver are unequal in size and bear only little relevance to operative anatomy.

The traditional eight segment anatomy of the liver relates to the hepatic arterial, portal, and biliary drainage of these segments (Fig. 4.70).

The caudate lobe is defined as segment I; the remaining segments are numbered in a clockwise fashion up to segment VIII. The features are extremely consistent among individuals.

From a surgical perspective, a right hepatectomy would involve division of the liver in the principal plane in which segments V, VI, VII, and VIII would be removed, leaving segments I, II, III, and IV.

Fig. 4.70 Division of the liver into segments based on the distributions of the bile ducts and hepatic vessels (Couinaud's segments).

Gallbladder

The **gallbladder** is a pear-shaped sac lying on the visceral surface of the right lobe of the liver in a fossa between the right and quadrate lobes (see Fig. 4.67). It has:

- a rounded end (**fundus of gallbladder**), which may project from the inferior border of the liver;
- a major part in the fossa (**body of gallbladder**), which may be against the transverse colon and the superior part of the duodenum; and
- a narrow part (**neck of gallbladder**) with mucosal folds forming the spiral fold.

The arterial supply to the gallbladder (see Fig. 4.69) is the cystic artery from the right hepatic artery (a branch of the hepatic artery proper).

The gallbladder receives, concentrates, and stores bile from the liver.

Pancreas

The pancreas lies mostly posterior to the stomach (Figs. 4.71, 4.73). It extends across the posterior abdominal wall from the duodenum on the right to the spleen on the left.

The pancreas is (secondarily) retroperitoneal except for a small part of its tail and consists of a head, uncinate process, neck, body, and tail (Fig. 4.71).

- The **head of pancreas** lies within the C-shaped concavity of the duodenum.
- Projecting from the lower part of the head is the **uncinate process,** which passes posterior to the superior mesenteric vessels.

- The **neck of pancreas** is anterior to the superior mesenteric vessels. Posterior to the neck of the pancreas, the superior mesenteric and the splenic veins join to form the portal vein.
- The **body of pancreas** is elongate and extends from the neck to the tail of the pancreas.
- The **tail of pancreas** passes between layers of the splenorenal ligament.

Fig. 4.71 Pancreas.

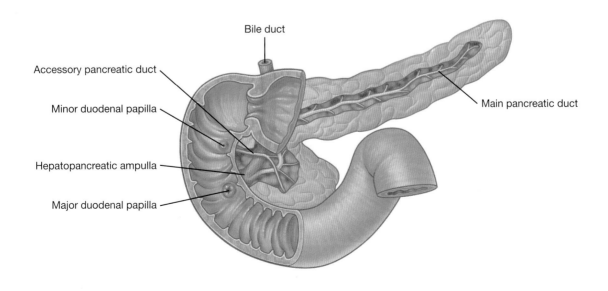

Fig. 4.72 Pancreatic duct system.

The **pancreatic duct** begins in the tail of the pancreas (Fig. 4.72). It passes to the right through the body of the pancreas and, after entering the head of the pancreas, turns inferiorly. In the lower part of the head of pancreas, the pancreatic duct joins the bile duct. The joining of these two structures forms the **hepatopancreatic ampulla** (ampulla of Vater), which enters the descending (second) part of the duodenum at the **major duodenal papilla.** Surrounding the ampulla is the **sphincter of ampulla** (sphincter of Oddi), which is a collection of smooth muscle cells.

The **accessory pancreatic duct** empties into the duodenum just above the major duodenal papilla at the **minor duodenal papilla** (Fig. 4.72). If the accessory duct is followed from the minor papilla into the head of the pancreas, a branch point is discovered:

- One branch continues to the left through the head of the pancreas and may connect with the pancreatic duct at the point where it turns inferiorly.
- A second branch descends into the lower part of the head of the pancreas, anterior to the pancreatic duct, and ends in the uncinate process.

The main and accessory pancreatic ducts usually communicate with each other. The presence of these two ducts reflects the embryological origin of the pancreas from dorsal and ventral buds from the foregut.

The arterial supply to the pancreas (Fig. 4.74) includes the:

- gastroduodenal artery from the common hepatic artery (a branch of the celiac trunk),
- anterior superior pancreaticoduodenal artery from the gastroduodenal artery,
- posterior superior pancreaticoduodenal artery from the gastroduodenal artery,
- dorsal pancreatic artery from the inferior pancreatic artery (a branch of the splenic artery),
- great pancreatic artery from the inferior pancreatic artery (a branch of the splenic artery),
- dorsal pancreatic and greater pancreatic arteries (branches of the splenic artery),
- anterior inferior pancreaticoduodenal artery from the inferior pancreaticoduodenal artery (a branch of the superior mesenteric artery), and
- posterior inferior pancreaticoduodenal artery from the inferior pancreaticoduodenal artery (a branch of the superior mesenteric artery).

Clinical app

Anular pancreas

The pancreas develops from ventral and dorsal buds from the foregut. The dorsal bud forms most of the head, neck, and body of pancreas. The ventral bud, which consists of right and left portions that normally fuse, rotates posteriorly around the bile duct to form part of the head and the uncinate process. If the two components of the ventral bud fail to fuse, they may encircle the duodenum. The duodenum is therefore constricted and may even undergo atresia and be absent at birth because of developmental problems. After birth, the child may fail to thrive and vomit due to poor gastric emptying.

Sometimes an anular pancreas is diagnosed in utero by ultrasound scanning. The obstruction of the duodenum may prevent the fetus from swallowing enough amniotic fluid, which may increase the overall volume of amniotic fluid in the amniotic sac surrounding the fetus **(polyhydramnios).**

Imaging app

Visualizing the pancreas

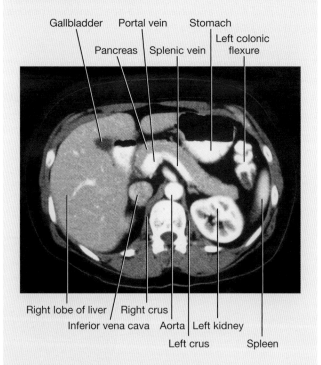

Fig. 4.73 Abdominal computed tomogram with contrast in the axial plane.

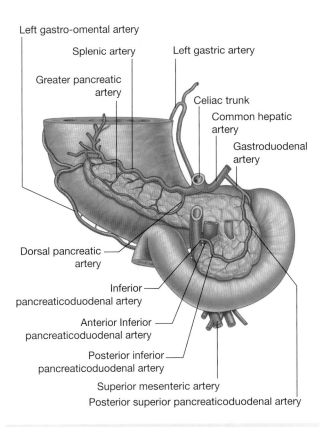

Fig. 4.74 Arterial supply to the pancreas. Posterior view.

Clinical app

Pancreatic cancer

Pancreatic cancer accounts for a significant number of deaths and is often referred to as the *silent killer*. Malignant tumors of the pancreas may occur anywhere within the pancreas but are most frequent within the head and the neck. There are a number of nonspecific findings in patients with pancreatic cancer, including upper abdominal pain, loss of appetite, and weight loss. Depending on the exact site of the cancer, obstruction of the common bile duct may occur, which can produce obstructive jaundice. Although surgery is indicated in patients where there is a possibility of cure, most detected cancers have typically spread locally, invading the portal vein and superior mesenteric vessels and may extend into the porta hepatis. Lymph node spread also is common, and these factors would preclude curative surgery.

Given the position of the pancreas, a surgical resection is a complex procedure involving resection of the region of pancreatic tumor usually with part of the duodenum necessitating a complex bypass procedure.

Duct system for bile

The duct system for the passage of bile extends from the liver, connects with the gallbladder, and empties into the descending part of the duodenum (Fig. 4.75). The coalescence of

Fig. 4.75 Bile drainage. **A.** Duct system for passage of bile. **B.** Percutaneous transhepatic cholangiogram demonstrating the bile duct system.

ducts begins in the liver parenchyma and continues until the **right** and **left hepatic ducts** are formed. These drain the respective lobes of the liver.

The two hepatic ducts combine to form the **common hepatic duct,** which runs near the liver with the hepatic artery proper and portal vein in the free margin of the lesser omentum.

As the common hepatic duct continues to descend, it is joined by the **cystic duct** from the gallbladder. This completes the formation of the **bile duct.** At this point, the bile duct lies to the right of the hepatic artery proper and usually to the right of and anterior to the portal vein in the free margin of the lesser omentum (see Fig. 4.35). The **omental foramen** is posterior to these structures at this point.

The bile duct continues to descend, passing posteriorly to the superior part of the duodenum before joining with the pancreatic duct to enter the descending part of the duodenum at the major duodenal papilla (Fig. 4.75).

Clinical app

Gallstones

Gallstones are present in approximately 10% of people over the age of 40 and are more common in women. They consist of a variety of components, but are predominantly a mixture of cholesterol and bile pigment. They may undergo calcification, which can be demonstrated on plain radiographs. From time to time, gallstones lodge in the neck of the gallbladder. The gallbladder cannot empty normally and contractions of the gallbladder wall produce severe pain. If this persists, a **cholecystectomy** (removal of the gallbladder) may be necessary.

Sometimes the gallbladder may become inflamed (**cholecystitis**). If the inflammation involves the related parietal peritoneum of the diaphragm, pain may not only occur in the right upper quadrant of the abdomen but may also be referred to the shoulder on the right side (phrenic nerve, C3-C5, innervation of diaphragm).

From time to time, small gallstones pass into the bile duct and are trapped in the region of the sphincter of the ampulla, which obstructs the flow of bile into the duodenum. This, in turn, produces jaundice.

Clinical app

Jaundice

Jaundice is a yellow discoloration of the skin caused by excess bile pigment (bilirubin) within the plasma. The yellow color is best appreciated by looking at the normally white sclerae of the eyes, which turn yellow.

Any obstruction to the biliary tree can produce jaundice, but the two most common causes are gallstones within the bile duct and an obstructing tumor at the head of the pancreas.

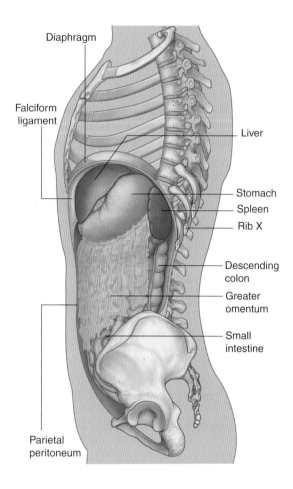

Fig. 4.76 Location of the spleen in a lateral view.

Spleen

The spleen develops as part of the vascular system in the part of the dorsal mesentery that suspends the developing stomach from the body wall. In the adult, the spleen lies against the diaphragm in the area of rib IX to rib X (Fig. 4.76). It is therefore in the left upper quadrant, or left hypochondrium, of the abdomen.

The spleen is connected to the:

- greater curvature of the stomach by the gastrosplenic ligament, which contains the short gastric and gastro-omental vessels; and
- left kidney by the splenorenal ligament (Fig. 4.77), which contains the splenic vessels.

Both these ligaments are parts of the greater omentum.

The spleen is surrounded by visceral peritoneum except in the area of the hilum on the medial surface of the spleen (Fig. 4.78). The **splenic hilum** is the entry point for the splenic vessels, and, occasionally, the tail of the pancreas reaches this area.

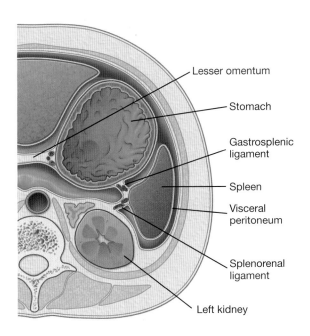

Fig. 4.77 Splenic ligaments and related vasculature.

The arterial supply to the spleen (Fig. 4.79) is the splenic artery from the celiac trunk.

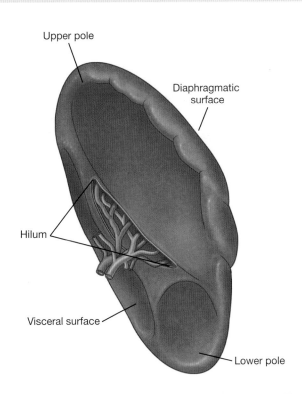

Fig. 4.78 Surfaces and hilum of the spleen.

Clinical app

Spleen disorders
From a clinical point of view, there are two main categories of spleen disorders: rupture and enlargement.

Rupture
This tends to occur when there is localized trauma to the left upper quadrant. It may be associated with left lower rib fractures. Because the spleen has such an extremely thin capsule, it is susceptible to injury even when there is no damage to surrounding structures, and because the spleen is highly vascular, when ruptured, it bleeds profusely into the peritoneal cavity.

Splenic enlargement
The spleen is an organ of the reticuloendothelial system involved in hematopoiesis and immunological surveillance. Diseases that affect the reticuloendothelial system (e.g., leukemia or lymphoma) may produce generalized lymphadenopathy and enlargement of the spleen (**splenomegaly**).

Arterial supply to the gastrointestinal tract

The **abdominal aorta** begins at the aortic hiatus of the diaphragm, anterior to the lower border of vertebra TXII (Fig. 4.80). It descends through the abdomen anterior to the

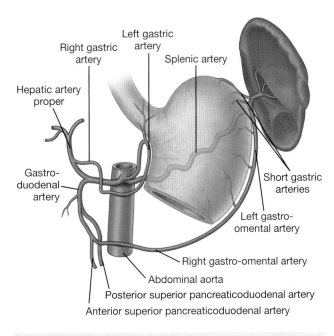

Fig. 4.79 Arterial supply to the spleen.

vertebral bodies, and by the time it ends at the level of vertebra LIV, it is slightly to the left of midline. The terminal branches of the abdominal aorta are the two **common iliac arteries**.

Anterior branches of the abdominal aorta

The abdominal aorta has anterior, lateral, and posterior branches as it passes through the abdominal cavity. The three anterior branches supply the gastrointestinal viscera:

Anterior branches

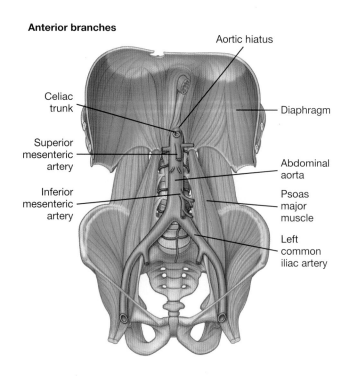

Fig. 4.80 Anterior branches of the abdominal aorta.

the **celiac trunk** and the **superior mesenteric** and **inferior mesenteric arteries** (Fig. 4.80).

The primitive gut tube can be divided into foregut, midgut, and hindgut regions. The boundaries of these regions are directly related to the areas of distribution of the three anterior branches of the abdominal aorta (Fig. 4.81).

- The **foregut** begins with the abdominal esophagus and ends just inferior to the major duodenal papilla midway along the descending part of the duodenum. It includes the abdominal esophagus, stomach, duodenum (superior to the major papilla), liver, pancreas, and gallbladder. The spleen also develops in relation to the foregut region. The foregut is supplied by the celiac trunk (Fig. 4.81).
- The **midgut** begins just inferior to the major duodenal papilla in the descending part of the duodenum and ends at the junction between the proximal two-thirds and distal one-third of the transverse colon. It includes the duodenum (inferior to the major duodenal papilla), jejunum, ileum, cecum, appendix, ascending colon, and the right two-thirds of the transverse colon. The midgut is supplied by the superior mesenteric artery (Fig. 4.81).
- The **hindgut** begins just before the left colic flexure (the junction between the proximal two-thirds and distal one-third of the transverse colon) and ends midway through the anal canal. It includes the left one-third of the transverse colon, descending colon, sigmoid colon, rectum, and upper part of the anal canal. The hindgut is supplied by the inferior mesenteric artery (Fig. 4.81).

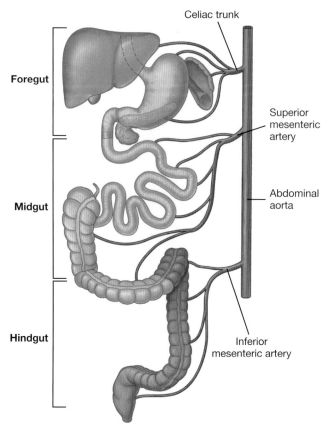

Fig. 4.81 Divisions of the gastrointestinal tract into the foregut, midgut, and hindgut, summarizing the primary arterial supply to each segment.

Celiac trunk

The celiac trunk is the anterior branch of the abdominal aorta supplying the foregut. It arises from the abdominal aorta immediately below the aortic hiatus of the diaphragm (Fig. 4.82) anterior to the upper part of vertebra LI. It immediately divides into the left gastric, splenic, and common hepatic arteries.

Left gastric artery

The left gastric artery is the smallest branch of the celiac trunk. It ascends to the cardioesophageal junction and sends **esophageal branches** upward to the abdominal part of the esophagus (Fig. 4.82). Some of these branches continue through the esophageal hiatus of the diaphragm and anastomose with esophageal branches from the thoracic aorta. The left gastric artery itself turns to the right and descends along the lesser curvature of the stomach in the lesser omentum. It supplies both surfaces of the stomach in this area and anastomoses with the right gastric artery.

Splenic artery

The **splenic artery,** the largest branch of the celiac trunk, takes a tortuous course to the left along the superior border of the pancreas (Fig. 4.82). It travels in the splenorenal ligament and divides into numerous branches, which enter the hilum of the spleen.

As the splenic artery passes along the superior border of the pancreas, it gives off numerous small branches to supply the neck, body, and tail of the pancreas (Fig. 4.83).

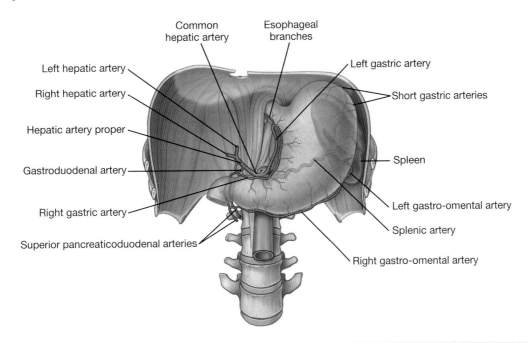

Fig. 4.82 Distribution of the celiac trunk.

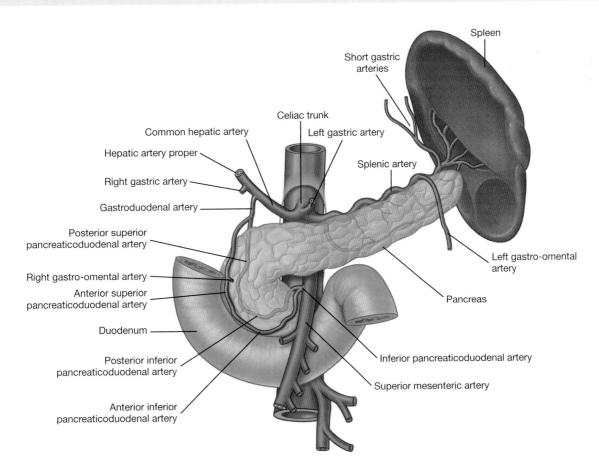

Fig. 4.83 Branches of the gastroduodenal artery.

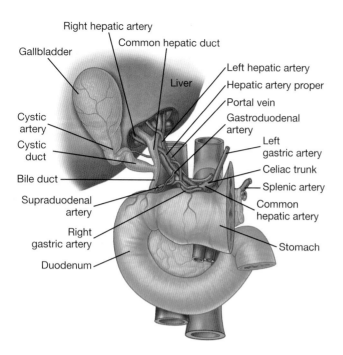

Fig. 4.84 Distribution of the common hepatic artery.

Approaching the spleen, the splenic artery gives off **short gastric arteries,** which pass through the gastrosplenic ligament to supply the fundus of the stomach. It also gives off the **left gastro-omental artery,** which runs to the right along the greater curvature of the stomach and anastomoses with the right gastro-omental artery.

Common hepatic artery

The **common hepatic artery** is a medium-sized branch of the celiac trunk that runs to the right and divides into its two terminal branches, the **hepatic artery proper** and the **gastroduodenal artery** (Figs. 4.82, 4.83).

The hepatic artery proper ascends toward the liver in the free edge of the lesser omentum. It runs to the left of the bile duct and anterior to the portal vein and divides into **right** and **left hepatic arteries** near the porta hepatis (Fig. 4.84). As the right hepatic artery nears the liver, it gives off the cystic artery to the gallbladder.

A right gastric artery often originates from the hepatic artery proper but can also arise from the common hepatic artery or from the left hepatic, gastroduodenal, or supraduodenal arteries. It courses to the left and ascends along the lesser curvature of the stomach in the lesser omentum, supplies adjacent areas of the stomach, and anastomoses with the left gastric artery.

The gastroduodenal artery may give off the **supraduodenal artery** and does give off the **posterior superior pancreaticoduodenal artery** near the upper border of the superior part of the duodenum. After these branches the gastroduodenal artery continues descending posterior to the superior

part of the duodenum. Reaching the lower border of the superior part of the duodenum, the gastroduodenal artery divides into its terminal branches, the **right gastro-omental artery** and the **anterior superior pancreaticoduodenal artery** (Fig. 4.83).

The right gastro-omental artery passes to the left along the greater curvature of the stomach, eventually anastomosing with the left gastro-omental artery from the splenic artery. The right gastro-omental artery sends branches to both surfaces of the stomach, and additional branches descend into the greater omentum.

The anterior superior pancreaticoduodenal artery descends and, along with the posterior superior pancreaticoduodenal artery, supplies the head of the pancreas and the duodenum (Fig. 4.83). These vessels eventually anastomose with the anterior and posterior branches of the inferior pancreaticoduodenal artery.

Superior mesenteric artery

The superior mesenteric artery is the anterior branch of the abdominal aorta supplying the midgut. It arises from the abdominal aorta immediately below the celiac artery (Fig. 4.85) anterior to the lower part of vertebra LI.

The superior mesenteric artery is crossed anteriorly by the splenic vein and the neck of pancreas. Posterior to the artery are the left renal vein, the uncinate process of the pancreas, and the inferior part of the duodenum (Fig. 4.85). After giving off its first branch (the **inferior pancreaticoduodenal artery**), the superior mesenteric artery gives off **jejunal** and **ileal arteries** on its left (Figs. 4.85, 4.86). Branching from the right side of the main trunk of the superior mesenteric artery are three vessels—the **middle colic, right colic,** and **ileocolic arteries**—that supply the terminal ileum, cecum, ascending colon, and two-thirds of the transverse colon (Fig. 4.86).

Inferior pancreaticoduodenal artery

The inferior pancreaticoduodenal artery is the first branch of the superior mesenteric artery (Fig. 4.85). It divides immediately into anterior and posterior branches, which ascend on the corresponding sides of the head of the pancreas. Superiorly, these arteries anastomose with anterior and posterior superior pancreaticoduodenal arteries (Figs. 4.83, 4.85). This arterial network supplies the head and uncinate process of the pancreas and the duodenum.

Jejunal and ileal arteries

Distal to the inferior pancreaticoduodenal artery, the superior mesenteric artery gives off numerous branches. Arising on the left is a large number of jejunal and ileal arteries supplying the jejunum and most of the ileum (Fig. 4.86). These branches leave the main trunk of the artery, pass between

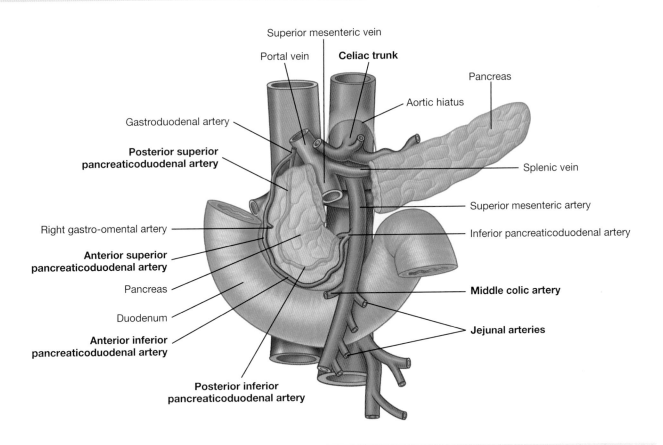

Fig. 4.85 Initial branching and relationships of the superior mesenteric artery.

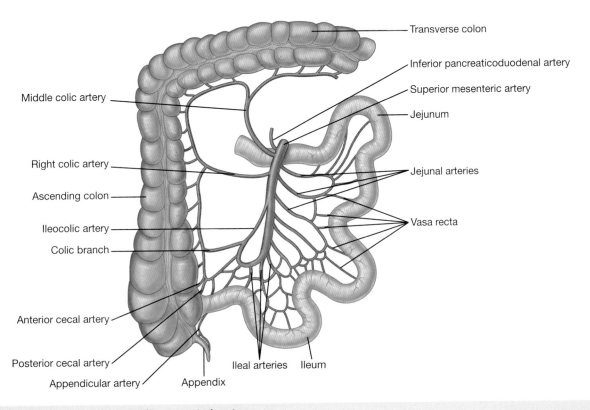

Fig. 4.86 Distribution of the superior mesenteric artery.

two layers of the mesentery, and form anastomosing arches or arcades as they pass outward to supply the small intestine. The number of arterial arcades increases distally along the gut.

There may be single and then double arcades in the area of the jejunum with a continued increase in the number of arcades moving into and through the area of the ileum (Fig. 4.86). Extending from the terminal arcade are **vasa recta** (straight arteries), which provide the final direct vascular supply to the walls of the small intestine. The vasa recta supplying the jejunum are usually long and close together, forming narrow windows visible in the mesentery. The vasa recta supplying the ileum are generally short and far apart, forming low broad windows.

Middle colic artery

The middle colic artery is the first of the three branches from the right side of the main trunk of the superior mesenteric artery (Fig. 4.86). Arising as the superior mesenteric artery emerges from beneath the pancreas, the middle colic artery enters the transverse mesocolon and divides into right and left branches. The right branch anastomoses with the right colic artery, and the left branch anastomoses with the left colic artery, which is a branch of the inferior mesenteric artery.

Right colic artery

Continuing distally along the main trunk of the superior mesenteric artery, the right colic artery is the second of the three branches from the right side of the main trunk of the superior mesenteric artery (Fig. 4.86). It is an inconsistent branch and passes to the right in a retroperitoneal position to supply the ascending colon. Nearing the colon, it divides into a descending branch, which anastomoses with the ileocolic artery and an ascending branch, which anastomoses with the middle colic artery.

Ileocolic artery

The final branch arising from the right side of the superior mesenteric artery is the ileocolic artery (Fig. 4.86). This passes downward and to the right toward the right iliac fossa where it divides into superior and inferior branches:

- The superior branch passes upward along the ascending colon to anastomose with the right colic artery.
- The inferior branch continues toward the ileocolic junction, dividing into **colic, cecal, appendicular,** and **ileal branches** (Fig. 4.86).

The specific pattern of distribution and origin of these branches are variable:

- The colic branch crosses to the ascending colon and passes upward to supply the first part of the ascending colon.
- Anterior and posterior cecal branches, arising either as a common trunk or as separate branches, supply corresponding sides of the cecum.
- The appendicular branch enters the free margin of and supplies the mesoappendix and the appendix.
- The ileal branch passes to the left and ascends to supply the final part of the ileum before anastomosing with the superior mesenteric artery.

Inferior mesenteric artery

The inferior mesenteric artery is the anterior branch of the abdominal aorta that supplies the hindgut. It is the smallest of the three anterior branches of the abdominal aorta and arises anterior to the body of vertebra LIII. Initially, the inferior mesenteric artery descends anteriorly to the aorta and then passes to the left as it continues inferiorly (Fig. 4.87). Its branches include the **left colic artery, several sigmoid arteries,** and the **superior rectal artery.**

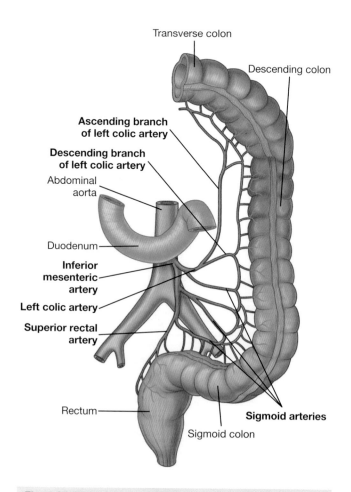

Fig. 4.87 Distribution of the inferior mesenteric artery.

Left colic artery

The left colic artery is the first branch of the inferior mesenteric artery (Fig. 4.87). It ascends retroperitoneally, dividing into ascending and descending branches:

- The ascending branch passes anteriorly to the left kidney, then enters the transverse mesocolon, and passes superiorly to supply the upper part of the descending colon and the distal part of the transverse colon; it anastomoses with branches of the middle colic artery.
- The descending branch passes inferiorly, supplying the lower part of the descending colon and anastomoses with the first sigmoid artery.

Sigmoid arteries

The sigmoid arteries consist of two to four branches, which descend to the left in the sigmoid mesocolon to supply the lowest part of the descending colon and the sigmoid colon (Fig. 4.87). These branches anastomose superiorly with branches from the left colic artery and inferiorly with branches from the superior rectal artery.

Superior rectal artery

The terminal branch of the inferior mesenteric artery is the superior rectal artery (Fig. 4.87). This vessel descends into the pelvic cavity in the sigmoid mesocolon, crossing the left common iliac vessels. Opposite vertebra SIII, the superior rectal artery divides. The two terminal branches descend on each side of the rectum, dividing into smaller branches in the wall of the rectum. These smaller branches continue inferiorly to the level of the internal anal sphincter, anastomosing along the way with branches from the middle rectal arteries (from the internal iliac artery) and the inferior rectal arteries (from the internal pudendal artery).

Clinical app

Vascular supply to the gastrointestinal system

Arteriosclerosis may occur throughout the abdominal aorta and at the openings of the celiac trunk and the superior mesenteric and inferior mesenteric arteries. Not infrequently, the inferior mesenteric artery becomes occluded. Interestingly, many of these patients do not suffer any complications because anastomoses between the right, middle, and left colic arteries gradually enlarge, forming a continuous **marginal artery.** The distal large bowel therefore becomes supplied by this enlarged marginal artery (marginal artery of Drummond), which replaces the blood supply of the inferior mesenteric artery.

Venous drainage

Venous drainage of the spleen, pancreas, gallbladder, and the abdominal part of the gastrointestinal tract, except for the inferior part of the rectum, is through the portal system of veins, which delivers blood from these structures to the liver. Once blood passes through the hepatic sinusoids, it passes through progressively larger veins until it enters the hepatic veins, which return the venous blood to the inferior vena cava just inferior to the diaphragm.

Portal vein

The **portal vein** is the final common pathway for the transport of venous blood from the spleen, pancreas, gallbladder, and the abdominal part of the gastrointestinal tract. It is formed by the union of the **splenic vein** and the **superior mesenteric vein** posterior to the neck of the pancreas at the level of vertebra LII (Figs. 4.88, 4.89).

Ascending toward the liver, the portal vein passes posterior to the superior part of the duodenum and enters the right margin of the lesser omentum. As it passes through this part of the lesser omentum, it is anterior to the omental foramen and posterior to both the bile duct, which is slightly to its right, and the hepatic artery proper, which is slightly to its left (see Fig. 4.84).

On approaching the liver, the portal vein divides into **right** and **left branches,** which enter the liver parenchyma. Tributaries to the portal vein include:

- **right** and **left gastric veins** draining the lesser curvature of the stomach and abdominal esophagus,
- **cystic veins** from the gallbladder, and
- **para-umbilical veins,** which are normally small veins associated with the obliterated umbilical vein and connect to veins on the anterior abdominal wall (Fig. 4.90).

Splenic vein

The splenic vein forms from numerous smaller vessels leaving the hilum of the spleen (Fig. 4.89). It passes to the right, passing through the splenorenal ligament with the splenic artery and the tail of pancreas. Continuing to the right, the large, straight splenic vein is in contact with the body of the pancreas as it crosses the posterior abdominal wall. Posterior to the neck of the pancreas, the splenic vein joins the superior mesenteric vein to form the portal vein.

Tributaries to the splenic vein include:

- **short gastric veins** from the fundus and left part of the greater curvature of the stomach,
- the **left gastro-omental vein** from the greater curvature of the stomach,

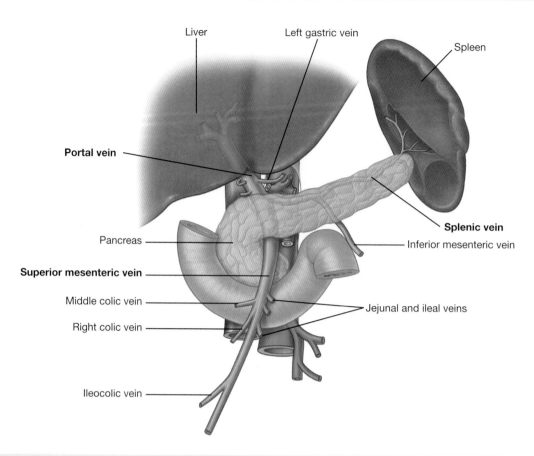

Liver   Left gastric vein   Spleen

Portal vein

Splenic vein

Pancreas   Inferior mesenteric vein

Superior mesenteric vein

Middle colic vein   Jejunal and ileal veins

Right colic vein

Ileocolic vein

Fig. 4.88 Portal vein.

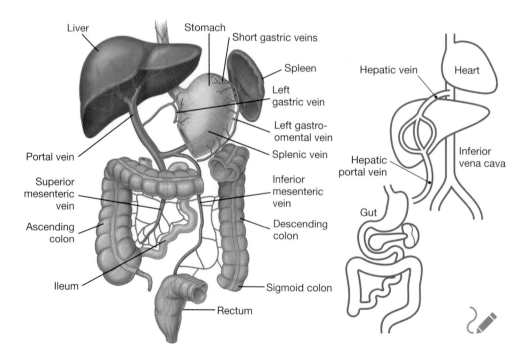

Liver   Stomach   Short gastric veins

Spleen

Left
gastric vein

Left gastro-
omental vein

Portal vein   Splenic vein

Superior
mesenteric
vein

Inferior
mesenteric
vein

Ascending
colon

Descending
colon

Ileum

Sigmoid colon

Rectum

Hepatic vein   Heart

Hepatic
portal vein

Inferior
vena cava

Gut

Fig. 4.89 Venous drainage of the abdominal portion of the gastrointestinal tract.

- **pancreatic veins** draining the body and tail of pancreas, and
- usually the **inferior mesenteric vein.**

Superior mesenteric vein

The superior mesenteric vein drains blood from the small intestine, cecum, ascending colon, and transverse colon (Fig. 4.89). It begins in the right iliac fossa as veins draining the terminal ileum, cecum, and appendix join and ascends in the mesentery to the right of the superior mesenteric artery.

Posterior to the neck of the pancreas, the superior mesenteric vein joins the splenic vein to form the portal vein (Fig. 4.88).

As a corresponding vein accompanies each branch of the superior mesenteric artery, tributaries to the superior mesenteric vein include jejunal, ileal, ileocolic, right colic, and middle colic veins. Additional tributaries include:

- the **right gastro-omental vein** draining the right part of the greater curvature of the stomach, and
- the **anterior** and **posterior inferior pancreaticoduodenal veins,** which pass alongside the arteries of the same

Clinical app

Hepatic cirrhosis

Cirrhosis is a complex disorder of the liver, the diagnosis of which is confirmed histologically. When a diagnosis is suspected, a liver biopsy is necessary.

Cirrhosis is characterized by widespread hepatic fibrosis interspersed with areas of nodular regeneration and abnormal reconstruction of preexisting lobular architecture. The presence of cirrhosis implies previous or continuing liver cell damage. The poorly functioning liver cells (hepatocytes) are unable to break down blood and blood products, leading to an increase in the serum bilirubin level, which manifests as jaundice.

As the cirrhosis progresses, the intrahepatic vasculature is distorted, which, in turn, leads to increased pressure in the portal vein and its draining tributaries (portal hypertension). Portal hypertension produces increased pressure in the splenic venules leading to splenic enlargement. At the sites of portosystemic anastomosis, large dilated varicose veins develop. These veins are susceptible to bleeding and may produce marked blood loss, which, in some instances, can be fatal.

Clinical app

Portosystemic anastomosis

The hepatic portal system drains blood from the visceral organs of the abdomen to the liver. In normal individuals, 100% of the portal venous blood flow can be recovered from the hepatic veins, whereas in patients with elevated portal vein pressure (e.g., portal hypertension from cirrhosis), there is significantly less blood flow to the liver. The rest of the blood enters collateral channels, which drain into the systemic circulation at specific points (Fig. 4.90). The largest of these collaterals occur at:

- the gastroesophageal junction around the cardia of the stomach—where the left gastric vein and its tributaries form a portosystemic anastomosis with tributaries to the azygos system of veins;
- the anus—the superior rectal vein of the portal system anastomoses with the middle and inferior rectal veins of the systemic venous system; and
- the anterior abdominal wall around the umbilicus—the para-umbilical veins anastomose with veins on the anterior abdominal wall.

When the pressure in the portal vein is elevated, venous enlargement (varices) tends to occur at and around the sites of portosystemic anastomoses, and these enlarged veins are called:

- *varices at the anorectal junction,*
- *esophageal varices at the gastroesophageal junction,* and
- *caput medusae at the umbilicus.*

Fig. 4.90 Portosystemic anastomoses.

name; the anterior superior pancreaticoduodenal vein usually empties into the right gastro-omental vein, and the posterior superior pancreaticoduodenal vein usually empties directly into the portal vein.

Inferior mesenteric vein

The **inferior mesenteric vein** drains blood from the rectum, sigmoid colon, descending colon, and **splenic flexure** (Figs. 4.89, 4.90). It begins as the **superior rectal vein** and ascends, receiving tributaries from the sigmoid veins and the **left colic vein.** All these veins accompany arteries of the same name. Continuing to ascend, the inferior mesenteric vein passes posterior to the body of the pancreas and usually joins the splenic vein. Occasionally, it ends at the junction of the splenic and superior mesenteric veins or joins the superior mesenteric vein.

Lymphatics

Lymphatic drainage of the abdominal part of the gastrointestinal tract, as low as the inferior part of the rectum, as

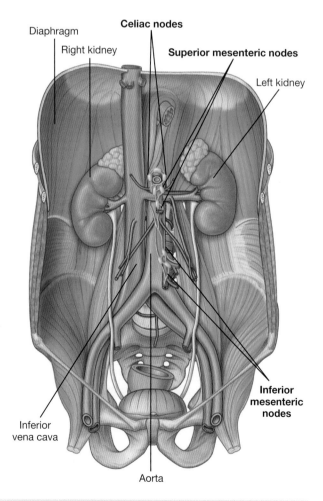

Fig. 4.91 Lymphatic drainage of the abdominal portion of the gastrointestinal tract.

well as the spleen, pancreas, gallbladder, and liver, is through vessels and nodes that eventually end in large collections of **pre-aortic lymph nodes** at the origins of the three anterior branches of the abdominal aorta, which supply these structures. These collections are therefore referred to as the **celiac, superior mesenteric,** and **inferior mesenteric** groups of pre-aortic lymph nodes. Lymph from viscera supplied by (Fig. 4.91):

- the celiac trunk (i.e., structures that are part of the abdominal foregut) drains to pre-aortic nodes near the origin of the celiac trunk (Fig. 4.91)—these celiac nodes also receive lymph from the superior mesenteric and inferior mesenteric groups of pre-aortic nodes, and lymph from the celiac nodes enters the **cisterna chyli;**
- the superior mesenteric artery (i.e., structures that are part of the abdominal midgut) drains to pre-aortic nodes near the origin of the superior mesenteric artery (Fig. 4.91)—these superior mesenteric nodes also receive lymph from the inferior mesenteric groups of pre-aortic nodes, and lymph from the superior mesenteric nodes drains to the celiac nodes; and
- the inferior mesenteric artery (i.e., structures that are part of the abdominal hindgut) drains to pre-aortic nodes near the origin of the inferior mesenteric artery (Fig. 4.91), and lymph from the inferior mesenteric nodes drains to the superior mesenteric nodes.

Innervation

Abdominal viscera are innervated by both extrinsic and intrinsic components of the nervous system:

- Extrinsic innervation involves receiving motor impulses from and sending sensory information to the central nervous system.
- Intrinsic innervation involves the regulation of digestive tract activities by a generally self-sufficient network of sensory and motor neurons (the **enteric nervous system**).

Abdominal viscera receiving extrinsic innervation include the abdominal part of the gastrointestinal tract, the spleen, the pancreas, the gallbladder, and the liver. These viscera send sensory information back to the central nervous system through visceral afferent fibers and receive motor impulses from the central nervous system through visceral efferent fibers.

The visceral efferent fibers are part of the sympathetic and parasympathetic parts of the autonomic division of the peripheral nervous system.

Structural components serving as conduits for these afferent and efferent fibers include posterior and anterior roots of the spinal cord, respectively; spinal nerves; anterior rami; white and gray rami communicantes; the sympathetic trunks; splanchnic nerves carrying sympathetic fibers (thoracic, lumbar, and sacral); parasympathetic fibers (pelvic); the prevertebral plexus and related ganglia; and the vagus nerves [X].

The enteric nervous system consists of motor and sensory neurons in two interconnected plexuses in the walls of the gastrointestinal tract. These neurons control the coordinated contraction and relaxation of intestinal smooth muscle and regulate gastric secretion and blood flow.

Sympathetic trunks

The sympathetic trunks are two parallel nerve cords extending on either side of the vertebral column from the base of the skull to the coccyx (Fig. 4.92). As they pass through the neck, they lie posterior to the carotid sheath. In the upper thorax, they are anterior to the necks of the ribs, whereas in the lower thorax they are on the lateral aspect of the vertebral bodies. In the abdomen, they are anterolateral to the lumbar vertebral bodies and, continuing into the pelvis, they are anterior to the sacrum. The two sympathetic trunks come together anterior to the coccyx to form the **ganglion impar.**

Throughout the extent of the sympathetic trunks, small raised areas are visible. These collections of neuronal cell bodies outside the central nervous system are the paravertebral sympathetic ganglia (Fig. 4.92). There are usually:

- 3 ganglia in the cervical region,
- 11 or 12 ganglia in the thoracic region,
- 3 ganglia in the lumbar region,
- 4 or 5 ganglia in the sacral region, and
- the ganglion impar anterior to the coccyx.

The ganglia and trunks are connected to adjacent spinal nerves by gray rami communicantes throughout the length of the sympathetic trunk and by white rami communicantes in the thoracic and upper lumbar parts of the trunk (T1 to L2). Neuronal fibers found in the sympathetic trunks include **preganglionic** and **postganglionic sympathetic fibers** and **visceral afferent fibers.**

Splanchnic nerves

The splanchnic nerves are important components in the innervation of the abdominal viscera. They pass from the sympathetic trunk or sympathetic ganglia associated with the trunk to the prevertebral plexus and ganglia anterior to the abdominal aorta.

There are two different types of splanchnic nerves, depending on the type of visceral efferent fiber they are carrying:

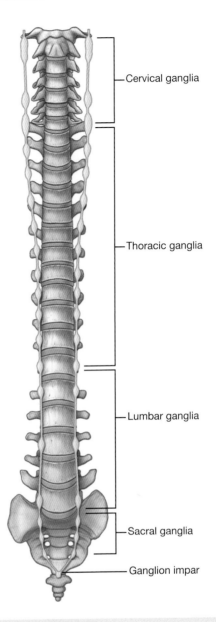

Cervical ganglia

Thoracic ganglia

Lumbar ganglia

Sacral ganglia

Ganglion impar

Fig. 4.92 Sympathetic trunks.

- The thoracic, lumbar, and sacral splanchnic nerves carry preganglionic sympathetic fibers from the sympathetic trunk to ganglia in the prevertebral plexus and visceral afferent fibers.
- The pelvic splanchnic nerves carry preganglionic parasympathetic fibers from anterior rami of S2, S3, and S4 spinal nerves to an extension of the prevertebral plexus in the pelvis (the **inferior hypogastric plexus** or **pelvic plexus**).

Thoracic splanchnic nerves

Three **thoracic splanchnic nerves** pass from sympathetic ganglia along the sympathetic trunk in the thorax to the prevertebral plexus and ganglia associated with the abdominal aorta in the abdomen (Fig. 4.93):

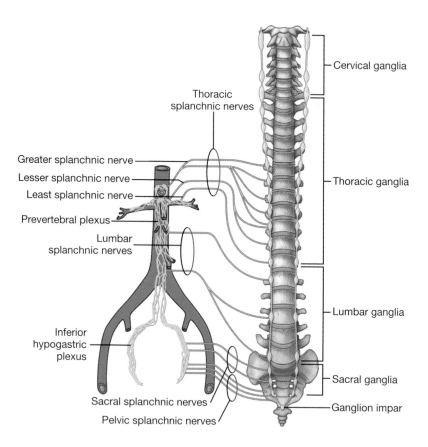

Fig. 4.93 Splanchnic nerves.

- The **greater splanchnic nerve** arises from the fifth to the ninth (or tenth) thoracic ganglia and travels to the celiac ganglion in the abdomen (a prevertebral ganglion associated with the celiac trunk).
- The **lesser splanchnic nerve** arises from the ninth and tenth (or tenth and eleventh) thoracic ganglia and travels to the aorticorenal ganglion.
- The **least splanchnic nerve** arises from the twelfth thoracic ganglion and travels to the renal plexus.

Lumbar and sacral splanchnic nerves

There are usually two to four **lumbar splanchnic nerves,** which pass from the lumbar part of the sympathetic trunk or associated ganglia and enter the prevertebral plexus (Fig. 4.93).

Similarly, the **sacral splanchnic nerves** pass from the sacral part of the sympathetic trunk or associated ganglia and enter the inferior hypogastric plexus, which is an extension of the prevertebral plexus into the pelvis.

Pelvic splanchnic nerves

The **pelvic splanchnic nerves (parasympathetic root)** are unique. They are the only splanchnic nerves that carry parasympathetic fibers. In other words, they do not originate from the sympathetic trunks. Rather, they originate directly from the anterior rami of S2 to S4. Preganglionic

parasympathetic fibers originating in the sacral spinal cord pass from the S2 to S4 spinal nerves to the inferior hypogastric plexus (Fig. 4.93). Once in this plexus, some of these fibers pass upward, enter the abdominal prevertebral plexus, and distribute with the arteries supplying the hindgut. This provides the pathway for innervation of the distal one-third of the transverse colon, the descending colon, and the sigmoid colon by preganglionic parasympathetic fibers.

Abdominal prevertebral plexus and ganglia

The abdominal prevertebral plexus is a collection of nerve fibers that surrounds the abdominal aorta and is continuous onto its major branches. Scattered throughout the length of the abdominal prevertebral plexus are cell bodies of postganglionic sympathetic fibers. Some of these cell bodies are organized into distinct ganglia, whereas others are more random in their distribution. The ganglia are usually associated with specific branches of the abdominal aorta and named after these branches.

The three major divisions of the abdominal prevertebral plexus and associated ganglia are the celiac, aortic, and superior hypogastric plexuses (Fig. 4.94).

- The **celiac plexus** is the large accumulation of nerve fibers and ganglia associated with the roots of the celiac trunk and superior mesenteric artery immediately below the aortic hiatus of the diaphragm. Ganglia associated with the

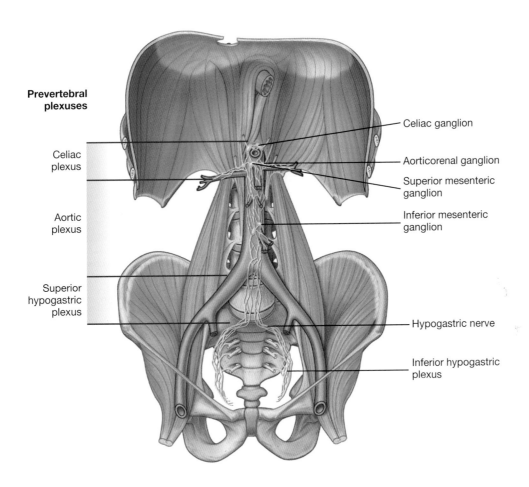

Fig. 4.94 Abdominal prevertebral plexus and ganglia.

celiac plexus include two celiac ganglia, a single superior mesenteric ganglion, and two aorticorenal ganglia.

■ The **aortic plexus** consists of nerve fibers and associated ganglia on the anterior and lateral surfaces of the abdominal aorta extending from just below the origin of the superior mesenteric artery to the bifurcation of the aorta and into the two common iliac arteries. The major ganglion in this plexus is the inferior mesenteric ganglion at the root of the inferior mesenteric artery.

■ The **superior hypogastric plexus** contains numerous small ganglia and is the final part of the abdominal prevertebral plexus before the prevertebral plexus continues into the pelvic cavity.

Each of these major plexuses gives origin to a number of secondary plexuses, which may also contain small ganglia. These plexuses are usually named after the vessels with which they are associated. For example, the celiac plexus is usually described as giving origin to the superior mesenteric plexus and the renal plexus, as well as other plexuses that extend out along the various branches of the celiac trunk.

Similarly, the aortic plexus has secondary plexuses consisting of the inferior mesenteric plexus, the spermatic plexus, and the external iliac plexus.

Inferiorly, the superior hypogastric plexus divides into the **hypogastric nerves,** which descend into the pelvis and contribute to the formation of the inferior hypogastric or pelvic plexus (Fig. 4.94).

The abdominal prevertebral plexus receives:

■ preganglionic parasympathetic and visceral afferent fibers from the vagus nerves [X],

■ preganglionic sympathetic and visceral afferent fibers from the thoracic and lumbar splanchnic nerves, and

■ preganglionic parasympathetic fibers from the pelvic splanchnic nerves.

Parasympathetic innervation

Parasympathetic innervation of the abdominal part of the gastrointestinal tract and of the spleen, pancreas, gallbladder, and liver is from two sources—the vagus nerves [X] and the pelvic splanchnic nerves.

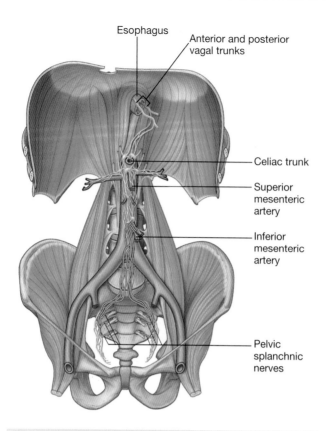

Fig. 4.95 Parasympathetic innervation of the abdominal portion of the gastrointestinal tract.

Fig. 4.96 The enteric system.

Vagus nerves

The **vagus nerves** [X] enter the abdomen associated with the esophagus as the esophagus passes through the diaphragm (Fig. 4.95) and provide parasympathetic innervation to the foregut and midgut.

After entering the abdomen as the **anterior** and **posterior vagal trunks,** they send branches to the abdominal prevertebral plexus. These branches contain preganglionic parasympathetic fibers and visceral afferent fibers, which are distributed with the other components of the prevertebral plexus along the branches of the abdominal aorta.

Pelvic splanchnic nerves

The **pelvic splanchnic nerves,** carrying preganglionic parasympathetic fibers from S2 to S4 spinal cord levels, enter the inferior hypogastric plexus in the pelvis. Some of these fibers move upward into the inferior mesenteric part of the prevertebral plexus in the abdomen (Fig. 4.95). Once there, these fibers are distributed with branches of the inferior mesenteric artery and provide parasympathetic innervation to the hindgut.

Enteric system

The enteric system is a division of the visceral part of the nervous system and is a local neuronal circuit in the wall of the gastrointestinal tract. It consists of motor and sensory neurons

organized into two interconnected plexuses (the **myenteric** and **submucosal plexuses**) between the layers of the gastrointestinal wall, and the associated nerve fibers that pass between the plexuses and from the plexuses to the adjacent tissue (Fig. 4.96).

The enteric system regulates and coordinates numerous gastrointestinal tract activities, including gastric secretory activity, gastrointestinal blood flow, and the contraction and relaxation cycles of smooth muscle **(peristalsis).**

Although the enteric system is generally independent of the central nervous system, it does receive input from postganglionic sympathetic and preganglionic parasympathetic neurons that modifies its activities.

Example—sympathetic innervation of stomach

The pathway of sympathetic innervation of the stomach is as follows:

- A preganglionic sympathetic fiber originating at the T6 level of the spinal cord enters an anterior root to leave the spinal cord.
- At the level of the intervertebral foramen, the anterior root (which contains the preganglionic fiber) and a posterior root join to form a spinal nerve.
- Outside the vertebral column, the preganglionic fiber leaves the anterior ramus of the spinal nerve through the white ramus communicans.
- The white ramus communicans, containing the preganglionic fiber, connects to the sympathetic trunk.
- Entering the sympathetic trunk, the preganglionic fiber does not synapse but passes through the trunk and enters the greater splanchnic nerve.
- The greater splanchnic nerve passes through the crura of the diaphragm and enters the celiac ganglion.

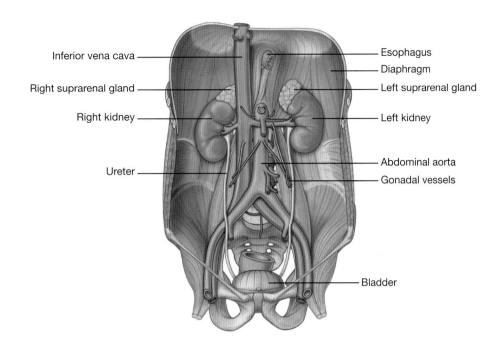

Inferior vena cava

Right suprarenal gland

Right kidney

Ureter

Esophagus

Diaphragm

Left suprarenal gland

Left kidney

Abdominal aorta

Gonadal vessels

Bladder

Fig. 4.97 Posterior abdominal region.

- In the celiac ganglion, the preganglionic fiber synapses with a postganglionic neuron.
- The postganglionic fiber joins the plexus of nerve fibers surrounding the celiac trunk and continues along its branches.
- The postganglionic fiber travels through the plexus of nerves accompanying the branches of the celiac trunk, supplying the stomach, and eventually reaches its point of distribution.
- This input from the sympathetic system may modify the activities of the gastrointestinal tract controlled by the enteric nervous system.

POSTERIOR ABDOMINAL REGION

The posterior abdominal region is posterior to the abdominal part of the gastrointestinal tract, the spleen, and the pancreas (Fig. 4.97). This area, bounded by bones and muscles making up the posterior abdominal wall, contains numerous structures that not only are directly involved in the activities of the abdominal contents but also use this area as a conduit between body regions. Examples include the abdominal aorta and its associated nerve plexuses, the inferior vena cava, the sympathetic trunks, and lymphatics. There are also structures originating in this area that are critical to the normal function of other regions of the body (i.e., the lumbar plexus of nerves), and there are organs that associate with this area during development and remain in it in the adult (i.e., the kidneys and suprarenal glands).

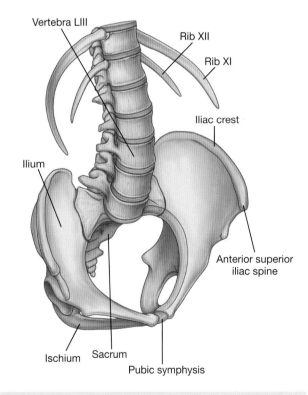

Vertebra LIII

Rib XII

Rib XI

Iliac crest

Ilium

Anterior superior iliac spine

Ischium   Sacrum

Pubic symphysis

Fig. 4.98 Osteology of the posterior abdominal wall.

Posterior abdominal wall

Bones

Lumbar vertebrae and the sacrum

Projecting into the midline of the posterior abdominal area are the bodies of the five lumbar vertebrae (Fig. 4.98). The

201

Abdomen

prominence of these structures in this region is due to the secondary curvature (a forward convexity) of the lumbar part of the vertebral column.

The lumbar vertebrae can be distinguished from cervical and thoracic vertebrae because of their size. They are much larger than any other vertebrae in any other region. The vertebral bodies are massive and progressively increase in size from vertebra LI to LV. The pedicles are short and stocky, the transverse processes are long and slender, and the spinous processes are large and stubby. The articular processes are large and oriented medially and laterally, which promotes flexion and extension in this part of the vertebral column.

Between each lumbar vertebra is an intervertebral disc, which completes this part of the midline boundary of the posterior abdominal wall.

The midline boundary of the posterior abdominal wall, inferior to the lumbar vertebrae, consists of the upper margin of the sacrum (Fig. 4.98). The sacrum is formed by the fusion of the five sacral vertebrae into a single, wedge-shaped, bony structure that is broad superiorly and narrows inferiorly. Its concave anterior surface and its convex posterior surface contain anterior and posterior sacral foramina for the anterior and posterior rami of spinal nerves to pass through.

Pelvic bones

The **ilia,** which are components of each pelvic bone, attach laterally to the sacrum at the sacro-iliac joints (Fig. 4.98). The upper part of each ilium expands outward into a thin wing-like area (the **iliac fossa**). The medial side of this region of each iliac bone and the related muscles are components of the posterior abdominal wall.

Ribs

Superiorly, ribs XI and XII complete the bony framework of the posterior abdominal wall (Fig. 4.98). These ribs are unique in that they do not articulate with the sternum, they have a single articular facet on their heads, and they do not have necks or tubercles.

Rib XI is posterior to the superior part of the left kidney, and rib XII is posterior to the superior part of both kidneys. Also, rib XII serves as a point of attachment for numerous muscles and ligaments.

Muscles

Muscles forming the medial, lateral, inferior, and superior boundaries of the posterior abdominal region fill in the bony framework of the posterior abdominal wall (Table 4.2). Medially are the psoas major and minor muscles, laterally is the quadratus lumborum muscle, inferiorly is the iliacus muscle, and superiorly is the diaphragm (Figs. 4.99, 4.100).

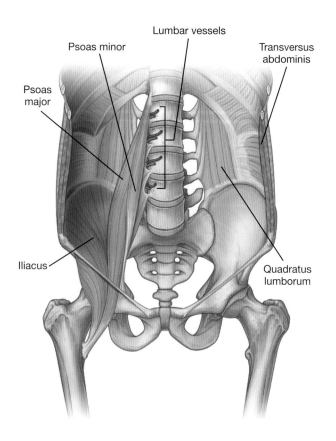

Fig. 4.99 Muscles of the posterior abdominal wall.

Psoas major and minor

Medially, the **psoas major** muscles cover the anterolateral surface of the bodies of the lumbar vertebrae, filling in the space between the vertebral bodies and the transverse processes (Table 4.2, Fig. 4.99). Associated with the psoas major muscle is the **psoas minor** muscle, which is sometimes absent.

Quadratus lumborum

Laterally, the quadratus lumborum muscles fill the space between ribs XII and the iliac crest on both sides of the vertebral column (Table 4.2, Fig. 4.99). They are overlapped medially by the psoas major muscles; along their lateral borders are the transversus abdominis muscles.

Iliacus

Inferiorly, an **iliacus** muscle fills the iliac fossa on each side (Table 4.2, Fig. 4.99). From this expansive origin covering the iliac fossa, the muscle passes inferiorly, joins with the psoas major muscle, and passes into the thigh. These combined muscles are referred to as the **iliopsoas** muscle.

Diaphragm

Superiorly, the diaphragm forms the boundary of the posterior abdominal region. This musculotendinous sheet also separates the abdominal cavity from the thoracic cavity.

Table 4.2 Posterior abdominal wall muscles

Muscle	Origin	Insertion	Innervation	Function
Psoas major	Lateral surface of bodies of TXII and LI to LV vertebrae, transverse processes of the lumbar vertebrae, and the intervertebral discs between TXII and LI to LV vertebrae	Lesser trochanter of the femur	Anterior rami of L1 to L3	Flexion of thigh at hip joint
Psoas minor	Lateral surface of bodies of TXII and LI vertebrae and intervening intervertebral disc	Pectineal line of the pelvic brim and iliopubic eminence	Anterior rami of L1	Weak flexion of lumbar vertebral column
Quadratus lumborum	Transverse process of LV vertebra, iliolumbar ligament, and iliac crest	Transverse processes of LI to LIV vertebrae and inferior border of rib XII	Anterior rami of T12 and L1 to L4	Depress and stabilize rib XII and some lateral bending of trunk
Iliacus	Upper two-`thirds of iliac fossa, anterior sacro-iliac and iliolumbar ligaments, and upper lateral surface of sacrum	Lesser trochanter of femur	Femoral nerve (L2 to L4)	Flexion of thigh at hip joint

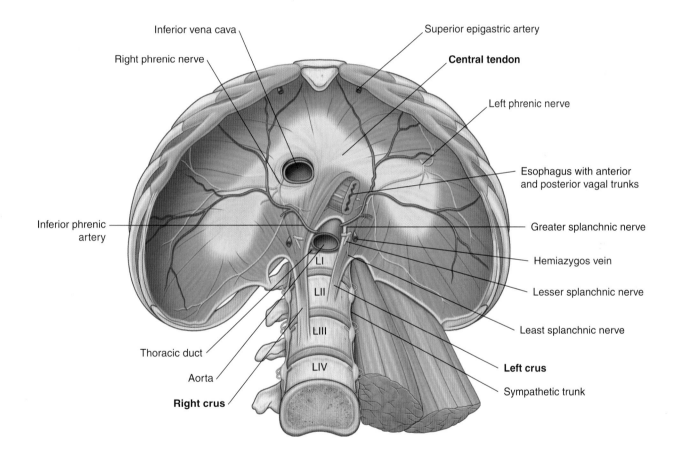

Fig. 4.100 Diaphragm.

Structurally, the diaphragm consists of a central tendinous part into which the circumferentially arranged muscle fibers attach (Fig. 4.100). The diaphragm is anchored to the lumbar vertebrae by musculotendinous crura, which blend with the anterior longitudinal ligament of the vertebral column.

■ The **right crus** is the longest and broadest of the **crura** and is attached to the bodies of vertebrae LI to LIII and the intervening intervertebral discs (Fig. 4.101).

■ Similarly, the **left crus** is attached to vertebrae LI and LII and the associated intervertebral disc (Fig. 4.101).

The crura are connected across the midline by a tendinous arch (the **median arcuate ligament**), which passes anterior to the aorta (Fig. 4.101).

Lateral to the crura, a second tendinous arch is formed by the fascia covering the upper part of the psoas major muscle. This is the **medial arcuate ligament,** which is attached

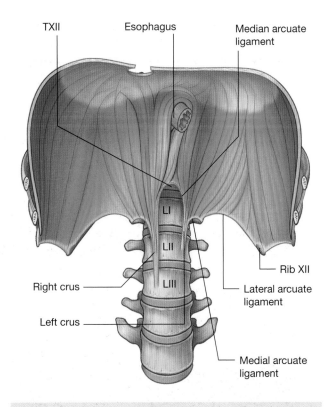

Fig. 4.101 Crura of the diaphragm.

medially to the sides of vertebrae LI and LII and laterally to the transverse process of vertebra LI (Fig. 4.101).

A third tendinous arch, the **lateral arcuate ligament,** is formed by a thickening in the fascia that covers the quadratus lumborum. It is attached medially to the transverse process of vertebra LI and laterally to rib XII (Fig. 4.101).

The medial and lateral arcuate ligaments serve as points of origin for some of the muscular components of the diaphragm.

Structures passing through or around the diaphragm

Numerous structures pass through or around the diaphragm (Fig. 4.100):

- The aorta passes posterior to the diaphragm and anterior to the vertebral bodies at the lower level of vertebra TXII; it is between the two crura of the diaphragm and posterior to the median arcuate ligament just to the left of midline.
- Accompanying the aorta through the aortic hiatus is the thoracic duct and, sometimes, the azygos vein.
- The esophagus passes through the musculature of the right crus of the diaphragm at the level of vertebra TX just to the left of the aortic hiatus.
- Passing through the esophageal hiatus with the esophagus are the anterior and posterior vagal trunks, the esophageal branches of the left gastric artery and vein, and a few lymphatic vessels.

- The third large opening in the diaphragm is the caval opening through which the inferior vena cava passes from the abdominal cavity to the thoracic cavity (Fig. 4.100) at approximately vertebra TVIII in the central tendinous part of the diaphragm.
- Accompanying the inferior vena cava through the caval opening is the right phrenic nerve.
- The left phrenic nerve passes through the muscular part of the diaphragm just anterior to the central tendon on the left side.

Additional structures pass through small openings either in or just outside the diaphragm as they pass from the thoracic cavity to the abdominal cavity (Fig. 4.100):

- The greater, lesser, and least (when present) splanchnic nerves pass through the crura on either side.
- The hemiazygos vein passes through the left crus.
- Passing posterior to the medial arcuate ligament on either side are the sympathetic trunks.
- Passing anterior to the diaphragm just deep to the ribs are the superior epigastric vessels.
- Other vessels and nerves (i.e., the musculophrenic vessels and intercostal nerves) also pass through the diaphragm at various points.

Domes

The classic appearance of the right and left domes of the diaphragm is caused by the underlying abdominal contents pushing these lateral areas upward and by the fibrous pericardium, which is attached centrally, causing a flattening of the diaphragm in this area (Fig. 4.102).

The domes are produced by:

- the liver on the right, with some contribution from the right kidney and the right suprarenal gland, and
- the fundus of the stomach and spleen on the left, with contributions from the left kidney and the left suprarenal gland.

Although the height of these domes varies during breathing, a reasonable estimate in normal expiration places the left dome at the fifth intercostal space and the right dome at rib V. This is important to remember when percussing the thorax.

During inspiration, the muscular part of the diaphragm contracts, causing the central tendon of the diaphragm to be drawn inferiorly. This results in some flattening of the domes, enlargement of the thoracic cavity, and a reduction in intrathoracic pressure. The physiological effects of these changes are that air enters the lungs and venous return to the heart is enhanced.

Imaging app

Visualizing the diaphragm

Right dome of diaphragm   Left dome of diaphragm

Heart

Fig. 4.102 Right and left domes of the diaphragm. Chest radiograph.

Blood supply

There is blood supply to the diaphragm on its superior and inferior surfaces:

- superiorly, the **musculophrenic** and **pericardiacophrenic arteries,** both branches of the **internal thoracic artery,** and the **superior phrenic artery,** a branch of the **thoracic aorta,** supply the diaphragm;
- inferiorly, the **inferior phrenic arteries,** branches of the **abdominal aorta,** supply the diaphragm (see Fig. 4.100).

Venous drainage is through companion veins to these arteries.

Innervation

Innervation of the diaphragm is primarily by the **phrenic nerves.** These nerves, from the C3 to C5 spinal cord levels, provide all motor innervation to the diaphragm and sensory fibers to the central part. They pass through the thoracic cavity, deep to the mediastinal pleura in the fibrous pericardium, to the superior surface of the diaphragm. At

this point, the right phrenic nerve accompanies the inferior vena cava through the diaphragm and the left phrenic nerve passes through the diaphragm by itself (see Fig. 4.100). Additional sensory fibers are supplied to the peripheral areas of the diaphragm by intercostal nerves.

Clinical app

Psoas muscle abscess

At first glance, it is difficult to appreciate why the psoas muscle sheath is of greater importance than any other muscle sheath. The psoas muscle and its sheath arise not only from the lumbar vertebrae but also from the intervertebral discs between each vertebra. This disc origin is of critical importance. In certain types of infection, the intervertebral disc is preferentially affected (e.g., tuberculosis and salmonella discitis). As the infection of the disc progresses, the infection spreads anterolaterally and passes into the psoas muscle sheath. The infection spreads inferiorly in the sheath and may appear below the inguinal ligament as a mass.

Clinical app

Diaphragmatic hernias

To understand why a hernia occurs through the diaphragm, it is necessary to consider the embryology of the diaphragm.

The diaphragm is formed from four structures—the septum transversum, the posterior esophageal mesentery, the pleuroperitoneal membrane, and the peripheral rim—which eventually fuse together, separating the abdominal cavity from the thoracic cavity. The septum transversum forms the central tendon, which develops from a mesodermal origin superior to the embryo's head and then moves to its more adult position during folding of the cephalic portion of the embryo.

Fusion of the various components of the diaphragm may fail, and hernias may occur through the failed points of fusion. The commonest sites are:

- between the xiphoid process and the costal margins on the right (Morgagni's hernia), and
- through an opening on the left when the pleuroperitoneal membrane fails to close the pericardioperitoneal canal (Bochdalek's hernia).

Hernias may also occur through the central tendon and through a congenitally large esophageal hiatus.

Morgagni's and Bochdalek's hernias tend to appear at or around the time of birth or in early infancy. They allow abdominal bowel to enter the thoracic cavity, which may compress the lungs and reduce respiratory function. Most of these hernias require surgical closure of the diaphragmatic defect.

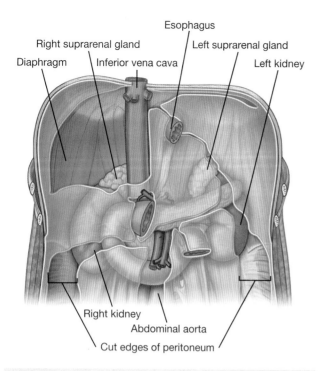

Fig. 4.103 Retroperitoneal position of the kidneys in the posterior abdominal region.

Viscera

Kidneys

The bean-shaped kidneys are retroperitoneal in the posterior abdominal region (Fig. 4.103). They lie in the extraperitoneal connective tissue immediately lateral to the vertebral column. In the supine position, the kidneys extend from approximately vertebra TXII superiorly to vertebra LIII inferiorly, with the right kidney somewhat lower than the left because of its relationship with the liver. Although they are similar in size and shape, the left kidney is a longer and more slender organ than the right kidney, and nearer to the midline.

Relationships to other structures

The anterior surface of the right kidney is related to numerous structures, some of which are separated from the kidney by a layer of peritoneum and some of which are directly against the kidney (Fig. 4.104):

- A small part of the **superior pole** is covered by the right suprarenal gland.
- Moving inferiorly, a large part of the rest of the upper part of the **anterior surface** is against the liver and is separated from it by a layer of peritoneum.
- Medially, the descending part of the duodenum is retroperitoneal and contacts the kidney.
- The **inferior pole** of the kidney, on its lateral side, is directly associated with the right colic flexure and, on its medial side, is covered by a segment of the intraperitoneal small intestine.

The anterior surface of the left kidney is also related to numerous structures, some with an intervening layer of peritoneum and some directly against the kidney (Fig. 4.104):

- A small part of the superior pole, on its medial side, is covered by the left suprarenal gland.
- The rest of the superior pole is covered by the intraperitoneal stomach and spleen.
- Moving inferiorly, the retroperitoneal pancreas covers the middle part of the kidney.
- On its lateral side, the lower half of the kidney is covered by the left colic flexure and the beginning of the descending colon and, on its medial side, by the parts of the intraperitoneal jejunum.

Posteriorly, the right and left kidneys are related to similar structures (Fig. 4.105). Superiorly is the diaphragm and inferior to this, moving in a medial to lateral direction, are psoas major, quadratus lumborum, and transversus abdominis muscles.

The superior pole of the right kidney is anterior to rib XII, whereas the same region of the left kidney is anterior to ribs XI and XII. The pleural sacs, and specifically, the costodiaphragmatic recesses, therefore extend posterior to the kidneys.

Also passing posterior to the kidneys are the subcostal vessels and nerves and the iliohypogastric and ilio-inguinal nerves.

Renal fat and fascia

The kidneys are enclosed in and associated with a unique arrangement of fascia and fat. Immediately outside the renal capsule there is an accumulation of extraperitoneal fat—the **perinephric fat (perirenal fat)**, which completely surrounds the kidney (Fig. 4.106). Enclosing the perinephric fat is a membranous condensation of the extraperitoneal fascia (the **renal**, or **Gerota's, fascia**). The suprarenal glands are also enclosed in this fascial compartment, usually separated from the kidneys by a thin septum. The renal fascia must be incised in any surgical approach to this organ.

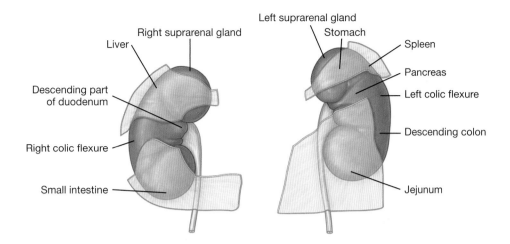

Fig. 4.104 Structures related to the anterior surface of each kidney.

At the lateral margins of each kidney, the anterior and posterior layers of the renal fascia fuse (Fig. 4.106). This fused layer may connect with the transversalis fascia on the lateral abdominal wall.

Above each suprarenal gland, the anterior and posterior layers of the renal fascia fuse and blend with the fascia that covers the diaphragm.

Medially, the anterior layer of the renal fascia continues over the vessels in the hilum and fuses with the connective tissue associated with the abdominal aorta and the inferior vena cava (Fig. 4.106). In some cases, the anterior layer may cross the midline to the opposite side and blend with its companion layer.

The posterior layer of the renal fascia passes medially between the kidney and the fascia covering the quadratus lumborum muscle to fuse with the fascia covering the psoas major muscle.

Inferiorly, the anterior and posterior layers of the renal fascia enclose the ureters.

In addition to perinephric fat and the renal fascia, a final layer of **paranephric fat (pararenal fat)** completes the fat and fascias associated with the kidney (Fig. 4.106). This fat accumulates posterior and posterolateral to each kidney.

Kidney structure

Each kidney has a smooth anterior and posterior surface covered by a fibrous capsule, which is easily removable except during disease.

On the medial margin of each kidney is the **hilum of kidney,** which is a deep vertical slit through which renal vessels, lymphatics, and nerves enter and leave the substance of the kidney (Fig. 4.107). Internally, the hilum is continuous with the renal sinus. Perinephric fat continues into the hilum and sinus and surrounds all structures.

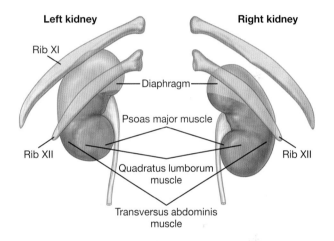

Fig. 4.105 Structures related to the posterior surface of each kidney.

Each kidney consists of an outer **renal cortex** and an inner **renal medulla** (Fig. 4.107). The renal cortex is a continuous band of pale tissue that completely surrounds the renal medulla. Extensions of the renal cortex (the **renal columns**) project into the inner aspect of the kidney, dividing the renal medulla into discontinuous aggregations of triangular-shaped tissue (the **renal pyramids**).

The bases of the renal pyramids are directed outward toward the renal cortex, whereas the apex of each renal pyramid projects inward toward the **renal sinus.** The apical projection **(renal papilla)** contains the openings of the papillary ducts draining the renal tubules and is surrounded by a **minor calyx.**

The minor calices receive urine from the papillary ducts and represent the proximal parts of the tube that will eventually form the ureter (Fig. 4.107). In the renal sinus, several minor calices unite to form a **major calyx,** and two or three major calices unite to form the **renal pelvis,** which is the funnel-shaped superior end of the ureters.

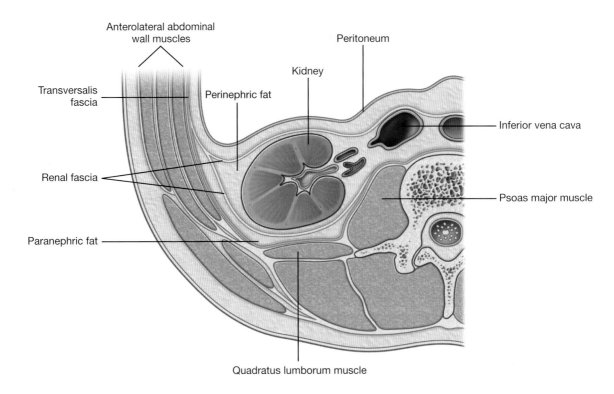

Fig. 4.106 Organization of fat and fascia surrounding the kidney.

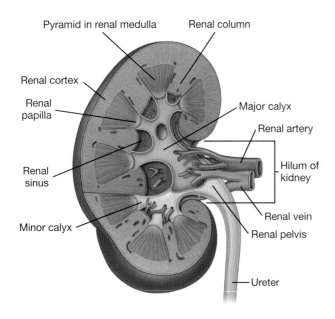

Fig. 4.107 Internal structure of the kidney.

Renal vasculature and lymphatics

A single large **renal artery,** a lateral branch of the abdominal aorta, supplies each kidney. These vessels usually arise just inferior to the origin of the superior mesenteric artery between vertebrae LI and LII (Fig. 4.108). The **left renal artery** usually arises a little higher than the right, and the **right renal artery** is longer and passes posterior to the inferior vena cava.

As each renal artery approaches the renal hilum, it divides into anterior and posterior branches, which supply the renal parenchyma. Accessory renal arteries are common. They originate from the lateral aspect of the abdominal aorta either above or below the primary renal arteries, enter the hilum with the primary arteries or pass directly into the kidney at some other level, and are commonly called **extrahilar arteries.**

Multiple renal veins contribute to the formation of the left and **right renal veins,** both of which are anterior to the renal arteries (Fig. 4.108). Importantly, the longer left renal vein crosses the midline anterior to the abdominal aorta and posterior to the superior mesenteric artery and can be compressed by an aneurysm in either of these two vessels.

The lymphatic drainage of each kidney is to the **lateral aortic (lumbar) nodes** around the origin of the renal artery.

Ureters

The ureters are muscular tubes that transport urine from the kidneys to the bladder. They are continuous superiorly with the renal pelvis, which is a funnel-shaped structure in the renal sinus. The renal pelvis is formed from a condensation of two or three major calices, which, in turn, are formed by the condensation of several minor calices (see Fig. 4.107). The minor calices surround a renal papilla.

Fig. 4.108 Renal vasculature.

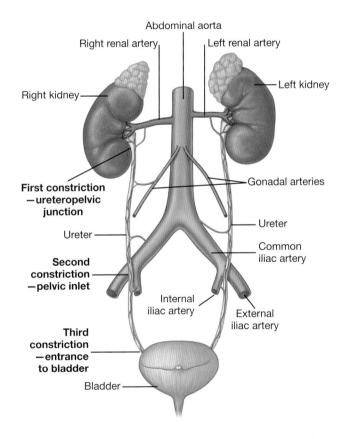

Fig. 4.109 Ureters.

The renal pelvis narrows as it passes inferiorly through the hilum of the kidney and becomes continuous with the ureter at the **ureteropelvic junction** (Fig. 4.109). Inferior to this junction, the ureters descend retroperitoneally on the medial aspect of the psoas major muscle. At the pelvic brim, the ureters cross either the end of the common iliac or the

beginning of the external iliac arteries, enter the pelvic cavity, and continue their journey to the bladder.

At three points along their course the ureters are constricted (Fig. 4.109):

- the first point is at the ureteropelvic junction,
- the second point is where the ureters cross the common iliac vessels at the pelvic brim, and
- the third point is where the ureters enter the wall of the bladder.

Kidney stones can become lodged at these constrictions.

Ureteric vasculature and lymphatics

The ureters receive arterial branches from adjacent vessels as they pass toward the bladder (Fig. 4.109):

- The renal arteries supply the upper end.
- The middle part may receive branches from the abdominal aorta, the testicular or ovarian arteries, and the common iliac arteries.
- In the pelvic cavity, the ureters are supplied by one or more arteries from branches of the internal iliac arteries.

In all cases, arteries reaching the ureters divide into ascending and descending branches, which form longitudinal anastomoses.

Lymphatic drainage of the ureters follows a pattern similar to that of the arterial supply. Lymph from:

- the upper part of each ureter drains to the lateral aortic (lumbar) nodes,
- the middle part of each ureter drains to lymph nodes associated with the common iliac vessels, and
- the inferior part of each ureter drains to lymph nodes associated with the external and internal iliac vessels.

Ureteric innervation

Ureteric innervation is from the renal, aortic, superior hypogastric, and inferior hypogastric plexuses through nerves that follow the blood vessels.

Visceral efferent fibers come from both sympathetic and parasympathetic sources, whereas visceral afferent fibers return to T11 to L2 spinal cord levels. Ureteric pain, which is usually related to distention of the ureter, is therefore referred to cutaneous areas supplied by T11 to L2 spinal cord levels. These areas would most likely include the posterior and lateral abdominal wall below the ribs and above the iliac crest, the pubic region, the scrotum in males, the labia majora in females, and the proximal anterior aspect of the thigh.

Clinical app

Urinary tract stones

Urinary tract stones (calculi) occur more frequently in men than in women, are most common in people aged between 20 and 60 years, and are usually associated with sedentary lifestyles. The stones are polycrystalline aggregates of calcium, phosphate, oxalate, urate, and other soluble salts within an organic matrix. The urine becomes saturated with these salts, and small variations in the pH cause the salts to precipitate.

Typically the patient has pain that radiates from the infrascapular region (loin) into the groin and even into the scrotum or labia majora. Blood in the urine **(hematuria)** may also be noticed.

Clinical app

Urinary tract cancer

Most tumors that arise in the kidney are renal cell carcinomas. These tumors develop from the proximal tubular epithelium. Approximately 5% of tumors within the kidney are transitional cell tumors, which arise from the urothelium of the renal pelvis. Most patients typically have blood in the urine (hematuria), pain in the infrascapular region (loin), and a mass.

Renal cell tumors are unusual because not only do they grow outward from the kidney, invading the fat and fascia, but they also spread into the renal vein. This venous extension is rare for any other type of tumor, so when seen, renal cell carcinoma should be suspected. Transitional cell carcinoma arises from the urothelium. The urothelium is present from the calices to the urethra and behaves as a "single unit." Therefore when patients develop transitional carcinomas within the bladder, similar tumors may also be present within upper parts of the urinary tract.

Clinical app

Kidney transplant

Renal transplantation is a common procedure undertaken in patients with end-stage renal failure.

An ideal place to situate the transplant kidney is in the left or the right iliac fossa (Fig. 4.110). A curvilinear incision is made paralleling the iliac crest and pubic symphysis. The external oblique muscle, internal oblique muscle, transverse abdominis muscle, and transversalis fascia are divided. The surgeon identifies the parietal peritoneum but does not enter the peritoneal cavity. The

Clinical app—cont'd

parietal peritoneum is medially retracted to reveal the external iliac artery, external iliac vein, and the bladder. In some instances the internal iliac artery of the recipient is mobilized and anastomosed directly as an end-to-end procedure onto the renal artery of the donor kidney. Similarly the internal iliac vein is anastomosed to the donor vein. The ureter is easily tunneled obliquely through the bladder wall with a straightforward anastomosis.

The left and right iliac fossae are ideal locations for the transplant kidney, because a new space can be created without compromise to other structures. The extraperitoneal approach enables patients to make a swift recovery.

Fig. 4.110 Abdominal computed tomogram in the axial plane showing the transplanted kidney in the left iliac fossa.

Suprarenal glands

The suprarenal glands are associated with the superior pole of each kidney (Fig. 4.112). They consist of an outer cortex and an inner medulla. The right gland is shaped like a pyramid, whereas the left gland is semilunar in shape and the larger of the two.

Anterior to the right suprarenal gland is part of the right lobe of the liver and the inferior vena cava, whereas anterior to the left suprarenal gland is part of the stomach, pancreas, and, on occasion, the spleen. Parts of the diaphragm are posterior to both glands.

The suprarenal glands are surrounded by the perinephric fat and enclosed in the renal fascia, although a thin septum separates each gland from its associated kidney.

Imaging app

Investigation of the urinary tract

After an appropriate history and examination of the patient, including a digital rectal examination to assess the prostate in men, special investigations are required.

Intravenous urogram (IVU)

An IVU is one of the most important and commonly carried out radiological investigations (Fig. 4.111A). The patient is injected with iodinated contrast medium. Most contrast media contain three iodine atoms spaced around a benzene ring. The relatively high atomic number of iodine compared with the atomic number of carbon, hydrogen, and oxygen attenuates the radiation beam. After intravenous injection, contrast media are excreted predominantly by glomerular filtration, although some are secreted by the renal tubules. This allows visualization of the collecting system as well as the ureters and bladder.

Ultrasound

Ultrasound can be used to assess kidney size and the size of the calices, which may be dilated when obstructed. Although the ureters are poorly visualized using ultrasound, the bladder can be easily seen when full. Ultrasound measurements of bladder volume can be obtained before and after micturition.

Computed tomography

Computed tomography can be used to assess the kidneys, ureters, bladder, and adjacent structures and is a powerful tool for staging primary urinary tract tumors (Fig. 4.111,B).

Nuclear medicine

Nuclear medicine is an extremely useful tool for investigating the urinary tract, because radioisotope compounds can be used to estimate renal cell mass and function, and assess the parenchyma for renal scarring. These tests are often very useful in children when renal scarring and reflux disease are suspected.

Fig. 4.111 A. Pathway of ureter in relation to other structures. Coronal view of 3-D urogram using multidetector computed tomography (CT). **B.** Renal pelvis. CT image with contrast in axial plane.

Suprarenal vasculature

The arterial supply to the suprarenal glands is extensive and arises from three primary sources (Fig. 4.112):

- As the bilateral **inferior phrenic arteries** pass upward from the abdominal aorta to the diaphragm, they give off multiple branches (**superior suprarenal arteries**) to the suprarenal glands.
- A middle branch (**middle suprarenal artery**) to the suprarenal glands usually arises directly from the abdominal aorta.
- Inferior branches (**inferior suprarenal arteries**) from the renal arteries pass upward to the suprarenal glands.

In contrast to this multiple arterial supply is the venous drainage, which usually consists of a single vein leaving the

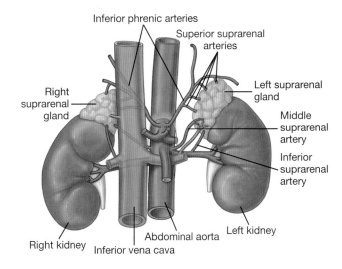

Fig. 4.112 Arterial supply to the suprarenal glands.

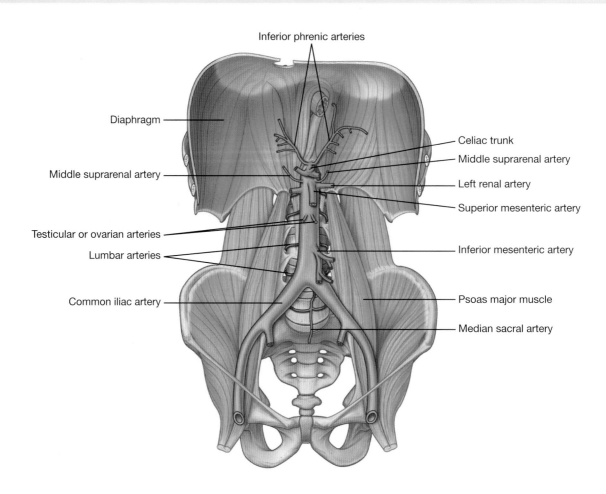

Inferior phrenic arteries

Diaphragm

Middle suprarenal artery

Testicular or ovarian arteries

Lumbar arteries

Common iliac artery

Celiac trunk

Middle suprarenal artery

Left renal artery

Superior mesenteric artery

Inferior mesenteric artery

Psoas major muscle

Median sacral artery

Fig. 4.113 Abdominal aorta.

hilum of each gland. On the right side, the **right suprarenal vein** is short and almost immediately enters the inferior vena cava; whereas on the left side, the **left suprarenal vein** passes inferiorly to enter the left renal vein.

Suprarenal Innervation

The suprarenal gland is mainly innervated by preganglionic sympathetic fibers from spinal levels T8 to L1 that pass through both the sympathetic trunk and the prevertebral plexus without synapsing. These preganglionic fibers directly innervate cells of the adrenal medulla.

Vasculature
Abdominal aorta

The abdominal aorta begins at the aortic hiatus of the diaphragm as a midline structure at approximately the lower level of vertebra TXII (Fig. 4.113). It passes downward on the anterior surface of the bodies of vertebrae LI to LIV, ending just to the left of midline at the lower level of vertebra LIV. At this point, it divides into the **right** and **left common iliac arteries.** This bifurcation can be visualized on the anterior abdominal wall at

a point approximately 2.6 cm below the umbilicus or even with a line extending between the highest points of the iliac crest.

As the abdominal aorta passes through the posterior abdominal region, the prevertebral plexus of nerves and ganglia covers its anterior surface. It is also related to numerous other structures:

■ Anterior to the abdominal aorta, as it descends, are the pancreas and splenic vein, the left renal vein, and the inferior part of the duodenum.
■ Several lumbar veins cross it posteriorly as they pass to the inferior vena cava.
■ On its right side are the cisterna chyli, thoracic duct, azygos vein, right crus of the diaphragm, and the inferior vena cava.
■ On its left side is the left crus of the diaphragm.

Branches of the abdominal aorta (Table 4.3) can be classified as:
■ visceral branches supplying organs,
■ posterior branches supplying the diaphragm or body wall, or
■ terminal branches.

Table 4.3 Branches of the abdominal aorta

Artery	Branch	Origin	Parts supplied
Celiac trunk	Anterior	Immediately inferior to the aortic hiatus of the diaphragm	Abdominal foregut
Superior mesenteric artery	Anterior	Immediately inferior to the celiac trunk	Abdominal midgut
Inferior mesenteric artery	Anterior	Inferior to the renal arteries	Abdominal hindgut
Middle suprarenal arteries	Lateral	Immediately superior to the renal arteries	Suprarenal glands
Renal arteries	Lateral	Immediately inferior to the superior mesenteric artery	Kidneys
Testicular or ovarian arteries	Paired anterior	Inferior to the renal arteries	Testes in male and ovaries in female
Inferior phrenic arteries	Lateral	Immediately inferior to the aortic hiatus	Diaphragm
Lumbar arteries	Posterior	Usually four pairs	Posterior abdominal wall and spinal cord
Median sacral artery	Posterior	Just superior to the aortic bifurcation, passes inferiorly across lumbar vertebrae, sacrum, and coccyx	
Common iliac arteries	Terminal	Bifurcation usually occurs at the level of LIV vertebra	

Visceral branches

The visceral branches are either unpaired or paired vessels.

The three unpaired visceral branches that arise from the anterior surface of the abdominal aorta (Table 4.3, Fig. 4.113) are:

- the celiac trunk, which supplies the abdominal foregut,
- the superior mesenteric artery, which supplies the abdominal midgut, and
- the inferior mesenteric artery, which supplies the abdominal hindgut.

The paired visceral branches of the abdominal aorta (Table 4.3; also see Fig. 4.113) include:

- the **middle suprarenal arteries**—small, lateral branches of the abdominal aorta arising just above the renal arteries that are part of the multiple vascular supply to the suprarenal gland,
- the **renal arteries**—lateral branches of the abdominal aorta that arise just inferior to the origin of the superior mesenteric artery between vertebrae LI and LII and supply the kidneys, and
- the **testicular** or **ovarian arteries**—anterior branches of the abdominal aorta that arise below the origin of the renal arteries and pass downward and laterally on the anterior surface of the psoas major muscle.

Posterior branches

The posterior branches of the abdominal aorta are vessels supplying the diaphragm or body wall and are (Table 4.3; also see Fig. 4.113):

- the **inferior phrenic arteries** arising immediately inferior to the aortic hiatus of the diaphragm, either directly from the abdominal aorta as a common trunk from the

abdominal aorta or from the base of the celiac trunk (see Fig. 4.113). Whatever their origin, they pass upward, provide some arterial supply to the suprarenal gland, and continue onto the inferior surface of the diaphragm.

- four pairs of **lumbar arteries** from the posterior surface of the abdominal aorta (see Fig. 4.113). They run laterally and posteriorly over the bodies of the lumbar vertebrae, continue laterally, passing posterior to the sympathetic trunks and between the transverse processes of adjacent lumbar vertebrae, and reach the abdominal wall. From this point onward, they demonstrate a branching pattern similar to a posterior intercostal artery, which includes providing segmental branches that supply the spinal cord.

- the **median sacral artery** (see Fig. 4.113). This vessel arises from the posterior surface of the abdominal aorta just superior to the bifurcation and passes in an inferior direction, first over the anterior surface of the lower lumbar vertebrae and then over the anterior surface of the sacrum and coccyx.

Clinical app

Abdominal aortic stent graft

An abdominal aortic aneurysm is a dilation of the aorta and generally tends to occur in the infrarenal region (the region at or below the renal arteries). As the aorta expands, the risk of rupture increases, and it is now generally accepted that when an aneurysm reaches 5.6 cm or greater, an operation will significantly benefit the patient.

Treatment of aneurysms prior to rupture can involve inserting an endovascular graft (Fig. 4.114). The technique involves surgically dissecting the femoral artery below the inguinal ligament. A small incision is made in the femoral artery and the pre-loaded compressed graft with metal support struts is passed on a large catheter into the abdominal aorta through the femoral artery. Using X-ray for guidance the graft is opened so that it lines

Clinical app—cont'd

the inside of the aorta. Attachments are made to the graft that extend into the common iliac vessels. This bifurcated tube device effectively excludes the abdominal aortic aneurysm.

Fig. 4.114 Volume-rendered reconstruction using multidetector computed tomography of a patient with an infrarenal abdominal aortic aneurysm before (**A**) and after (**B**) endovascular aneurysm repair. Note the images only demonstrate the intraluminal contrast and not the entire vessel. White patches in the aorta (**A**) represent intramural calcium.

Inferior vena cava

The inferior vena cava returns blood from all structures below the diaphragm to the right atrium of the heart (Fig. 4.115). It is formed when the two common iliac veins come together at the level of vertebra LV just to the right of the midline. It ascends through the posterior abdominal region anterior to the vertebral column immediately to the right of the abdominal aorta (Fig. 4.115), continues in a superior direction, and leaves the abdomen by piercing the central tendon of the diaphragm at the level of vertebra TVIII.

During its course, the anterior surface of the inferior vena cava is crossed by the right common iliac artery, the root of the mesentery, the right testicular or ovarian artery, the

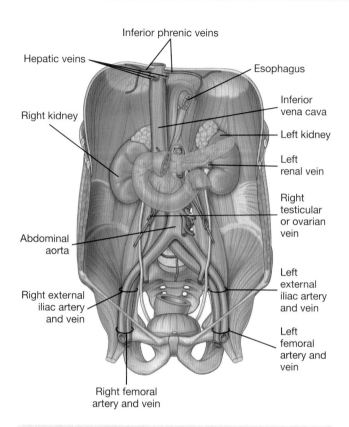

Fig. 4.115 Inferior vena cava.

inferior part of the duodenum, the head of the pancreas, the superior part of the duodenum, the bile duct, the portal vein, and the liver, which overlaps and on occasion completely surrounds the vena cava (Fig. 4.115).

Tributaries to the inferior vena cava include the:

- common iliac veins,
- lumbar veins,
- right testicular or ovarian vein,
- renal veins,
- right suprarenal vein,
- inferior phrenic veins, and
- hepatic veins.

There are no tributaries from the abdominal part of the gastrointestinal tract, the spleen, the pancreas, or the gallbladder, because veins from these structures are components of the portal venous system, which first passes through the liver.

Of the venous tributaries mentioned above, the **lumbar veins** are unique in their connections and deserve special attention. Not all of the lumbar veins drain directly into the inferior vena cava:

- The fifth lumbar vein generally drains into the **iliolumbar vein,** a tributary of the common iliac vein.
- The third and fourth lumbar veins usually drain into the inferior vena cava.

■ The first and second lumbar veins may empty into the ascending lumbar veins.

The **ascending lumbar veins** are long, anastomosing, venous channels that connect the common iliac, iliolumbar,

and lumbar veins with the azygos and hemiazygos veins of the thorax (Fig. 4.116).

If the inferior vena cava becomes blocked, the ascending lumbar veins become important collateral channels between the lower and upper parts of the body.

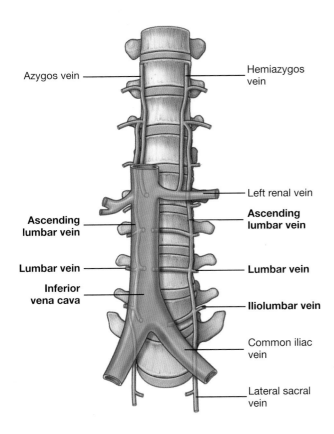

Fig. 4.116 Lumbar veins.

Clinical app

Inferior vena cava filter

Deep vein thrombosis is a potentially fatal condition in which a clot (thrombus) is formed in the deep venous system of the legs and the veins of the pelvis. Common predisposing factors include hospitalization, surgery, oral contraceptives, smoking, and air travel. Other factors include clotting abnormalities (e.g., protein S and protein C deficiency).

The diagnosis of deep vein thrombosis may be difficult to establish with symptoms including leg swelling and pain and discomfort in the calf.

Occasionally the clot may dislodge and pass into the venous system through the right side of the heart and into the main pulmonary arteries. If the clots are of significant size they obstruct blood flow to the lung and may produce instantaneous death.

Other complications include destruction of the normal valvular system in the legs, which may lead to venous incompetency and chronic leg swelling with ulceration.

In certain situations it is not possible to optimize the patient with prophylactic treatment, and it may be necessary to insert a filter into the inferior vena cava that traps any large clots. It may be removed after the risk period has ended.

Surface anatomy

Visualizing the position of major blood vessels

Each of the vertebral levels in the abdomen is related to the origin of major blood vessels (Fig. 4.117):

- The celiac trunk originates from the aorta at the upper border of the LI vertebra.
- The superior mesenteric artery originates at the lower border of the LI vertebra.
- The renal arteries originate at approximately the LII vertebra.
- The inferior mesenteric artery originates at the LIII vertebra.
- The aorta bifurcates into the right and left common iliac arteries at the level of the LIV vertebra.
- The left and right common iliac veins join to form the inferior vena cava at the LV vertebral level.

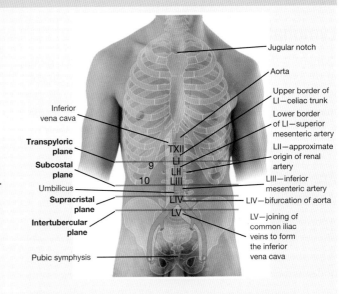

Fig. 4.117 Major vessels projected onto the body's surface. Anterior view of the abdominal region of a man.

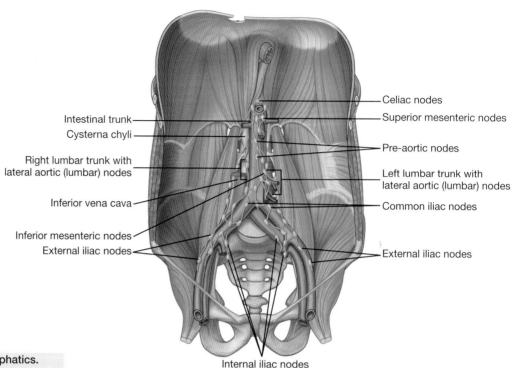

Fig. 4.118 Abdominal lymphatics.

Labels (clockwise from left):
- Intestinal trunk
- Cysterna chyli
- Right lumbar trunk with lateral aortic (lumbar) nodes
- Inferior vena cava
- Inferior mesenteric nodes
- External iliac nodes
- Celiac nodes
- Superior mesenteric nodes
- Pre-aortic nodes
- Left lumbar trunk with lateral aortic (lumbar) nodes
- Common iliac nodes
- External iliac nodes
- Internal iliac nodes

Table 4.4 Summary of lymphatic drainage in the body

Lymphatic vessel	Area drained
Right jugular trunk	Right side of head and neck
Left jugular trunk	Left side of head and neck
Right subclavian trunk	Right upper limb, superficial regions of thoracic and upper abdominal wall
Left subclavian trunk	Left upper limb, superficial regions of thoracic and upper abdominal wall
Right bronchomediastinal trunk	Right lung and bronchi, mediastinal structures, thoracic wall
Left bronchomediastinal trunk	Left lung and bronchi, mediastinal structures, thoracic wall
Thoracic duct	Lower limbs, abdominal walls and viscera, pelvic walls and viscera, thoracic wall

Lymphatic system

Lymphatic drainage from most deep structures and regions of the body below the diaphragm converges mainly on collections of lymph nodes and vessels associated with the major blood vessels of the posterior abdominal region (Fig. 4.118). The lymph then predominantly drains into the thoracic duct (Table 4.4).

Pre-aortic and lateral aortic or lumbar nodes (para-aortic nodes)

Approaching the aortic bifurcation, the collections of lymphatics associated with the two common iliac arteries and veins merge, and multiple groups of lymphatic vessels and nodes associated with the abdominal aorta and inferior vena cava pass superiorly. These collections may be subdivided into **pre-aortic nodes,** which are anterior to the abdominal aorta, and **right** and **left lateral aortic** or **lumbar nodes**

(para-aortic nodes), which are positioned on either side of the abdominal aorta (Table 4.4, Fig. 4.118).

As these collections of lymphatics pass through the posterior abdominal region, they continue to collect lymph from a variety of structures. The lateral aortic or lumbar lymph nodes (para-aortic nodes) receive lymphatics from the body wall, the kidneys, the suprarenal glands, and the testes or ovaries.

The pre-aortic nodes are organized around the three anterior branches of the abdominal aorta that supply the abdominal part of the gastrointestinal tract, as well as the spleen, pancreas, gallbladder, and liver. They are divided into celiac, superior mesenteric, and inferior mesenteric nodes and receive lymph from the organs supplied by the similarly named arteries.

Finally, the lateral aortic or lumbar nodes form the right and left lumbar trunks, whereas the pre-aortic nodes form the intestinal trunk (Fig. 4.118). These trunks come together and form a confluence that, at times, appears as a saccular dilation (the cisterna chyli). This confluence of lymph trunks nerves and ganglia associated with the abdominal aorta, and the lumbar plexus of nerves.

Clinical app

Retroperitoneal lymph node surgery

From a clinical perspective, retroperitoneal lymph nodes are arranged in two groups. The pre-aortic lymph node group drains lymph from the embryological midline structures, such as the liver, bowel, and pancreas. The para-aortic lymph node group (the lateral aortic or lumbar nodes), on either side of the aorta, drain lymph from bilateral structures, such as the kidneys and adrenal glands. Organs embryologically derived from the posterior abdominal wall also drain lymph to these nodes. These organs include the ovaries and the testes (importantly, the testes do not drain lymph to the inguinal regions).

There are a number of causes for enlarged retroperitoneal lymph nodes. Massively enlarged lymph nodes are a feature of lymphoma, and smaller lymph node enlargement is observed in the presence of infection and metastatic malignant spread of disease (e.g., colon cancer).

The surgical approach to retroperitoneal lymph node resection involves a lateral paramedian incision in the midclavicular line. The three layers of the anterolateral abdominal wall (external oblique, internal oblique, and transversus abdominis) are opened and the transversalis fascia is divided. The next structure the surgeon sees is the parietal peritoneum. Instead of entering the parietal peritoneum, which is standard procedure for most intra-abdominal surgical operations, the surgeon gently pushes the parietal peritoneum toward the midline, which moves the intra-abdominal contents and allows a clear view of the retroperitoneal structures. On the left, the para-aortic lymph node group (lateral aortic or lumbar nodes) are easily demonstrated with a clear view of the abdominal aorta and kidney. On the right the inferior vena cava is demonstrated, which has to be retracted to access to the right para-aortic lymph node chain (lateral aortic or lumbar nodes).

The procedure of the retroperitoneal lymph node dissection is extremely well tolerated and lacks the problems of entering the peritoneal cavity (e.g., paralytic ileus). Unfortunately, the complication of a vertical incision in the midclavicular line is to divide the segmental nerve supply to the rectus abdominis muscle. This produces muscle atrophy and asymmetrical proportions to the anterior abdominal wall.

is posterior to the right side of the abdominal aorta and anterior to the bodies of vertebrae LI and LII. It marks the beginning of the thoracic duct.

Nervous system in the posterior abdominal region

Several important components of the nervous system are in the posterior abdominal region. These include the sympathetic trunks and associated splanchnic nerves, the plexus of

Sympathetic trunks and splanchnic nerves

The sympathetic trunks pass through the posterior abdominal region anterolateral to the lumbar vertebral bodies before continuing across the sacral promontory and into the pelvic cavity (Fig. 4.119). Along their course, small raised areas are visible. These represent collections of neuronal cell bodies—primarily postganglionic neuronal cell bodies—which are located outside the central nervous system. They are sympathetic paravertebral ganglia. There are usually four ganglia along the sympathetic trunks in the posterior abdominal (lumbar) region.

Also associated with the sympathetic trunks in the posterior abdominal region are the lumbar splanchnic nerves (Fig. 4.119). These components of the nervous system pass from the sympathetic trunks to the plexus of nerves and ganglia associated with the abdominal aorta. Usually two to four lumbar splanchnic nerves carry preganglionic sympathetic fibers and visceral afferent fibers.

Abdominal prevertebral plexus and ganglia

The abdominal prevertebral plexus is a network of nerve fibers surrounding the abdominal aorta. It extends from the aortic hiatus of the diaphragm to the bifurcation of the aorta into the right and left common iliac arteries. Along its route, it is subdivided into smaller, named plexuses (Fig. 4.119):

- Beginning at the diaphragm and moving inferiorly, the initial accumulation of nerve fibers is referred to as the **celiac plexus**—this subdivision includes nerve fibers associated with the roots of the celiac trunk and superior mesenteric artery.
- Continuing inferiorly, the plexus of nerve fibers extending from just below the superior mesenteric artery to the aortic bifurcation is the **abdominal aortic plexus** (Fig. 4.119).
- At the bifurcation of the abdominal aorta, the abdominal prevertebral plexus continues inferiorly as the **superior hypogastric plexus** (Fig. 4.119).

Throughout its length, the abdominal prevertebral plexus is a conduit for:

- preganglionic sympathetic and visceral afferent fibers from the thoracic and lumbar splanchnic nerves (Fig. 4.120),
- preganglionic parasympathetic and visceral afferent fibers from the vagus nerves [X] (Fig. 4.120), and
- preganglionic parasympathetic fibers from the pelvic splanchnic nerves.

Associated with the abdominal prevertebral plexus are clumps of nervous tissue (the **prevertebral ganglia**), which

217

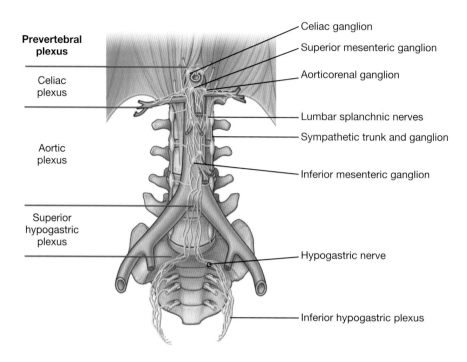

Fig. 4.119 Prevertebral plexus and ganglia in the posterior abdominal region.

Fig. 4.120 Nerve fibers passing through the abdominal prevertebral plexus and ganglia.

Table 4.5   Referred pain pathways (visceral afferents)

Organ	Afferent pathway	Spinal cord level	Referral area
Heart	Thoracic splanchnic nerves	T1 to T4	Upper thorax and medial arm
Foregut (organs supplied by celiac trunk)	Greater splanchnic nerve	T5 to T9 (or T10)	Lower thorax and epigastric region
Midgut (organs supplied by superior mesenteric artery)	Lesser splanchnic nerve	T9, T10 (or T10, T11)	Umbilical region
Kidneys and upper ureter	Least splanchnic nerve	T12	Flanks (lateral regions) and pubic region
Hindgut (organs supplied by inferior mesenteric artery)	Lumbar splanchnic nerves	L1, L2	Left and right flanks and groins, lateral and anterior thighs

Table 4.6   Branches of the lumbar plexus

Branch	Origin	Spinal segments	Function: motor	Function: sensory
Iliohypogastric	Anterior ramus L1	L1	Internal oblique and transversus abdominis	Posterolateral gluteal skin and skin in pubic region
Ilio-inguinal	Anterior ramus L1	L1	Internal oblique and transversus abdominis	Skin in the upper medial thigh, and either the skin over the root of the penis and anterior scrotum or the mons pubis and labium majus
Genitofemoral	Anterior rami L1 and L2	L1, L2	Genital branch—male cremasteric muscle	Genital branch—skin of anterior scrotum or skin of mons pubis and labium majus; femoral branch—skin of upper anterior thigh
Lateral cutaneous nerve of thigh	Anterior rami L2 and L3	L2, L3		Skin on anterior and lateral thigh to the knee
Obturator	Anterior rami L2 to L4	L2 to L4	Obturator externus, pectineus, and muscles in medial compartment of thigh	Skin on medial aspect of the thigh
Femoral	Anterior rami L2 to L4	L2 to L4	Iliacus, pectineus, and muscles in anterior compartment of thigh	Skin on anterior thigh and medial surface of leg

are collections of postganglionic sympathetic neuronal cell bodies in recognizable aggregations along the abdominal prevertebral plexus; they are usually named after the nearest branch of the abdominal aorta. They are therefore referred to as **celiac, superior mesenteric, aorticorenal, and inferior mesenteric ganglia** (Fig. 4.119). These structures, along with the abdominal prevertebral plexus, play a critical role in the innervation of the abdominal viscera.

Common sites for pain referred from the abdominal viscera are given in Table 4.5.

Lumbar plexus

The lumbar plexus is formed by the anterior rami of nerves L1 to L3 and most of the anterior ramus of L4 (Table 4.6, Fig. 4.121). It also receives a contribution from the T12 (subcostal) nerve.

Branches of the lumbar plexus include the iliohypogastric, ilio-inguinal, genitofemoral, lateral cutaneous nerve of thigh (lateral femoral cutaneous), femoral, and obturator nerves. The lumbar plexus forms in the substance of the psoas major muscle anterior to its attachment to the transverse processes of the lumbar vertebrae (Fig. 4.122). Therefore relative to the psoas major muscle, the various branches emerge either:

Fig. 4.121 Lumbar plexus.

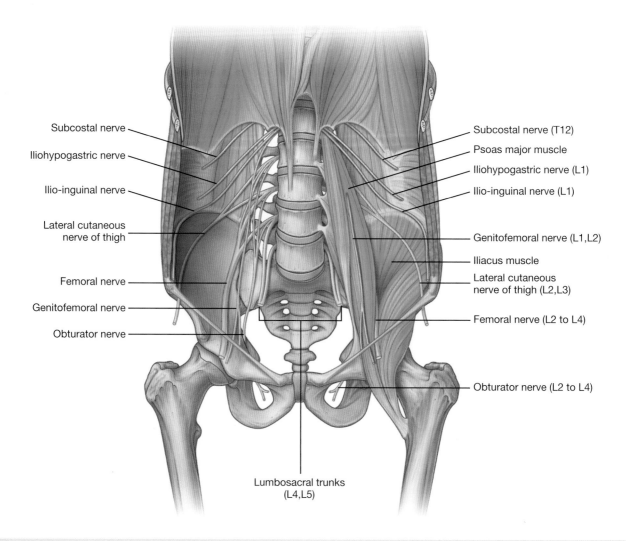

Subcostal nerve

Iliohypogastric nerve

Ilio-inguinal nerve

Lateral cutaneous
nerve of thigh

Femoral nerve

Genitofemoral nerve

Obturator nerve

Subcostal nerve (T12)

Psoas major muscle

Iliohypogastric nerve (L1)

Ilio-inguinal nerve (L1)

Genitofemoral nerve (L1,L2)

Iliacus muscle

Lateral cutaneous
nerve of thigh (L2,L3)

Femoral nerve (L2 to L4)

Obturator nerve (L2 to L4)

Lumbosacral trunks
(L4,L5)

Fig. 4.122 Lumbar plexus in the posterior abdominal region.

- anterior—genitofemoral nerve,
- medial—obturator nerve, or
- lateral—iliohypogastric, ilio-inguinal, and femoral nerves and the lateral cutaneous nerve of the thigh.

Iliohypogastric and ilio-inguinal nerves (L1)

The iliohypogastric and ilio-inguinal nerves arise as a single trunk from the anterior ramus of nerve L1 (Fig. 4.122). Either before or soon after emerging from the lateral border of the psoas major muscle, this single trunk divides into the iliohypogastric and the ilio-inguinal nerves.

Iliohypogastric nerve

The **iliohypogastric nerve** passes across the anterior surface of the quadratus lumborum muscle posterior to the kidney. It pierces the transversus abdominis muscle and continues anteriorly around the body between the transversus abdominis and internal oblique muscles. Above the iliac crest, a **lateral cutaneous branch** pierces the internal and external oblique muscles to supply the posterolateral gluteal skin (Fig. 4.123).

The remaining part of the iliohypogastric nerve (the **anterior cutaneous branch**) continues in an anterior direction, piercing the internal oblique just medial to the anterior superior iliac spine as it continues in an obliquely downward and medial direction. Becoming cutaneous just above the superficial inguinal ring after piercing the aponeurosis of the external oblique, it distributes to the skin in the pubic region (Fig. 4.123). Throughout its course, it also supplies branches to the abdominal musculature.

Ilio-inguinal nerve

The ilio-inguinal nerve is smaller than, and inferior to, the iliohypogastric nerve as it crosses the quadratus lumborum muscle (Fig. 4.122). Its course is more oblique than that of the iliohypogastric nerve, and it usually crosses part of the iliacus muscle on its way to the iliac crest. Near the anterior end of the iliac crest, it pierces the transversus abdominis

Fig. 4.123 Cutaneous distribution of the nerves from the lumbar plexus.

muscle and then pierces the internal oblique muscle and enters the inguinal canal.

The ilio-inguinal nerve emerges through the superficial inguinal ring, along with the spermatic cord, and provides cutaneous innervation to the upper medial thigh, the root of the penis, and the anterior surface of the scrotum in men or the mons pubis and labium majus in women (Fig. 4.123). Throughout its course, it also supplies branches to the abdominal musculature.

Genitofemoral nerve (L1 and L2)

The genitofemoral nerve arises from the anterior rami of the nerves L1 and L2 (Fig. 4.121). It passes downward in the substance of the psoas major muscle until it emerges on the anterior surface of psoas major. It then descends on the surface of the muscle in a retroperitoneal position, passing posterior to the ureter. It eventually divides into genital and femoral branches.

The **genital branch** continues downward and enters the inguinal canal through the deep inguinal ring. It continues through the canal and:

- in men, innervates the cremasteric muscle and terminates on the skin in the upper anterior part of the scrotum and
- in women, accompanies the round ligament of the uterus and terminates on the skin of the mons pubis and labium majus.

The **femoral branch** descends on the lateral side of the external iliac artery and passes posterior to the inguinal ligament, entering the femoral sheath lateral to the femoral artery. It pierces the anterior layer of the femoral sheath and the fascia lata to supply the skin of the upper anterior thigh (Fig. 4.123).

Lateral cutaneous nerve of thigh (L2 and L3)

The lateral cutaneous nerve of thigh arises from the anterior rami of nerves L2 and L3 (see Fig. 4.121). It emerges from the lateral border of the psoas major muscle, passing obliquely downward across the iliacus muscle toward the anterior superior iliac spine (see Fig. 4.122). It passes posterior to the inguinal ligament and enters the thigh.

The lateral cutaneous nerve of thigh supplies the skin on the anterior and lateral thigh to the level of the knee (Fig. 4.123).

Obturator nerve (L2 to L4)

The obturator nerve arises from the anterior rami of the nerves L2 to L4 (see Fig. 4.121). It descends in the psoas major muscle, emerging from its medial side near the pelvic brim (see Fig. 4.122).

The obturator nerve continues posterior to the common iliac vessels, passes across the lateral wall of the pelvic cavity, and enters the obturator canal, through which the obturator nerve gains access to the medial compartment of the thigh (see Fig. 4.122).

In the area of the obturator canal, the obturator nerve divides into **anterior** and **posterior branches.** On entering the medial compartment of the thigh, the two branches are separated by the obturator externus and adductor brevis muscles. Throughout their course through the medial compartment, these two branches supply:

- articular branches to the hip joint,
- muscular branches to obturator externus, pectineus, adductor longus, gracilis, adductor brevis, and adductor magnus muscles,
- cutaneous branches to the medial aspect of the thigh, and
- in association with the saphenous nerve, cutaneous branches to the medial aspect of the upper part of the leg and articular branches to the knee joint (Fig. 4.123).

Femoral nerve (L2 to L4)

The femoral nerve arises from the anterior rami of nerves L2 to L4 (see Fig. 4.121). It descends through the substance of the psoas major muscle, emerging from the lower lateral border of the psoas major (see Fig. 4.122). Continuing its descent, the femoral nerve lies between the lateral border of the psoas major and the anterior surface of the iliacus muscle. It is deep to the iliacus fascia and lateral to the femoral artery as it passes posterior to the inguinal ligament and enters the anterior compartment of the thigh. Upon entering the thigh, it immediately divides into multiple branches.

Cutaneous branches of the femoral nerve include (Fig. 4.123):

- medial and intermediate cutaneous nerves supplying the skin on the anterior surface of the thigh and
- the **saphenous nerve** supplying the skin on the medial surface of the leg (Fig. 4.123).

Muscular branches innervate the iliacus, pectineus, sartorius, rectus femoris, vastus medialis, vastus intermedius, and vastus lateralis muscles. Articular branches supply the hip and knee joints.

5

Pelvis and Perineum

Regional anatomy   224

Pelvis   224
    Bones   224
    Joints   227
    Orientation   229
    Differences between men and women   229
    True pelvis   230
    Viscera   236
    Fascia   247
    Peritoneum   248
    Nerves   251
    Blood vessels   258
    Lymphatics   262
Perineum   262
    Borders and ceiling   263
    Ischio-anal fossae and their anterior recesses   264
    Anal triangle   265
    Urogenital triangle   265
    Somatic nerves   271
    Visceral nerves   271
    Blood vessels   272
    Veins   274
    Lymphatics   274

Regional anatomy

The pelvis and perineum are interrelated regions associated with the pelvic bones and the terminal parts of the vertebral column. The pelvis is divided into two regions (Fig. 5.1):

- The superior region related to upper parts of the pelvic bones and lower lumbar vertebrae is the **false** pelvis (greater pelvis) and is generally considered part of the abdominal cavity.
- The **true pelvis** (lesser pelvis) is related to the inferior parts of the pelvic bones, sacrum, and coccyx and has an inlet and an outlet.

The bowl-shaped **pelvic cavity** (Fig. 5.1) enclosed by the true pelvis consists of the pelvic inlet, walls, and floor. This cavity is continuous superiorly with the abdominal cavity and contains and supports elements of the urinary, gastrointestinal, and reproductive systems.

The **perineum** (Fig. 5.1) is inferior to the floor of the pelvic cavity; its boundaries form the **pelvic outlet.** The perineum contains and supports the external genitalia and external openings of the genitourinary and gastrointestinal systems.

PELVIS
Bones

The bones of the pelvis consist of the right and left pelvic (hip) bones, the sacrum, and the coccyx. The sacrum articulates superiorly with vertebra LV at the lumbosacral joint. The pelvic bones articulate posteriorly with the sacrum at the sacro-iliac joints and with each other anteriorly at the pubic symphysis.

Pelvic bone

The pelvic bone is irregular in shape and has two major parts separated by an oblique line on the medial surface of the bone (Fig. 5.2A):

- The pelvic bone above this line represents the lateral wall of the false pelvis, which is part of the abdominal cavity.

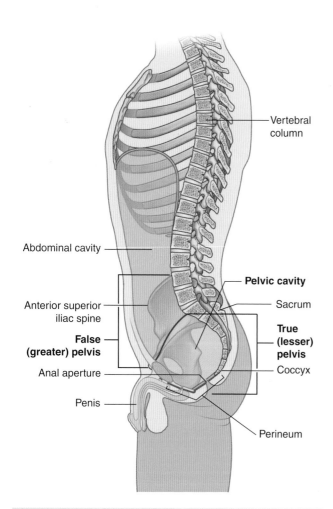

Fig. 5.1 Pelvis and perineum.

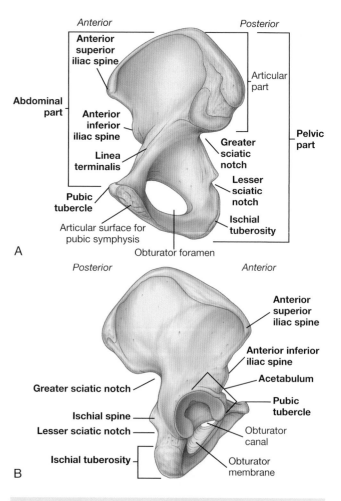

Fig. 5.2 Right pelvic bone. **A.** Medial view. **B.** Lateral view.

■ The pelvic bone below this line represents the lateral wall of the true pelvis, which contains the pelvic cavity.

The **linea terminalis** is the lower two-thirds of this line and contributes to the margin of the pelvic inlet.

The lateral surface of the pelvic bone has a large articular socket, the **acetabulum,** which, together with the head of the femur, forms the hip joint (Fig. 5.2B).

Inferior to the acetabulum is the large **obturator foramen,** most of which is closed by a flat connective tissue membrane, the **obturator membrane.** A small obturator canal remains open superiorly between the membrane and adjacent bone, providing a route of communication between the lower limb and the pelvic cavity.

The posterior margin of the bone is marked by two notches separated by the **ischial spine** (Fig. 5.2):

■ the **greater sciatic notch,** and
■ the **lesser sciatic notch.**

The posterior margin terminates inferiorly as the large **ischial tuberosity.**

The irregular anterior margin of the pelvic bone is marked by the **anterior superior iliac spine,** the **anterior inferior iliac spine,** and the **pubic tubercle.**

Components of the pelvic bone

Each pelvic bone is formed by three elements: the ilium, pubis, and ischium (Fig. 5.3). At birth, these bones are connected by cartilage in the area of the acetabulum; later, between 16 and 18 years of age, they fuse into a single bone.

Ilium

Of the three components of the pelvic bone, the **ilium** is the most superior in position.

The ilium is separated into upper and lower parts by a ridge on the medial surface (Fig. 5.4A).

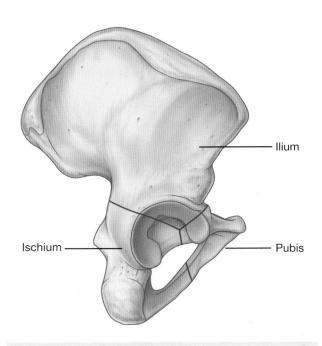

Fig. 5.3 Ilium, ischium, and pubis.

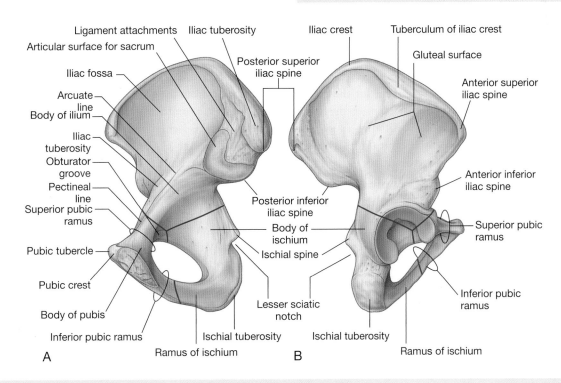

Fig. 5.4 Components of the pelvic bone. **A.** Medial surface. **B.** Lateral surface.

- Posteriorly, the ridge is sharp and lies immediately superior to the surface of the bone that articulates with the sacrum. This sacral surface has a large L-shaped facet for articulating with the sacrum and an expanded, posterior, roughened area for the attachment of the strong ligaments that support the sacro-iliac joint (Fig. 5.4).
- Anteriorly, the ridge separating the upper and lower parts of the ilium is rounded and termed the **arcuate line** (Fig. 5.4).

The arcuate line forms part of the linea terminalis and the pelvic brim.

The portion of the ilium lying inferiorly to the arcuate line is the pelvic part of the ilium and contributes to the wall of the lesser or true pelvis.

The upper part of the ilium expands to form a flat, fan-shaped "wing," which provides bony support for the lower abdomen, or false pelvis (Fig. 5.4). This part of the ilium provides attachment for muscles functionally associated with the lower limb. The anteromedial surface of the wing is concave and forms the **iliac fossa.** The external (gluteal surface) of the wing is marked by lines and roughenings and is related to the gluteal region of the lower limb (Fig. 5.4B).

The entire superior margin of the ilium is thickened to form a prominent crest (the **iliac crest**), which is the site of attachment for muscles and fascia of the abdomen, back, and lower limb and terminates anteriorly as the **anterior superior iliac spine** and posteriorly as the **posterior superior iliac spine** (Fig. 5.4).

A prominent tubercle, **tuberculum of iliac crest,** projects laterally near the anterior end of the crest; the posterior end of the crest thickens to form the **iliac tuberosity** (Fig. 5.4).

Inferior to the anterior superior iliac spine of the crest, on the anterior margin of the ilium, is a rounded protuberance called the **anterior inferior iliac spine** (Fig 5.4). This structure serves as the point of attachment for the rectus femoris muscle of the anterior compartment of the thigh and the iliofemoral ligament associated with the hip joint. A less prominent **posterior inferior iliac spine** (Fig 5.4) occurs along the posterior border of the sacral surface of the ilium where the bone angles forward to form the superior margin of the greater sciatic notch.

Clinical app

Bone marrow biopsy

In certain diseases (e.g., leukemia), a sample of bone marrow must be obtained to assess the stage and severity of the problem. The iliac crest is often used for such bone marrow biopsies. The iliac crest lies close to the surface, is palpable, and is easily accessed.

Pubis

The anterior and inferior part of the pelvic bone is the **pubis** (Fig. 5.4). It has a body and two arms (rami).

- The **body** is flattened dorsoventrally and articulates with the body of the pubic bone on the other side at the **pubic symphysis.** The body has a rounded pubic crest on its superior surface that ends laterally as the prominent **pubic tubercle.**
- The **superior pubic ramus** projects posterolaterally from the body and joins with the ilium and ischium at its base, which is positioned toward the acetabulum. The sharp superior margin of this triangular surface is termed the **pecten pubis (pectineal line),** which forms part of the linea terminalis of the pelvic bone and the pelvic inlet. Anteriorly, this line is continuous with the **pubic crest,** which also is part of the linea terminalis and pelvic inlet. The **superior pubic ramus** is marked on its inferior surface by the **obturator groove,** which forms the upper margin of the obturator canal.
- The **inferior ramus** projects laterally and inferiorly to join with the ramus of the ischium.

Ischium

The ischium is the posterior and inferior part of the pelvic bone (Fig. 5.4). It has:

- a large body that projects superiorly to join with the ilium and the superior ramus of the pubis; and
- a ramus that projects anteriorly to join with the inferior ramus of the pubis.

The posterior margin of the bone is marked by a prominent **ischial spine** (Fig. 5.4) that separates the lesser sciatic notch below from the greater sciatic notch above.

The most prominent feature of the ischium is a large tuberosity (the **ischial tuberosity**) on the posteroinferior aspect of the bone (Fig. 5.4). This tuberosity is an important site for the attachment of lower limb muscles and for supporting the body when sitting.

Sacrum

The sacrum, which has the appearance of an inverted triangle, is formed by the fusion of the five sacral vertebrae (Fig. 5.5). The base of the sacrum articulates with vertebra LV, and its apex articulates with the coccyx. Each of the lateral surfaces of the bone bears a large L-shaped facet for articulation with the ilium of the pelvic bone. Posterior to the facet is a large roughened area for the attachment of ligaments that support the sacro-iliac joint. The superior surface of the sacrum is characterized by the superior aspect of the body of vertebra SI

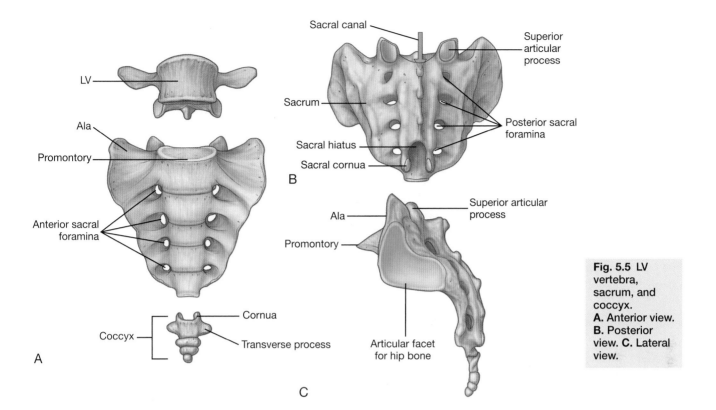

Sacral canal

Superior articular process

LV

Sacrum

Ala

Promontory

Posterior sacral foramina

Sacral hiatus

Sacral cornua

B

Anterior sacral foramina

Superior articular process

Ala

Promontory

Fig. 5.5 LV vertebra, sacrum, and coccyx. **A.** Anterior view. **B.** Posterior view. **C.** Lateral view.

Coccyx

Cornua

Transverse process

Articular facet for hip bone

A

C

and is flanked on each side by an expanded wing-like transverse process termed the **ala** (Fig. 5.5A). The anterior edge of the vertebral body projects forward as the **promontory.** The anterior surface of the sacrum is concave; the posterior surface is convex. Because the transverse processes of adjacent sacral vertebrae fuse laterally to the position of the intervertebral foramina and laterally to the bifurcation of spinal nerves into posterior and anterior rami, the posterior and anterior rami of spinal nerves S1 to S4 emerge from the sacrum through separate foramina. There are four pairs of **anterior sacral foramina** on the anterior surface of the sacrum for anterior rami (Fig. 5.5A) and four pairs of **posterior sacral foramina** on the posterior surface for the posterior rami (Fig. 5.5B). The **sacral canal** is a continuation of the vertebral canal that terminates as the **sacral hiatus.**

Coccyx

The small terminal part of the vertebral column is the coccyx, which consists of four fused coccygeal vertebrae (Fig. 5.5A) and, like the sacrum, has the shape of an inverted triangle. The base of the coccyx is directed superiorly. The superior surface bears a facet for articulation with the sacrum and two **horns,** or **cornua,** one on each side, that project upward to articulate or fuse with similar downward-projecting cornua from the sacrum. These processes are modified superior and inferior articular processes that are

present on other vertebrae. Each lateral surface of the coccyx has a small rudimentary transverse process extending from the first coccygeal vertebra. Vertebral arches are absent from coccygeal vertebrae; therefore no bony vertebral canal is present in the coccyx.

Joints
Lumbosacral joints

The sacrum articulates superiorly with the lumbar part of the vertebral column. The lumbosacral joints are formed between vertebra LV and the sacrum and consist of (Fig. 5.6A):

- the two **zygapophyseal joints,** which occur between adjacent inferior and superior articular processes; and
- an intervertebral disc that joins the bodies of vertebrae LV and SI.

These joints are similar to those between other vertebrae, with the exception that the sacrum is angled posteriorly on vertebra LV. As a result, the anterior part of the intervertebral disc between the two bones is thicker than the posterior part.

The lumbosacral joints are reinforced by strong iliolumbar and lumbosacral ligaments that extend from the expanded transverse processes of vertebra LV to the ilium and the sacrum, respectively (Fig. 5.6B).

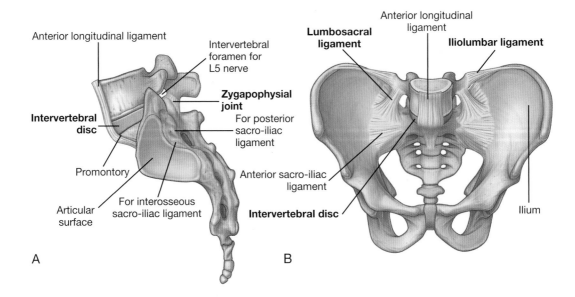

Fig. 5.6 Lumbosacral joints and associated ligaments. **A.** Lateral view. **B.** Anterior view.

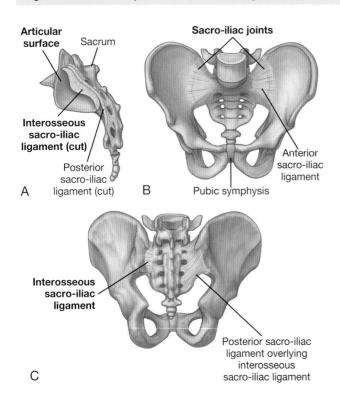

Fig. 5.7 Sacro-iliac joints and associated ligaments.
A. Lateral view. **B.** Anterior view. **C.** Posterior view.

Sacro-iliac joints

The sacro-iliac joints transmit forces from the lower limbs to the vertebral column. They are synovial joints between the L-shaped articular facets on the lateral surfaces of the sacrum and similar facets on the iliac parts of the pelvic bones (Figs. 5.6A, 5.7A). The joint surfaces have an irregular contour and interlock to resist movement. The joints often become fibrous with age and may become completely ossified.

Each sacro-iliac joint is stabilized by three ligaments:

- the **anterior sacro-iliac ligament,** which is a thickening of the fibrous membrane of the joint capsule and runs anteriorly and inferiorly to the joint (Figs. 5.6B, 5.7B);
- the **interosseous sacro-iliac ligament,** which is the largest, strongest ligament of the three, is positioned immediately posterosuperior to the joint, and attaches to adjacent expansive roughened areas on the ilium and sacrum, thereby filling the gap between the two bones (Fig. 5.7A and 5.7C); and
- the **posterior sacro-iliac ligament,** which covers the interosseous sacro-iliac ligament (Fig. 5.7C).

Clinical app

Common problems with the sacro-iliac joints

As with many weight-bearing joints, degenerative changes may occur with the sacro-iliac joints and cause pain and discomfort in the region. In addition, disorders associated with the major histocompatibility complex antigen HLA B27, such as ankylosing spondylitis, psoriatic arthritis, inflammatory arthritis associated with inflammatory bowel disease, or reactive arthritis (the group referred to as *seronegative spondyloarthropathies),* can produce specific inflammatory changes within these joints.

Pubic symphysis joint

The pubic symphysis lies anteriorly between the adjacent surfaces of the pubic bones (Fig. 5.8). Each of the joint's surfaces is covered by hyaline cartilage and is linked across the midline to adjacent surfaces by fibrocartilage. The joint is surrounded by interwoven layers of collagen fibers, and the two major ligaments associated with it are (Fig. 5.8):

- the **superior pubic ligament,** located above the joint, and
- the **inferior pubic ligament,** located below it.

Orientation

In the anatomical position, the pelvis is oriented so that the front edge of the top of the pubic symphysis and the anterior superior iliac spines lie in the same vertical plane (Fig. 5.9). As a consequence, the pelvic inlet, which marks the entrance to the pelvic cavity, is tilted to face anteriorly, and the bodies of the pubic bones and the pubic arch are positioned in a nearly horizontal plane facing the ground.

Differences between men and women

The pelvises of women and men differ in a number of ways, many of which have to do with the passing of a baby through a woman's pelvic cavity during childbirth.

- The pelvic inlet in women is circular (Fig. 5.10A) compared with the more heart-shaped pelvic inlet (Fig. 5.10B) in

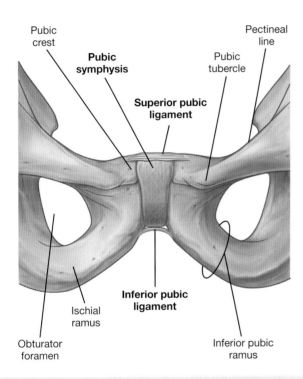

Fig. 5.8 Pubic symphysis and associated ligaments.

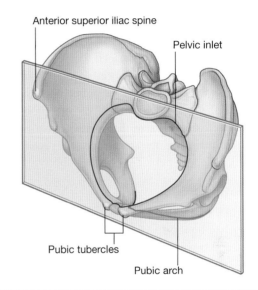

Fig. 5.9 Orientation of the pelvis (anatomical position).

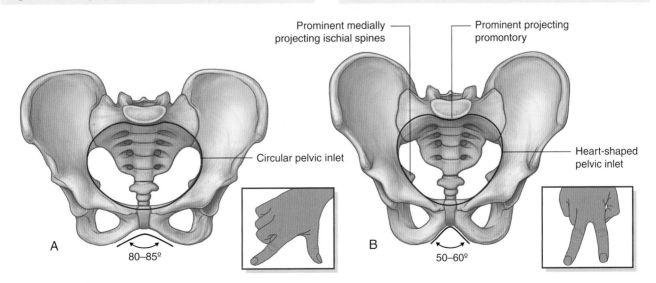

Fig. 5.10 Structure of the bony pelvis. **A.** In women. **B.** In men. The angle formed by the pubic arch can be approximated by the angle between the thumb and index finger for women and the angle between the index finger and middle finger for men, as shown in the insets.

men. The more circular shape is partly caused by the less distinct promontory and broader alae in women.

- The angle formed by the two arms of the pubic arch is larger in women (80° to 85°) than it is in men (50° to 60°) (Fig. 5.10).
- The ischial spines generally do not project as far medially into the pelvic cavity in women as they do in men.

True pelvis

The true pelvis is cylindrical and has an inlet, a wall, and an outlet. The inlet is open, whereas the pelvic floor closes the outlet and separates the pelvic cavity above from the perineum below.

Pelvic inlet

The pelvic inlet is the circular opening between the abdominal cavity and the pelvic cavity through which structures traverse between the abdomen and pelvic cavity. It is completely surrounded by bones and joints (Fig. 5.11). The promontory of the sacrum protrudes into the inlet, forming its posterior margin in the midline. On either side of the promontory, the margin is formed by the alae of the sacrum. The margin of the pelvic inlet then crosses the sacro-iliac joint and continues along the linea terminalis (i.e., the arcuate line, the pecten pubis or pectineal line, and the pubic crest) to the pubic symphysis.

Pelvic wall

The walls of the pelvic cavity consist of the sacrum, the coccyx, the pelvic bones inferior to the linea terminalis, two ligaments, and two muscles.

Clinical app

Pelvic fracture

The pelvis can be viewed as a series of anatomical rings. There are three bony rings and four fibro-osseous rings. The major bony pelvic ring consists of parts of the sacrum, ilium, and pubis, which forms the pelvic inlet. Two smaller subsidiary bony rings are the obturator foraminae. The greater and lesser sciatic foraminae, formed by the greater and lesser sciatic notches and the sacrospinous and sacrotuberous ligaments, form the four fibro-osseous rings. It is not possible to break one side of a bony ring without breaking the other side of the ring, which in clinical terms means that if a fracture is demonstrated on one side, a second fracture should always be suspected.

Ligaments of the pelvic wall

The **sacrospinous and sacrotuberous ligaments** (Fig. 5.12A) are major components of the lateral pelvic walls that help define the apertures between the pelvic cavity and adjacent regions through which structures pass.

Fig. 5.11 Pelvic inlet.

- The smaller of the two, the sacrospinous ligament, is triangular, with its apex attached to the ischial spine and its base attached to the related margins of the sacrum and the coccyx (Fig. 5.12A).
- The sacrotuberous ligament is also triangular and is superficial to the sacrospinous ligament. Its base has a broad attachment that extends from the posterior superior iliac spine of the pelvic bone, along the dorsal aspect and the lateral margin of the sacrum, and onto the dorsolateral surface of the coccyx. Laterally, the apex of the ligament is attached to the medial margin of the ischial tuberosity (Fig. 5.12A).

These ligaments stabilize the sacrum on the pelvic bones by resisting the upward tilting of the inferior aspect of the sacrum (Fig. 5.12B). They also convert the greater and lesser sciatic notches of the pelvic bone into foramina (Fig. 5.12A,B).

- The **greater sciatic foramen** lies superior to the sacrospinous ligament and the ischial spine.
- The **lesser sciatic foramen** lies inferior to the ischial spine and sacrospinous ligament between the sacrospinous and sacrotuberous ligaments.

Muscles of the pelvic wall

Two muscles, the **obturator internus** and the **piriformis,** contribute to the lateral walls of the pelvic cavity. These muscles originate in the pelvic cavity but attach peripherally to the femur (Table 5.1, Fig. 5.13).

Apertures in the pelvic wall

Each lateral pelvic wall has three major apertures through which structures pass between the pelvic cavity and other regions (Fig. 5.14):

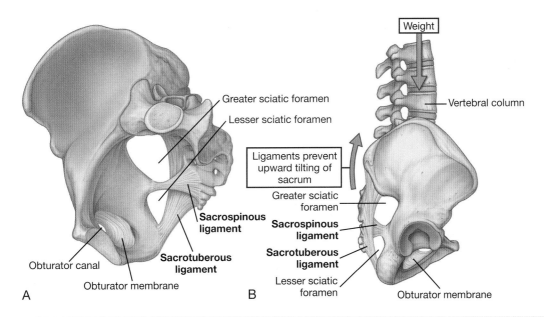

Fig. 5.12 Sacrospinous and sacrotuberous ligaments. **A.** Medial view of right side of pelvis. **B.** Function of the ligaments.

Table 5.1 Muscles of the pelvic walls (spinal segments in bold are the major segments innervating the muscle)

Muscles	Origin	Insertion	Innervation	Function
Obturator internus	Anterolateral wall of true pelvis (deep surface of obturator membrane and surrounding bone). The muscle fibers of the obturator internus converge to form a tendon that leaves the pelvic cavity through the lesser sciatic foramen, makes a 90° bend around the ischium between the ischial spine and ischial tuberosity, and then passes posterior to the hip joint to reach its insertion	Medial surface of greater trochanter of femur	Nerve to obturator internus **L5, S1**	Lateral rotation of the extended hip joint; abduction of flexed hip
Piriformis	Anterior surface of sacrum between anterior sacral foramina	Medial side of superior border of greater trochanter of femur	Branches from L5, **S1**, and **S2**	Lateral rotation of the extended hip joint; abduction of flexed hip

- the obturator canal,
- the greater sciatic foramen, and
- the lesser sciatic foramen.

Obturator canal

At the top of the obturator foramen is the obturator canal, which is bordered by the obturator membrane, the associated obturator muscles, and the superior pubic ramus (Fig. 5.14). The obturator nerve and vessels pass from the pelvic cavity to the thigh through this canal.

Greater sciatic foramen

The greater sciatic foramen is a major route of communication between the pelvic cavity and the lower limb (Fig. 5.14). It is formed by the greater sciatic notch in the pelvic bone, the sacrotuberous and the sacrospinous ligaments, and the spine of the ischium.

The piriformis muscle passes through the greater sciatic foramen, dividing it into two parts.

- The superior gluteal nerves and vessels pass through the foramen above the piriformis.
- Passing through the foramen below the piriformis are the inferior gluteal nerves and vessels, the sciatic nerve, the pudendal nerve, the internal pudendal vessels, the posterior femoral cutaneous nerves, and the nerves to the obturator internus and quadratus femoris muscles.

Lesser sciatic foramen

The lesser sciatic foramen is formed by the lesser sciatic notch of the pelvic bone, the ischial spine, the sacrospinous ligament, and the sacrotuberous ligament (Fig. 5.14). The tendon of the obturator internus muscle passes through this foramen to enter the gluteal region of the lower limb.

Because the lesser sciatic foramen is positioned below the attachment of the pelvic floor, it acts as a route of communication between the perineum and the gluteal region. The pudendal nerve and internal pudendal vessels pass between the pelvic cavity (above the pelvic floor) and the perineum

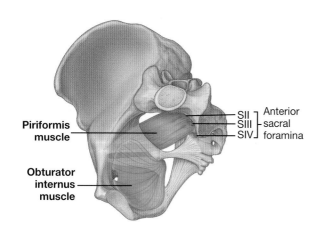

Fig. 5.13 Obturator internus and piriformis muscles (medial view of right side of pelvis).

Piriformis muscle

Obturator internus muscle

SII ⎤ Anterior
SIII ⎬ sacral
SIV ⎦ foramina

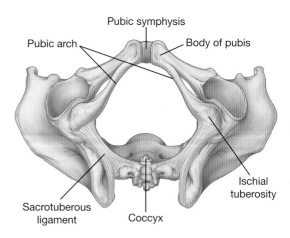

Fig. 5.15 Pelvic outlet.

Pubic symphysis

Pubic arch

Body of pubis

Sacrotuberous ligament

Coccyx

Ischial tuberosity

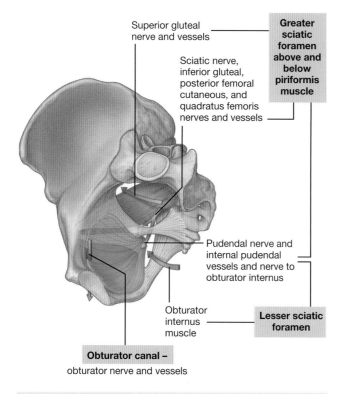

Fig. 5.14 Apertures in the pelvic wall.

Superior gluteal nerve and vessels

Greater sciatic foramen above and below piriformis muscle

Sciatic nerve, inferior gluteal, posterior femoral cutaneous, and quadratus femoris nerves and vessels

Pudendal nerve and internal pudendal vessels and nerve to obturator internus

Obturator internus muscle

Lesser sciatic foramen

Obturator canal –
obturator nerve and vessels

Extending laterally and posteriorly, the boundary on each side is the inferior border of the body of the pubis, the inferior ramus of the pubis, the ramus of the ischium, and the ischial tuberosity. Together, the elements on both sides form the pubic arch.

From the ischial tuberosities, the boundaries continue posteriorly and medially along the sacrotuberous ligament on both sides to the coccyx.

Terminal parts of the urinary and gastrointestinal tracts and the vagina pass through the pelvic outlet.

Clinical app

Pelvic measurements in obstetrics
Accurate measurements of a women's pelvic inlet and outlet can help in predicting the likelihood of a successful vaginal delivery during childbirth. These measurements include:
- the sagittal inlet (between the promontory and the top of the pubic symphysis);
- the maximum transverse diameter of the inlet;
- the bispinous outlet (the distance between ischial spines); and
- the sagittal outlet (the distance between the tip of the coccyx and the inferior margin of the pubic symphysis).

The area enclosed by the boundaries of the pelvic outlet and below the pelvic floor is the **perineum.**

Pelvic floor

The pelvic floor is formed by the **pelvic diaphragm** and, in the anterior midline, the **perineal membrane** and the muscles in the **deep perineal pouch**. The pelvic diaphragm is formed by the **levator ani** and the **coccygeus muscles** from both sides. The pelvic floor separates the pelvic cavity above from the perineum below.

(below the pelvic floor) by first passing out of the pelvic cavity through the greater sciatic foramen and then looping around the ischial spine and sacrospinous ligament to pass through the lesser sciatic foramen to enter the perineum. The nerve to obturator internus follows a similar course.

Pelvic outlet

The pelvic outlet is diamond shaped, with the anterior part of the diamond defined predominantly by bone and the posterior part mainly by ligaments (Fig. 5.15). In the midline anteriorly, the boundary of the pelvic outlet is the pubic symphysis.

Table 5.2   Muscles of the pelvic diaphragm

Muscles	Origin	Insertion	Innervation	Function
Levator ani	In a line around the pelvic wall beginning on the posterior aspect of the pubic bone and extending across the obturator internus muscle as a tendinous arch (thickening of the obturator internus fascia) to the ischial spine	The anterior part is attached to the superior surface of the perineal membrane; the posterior part meets its partner on the other side at the perineal body, around the anal canal, and along the anococcygeal ligament	Branches direct from the anterior ramus of S4 and by the inferior rectal branch of the pudendal nerve (S2 to S4)	Contributes to the formation of the pelvic floor, which supports the pelvic viscera; maintains an angle between the rectum and anal canal. Reinforces the external anal sphincter and, in women, functions as a vaginal sphincter
Coccygeus	Ischial spine and pelvic surface of the sacrospinous ligament	Lateral margin of coccyx and related border of sacrum	Branches from the anterior rami of S3 and S4	Contributes to the formation of the pelvic floor, which supports the pelvic viscera; pulls the coccyx forward after defecation

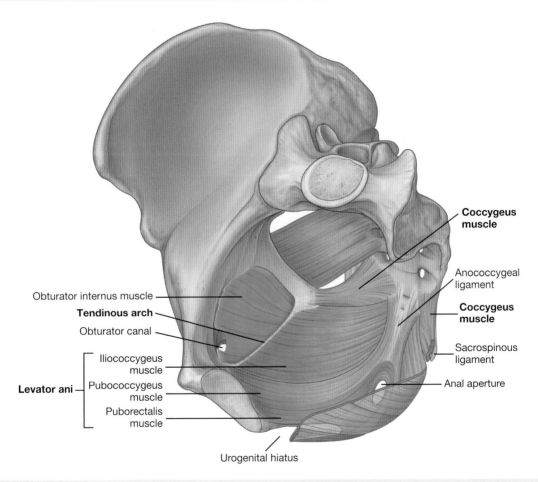

Fig. 5.16 Pelvic diaphragm.

The pelvic diaphragm

The pelvic diaphragm is the muscular part of the pelvic floor. Shaped like a bowl or funnel and attached superiorly to the pelvic walls, it consists of the levator ani and the coccygeus muscles (Table 5.2, Fig. 5.16).

The pelvic diaphragm's circular line of attachment to the cylindrical pelvic wall passes, on each side, between the greater sciatic foramen and the lesser sciatic foramen. Thus:

- the greater sciatic foramen is situated above the level of the pelvic floor and is a route of communication between

the pelvic cavity and the gluteal region of the lower limb; and

- the lesser sciatic foramen is situated below the pelvic floor, providing a route of communication between the gluteal region of the lower limb and the perineum.

Levator ani

The two levator ani muscles originate from each side of the pelvic wall, course medially and inferiorly, and join together in the midline. The attachment to the pelvic wall follows the circular contour of the wall and includes (Fig. 5.16):

- the posterior aspect of the body of the pubic bone,
- a linear thickening called the **tendinous arch** in the fascia covering the obturator internus muscle, and
- the spine of the ischium.

At the midline, the muscles blend together posterior to the vagina in women and around the anal aperture in both sexes. Posterior to the anal aperture, the muscles come together as a ligament or raphe called the **anococcygeal ligament (anococcygeal body)** and attaches to the coccyx (Fig. 5.16). Anteriorly, the muscles are separated by a U-shaped defect or gap termed the **urogenital hiatus.** The margins of this hiatus merge with the walls of the associated viscera and with muscles in the deep perineal pouch below. The hiatus allows the urethra (in both men and women) and the vagina (in women) to pass through the pelvic diaphragm (Fig. 5.16).

The levator ani muscles are divided into at least three collections of muscle fibers based on site of origin and relationship to viscera in the midline: the pubococcygeus, the puborectalis, and the iliococcygeus muscles (Fig. 5.16).

- The **pubococcygeus** originates from the body of the pubis and courses posteriorly to attach along the midline as far back as the coccyx. This part of the muscle is further subdivided on the basis of association with structures in the midline into the **puboprostaticus (levator prostatae),** the **pubovaginalis,** and the **puboanalis muscles.**
- A second major collection of muscle fibers, the **puborectalis** portion of the levator ani muscles, originates, in association with the pubococcygeus muscle, from the pubis and passes inferiorly on each side to form a sling around the terminal part of the gastrointestinal tract. This muscular sling maintains an angle or flexure, called the **perineal flexure,** at the anorectal junction. This angle functions as part of the mechanism that keeps the end of the gastrointestinal system closed.
- The final part of the levator ani muscle is the **iliococcygeus.** This part of the muscle originates from the fascia that covers the obturator internus muscle. It joins the same muscle on the other side in the midline to form a ligament or raphe that extends from the anal aperture to the coccyx.

The levator ani muscles help support the pelvic viscera and maintain closure of the rectum and vagina.

Clinical app

Defecation

At the beginning of defecation, closure of the larynx stabilizes the diaphragm and intra-abdominal pressure is increased by contraction of abdominal wall muscles. As defecation proceeds, the puborectalis muscle surrounding the anorectal junction relaxes, which straightens the anorectal angle. Both the internal and the external anal sphincters also relax to allow feces to move through the anal canal. Normally, the puborectal sling maintains an angle of about 90° between the rectum and the anal canal and acts as a "pinch valve" to prevent defecation. When the puborectalis muscle relaxes, the anorectal angle increases to about 130° to 140°.

The fatty tissue of the ischio-anal fossa allows for changes in the position and size of the anal canal and anus during defecation. During evacuation, the anorectal junction moves down and back and the pelvic floor usually descends slightly.

During defecation, the circular muscles of the rectal wall undergo a wave of contraction to push feces toward the anus. As feces emerge from the anus, the longitudinal muscles of the rectum and levator ani bring the anal canal back up, the feces are expelled, and the anus and rectum return to their normal positions.

The perineal membrane and deep perineal pouch

The **perineal membrane** is a thick fascial, triangular structure attached to the bony framework of the pubic arch (Fig. 5.17A). It is oriented in the horizontal plane and has a free posterior margin. Anteriorly, there is a small gap between the membrane and the **inferior pubic ligament** (a ligament associated with the pubic symphysis).

The perineal membrane is related above to a thin space called the **deep perineal pouch (deep perineal space)** (Fig. 5.17B) which contains a layer of skeletal muscle and various neurovascular elements.

The deep perineal pouch is open above and is not separated from more superior structures by a distinct layer of fascia. The parts of perineal membrane and structures in the deep perineal pouch, enclosed by the urogenital hiatus above therefore contribute to the pelvic floor and support elements of the urogenital system in the pelvic cavity, even though the perineal membrane and deep perineal pouch are usually considered parts of the perineum.

The perineal membrane and adjacent pubic arch provide attachment for the roots of the external genitalia and the muscles associated with them (Fig. 5.17C).

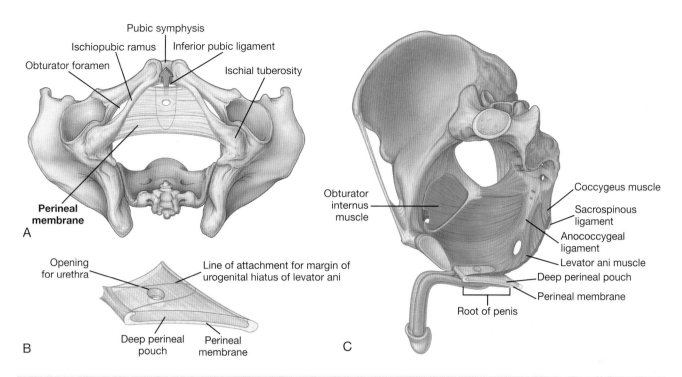

Fig. 5.17 Perineal membrane and deep perineal pouch. **A.** Inferior view. **B.** Superolateral view. **C.** Medial view.

Table 5.3 Muscles within the deep perineal pouch

Muscles	Origin	Insertion	Innervation	Function
External urethral sphincter	From the inferior ramus of the pubis on each side and adjacent walls of the deep perineal pouch	Surrounds membranous part of urethra	Perineal branches of the pudendal nerve (S2 to S4)	Compresses the membranous urethra; relaxes during micturition
Deep transverse perineal	Medial aspect of ischial ramus	Perineal body	Perineal branches of the pudendal nerve (S2 to S4)	Stabilizes the position of the perineal body
Compressor urethrae (in women only)	Ischiopubic ramus on each side	Blends with partner on other side anterior to the urethra	Perineal branches of the pudendal nerve (S2 to S4)	Functions as an accessory sphincter of the urethra
Sphincter urethrovaginalis (in women only)	Perineal body	Passes forward lateral to the vagina to blend with partner on other side anterior to the urethra	Perineal branches of the pudendal nerve (S2 to S4)	Functions as an accessory sphincter of the urethra (also may facilitate closing the vagina)

The urethra penetrates vertically through a circular hiatus in the perineal membrane as it passes from the pelvic cavity above to the perineum below. In women, the vagina also passes through a hiatus in the perineal membrane just posterior to the urethral hiatus.

Within the deep perineal pouch, a sheet of skeletal muscle functions as a sphincter, mainly for the urethra, and as a stabilizer of the posterior edge of the perineal membrane (Table 5.3, Fig. 5.18).

- Anteriorly, a group of muscle fibers surround the urethra and collectively form the **external urethral sphincter** (Fig. 5.18).

- Two additional groups of muscle fibers are associated with the urethra and vagina in women (Fig. 5.18A). One group forms the **sphincter urethrovaginalis,** which surrounds the urethra and vagina as a unit. The second group forms the **compressor urethrae** on each side, which originate from the ischiopubic rami and meet anterior to the urethra. Together with the external urethral sphincter, the sphincter urethrovaginalis and compressor urethrae facilitate closing of the urethra.

- In both men and women, a **deep transverse perineal muscle** on each side parallels the free margin of the perineal membrane and joins with its partner at the midline. These muscles are thought to stabilize the position of the perineal body, which is a midline structure along the posterior edge of the perineal membrane.

Perineal body

The perineal body is an ill-defined but important connective tissue structure into which muscles of the pelvic floor and the perineum attach (Fig. 5.19). It is positioned in the midline along the posterior border of the perineal membrane to which it attaches. The posterior end of the urogenital hiatus in the levator ani muscles is also connected to it.

The deep transverse perineal muscles intersect at the perineal body; in women, the sphincter urethrovaginalis also attaches to the perineal body. Other muscles that connect to the perineal body include the external anal sphincter, the superficial transverse perineal muscles, and the bulbospongiosus muscles of the perineum.

Clinical app

Episiotomy

During childbirth the perineal body may be stretched and torn. Traditionally it was felt that if a perineal tear is likely, the obstetrician may proceed with an episiotomy. This is a procedure in which an incision is made in the perineal body to allow the head of the fetus to pass through the vagina. There are two types of episiotomies: a median episiotomy cuts through the perineal body, while a mediolateral episiotomy is an incision 45° from the midline. The maternal benefits of this procedure have been thought to be less trauma to the perineum and decreased pelvic floor dysfunction. However, more recent evidence suggests that an episiotomy should not be performed routinely. Review of data has failed to show a decrease in pelvic floor damage with routine use of episiotomies.

Viscera

The pelvic viscera include parts of the gastrointestinal system, the urinary system, and the reproductive system. The viscera are arranged in the midline, from front to back; the neurovascular supply is through branches that pass medially from vessels and nerves associated with the pelvic walls.

Gastrointestinal system

Pelvic parts of the gastrointestinal system consist mainly of the rectum and the anal canal, although the terminal part of the sigmoid colon is also in the pelvic cavity (Fig. 5.20).

Rectum

The **rectum** is continuous:

- above, with the sigmoid colon at about the level of vertebra SIII; and
- below, with the anal canal as this structure penetrates the pelvic floor and passes through the perineum to end as the anus.

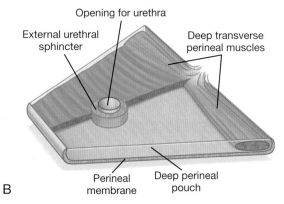

Fig. 5.18 Muscles in the deep perineal pouch. **A.** In women. **B.** In men.

Fig. 5.19 Perineal body.

The rectum, the most posterior element of the pelvic viscera, is immediately anterior to and follows the concave contour of the sacrum (Fig. 5.20A).

The anorectal junction is pulled forward (perineal flexure) by the action of the puborectalis part of the levator ani muscle, so the anal canal moves in a posterior direction as it passes inferiorly through the pelvic floor.

In addition to conforming to the general curvature of the sacrum in the anteroposterior plane, the rectum has three lateral curvatures; the upper and lower curvatures to the right and the middle curvature to the left. The lower part of the rectum is expanded to form the **rectal ampulla.** Finally, unlike the colon, the rectum lacks distinct taeniae coli muscles, omental appendices, and sacculations (haustra of the colon).

Clinical app

Digital rectal examination

A digital rectal examination (DRE) is performed by placing the gloved and lubricated index finger into the rectum through the anus. The anal mucosa can be palpated for abnormal masses, and in women, the posterior wall of the vagina and the cervix can be palpated. In men, the prostate can be evaluated for any extraneous nodules or masses. In persons who have undergone vaginoplasty, such as is common with transgender women, the prostate is not removed and the vaginal cavity is constructed between the prostate and rectum. The examination of the prostate in these individuals is easier to palpate transvaginally, along the anterior wall of the vagina, rather than rectally.

Anal canal

The **anal canal** begins at the terminal end of the rectal ampulla where it narrows at the pelvic floor (Fig. 5.20B). It terminates as the anus after passing through the perineum. As it passes through the pelvic floor, the anal canal is surrounded along its entire length by the internal and external anal sphincters, which normally keep it closed (Fig. 5.20B).

The lining of the anal canal bears a number of characteristic structural features that reflect the approximate position of the anococcygeal membrane in the fetus (which closes the terminal end of the developing gastrointestinal system in the fetus) and the transition from gastrointestinal mucosa to skin in the adult (Fig. 5.20B).

- The upper part of the anal canal is lined by mucosa similar to that lining the rectum and is distinguished by a number of longitudinally oriented folds known as **anal columns,** which are united inferiorly by crescentic folds termed **anal valves.** Superior to each valve is a depression termed an **anal sinus.** The anal valves together form a circle around the anal canal at a location known as the **pectinate line,** which marks the approximate position of the anal membrane in the fetus.
- Inferior to the pectinate line is a transition zone known as the *anal pecten,* which is lined by nonkeratinized, stratified,

squamous epithelium. The anal pecten ends inferiorly at the anocutaneous line ("white line"), or where the lining of the anal canal becomes true skin.

Clinical app

Carcinoma of the colon and rectum

Carcinoma of the colon and rectum (colorectum) is a common disease.

Given the position of the colon and rectum in the abdominopelvic cavity and its proximity to other organs, it is extremely important to accurately stage colorectal tumors: a tumor in the pelvis, for example, could invade the uterus or bladder.

Urinary system

The pelvic parts of the urinary system consist of the terminal parts of the ureters, the bladder, and the proximal part of the urethra (Fig. 5.21).

Ureters

The ureters enter the pelvic cavity from the abdomen by passing through the pelvic inlet (Fig. 5.21). On each side, the ureter crosses the pelvic inlet and enters the pelvic cavity in the area anterior to the bifurcation of the common iliac artery. From this point, it continues along the pelvic wall and floor to join the base of the bladder.

In the pelvis, the ureter is crossed by:

- the ductus deferens in men, and
- the uterine artery in women.

Bladder

The bladder is the most anterior element of the pelvic viscera. Although it is entirely situated in the pelvic cavity when empty, it expands superiorly into the abdominal cavity when full (Fig. 5.21).

The empty bladder is shaped like a three-sided pyramid that has tipped over to lie on one of its margins (Fig. 5.22A). It has an apex, a base, a superior surface, and two inferolateral surfaces (Fig. 5.22A).

- The **apex** of the bladder is directed toward the top of the pubic symphysis; a structure known as the **median umbilical ligament** (a remnant of the embryological urachus that contributes to the formation of the bladder) continues from it superiorly up the anterior abdominal wall to the umbilicus.
- The **base** of the bladder is shaped like an inverted triangle and faces posteroinferiorly. The two ureters enter the

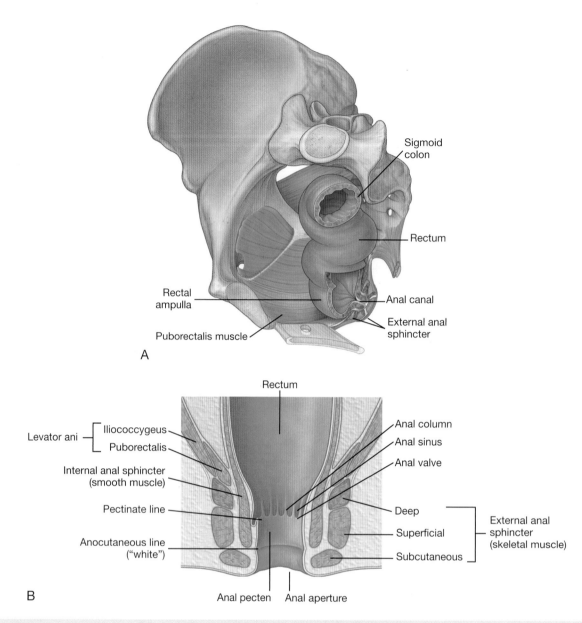

Fig. 5.20 Rectum and anal canal. A. Left pelvic bone removed. **B.** Longitudinal section.

bladder at each of the upper corners of the base, and the urethra drains inferiorly from the lower corner of the base (Fig. 5.22A, B). Inside, the mucosal lining on the base of the bladder is smooth and firmly attached to the underlying smooth muscle coat of the wall—unlike elsewhere in the bladder in which the mucosa is folded and loosely attached to the wall. The smooth triangular area between the openings of the ureters and urethra on the inside of the bladder is known as the **trigone** (Fig. 5.22B).

■ The **inferolateral surfaces** of the bladder are cradled between the levator ani muscles of the pelvic diaphragm and the adjacent obturator internus muscles above the attachment of the pelvic diaphragm. The superior surface is slightly domed when the bladder is empty; it balloons upward as the bladder fills.

Neck of bladder

The neck of the bladder surrounds the origin of the urethra at the point where the two inferolateral surfaces and the base intersect (see Fig. 5.21).

The neck is the most inferior part of the bladder and the most "fixed" part. It is anchored into position by a pair of tough fibromuscular bands, which connect the neck and pelvic part of the urethra to the posteroinferior aspect of each pubic bone.

■ In women, these fibromuscular bands are termed **pubovesical ligaments** (Fig. 5.23A). Together with the perineal membrane and associated muscles, the levator ani muscles, and the pubic bones, these ligaments help support the bladder.

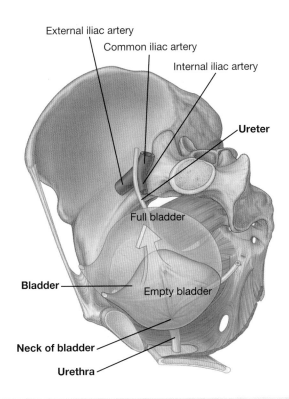

Fig. 5.21 Pelvic parts of the urinary system.

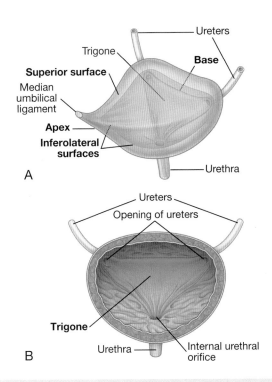

Fig. 5.22 Bladder. **A.** Superolateral view. **B.** The trigone. Anterior view with the anterior part of the bladder cut away.

■ In men, the paired fibromuscular bands are known as **puboprostatic ligaments** because they blend with the fibrous capsule of the prostate, which surrounds the neck of the bladder and adjacent part of the urethra (Fig. 5.23B).

Although the bladder is considered to be pelvic in the adult, it has a higher position in children. At birth, the bladder is almost entirely abdominal; the urethra begins approximately at the upper margin of the pubic symphysis. With age, the bladder descends until after puberty when it assumes the adult position.

Clinical app

Bladder cancer

Bladder cancer is the most common tumor of the urinary tract and is usually a disease of the sixth and seventh decades, although there is an increasing trend for younger patients to develop this disease.

Bladder tumors may spread through the bladder wall and invade local structures, including the rectum, uterus (in women), and the lateral walls of the pelvic cavity. Prostatic involvement is not uncommon in male patients.

Large bladder tumors may produce complications, including invasion and obstruction of the ureters. Ureteric obstruction can then obstruct the kidneys and induce kidney failure.

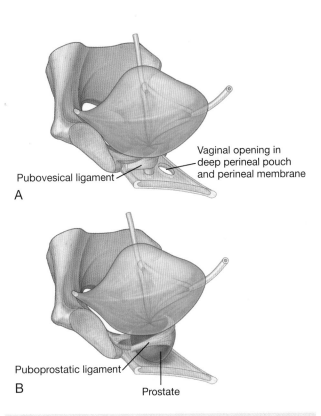

Fig. 5.23 Ligaments that anchor the neck of the bladder and pelvic part of the urethra to the pelvic bones. **A.** In women. **B.** In men.

Urethra

The urethra begins at the base of the bladder and ends with an external opening in the perineum. The paths taken by the urethra differ significantly in women and men.

In women

In women, the urethra is short, being about 4 cm long. It travels a slightly curved course as it passes inferiorly through the pelvic floor into the perineum where it passes through the deep perineal pouch and perineal membrane before opening in the vestibule that lies between the labia minora (Fig. 5.24A).

The urethral opening is anterior to the vaginal opening in the vestibule. The inferior aspect of the urethra is bound to the anterior surface of the vagina. Two small para-urethral mucous glands (**Skene's glands**) are associated with the lower end of the urethra. Each drains via a duct that opens onto the lateral margin of the external urethral orifice.

In men

In men, the urethra is long, about 20 cm, and bends twice along its course (Fig. 5.24B). Beginning at the base of the bladder and passing inferiorly through the prostate, it passes through the deep perineal pouch and perineal membrane and immediately enters the root of the penis. As the urethra exits the deep perineal pouch, it bends forward to course anteriorly in the root of the penis. When the penis is flaccid, the urethra makes another bend, this time inferiorly, when passing from the root to the body of the penis. During erection, the bend between the root and body of the penis disappears.

The urethra in men is divided into preprostatic, prostatic, membranous, and spongy parts (Fig. 5.24B).

Preprostatic part. The preprostatic part of the urethra is about 1 cm long, extends from the base of the bladder to the prostate, and is associated with a circular cuff of smooth muscle fibers (the **internal urethral sphincter**) (Fig. 5.24B). Contraction of this sphincter prevents retrograde movement of semen into the bladder during ejaculation.

Prostatic part. The prostatic part of the urethra (Fig. 5.24C) is 3 to 4 cm long and is surrounded by the prostate. In this region, the lumen of the urethra is marked by a longitudinal midline fold of mucosa (the **urethral crest**). The depression on each side of the crest is the **prostatic sinus;** the ducts of the prostate empty into these two sinuses.

Midway along its length, the urethral crest is enlarged to form a somewhat circular elevation (the seminal colliculus) (Fig. 5.24C). In men, the seminal colliculus is used to determine the position of the prostate gland during transurethral transection of the prostate.

A small blind-ended pouch—the **prostatic utricle** (thought to be the homologue of the uterus in women)—opens onto the center of the seminal colliculus (Fig. 5.24C). On each side of the prostatic utricle is the opening of the ejaculatory duct of the male reproductive system. Therefore the connection between the urinary and reproductive tracts in men occurs in the prostatic part of the urethra.

Membranous part. The membranous part of the urethra is narrow and passes through the deep perineal pouch (Fig. 5.24B). During its transit through this pouch, the urethra, in both men and women, is surrounded by skeletal muscle of the **external urethral sphincter.**

Spongy urethra. The spongy urethra is surrounded by erectile tissue (the **corpus spongiosum**) of the penis. It is enlarged to form a bulb at the base of the penis and again at the end of the penis to form the **navicular fossa** (Fig. 5.24B). The two bulbourethral glands in the deep perineal pouch are part of the male reproductive system and open into the bulb of the spongy urethra. The external urethral orifice is the sagittal slit at the end of the penis.

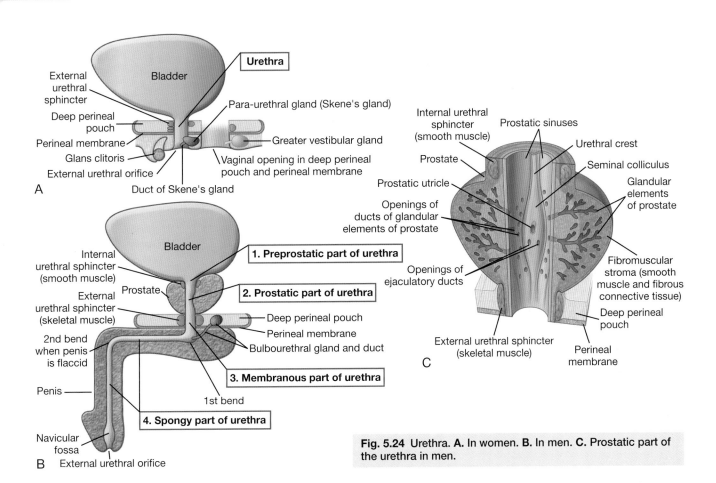

Fig. 5.24 Urethra. **A.** In women. **B.** In men. **C.** Prostatic part of the urethra in men.

Clinical app

Bladder infection

The relatively short length of the urethra in women makes them more susceptible than men to bladder infection. Similarly, transgender women who have undergone vaginoplasty will have a shortened urethra and are also at increased risk of urinary tract infection. Transgender men who have undergone metoidioplasty or phalloplasty will have lengthened urethras, but the neourethra lacks muscular and elastic tissue, reducing clearance of urine. This may also increase the risk of urinary tract infection. The primary symptoms of urinary tract infection in any individual is usually inflammation of the bladder (cystitis). In children younger than 1 year of age, infection from the bladder may spread via the ureters to the kidneys, where it can produce renal damage and ultimately lead to renal failure. Early diagnosis and treatment are necessary.

Reproductive system

In men

The reproductive system in men has components in the abdomen, pelvis, and perineum (Fig. 5.25A). The major

Clinical app

Urethral catheterization

Urethral catheterization is often performed to drain urine from a patient's bladder when the patient is unable to micturate. When inserting urinary catheters, it is important to appreciate the gender anatomy of the patient.

In men the spongy urethra angles superiorly to pass through the perineal membrane and into the pelvis. Just inferior to the perineal membrane, the wall of the urethral bulb is relatively thin and can be damaged when inserting catheters or doing cystoscopy. In women, these procedures are much simpler because the urethra is short and straight.

components are a testis, epididymis, ductus deferens, and ejaculatory duct on each side, and the urethra and penis in the midline. In addition, three types of accessory glands are associated with the system:

- a single prostate,
- a pair of seminal vesicles, and
- a pair of bulbourethral glands.

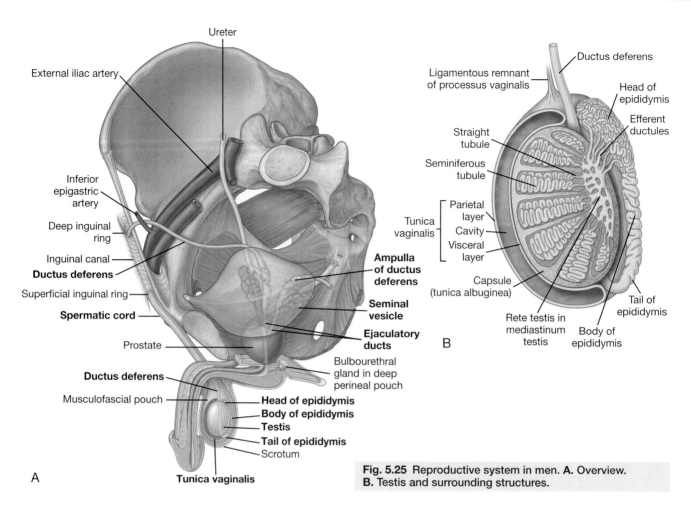

Fig. 5.25 Reproductive system in men. **A.** Overview. **B.** Testis and surrounding structures.

The design of the reproductive system in men is basically a series of ducts and tubules. The arrangement of parts and linkage to the urinary tract reflects its embryological development.

Testes

The **testes** originally develop high on the posterior abdominal wall and then descend, normally before birth, through the inguinal canal in the anterior abdominal wall and into the scrotum of the perineum. During descent, the testes carry their vessels, lymphatics, and nerves, as well as their principal drainage ducts, the **ductus deferens (vas deferens)** with them. The lymph drainage of the testes is therefore to the lateral aortic or lumbar nodes and pre-aortic nodes in the abdomen and not to the inguinal or pelvic lymph nodes.

Each ellipsoid-shaped testis is enclosed within the end of an elongated musculofascial pouch, which is continuous with the anterior abdominal wall and projects into the scrotum. The **spermatic cord** is the tube-shaped connection between the pouch in the scrotum and the abdominal wall (Fig. 5.25A).

The sides and anterior aspect of the testis are covered by a closed sac of peritoneum (the **tunica vaginalis**), which originally connected to the abdominal cavity (Fig. 5.25B).

Normally after testicular descent, the connection closes, leaving a fibrous remnant.

Each testis (Fig. 5.25B) is composed of seminiferous tubules and interstitial tissue surrounded by a thick connective tissue capsule (the **tunica albuginea**). Spermatozoa are produced by the seminiferous tubules. The 400 to 600 highly coiled seminiferous tubules are modified at each end to become straight tubules, which connect to a collecting chamber (the **rete testis**) in a thick, vertically oriented linear wedge of connective tissue (the **mediastinum testis**), projecting from the capsule into the posterior aspect of the

Clinical app

Undescended testes
Around the seventh month of gestation, the testes begin their descent from the posterior abdominal wall through the inguinal canal and into the scrotum. During the descent, the testes may arrest (undescended testes) or they may end up in an ectopic position. Undescended/ectopic testes are associated with infertility and increased risk of testicular tumors.

gonad (Fig. 5.25B). Approximately 12 to 20 **efferent ductules** originate from the upper end of the rete testis, penetrate the capsule, and connect with the epididymis.

Clinical app

Hydrocele of the testis
A hydrocele of the testis is an accumulation of fluid within the cavity of the tunica vaginalis. Hydroceles are typically unilateral and in most cases their cause is unknown, although they may occur secondary to physical trauma, infection, or tumor.

Clinical app

Testicular tumors
Tumors of the testis account for a small percentage of malignancies in men. However, they generally occur in younger patients (between 20 and 40 years of age).

Early diagnosis of testicular tumor is extremely important. Abnormal lumps can be detected by palpation and diagnosis can be made using ultrasound.

Surgical removal of the malignant testis is often carried out using an inguinal approach. The testis is not usually removed through a scrotal incision because it is possible to spread tumor cells into the subcutaneous tissues of the scrotum, which has a different lymphatic drainage than the testis.

Epididymis

The **epididymis** is a single, long coiled duct that courses along the posterolateral side of the testis (Fig. 5.25B). It has two distinct components:

- the **efferent ductules,** which form an enlarged coiled mass that sits on the posterior superior pole of the testis and forms the **head of the epididymis;** and
- the **true epididymis,** which is a single, long, coiled duct into which the efferent ductules all drain and that continues inferiorly along the posterolateral margin of the testis as the **body of epididymis** and enlarges to form the **tail of epididymis** at the inferior pole of the testis.

During passage through the epididymis, spermatozoa acquire the ability to move and fertilize an egg. The epididymis also stores spermatozoa until ejaculation. The end of the epididymis is continuous with the ductus deferens.

Ductus deferens

The ductus deferens is a long muscular duct that transports spermatozoa from the tail of the epididymis in the scrotum to the ejaculatory duct in the pelvic cavity (Fig. 5.25A). It ascends in the scrotum as a component of the spermatic cord and passes through the inguinal canal in the anterior abdominal wall.

After passing through the deep inguinal ring, the ductus deferens bends medially around the lateral side of the inferior epigastric artery and crosses the external iliac artery and the external iliac vein at the pelvic inlet to enter the pelvic cavity (Fig. 5.25A).

The duct descends medially on the pelvic wall deep to the peritoneum and crosses the ureter posterior to the bladder. It continues inferomedially along the base of the bladder, anterior to the rectum, almost to the midline where it is joined by the duct of the seminal vesicle to form the ejaculatory duct (Fig. 5.25A).

Between the ureter and ejaculatory duct, the ductus deferens expands to form the ampulla of the ductus deferens. The ejaculatory duct penetrates through the prostate gland to connect with the prostatic urethra.

Clinical app

Vasectomy
The ductus deferens transports spermatozoa from the tail of the epididymis in the scrotum to the ejaculatory duct in the pelvic cavity. Because it has a thick smooth muscle wall, it can be easily palpated in the spermatic cord between the testes and the superficial inguinal ring. Also, because it can be accessed through skin and superficial fascia, it is amenable to surgical dissection and surgical division. When this is carried out bilaterally (vasectomy), the patient is rendered sterile—this is a useful method for male contraception.

Seminal vesicle

Each **seminal vesicle** is an accessory gland of the male reproductive system that develops as a blind-ended tubular outgrowth from the ductus deferens (Fig. 5.25A). The tube is coiled with numerous pocket-like outgrowths and is encapsulated by connective tissue to form an elongate structure situated between the bladder and rectum. The gland is immediately lateral to and follows the course of the ductus deferens at the base of the bladder.

The duct of the seminal vesicle joins the ductus deferens to form the **ejaculatory duct** (Fig. 5.25A). Secretions from the seminal vesicle contribute significantly to the volume of the ejaculate (semen).

Prostate

The **prostate** is an unpaired accessory structure of the male reproductive system that surrounds the urethra in the pelvic cavity (Fig. 5.25A). It lies immediately inferior to the bladder, posterior to the pubic symphysis, and anterior to the rectum.

The prostate is shaped like an inverted rounded cone with a larger base, which is continuous above with the neck of the bladder, and a narrower apex, which rests below on the pelvic floor. The inferolateral surfaces of the prostate are in contact with the levator ani muscles that together cradle the prostate between them.

The prostate develops as 30 to 40 individual complex glands, which grow from the urethral epithelium into the surrounding wall of the urethra. Collectively, these glands enlarge the wall of the urethra into what is known as the *prostate;* however, the individual glands retain their own ducts, which empty independently into the prostatic sinuses on the posterior aspect of the urethral lumen.

Secretions from the prostate, together with secretions from the seminal vesicles, contribute to the formation of semen during ejaculation.

The ejaculatory ducts pass almost vertically in an antero-inferior direction through the posterior aspect of the prostate to open into the prostatic urethra.

Clinical app

Prostate problems

Prostate cancer is one of the most commonly diagnosed malignancies in men, and often the disease is advanced at diagnosis. Prostate cancer typically occurs in the peripheral regions of the prostate and is relatively asymptomatic. In many cases it is diagnosed by either a digital rectal examination (cisgender men) or transvaginal examination (trasngender women having undergone vaginoplasty). Blood tests, which include serum acid phosphatase and serum prostate-specific antigen (PSA), are also used. Prostate volume and PSA is decreased with androgen suppression in transgender individuals on testosterone blockers. In rectal examinations, the tumorous prostate feels "rock" hard. The diagnosis is usually made by obtaining a number of biopsies of the prostate.

Benign prostatic hypertrophy is a disease of the prostate that occurs with increasing age in most men (Fig. 5.26). It generally involves the more central regions of the prostate, which gradually

Central zone of prostate   Pubic symphysis   Peripheral zone of prostate

Rectum   Obturator internus muscle

Fig. 5.26 Axial T2-weighted magnetic resonance image of benign prostatic hypertrophy.

enlarge. The prostate feels "bulky" on digital rectal examination. Owing to the more central hypertrophic change of the prostate, the urethra is compressed, and a urinary outflow obstruction develops in a number of patients. With time, the bladder may become hypertrophied in response to the urinary outflow obstruction. In some male patients, the obstruction becomes so severe that urine cannot be passed and transurethral or suprapubic catheterization is necessary. Despite being a benign disease, benign prostatic hypertrophy can therefore have a marked effect on the daily lives of many patients.

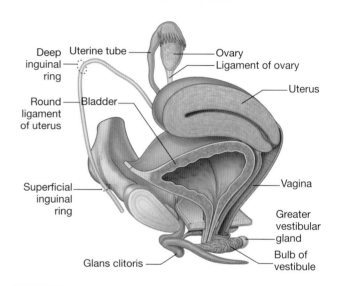

Deep inguinal ring — Uterine tube — Ovary — Ligament of ovary — Uterus

Round ligament of uterus — Bladder

Superficial inguinal ring — Vagina

Glans clitoris — Greater vestibular gland — Bulb of vestibule

Fig. 5.27 Reproductive system in women.

Bulbourethral glands

The **bulbourethral glands** (see Fig. 5.25A), one on each side, are small, pea-shaped mucous glands situated within the deep perineal pouch. They are lateral to the membranous part of the urethra. The duct from each gland passes infero-medially through the **perineal membrane** to open into the bulb of the spongy urethra at the root of the penis.

Together with small glands positioned along the length of the spongy urethra, the bulbourethral glands contribute to lubrication of the urethra and the pre-ejaculatory emission from the penis.

In women

The reproductive tract in women is contained mainly in the pelvic cavity and perineum, although during pregnancy, the uterus expands into the abdomen cavity. Major components of the system consist of (Fig. 5.27):

- an ovary on each side and
- a uterus, vagina, and clitoris in the midline.

In addition, a pair of accessory glands (the **greater vestibular glands**) are associated with the tract.

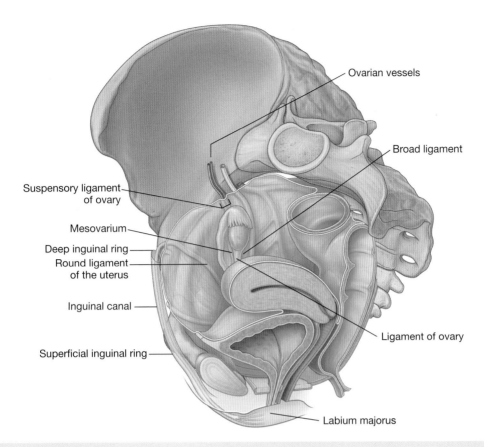

Ovarian vessels

Broad ligament

Suspensory ligament of ovary

Mesovarium

Deep inguinal ring

Round ligament of the uterus

Inguinal canal

Superficial inguinal ring

Ligament of ovary

Labium majorus

Fig. 5.28 Ovaries and broad ligament.

Ovaries

Like the testes in men, the **ovaries** develop high on the posterior abdominal wall and then descend before birth, bringing with them their vessels, lymphatics, and nerves. Unlike the testes, the ovaries do not migrate through the inguinal canal into the perineum but stop short and assume a position on the lateral wall of the pelvic cavity (Fig. 5.28).

The ovaries are the sites of egg production (oogenesis). Mature eggs are ovulated into the peritoneal cavity and normally directed into the adjacent openings of the uterine tubes by cilia on the ends of the uterine tubes.

Clinical app

Ovarian cancer

Ovarian cancer remains one of the major challenges in oncology. The ovaries contain numerous cell types, all of which can undergo malignant change and require different imaging and treatment protocols and ultimately have different prognoses. Ovarian cancer may occur at any age, but more typically it occurs in older women.

Many factors have been linked with the development of ovarian tumors, including a strong family history.

Cancer of the ovaries may spread via the blood and lymphatics and frequently metastasizes directly into the peritoneal cavity. Such direct peritoneal cavity spread allows the passage of tumor cells along the paracolic gutters and over the liver from where this disease may disseminate easily. Unfortunately, many patients already have metastatic and diffuse disease at the time of diagnosis. It is important to note that one or both ovaries may either be removed (oophorectomy) or retained in transgender men or nonbinary people as part of a spectrum of gender-affirming procedures. In any individual with ovaries, ovarian cancer risk remains and an investigation should proceed if deemed clinically appropriate. For cisgendered women, ovaries are imaged by transvaginal ultrasound. In those patients in whom vaginectomy has been performed (removal of the vagina) and an ultrasound is indicated, imaging can be done either transrectally or transabdominally.

The ovaries lie adjacent to the lateral pelvic wall just inferior to the pelvic inlet. Each of the two almond-shaped ovaries is about 3 cm long and is suspended by a mesentery (the **mesovarium**) that is a posterior extension of the broad ligament.

Uterus

The **uterus** is a thick-walled muscular organ in the midline between the bladder and rectum (see Fig. 5.28). It consists of a body and a cervix, and inferiorly it joins the vagina (Fig. 5.29). Superiorly, uterine tubes project laterally from the uterus and open into the peritoneal cavity immediately adjacent to the ovaries (Fig. 5.29).

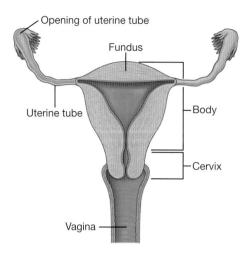

Fig. 5.29 Uterus. Anterior view. The anterior half of the uterus and vagina have been cut away.

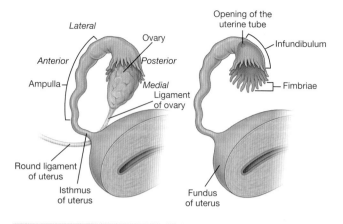

Fig. 5.30 Uterine tubes.

The body of the uterus is flattened anteroposteriorly and, above the level of origin of the uterine tubes (Fig. 5.29), has a rounded superior end **(fundus of uterus).** The cavity of the body of the uterus is a narrow slit when viewed laterally and is shaped like an inverted triangle when viewed anteriorly. Each of the superior corners of the cavity is continuous with the lumen of a uterine tube and the inferior corner is continuous with the central canal of the cervix.

Clinical app

Hysterectomy

A hysterectomy is the surgical removal of the uterus. This is usually a complete excision of the body, fundus, and cervix of the uterus, though occasionally the cervix may be left in situ. In some instances the uterine (fallopian) tubes and the ovaries also are removed. This procedure is called a *total abdominal hysterectomy* and *bilateral salpingo-oophorectomy*.

Hysterectomy, oophorectomy, and salpingo-oophorectomy may be performed in patients who have reproductive malignancy, such as uterine, cervical, and ovarian cancers. Other indications include strong family history of reproductive disorders, endometriosis, and excessive bleeding. Occasionally the uterus may need to be removed postpartum because of excessive postpartum bleeding. Hysterectomy is also indicated in transgender men who desire the procedure as a component of the gender-affirming process.

A hysterectomy is performed through a transverse suprapubic incision (Pfannenstiel's incision). During the procedure, tremendous care is taken to identify the distal ureters and to ligate the nearby uterine arteries without damage to the ureters.

Implantation of the blastocyst normally occurs in the body of the uterus. During pregnancy, the uterus dramatically expands superiorly into the abdominal cavity.

Uterine tubes

The **uterine tubes** extend from each side of the superior end of the body of the uterus to the lateral pelvic wall and are enclosed within the upper margins of the mesosalpinx portions of the broad ligaments. Because the ovaries are suspended from the posterior aspect of the broad ligaments, the uterine tubes pass superiorly over, and terminate laterally to, the ovaries.

Each uterine tube has an expanded trumpet-shaped end (the **infundibulum**), which curves around the superolateral pole of the related ovary (Fig. 5.30). The margin of the infundibulum is rimmed with small finger-like projections termed **fimbriae.** The lumen of the uterine tube opens into the peritoneal cavity at the narrowed end of the infundibulum. Medial to the infundibulum, the tube expands to form the **ampulla** and then narrows to form the **isthmus** before joining with the body of the uterus (Fig. 5.30).

The fimbriated infundibulum facilitates the collection of ovulated eggs from the ovary. Fertilization normally occurs in the ampulla.

Clinical app

Tubal ligation

A simple and effective method of birth control is to surgically ligate (clip) the uterine tubes, preventing spermatozoa from reaching the ampulla.

Cervix

The **cervix** forms the inferior part of the uterus and is shaped like a short, broad cylinder with a narrow central channel. The body of the uterus normally arches forward (anteflexed on the cervix) over the superior surface of the emptied bladder (Fig. 5.31A). In addition, the cervix is angled forward (anteverted) on the vagina so that the inferior end of the cervix projects into the upper anterior aspect of the vagina (Figs. 5.31A, 5.32). Because the end of the cervix is dome shaped, it bulges into the vagina, and a gutter, or fornix, is formed around the margin of the cervix where it joins the vaginal wall (Fig. 5.31B). The tubular central canal of the cervix opens below as the **external os** into the vaginal cavity and above as the **internal os** into the uterine cavity (Fig. 5.31B).

Clinical app

Carcinoma of the cervix and uterus

Carcinoma of the cervix and uterus is a common disease in any individual with a cervix and uterus, including women, transgender men, and some non-binary people who have not had a hysterectomy. Diagnosis is by inspection, cytology (examination of the cervical cells), imaging, biopsy, and dilatation and curettage (D&C) of the uterus.

Carcinoma of the cervix and uterus may be treated by local resection, removal of the uterus (hysterectomy), and adjuvant chemotherapy. The tumor spreads via lymphatics to the internal and common iliac lymph nodes.

Vagina

The **vagina** is the copulatory organ in women. It is a distensible fibromuscular tube that extends from the perineum through the pelvic floor and into the pelvic cavity (Fig. 5.32A). The internal end of the canal is enlarged to form a region called the **vaginal vault.**

The anterior wall of the vagina is related to the base of the bladder and to the urethra; in fact, the urethra is embedded in, or fused to, the anterior vaginal wall (Fig. 5.32A).

Posteriorly, the vagina is related principally to the rectum.

Inferiorly, the vagina opens into the vestibule of the perineum immediately posterior to the external opening of the urethra. From its external opening (the **introitus**), the vagina courses posterosuperiorly through the perineal membrane and into the pelvic cavity where it is attached by its anterior wall to the circular margin of the cervix.

The **vaginal fornix** is the recess formed between the margin of the cervix and the vaginal wall. Based on position, the fornix is subdivided into a posterior fornix, an anterior fornix, and two lateral fornices (Figs. 5.31B, 5.32B).

The vaginal canal is normally collapsed so that the anterior wall is in contact with the posterior wall. By using a speculum to open the vaginal canal, a physician can see the domed inferior end of the cervix, the vaginal fornices, and the external os of the cervical canal in a patient (Fig. 5.32B).

During intercourse, semen is deposited in the vaginal vault. Spermatozoa make their way into the external os of the cervical canal, pass through the cervical canal into the

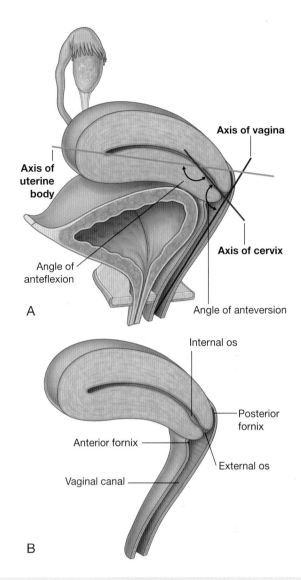

Fig. 5.31 Uterus and vagina. **A.** Angles of anteflexion and anteversion. **B.** The cervix protrudes into the vagina.

uterine cavity, and then continue through the uterine cavity into the uterine tubes.

Fascia

Fascia in the pelvic cavity lines the pelvic walls, surrounds the bases of the pelvic viscera, and forms sheaths around blood vessels and nerves that course medially from the pelvic walls to reach the viscera in the midline. This pelvic fascia is a continuation of the extraperitoneal connective tissue layer found in the abdomen.

In women

In women, a **rectovaginal septum** separates the posterior surface of the vagina from the rectum (Fig. 5.33A). Condensations of fascia form ligaments that extend from the cervix to the anterior (**pubocervical ligament)**, lateral

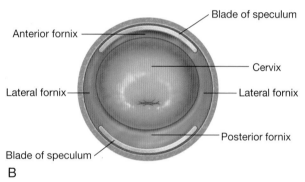

Fig. 5.32 Vagina. **A.** Left half of pelvis cut away. **B.** Vaginal fornices and cervix as viewed through a speculum.

(transverse cervical or **cardinal ligament),** and posterior **(uterosacral ligament)** pelvic walls. These ligaments, together with the perineal membrane, the levator ani muscles, and the perineal body are thought to stabilize the uterus in the pelvic cavity. The most important of these ligaments are the transverse cervical or cardinal ligaments, which extend laterally from each side of the cervix and vaginal vault to the related pelvic wall.

In men

In men, a condensation of fascia around the anterior and lateral region of the prostate **(prostatic fascia)** contains and surrounds the prostatic plexus of veins and is continuous posteriorly with the **rectovesical septum,** which separates the posterior surface of the prostate and base of the bladder from the rectum (Fig. 5.33B).

Peritoneum

The peritoneum of the pelvis is continuous at the pelvic inlet with the peritoneum of the abdomen. In the pelvis, the peritoneum drapes over the pelvic viscera in the midline, forming:

- pouches between adjacent viscera, and
- folds and ligaments between viscera and pelvic walls.

Anteriorly, median and medial umbilical folds of peritoneum cover the embryological remnants of the urachus and umbilical arteries, respectively (Fig. 5.34). These folds

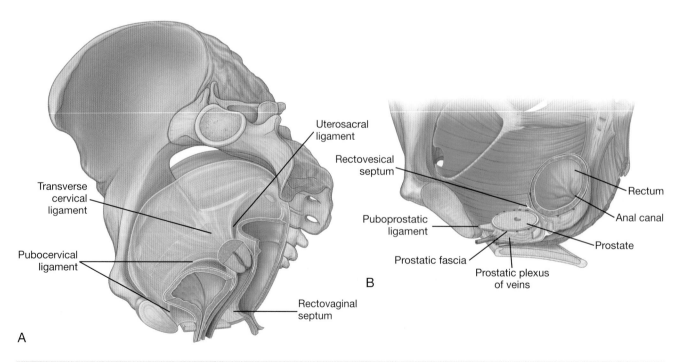

Fig. 5.33 Pelvic fascia. **A.** In women. **B.** In men.

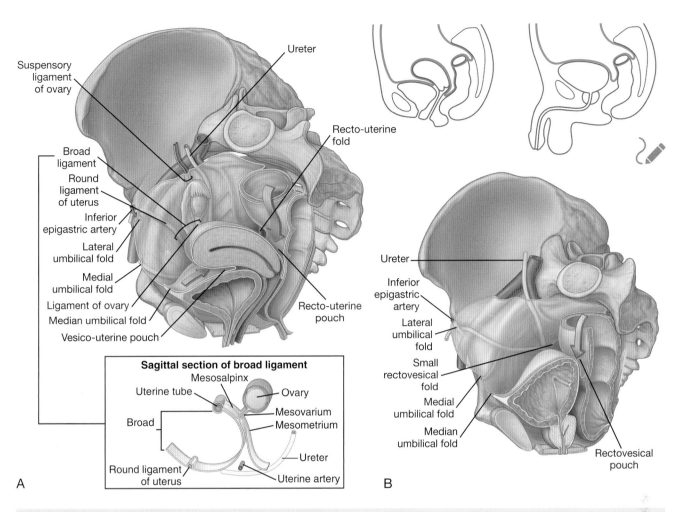

Fig. 5.34 Peritoneum in the pelvis. **A.** In women. **B.** In men.

ascend out of the pelvis and onto the anterior abdominal wall. Posteriorly, peritoneum drapes over the anterior and lateral aspects of the upper third of the rectum, but only the anterior surface of the middle third of the rectum is covered by peritoneum; the lower third of the rectum is not covered at all.

In women

In women, the uterus lies between the bladder and rectum, and the uterine tubes extend from the superior aspect of the uterus to the lateral pelvic walls (Fig. 5.34A). As a consequence, a shallow **vesico-uterine pouch** occurs anteriorly, between the bladder and uterus, and a deep **recto-uterine pouch** (pouch of Douglas) occurs posteriorly between the uterus and rectum. In addition, a large fold of peritoneum (the broad ligament), with a uterine tube enclosed in its superior margin and an ovary attached posteriorly, is located on each side of the uterus and extends to the lateral pelvic walls.

In the midline, the peritoneum descends over the posterior surface of the uterus and cervix and onto the vaginal wall adjacent to the posterior vaginal fornix. It then reflects onto the anterior and lateral walls of the rectum. The deep pouch of peritoneum formed between the anterior surface of the rectum and posterior surfaces of the uterus, cervix, and vagina is the recto-uterine pouch. A sharp sickle-shaped ridge of peritoneum (**recto-uterine fold**) occurs on each side near the base of the recto-uterine pouch. The **recto-uterine folds** overlie the **uterosacral ligaments,** which are condensations of pelvic fascia that extend from the cervix to the posterolateral pelvic walls.

Broad ligament

The **broad ligament** is a sheet-like fold of peritoneum oriented in the coronal plane that runs from the lateral pelvic wall to the uterus, encloses the uterine tube in its superior margin, and suspends the ovary from its posterior aspect (Fig. 5.34). The uterine arteries cross the ureters at the base of the broad ligaments, and the ligament of the ovary and round ligament of the uterus are enclosed within the parts of the broad ligament related to the ovary and uterus, respectively. The broad ligament has three parts (Fig. 5.34A):

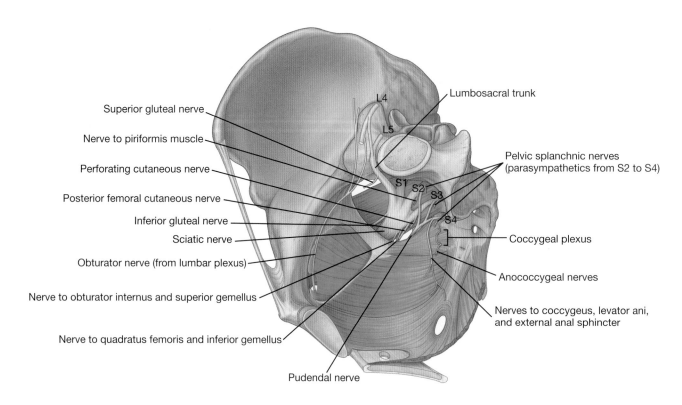

Superior gluteal nerve

Nerve to piriformis muscle

Perforating cutaneous nerve

Posterior femoral cutaneous nerve

Inferior gluteal nerve

Sciatic nerve

Obturator nerve (from lumbar plexus)

Nerve to obturator internus and superior gemellus

Nerve to quadratus femoris and inferior gemellus

Pudendal nerve

L4

L5

Lumbosacral trunk

S1 S2 S3

S4

Pelvic splanchnic nerves (parasympathetics from S2 to S4)

Coccygeal plexus

Anococcygeal nerves

Nerves to coccygeus, levator ani, and external anal sphincter

Fig. 5.35 Sacral and coccygeal plexuses.

- the **mesometrium,** the largest part of the broad ligament, which extends from the lateral pelvic walls to the body of the uterus;
- the **mesosalpinx,** the most superior part of the broad ligament, which suspends the uterine tube in the pelvic cavity; and
- the **mesovarium,** a posterior extension of the broad ligament, which attaches to the ovary.

The peritoneum of the mesovarium is continuous with the ovarian surface (germinal) epithelium (Fig. 5.34A). The ovaries are positioned with their long axis in the vertical plane. The ovarian vessels, nerves, and lymphatics enter the superior pole of the ovary from a lateral position and are covered by another raised fold of peritoneum, which, with the structures it contains, forms the **suspensory ligament of ovary (infundibulopelvic ligament)** (Fig. 5.34A).

The inferior pole of the ovary is attached to a fibromuscular band of tissue (the **ligament of ovary**), which courses medially in the margin of the mesovarium to the uterus and then continues anterolaterally as the **round ligament of uterus** (Fig. 5.34). The round ligament of uterus passes over the pelvic inlet to reach the deep inguinal ring and then courses through the inguinal canal to end in connective tissue related to the labium majus in the perineum. Both the

ligament of ovary and the round ligament of uterus are remnants of the gubernaculum, which attaches the gonad to the labioscrotal swellings in the embryo.

In men

In men, the visceral peritoneum drapes over the top of the bladder onto the superior poles of the seminal vesicles and then reflects onto the anterior and lateral surfaces of the rectum (Fig. 5.34B). A **rectovesical pouch** occurs between the bladder and rectum.

Clinical app

The recto-uterine pouch

The recto-uterine pouch (pouch of Douglas) is an extremely important clinical region situated between the rectum and uterus. When the patient is in the supine position, the recto-uterine pouch is the lowest portion of the abdominopelvic cavity and is a site where infection and fluids typically collect. It is impossible to palpate this region transabdominally, but it can be examined by transvaginal and transrectal digital palpation. If an abscess is suspected, it may be drained by a needle placed through the posterior fornix of the vagina or the anterior wall of the rectum.

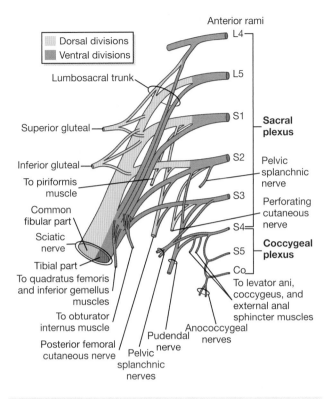

Fig. 5.36 Components and branches of the sacral and coccygeal plexuses.

Nerves

Somatic plexuses

Sacral and coccygeal plexuses

The sacral and coccygeal plexuses are situated on the posterolateral wall of the pelvic cavity and generally occur in the plane between the muscles and blood vessels. They are formed by the ventral rami of S1 to Co, with a significant contribution from L4 and L5, which enter the pelvis from the lumbar plexus (Figs. 5.35, 5.36). Nerves from these mainly somatic plexuses contribute to the innervation of the lower limb and muscles of the pelvis and perineum. Cutaneous branches supply skin over the lateral side of the foot, the posterior aspect of the lower limb, and most of the perineum.

Sacral plexus

The **sacral plexus** on each side is formed by the anterior rami of S1 to S4 and the lumbosacral trunk (L4 and L5) (Fig. 5.36). The plexus is formed in relation to the anterior surface of the piriformis muscle, which is part of the posterolateral pelvic wall. Sacral contributions to the plexus pass out of the anterior sacral foramina and course laterally and inferiorly on the pelvic wall. The lumbosacral trunk, consisting of part of the anterior ramus of L4 and all of the anterior ramus of L5, courses vertically into the pelvic cavity from the abdomen by passing immediately anterior to the sacro-iliac joint.

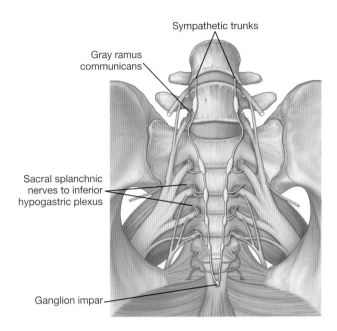

Fig. 5.37 Sympathetic trunks in the pelvis.

Gray rami communicantes from ganglia of the sympathetic trunk connect with each of the anterior rami and carry postganglionic sympathetic fibers destined for the periphery to the somatic nerves (Fig. 5.37). In addition, special visceral nerves (**pelvic splanchnic nerves**) originating from S2 to S4 deliver preganglionic parasympathetic fibers to the pelvic part of the prevertebral plexus (Fig. 5.38, p. 237).

Each anterior ramus has ventral and dorsal divisions that combine with similar divisions from other levels to form terminal nerves (Fig. 5.36). The anterior ramus of S4 has only a ventral division.

Branches of the sacral plexus include the sciatic nerve and gluteal nerves, which are major nerves of the lower limb, and the pudendal nerve, which is the nerve of the perineum (Table 5.4). Numerous smaller branches supply the pelvic wall, floor, and lower limb.

Most nerves originating from the sacral plexus leave the pelvic cavity by passing through the greater sciatic foramen inferior to piriformis muscle and enter the gluteal region of the lower limb. Other nerves leave the pelvic cavity using different routes; a few nerves do not leave the pelvic cavity and course directly into the muscles in the pelvic cavity. Finally, two nerves that leave the pelvic cavity through the greater sciatic foramen loop around the ischial spine and sacrospinous ligament and pass medially through the lesser sciatic foramen to supply structures in the perineum and lateral pelvic wall.

Sciatic nerve. The **sciatic nerve** is the largest nerve of the body and carries contributions from L4 to S3 (Table 5.4, Figs. 5.35, 5.36). It:

Table 5.4 Branches of the sacral and coccygeal plexuses (spinal segments in parentheses do not consistently participate)

BRANCH

Sacral plexus

Sciatic	Spinal segments	Motor function
Tibial part	L4 to S3	All muscles in the posterior or hamstring compartment of the thigh (including the hamstring part of the adductor magnus) except for the short head of the biceps
		All muscles in the posterior compartment of the leg
		All muscles in the sole of the foot
		Sensory (cutaneous) function
		Skin on posterolateral and lateral surfaces of foot and sole of foot
Common fibular part	L4 to S2	Motor function
		Short head of biceps in the posterior compartment of the thigh
		All muscles in the anterior and lateral compartments of the leg
		Extensor digitorum brevis in the foot (also contributes to the supply of the first dorsal interosseous muscle)
		Sensory (cutaneous) function
		Skin on the anterolateral surface of the leg and dorsal surface of the foot
Pudendal	S2 to S4	Motor function
		Skeletal muscles in the perineum including the external urethral and anal sphincters and levator ani (overlaps in supply of the levator ani and external sphincter with branches directly from ventral division of S4)
		Sensory (cutaneous) function
		Most skin of the perineum; penis and clitoris
Superior gluteal	L4 to S1	Motor function
		Gluteus medius, gluteus minimus, and tensor fasciae latae
Inferior gluteal	L5 to S2	Motor function
		Gluteus maximus
Nerve to obturator internus and superior gemellus	L5 to S2	Motor function
		Obturator internus and superior gemellus

Table 5.4 Branches of the sacral and coccygeal plexuses (spinal segments in parentheses do not consistently participate)—cont'd

BRANCH

Nerve to quadratus femoris and inferior gemellus	L4 to S1	Motor function Quadratus femoris and inferior gemellus
Posterior femoral cutaneous (posterior cutaneous nerve of thigh)	S1, S3	Sensory (cutaneous) function Skin on the posterior aspect of the thigh
Perforating cutaneous	S2, S3	Sensory (cutaneous) function Skin over gluteal fold (overlaps with posterior femoral cutaneous)
Nerve to piriformis	(L5), S1, S2	Motor function Piriformis muscle
Nerves to levator ani, coccygeus, and external anal sphincter	S4	Motor function Levator ani, coccygeus, and external anal sphincter (overlaps with pudendal nerve) Sensory (cutaneous) function Small patch of skin between anus and coccyx
Pelvic splanchnic nerves	S2, S3 (4)	Motor (visceral) function Visceral motor (preganglionic parasympathetic) to pelvic part of prevertebral plexus Stimulate erection, modulate mobility in gastrointestinal system distal to the left colic flexure, inhibitory to internal urethral sphincter Sensory (visceral) function Visceral afferents from pelvic viscera and distal parts of colon. Pain from cervix and possibly from bladder and proximal urethra
Coccygeal plexus		
Anococcygeal nerves	S4 to Co	Sensory (cutaneous) function Perianal skin

- forms on the anterior surface of the piriformis muscle and leaves the pelvic cavity through the greater sciatic foramen inferior to piriformis;
- passes through the gluteal region into the thigh where it divides into its two major branches: the common fibular nerve (common peroneal nerve) and the tibial nerve—dorsal divisions of L4, L5, S1, and S2 are carried in the common fibular part of the nerve, and the ventral divisions of L4, L5, S1, S2, and S3 are carried in the tibial part;
- innervates muscles in the posterior compartment of the thigh and muscles in the leg and foot; and
- carries sensory fibers from the skin of the foot and lateral leg.

Pudendal nerve. The **pudendal nerve** forms anteriorly to the lower part of piriformis muscle from ventral divisions of S2 to S4 (Table 5.4; also see Figs. 5.35, 5.36). It:

- leaves the pelvic cavity through the greater sciatic foramen, inferior to the piriformis muscle, and enters the gluteal region;
- courses into the perineum by immediately passing around the sacrospinous ligament where the ligament joins the ischial spine and through the lesser sciatic foramen (this course takes the nerve out of the pelvic cavity, around the peripheral attachment of the pelvic floor, and into the perineum);
- is accompanied throughout its course by the internal pudendal vessels; and
- innervates skin and skeletal muscles of the perineum, including the external anal and external urethral sphincters.

Other branches of the sacral plexus (see Table 5.4). Other branches of the sacral plexus include:

- motor branches to muscles of the gluteal region, pelvic wall, and pelvic floor (superior and inferior gluteal nerves, nerve to obturator internus and superior gemellus, nerve to quadratus femoris and inferior gemellus, nerve to piriformis, nerves to levator ani); and
- sensory nerves to skin over the inferior gluteal region and posterior aspects of the thigh and upper leg (perforating cutaneous nerve and posterior cutaneous nerve of the thigh) (see Figs. 5.35, 5.36).

The **superior gluteal nerve** leaves the pelvic cavity through the greater sciatic foramen superior to the piriformis muscle and supplies muscles in the gluteal region.

The **inferior gluteal nerve** leaves the pelvic cavity through the greater sciatic foramen inferior to the piriformis muscle and supplies the **gluteus maximus.**

The **nerve to the obturator internus** and the associated **superior gemellus** muscle leaves the pelvic cavity through the greater sciatic foramen inferior to the piriformis muscle. Like the pudendal nerve, it passes around the ischial spine and through the lesser sciatic foramen to enter the perineum and supply the obturator internus muscle from the medial side of the muscle inferior to the attachment of the levator ani muscle.

The **nerve to the quadratus femoris** muscle and the **inferior gemellus** muscle and the **posterior cutaneous nerve of the thigh (posterior femoral cutaneous nerve)** also leave the pelvic cavity through the greater sciatic foramen inferior to the piriformis muscle and course to muscles and skin, respectively, in the lower limb.

Unlike most of the other nerves originating from the sacral plexus, which leave the pelvic cavity through the greater sciatic foramen either above or below the piriformis muscle, the **perforating cutaneous nerve** leaves the pelvic cavity by penetrating directly through the sacrotuberous ligament and then courses to skin over the inferior aspect of the buttocks.

The **nerve to the piriformis** and a number of small nerves to the levator ani and coccygeus muscles originate from the sacral plexus and pass directly into their target muscles without leaving the pelvic cavity.

Coccygeal plexus

The small coccygeal plexus has a minor contribution from S4 and is formed mainly by the anterior rami of S5 and Co, which originate inferiorly to the pelvic floor. They penetrate the coccygeus muscle to enter the pelvic cavity and join with the anterior ramus of S4 to form a single trunk from which small **anococcygeal nerves** originate (see Table 5.4). These nerves penetrate the muscle and the overlying sacrospinous and sacrotuberous ligaments and pass superficially to innervate skin in the anal triangle of the perineum.

Visceral plexuses

Paravertebral sympathetic chain

The paravertebral part of the visceral nervous system is represented in the pelvis by the inferior ends of the sympathetic trunks (Fig. 5.38A). Each trunk enters the pelvic cavity from the abdomen by passing over the ala of the sacrum medially to the lumbosacral trunks and posteriorly to the iliac vessels. The trunks course inferiorly along the anterior surface of the sacrum where they are positioned medially to the anterior sacral foramina. Four ganglia occur along each trunk. Anteriorly to the coccyx, the two trunks join to form a single small terminal ganglion (the **ganglion impar**).

The principal function of the sympathetic trunks in the pelvis is to deliver postganglionic sympathetic fibers to the anterior rami of sacral nerves for distribution to the periphery, mainly to parts of the lower limb and perineum. This is accomplished by gray rami communicantes, which connect the trunks to the sacral anterior rami.

In addition to gray rami communicantes, other branches (the **sacral splanchnic nerves**) join and contribute to the pelvic part of the prevertebral plexus associated with innervating pelvic viscera.

Pelvic extensions of the prevertebral plexus

The pelvic parts of the prevertebral plexus carry sympathetic, parasympathetic, and visceral afferent fibers (see Fig. 5.38A). Pelvic parts of the plexus are associated with innervating pelvic viscera and erectile tissues of the perineum.

The prevertebral plexus enters the pelvis as two **hypogastric nerves,** one on each side, that cross the pelvic inlet medially to the internal iliac vessels. The hypogastric nerves are formed by the separation of the fibers in the **superior hypogastric plexus** into right and left bundles. The superior hypogastric plexus is situated anterior to vertebra LV between the promontory of the sacrum and the bifurcation of the aorta.

When the hypogastric nerves are joined by pelvic splanchnic nerves carrying preganglionic parasympathetic fibers from S2 to S4, the **pelvic plexuses (inferior hypogastric plexuses)** are formed (Fig. 5.38). The inferior hypogastric plexuses, one on each side, course in an inferior direction around the pelvic walls, medially to major vessels and somatic nerves. They give origin to the following subsidiary plexuses, which innervate the pelvic viscera:

- the **rectal plexus,**
- the **uterovaginal plexus,**
- the **prostatic plexus,** and
- the **vesical plexus.**

Terminal branches of the inferior hypogastric plexuses penetrate and pass through the deep perineal pouch and innervate erectile tissues of the penis and the clitoris in the perineum (Fig. 5.38B). In men, these nerves, called **cavernous nerves,** are extensions of the prostatic plexus. The pattern of distribution of similar nerves in women is not entirely clear, but they are likely extensions of the uterovaginal plexus.

Sympathetic fibers

Sympathetic fibers enter the inferior hypogastric plexuses from the hypogastric nerves and from branches (sacral splanchnic nerves) of the upper sacral parts of the sympathetic trunks (see Fig. 5.38A). Ultimately, these nerves are derived from preganglionic fibers that leave the spinal cord in the anterior roots, mainly of T10 to L2. These fibers:

- innervate blood vessels,
- cause contraction of smooth muscle in the internal urethral sphincter in men and the internal anal sphincters in both men and women,
- cause smooth muscle contraction associated with the reproductive tract and with the accessory glands of the reproductive system, and
- are important in moving secretions from the epididymis and associated glands into the urethra to form semen during ejaculation.

Parasympathetic fibers

Parasympathetic fibers enter the pelvic plexus in pelvic splanchnic nerves that originate from spinal cord levels S2 to S4 (Fig. 5.38). They:

- are generally vasodilatory,
- stimulate bladder contraction,
- stimulate erection, and
- modulate activity of the enteric nervous system of the colon distal to the left colic flexure (in addition to pelvic viscera, some of the fibers from the pelvic plexus course superiorly in the prevertebral plexus or as separate nerves and pass into the inferior mesenteric plexus of the abdomen).

Visceral afferent fibers

Visceral afferent fibers follow the course of the sympathetic and parasympathetic fibers to the spinal cord. Afferent fibers that enter the cord in lower thoracic levels and lumbar levels with sympathetic fibers generally carry pain; however, pain fibers from the cervix and some pain fibers from the bladder and urethra may accompany parasympathetic nerves to sacral levels of the spinal cord.

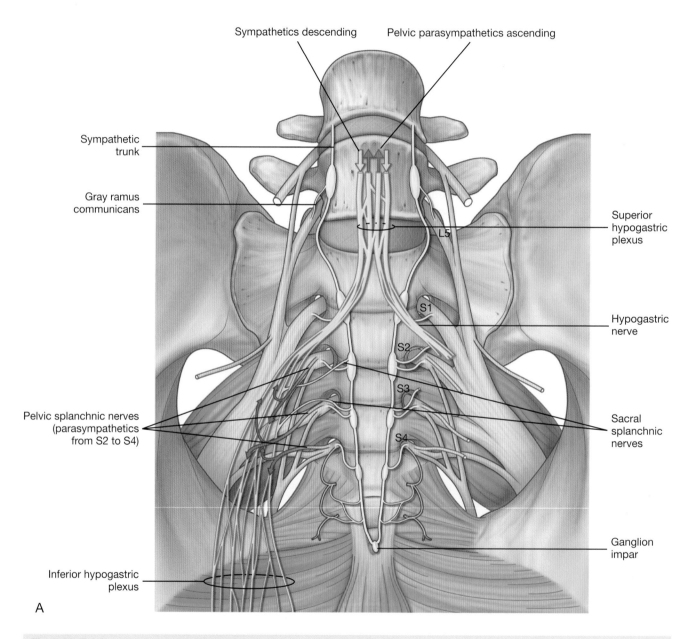

Sympathetics descending

Pelvic parasympathetics ascending

Sympathetic trunk

Gray ramus communicans

Superior hypogastric plexus

L5

S1

Hypogastric nerve

S2

S3

Pelvic splanchnic nerves (parasympathetics from S2 to S4)

Sacral splanchnic nerves

S4

Ganglion impar

Inferior hypogastric plexus

A

Fig. 5.38 Pelvic extensions of the prevertebral plexus. **A.** Anterior view.

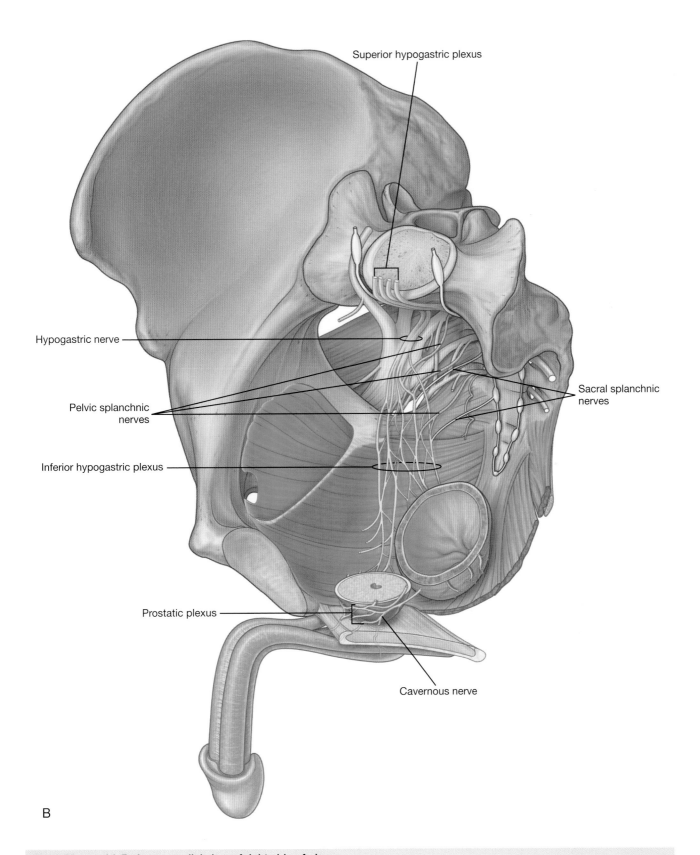

Superior hypogastric plexus

Hypogastric nerve

Pelvic splanchnic nerves

Inferior hypogastric plexus

Sacral splanchnic nerves

Prostatic plexus

Cavernous nerve

B

Fig. 5.38, cont'd B. Anteromedial view of right side of plexus.

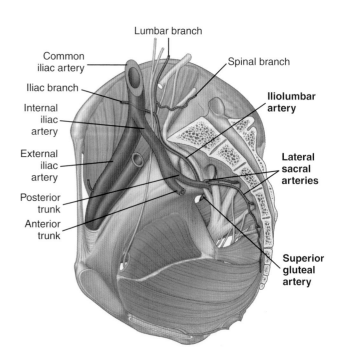

Fig. 5.39 Branches of the posterior trunk of the internal iliac artery.

Blood vessels

Arteries

The major artery of the pelvis and perineum is the internal iliac artery on each side (Figs. 5.39, 5.40). In addition to providing a blood supply to most of the pelvic viscera, pelvic walls and floor, and structures in the perineum, including erectile tissues of the clitoris and the penis, this artery gives rise to branches that follow nerves into the gluteal region of the lower limb. Other vessels that originate in the abdomen and contribute to the supply of pelvic structures include the median sacral artery and, in women, the ovarian arteries.

Internal iliac artery

The **internal iliac artery** originates from the common iliac artery on each side, approximately at the level of the intervertebral disc between LV and SI and lies anteromedial to the sacro-iliac joint (Fig. 5.39). The vessel courses inferiorly over the pelvic inlet, then divides into anterior and posterior trunks at the level of the superior border of the greater sciatic foramen. Branches from the posterior trunk contribute to the supply of the lower posterior abdominal wall, the posterior pelvic wall, and the gluteal region. Branches from the anterior trunk supply the pelvic viscera, the perineum, the gluteal region, the adductor region of the thigh, and, in the fetus, the placenta.

Posterior trunk

Branches of the posterior trunk include the following (Fig. 5.39):

■ The **iliolumbar artery** ascends laterally back out of the pelvic inlet and divides into a lumbar branch and an iliac branch. The lumbar branch contributes to the supply of the posterior abdominal wall, psoas, quadratus lumborum muscles, and cauda equina via a small spinal branch that passes through the intervertebral foramen between LV and SI. The iliac branch passes laterally into the iliac fossa to supply muscle and bone.

■ The **lateral sacral arteries,** usually two, originate from the posterior division of the internal iliac artery and course medially and inferiorly along the posterior pelvic wall. They give rise to branches that pass into the anterior sacral foramina to supply related bone and soft tissues, structures in the vertebral (sacral) canal, and skin and muscle posterior to the sacrum.

■ The **superior gluteal artery** is the largest branch of the internal iliac artery. It courses posteriorly, usually passing between the lumbosacral trunk and anterior ramus of S1, to leave the pelvic cavity through the greater sciatic foramen above the piriformis muscle and enter the gluteal region of the lower limb. This vessel makes a substantial contribution to the blood supply of muscles and skin in the gluteal region and supplies branches to adjacent muscles and bones of the pelvic walls.

Anterior trunk

Branches of the anterior trunk of the internal iliac artery include the following (Fig. 5.40):

■ The first branch of the anterior trunk is the **umbilical artery,** which gives origin to the superior vesical artery, then travels forward just inferior to the margin of the pelvic inlet. Anteriorly, the vessel leaves the pelvic cavity and

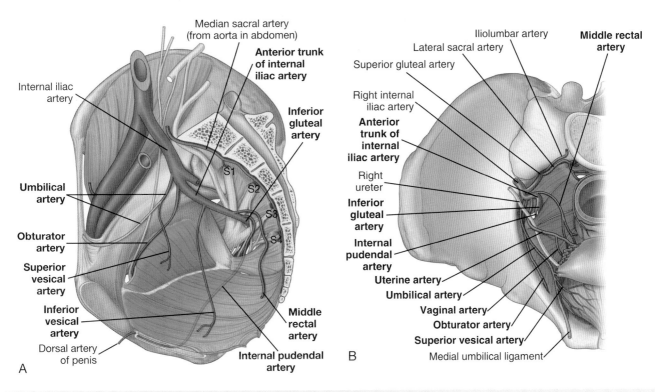

Fig. 5.40 Branches of the anterior trunk of the internal iliac artery. **A.** Male. **B.** Female.

ascends on the internal aspect of the anterior abdominal wall to reach the umbilicus. In the fetus, the umbilical artery is large and carries blood from the fetus to the placenta. After birth, the vessel closes distally to the origin of the superior vesical artery and eventually becomes a solid fibrous cord. On the anterior abdominal wall, the cord raises a fold of peritoneum termed the **medial umbilical fold.** The fibrous remnant of the umbilical artery itself is the **medial umbilical ligament.**

■ The **superior vesical artery** normally originates from the root of the umbilical artery and courses medially and inferiorly to supply the superior aspect of the bladder and distal parts of the ureter. In men, it also may give rise to an artery that supplies the ductus deferens.

■ The **inferior vesical artery** occurs in men and supplies branches to the bladder, ureter, seminal vesicle, and prostate. The **vaginal artery** in women is the equivalent of the inferior vesical artery in men and, descending to the vagina, supplies branches to the vagina and to adjacent parts of the bladder and rectum. The vaginal artery and uterine artery may originate together as a common branch from the anterior trunk, or the vaginal artery may arise independently.

■ The **middle rectal artery** courses medially to supply the rectum. The vessel anastomoses with the superior rectal artery, which originates from the inferior mesenteric artery in the abdomen, and the inferior rectal artery,

which originates from the internal pudendal artery in the perineum.

■ The **obturator artery** courses anteriorly along the pelvic wall and leaves the pelvic cavity via the obturator canal. Together with the obturator nerve above and the obturator vein below, it enters and supplies the adductor region of the thigh.

■ The **internal pudendal artery** courses inferiorly from its origin in the anterior trunk and leaves the pelvic cavity through the greater sciatic foramen inferior to the piriformis muscle. In association with the pudendal nerve on its medial side, the vessel passes laterally to the ischial spine and then through the lesser sciatic foramen to enter the perineum. The internal pudendal artery is the main artery of the perineum. Among the structures it supplies are the erectile tissues of the clitoris and the penis.

■ The **inferior gluteal artery** is a large terminal branch of the anterior trunk of the internal iliac artery. It passes between the anterior rami S1 and S2 or S2 and S3 of the sacral plexus and leaves the pelvic cavity through the greater sciatic foramen inferior to the piriformis muscle. It enters and contributes to the blood supply of the gluteal region and anastomoses with a network of vessels around the hip joint.

■ The **uterine artery** in women courses medially and anteriorly in the base of the broad ligament to reach the cervix (Figs. 5.40B, 5.41). Along its course, the vessel

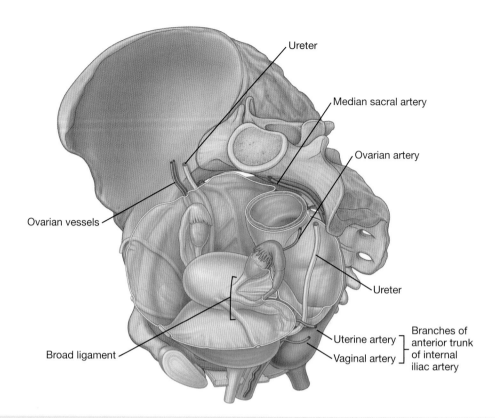

Fig. 5.41 Uterine and vaginal arteries.

crosses the ureter and passes superiorly to the lateral vaginal fornix. Once the vessel reaches the cervix, it ascends along the lateral margin of the uterus to reach the uterine tube where it curves laterally and anastomoses with the ovarian artery. The uterine artery is the major blood supply to the uterus and enlarges significantly during pregnancy. Through anastomoses with other arteries, the vessel contributes to the blood supply of the ovaries and vagina as well.

Ovarian arteries

In women, the gonadal (ovarian) vessels originate from the abdominal aorta and then descend to cross the pelvic inlet and supply the ovaries (see Fig. 5.41). They anastomose with terminal parts of the uterine arteries. On each side, the vessels travel in the **suspensory ligament of ovary** (the **infundibulopelvic ligament**) as they cross the pelvic inlet to the ovary. Branches pass through the mesovarium to reach the ovary and through the mesometrium of the broad ligament to anastomose with the uterine artery. The ovarian arteries enlarge significantly during pregnancy to augment uterine blood supply.

Median sacral artery

The median sacral artery (see Figs. 5.40A and 5.41) originates from the posterior surface of the aorta just superior to the aortic bifurcation at vertebral level LIV in the abdomen.

It descends in the midline, crosses the pelvic inlet, and then courses along the anterior surface of the sacrum and coccyx. It gives rise to the last pair of lumbar arteries and to branches that anastomose with the iliolumbar and lateral sacral arteries.

Veins

Pelvic veins follow the course of all branches of the internal iliac artery except for the umbilical artery and the iliolumbar artery (Fig. 5.42A). On each side, the veins drain into internal iliac veins, which leave the pelvic cavity to join common iliac veins situated just superior and lateral to the pelvic inlet.

Within the pelvic cavity, extensive interconnected venous plexuses are associated with the surfaces of the viscera (bladder, rectum, prostate, uterus, and vagina). Together, these plexuses form the pelvic plexus of veins. The part of the venous plexus surrounding the rectum and anal canal drains via superior rectal veins (tributaries of inferior mesenteric veins) into the hepatic portal system and via middle and inferior rectal veins into the caval system. This pelvic plexus is an important portacaval shunt when the hepatic portal system is blocked (Fig. 5.42B).

The inferior part of the rectal venous plexus around the anal canal has two parts, an internal and an external. The **internal rectal venous plexus** is in connective tissue between the internal anal sphincter and the epithelium lining the canal. This plexus connects superiorly with

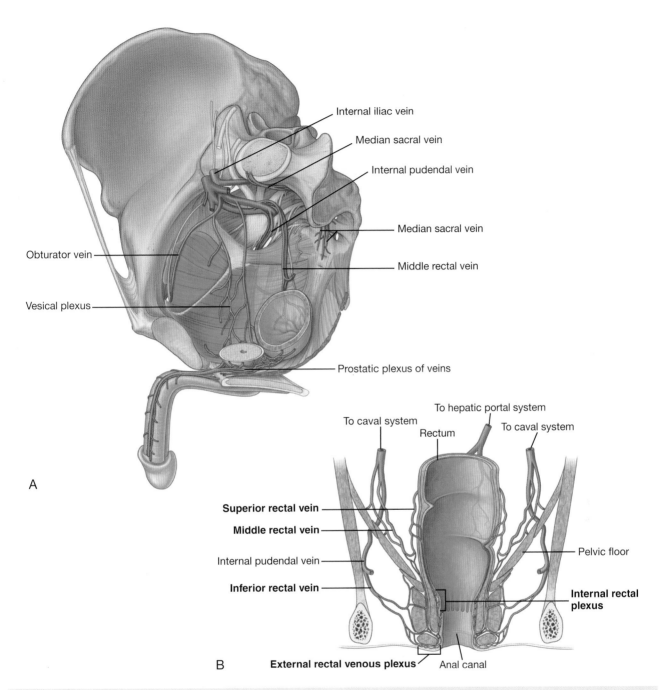

Fig. 5.42 Pelvic veins. **A.** In a man with the left side of the pelvis and most of the viscera removed. **B.** Veins associated with the rectum and anal canal.

longitudinally arranged branches of the superior rectal vein that lie one in each anal column. When enlarged, these branches form varices or internal hemorrhoids, which originate above the pectinate line and are covered by colonic mucosa. The **external rectal venous plexus** circles the external anal sphincter and is subcutaneous. Enlargement of vessels in the external rectal plexus results in external hemorrhoids.

The single **deep dorsal vein** that drains erectile tissues of the clitoris and the penis passes directly into the pelvic cavity through a gap formed between the arcuate

pubic ligament and the anterior margin of the perineal membrane. The vein joins the prostatic plexus of veins in men and the vesical (bladder) plexus of veins in women. Superficial veins that drain the skin of the penis and corresponding regions of the clitoris drain into the external pudendal veins, which are tributaries of the great saphenous vein in the thigh.

In addition to tributaries of the internal iliac vein, median sacral veins and ovarian veins parallel the courses of the median sacral artery and ovarian artery, respectively, and leave the pelvic cavity to join veins in the abdomen:

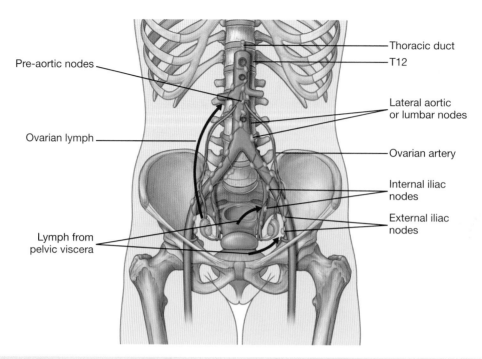

Thoracic duct
T12
Pre-aortic nodes
Lateral aortic or lumbar nodes
Ovarian lymph
Ovarian artery
Internal iliac nodes
External iliac nodes
Lymph from pelvic viscera

Fig. 5.43 Pelvic lymphatics.

- The **median sacral veins** coalesce to form a single vein that joins either the left common iliac vein or the junction of the two common iliac veins to form the inferior vena cava.
- The **ovarian veins** follow the course of the corresponding arteries; on the left they join the left renal vein, and on the right they join the inferior vena cava in the abdomen.

Lymphatics

Lymphatics from most pelvic viscera drain mainly into lymph nodes distributed along the internal iliac and external iliac arteries and their associated branches (Fig. 5.43), which drain into nodes associated with the common iliac arteries and then into the lateral aortic or lumbar nodes associated with the lateral surfaces of the abdominal aorta. In turn, these lateral aortic or lumbar nodes drain into the lumbar trunks, which continue to the origin of the thoracic duct at approximately vertebral level TXII.

Lymphatics from the ovaries and related parts of the uterus and uterine tubes leave the pelvic cavity superiorly and drain, via vessels that accompany the ovarian arteries, directly into lateral aortic or lumbar nodes and, in some cases, into the pre-aortic nodes on the anterior surface of the aorta.

In addition to draining pelvic viscera, nodes along the internal iliac artery also receive drainage from the gluteal region of the lower limb and from deep areas of the perineum.

Clinical app

Hemorrhoids

A hemorrhoid is an engorgement of veins related to the anal sphincter. Hemorrhoids have a slight genetic predisposition; however, straining during bowel movements, obesity, and sedentary life style can also produce hemorrhoids, as can portal hypertension. The symptoms include irritation, pain, and swelling. Internal hemorrhoids originate from the internal rectal venous plexus that occurs inside the rectum and have a tendency to bleed. Prolapsed hemorrhoids are internal hemorrhoids that pass outside the anal canal and form lumps, which may undergo thrombosis and become painful. External hemorrhoids originate from the external rectal plexus and occur at the distal boundary of the anal canal.

PERINEUM

The perineum is a diamond-shaped region positioned inferiorly to the pelvic floor between the thighs. Its peripheral boundary is the pelvic outlet; its ceiling is the pelvic diaphragm (the levator ani and coccygeus muscles); and its narrow lateral walls are formed by the walls of the pelvic cavity below the attachment of the levator ani muscle (Fig. 5.44A).

The perineum is divided into an anterior urogenital triangle and a posterior anal triangle.

- The urogenital triangle is associated with the openings of the urinary systems and the reproductive systems and functions to anchor the external genitalia.

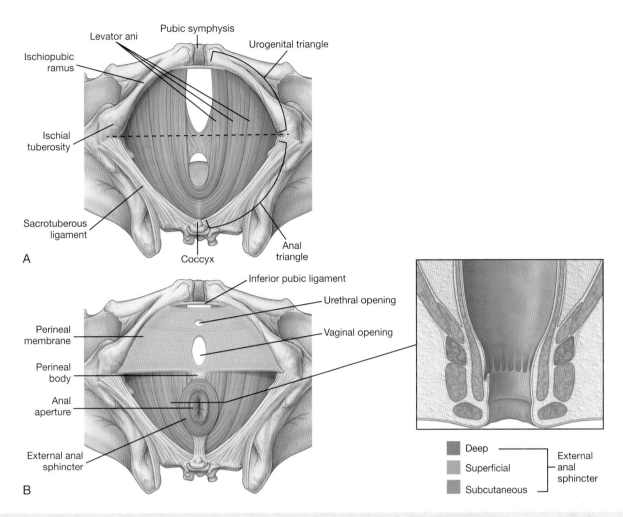

Fig. 5.44 Borders and ceiling of the perineum. **A.** Boundaries of the perineum. **B.** Perineal membrane.

■ The anal triangle contains the anus and the external anal sphincter.

The pudendal nerve (S2 to S4) and the internal pudendal artery are the major nerve and artery of the region.

Borders and ceiling

The margin of the perineum is marked by the inferior border of the pubic symphysis at its anterior point, the tip of the coccyx at its posterior point, and the ischial tuberosities at each of the lateral points (Fig. 5.44A). The lateral margins are formed by the ischiopubic rami anteriorly and by the sacrotuberous ligaments posteriorly.

The perineum is divided into two triangles by an imaginary line between the two ischial tuberosities (Fig. 5.44A). Anterior to the line is the urogenital triangle, and posterior to the line is the anal triangle. Significantly, the two triangles are not in the same plane. In the anatomical position, the urogenital triangle is oriented in the horizontal plane, whereas the anal triangle is tilted upward at the transtubercular line so that it faces more posteriorly.

The roof of the perineum is formed mainly by the levator ani muscles that separate the pelvic cavity above from the perineum below. These muscles, one on each side, form a cone- or funnel-shaped pelvic diaphragm, with the anal aperture at its inferior apex in the anal triangle.

Anteriorly, in the **urogenital triangle,** a U-shaped defect in the muscles, the **urogenital hiatus,** allows the passage of the urethra and vagina.

Perineal membrane and deep perineal pouch

The perineal membrane (see p. 218) is a thick fibrous sheet that fills the urogenital triangle (Fig. 5.44B). It has a free posterior border, which is anchored in the midline to the perineal body and is attached laterally to the pubic arch. Immediately superior to the perineal membrane is a thin region termed the *deep perineal pouch,* containing a layer of skeletal muscle and neurovascular tissues. Among the

263

Surface anatomy

Defining the margins of the perineum

The pubic symphysis, ischial tuberosities, and tip of the sacrum are palpable on patients and can be used to define the boundaries of the perineum. This is best done with patients lying on their backs with their thighs flexed and abducted in the lithotomy position (Fig. 5.45).

- The ischial tuberosities are palpable on each side as large bony masses near the crease of skin (gluteal fold) between the thigh and gluteal region. They mark the lateral corners of the diamond-shaped perineum.
- The tip of the coccyx is palpable in the midline posterior to the anal aperture and marks the most posterior limit of the perineum.
- The anterior limit of the perineum is the pubic symphysis. In women, this is palpable in the midline deep to the mons pubis. In men, the pubic symphysis is palpable immediately superior to where the body of the penis joins the lower abdominal wall.

Imaginary lines that join the ischial tuberosities with the pubic symphysis in front, and with the tip of the coccyx behind, outline the diamond-shaped perineum. An additional line between the ischial tuberosities divides the perineum into two triangles, the urogenital triangle anteriorly and anal triangle posteriorly. This line also approximates the position of the posterior margin of the perineal membrane. The midpoint of this line marks the location of the perineal body or central tendon of the perineum.

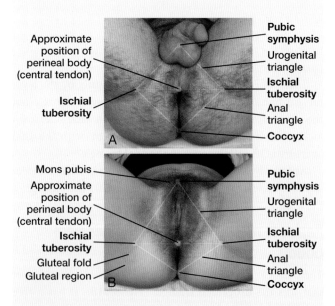

Fig. 5.45 Inferior view of the perineum in the lithotomy position. Boundaries, subdivisions, and palpable landmarks are indicated. **A.** In a man. **B.** In a woman.

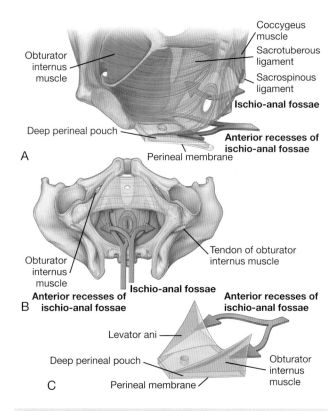

Fig. 5.46 Ischio-anal fossae and their anterior recesses. **A.** Anterolateral view with left pelvic wall removed. **B.** Inferior view. **C.** Anterolateral view with pelvic walls and diaphragm removed.

skeletal muscles in the pouch (see p. 218, Fig. 5.18) is the external urethral sphincter.

The perineal membrane and deep perineal pouch provide support for the external genitalia, which are attached to its inferior surface. Also, the parts of the perineal membrane and deep perineal pouch inferior to the urogenital hiatus in the levator ani provide support for pelvic viscera.

The urethra leaves the pelvic cavity and enters the perineum by passing through the deep perineal pouch and perineal membrane. In women, the vagina also passes through these structures posterior to the urethra.

Ischio-anal fossae and their anterior recesses

Because the levator ani muscles course medially from their origin on the lateral pelvic walls above to the anal aperture and urogenital hiatus below, inverted wedge-shaped gutters occur between the levator ani muscles and adjacent pelvic walls as the two structures diverge inferiorly (Fig. 5.46). In the anal triangle, these gutters, one on each side of the anal aperture, are termed **ischio-anal fossae.** The lateral wall of each fossa is formed mainly by the ischium, obturator

internus muscle, and the sacrotuberous ligament. The medial wall is the levator ani muscle. The medial and lateral walls converge superiorly where the levator ani muscle attaches to the fascia overlying the obturator internus muscle. The ischio-anal fossae allow movement of the pelvic diaphragm and expansion of the anal canal during defecation.

The ischio-anal fossae of the anal triangle are continuous anteriorly with recesses that project into the urogenital triangle superior to the deep perineal pouch. The ischio-anal fossae and their anterior recesses are normally filled with fat.

Clinical app

Abscesses in the ischio-anal fossae

The anal mucosa is particularly vulnerable to injury and may be easily torn by hard feces. Occasionally, patients develop inflammation and infection of the anal canal (sinuses or crypts), which can spread laterally into the ischio-anal fossae or superiorly into the pelvic cavity.

Anal triangle

The anal triangle of the perineum faces posteroinferiorly and is defined laterally by the medial margins of the sacrotuberous ligaments anteriorly by a horizontal line between the two ischial tuberosities and posteriorly by the coccyx. The ceiling of the anal triangle is the pelvic diaphragm, which is formed by the levator ani and coccygeus muscles. The anal aperture occurs centrally in the anal triangle and is related on either side to an ischio-anal fossa. The major muscle in the anal triangle is the external anal sphincter.

The **external anal sphincter,** which surrounds the anal canal, is formed by skeletal muscle and consists of three parts—deep, superficial, and subcutaneous—arranged sequentially along the canal from superior to inferior (Table 5.5, see Fig. 5.44B). The external anal sphincter is innervated by inferior rectal branches of the pudendal nerve and by branches directly from the anterior ramus of S4.

Urogenital triangle

The urogenital triangle of the perineum is the anterior half of the perineum and is oriented in the horizontal plane. It contains the roots of the external genitalia (Fig. 5.47) and the openings of the urogenital system.

The urogenital triangle is defined (see Fig. 5.44A):

- laterally by the ischiopubic rami,
- posteriorly by an imaginary line between the ischial tuberosities, and
- anteriorly by the inferior margin of the pubic symphysis.

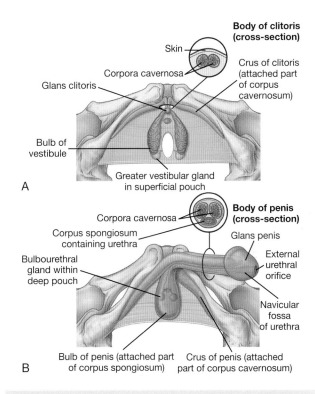

Fig. 5.47 Erectile tissues of clitoris and penis. A. Clitoris. B. Penis.

Table 5.5 Muscles of the anal triangle

Muscles of pelvic wall	Origin	Insertion	Innervation	Function
External anal sphincter				Closes anal canal
Deep part	Ring-shaped muscle that surrounds superior aspect of anal canal and blends with the fibers of levator ani muscle		Pudendal nerve (S2 and S3) and branches directly from S4	
Superficial part	Surrounds lower part of anal canal	Anchored anteriorly to the perineal body and posteriorly to the anococcygeal body		
Subcutaneous part	Horizontally flattened disc that surrounds the anal aperture just beneath the skin			

As with the anal triangle, the roof or ceiling of the urogenital triangle is the levator ani muscle.

Unlike the anal triangle, the urogenital triangle contains a strong fibromuscular support platform, the perineal membrane, and deep perineal pouch (see p. 218), which is attached to the pubic arch.

Anterior extensions of the ischio-anal fossae occur between the deep perineal pouch and the levator ani muscle on each side.

Between the perineal membrane and the membranous layer of superficial fascia is the **superficial perineal pouch.** The principal structures in this pouch are the erectile tissues of the penis and clitoris and associated skeletal muscles.

Structures in the superficial perineal pouch

The superficial perineal pouch contains (Figs. 5.47, 5.48):

- erectile structures that join together to form the penis in men and the clitoris in women and
- skeletal muscles that are associated mainly with parts of the erectile structures attached to the perineal membrane and adjacent bone.

Each erectile structure consists of a central core of expandable vascular tissue and its surrounding connective tissue capsule.

Erectile tissues

Two sets of erectile structures join to form the penis and the clitoris.

A pair of cylindrically shaped **corpora cavernosa,** one on each side of the urogenital triangle, are anchored by their proximal ends to the pubic arch (Fig. 5.47). These attached parts are often termed the **crura** (from the Latin for "legs") of the clitoris or the penis. The distal ends of the corpora, which are not attached to bone, form the body of the clitoris in women and the dorsal parts of the body of the penis in men.

The second set of erectile tissues surrounds the openings of the urogenital system.

- In women, a pair of erectile structures, termed the **bulbs of vestibule,** are situated one on each side at the vaginal opening and are firmly anchored to the perineal membrane (Fig. 5.47A). Small bands of erectile tissues connect the anterior ends of these bulbs to a single, small, pea-shaped erectile mass, the **glans clitoris,** which is positioned in the midline at the end of the body of the clitoris and anterior to the opening of the urethra.
- In men, a single large erectile mass, the **corpus spongiosum,** is the structural equivalent to the bulbs of the vestibule, the glans clitoris, and the interconnecting bands of erectile tissues in women (Fig. 5.47B). The corpus spongiosum is anchored at its base (bulb of penis) to the perineal membrane. Its

proximal end, which is not attached, forms the ventral part of the body of the penis and expands over the end of the body of the penis to form the glans penis. In men, the urethra is enclosed by the corpus spongiosum and opens at the end of the penis. This is unlike the situation in women in which the urethra is not enclosed by erectile tissue of the clitoris and opens directly into the vestibule of the perineum.

Clitoris

The clitoris is composed of two corpora cavernosa and the **glans clitoris** (Fig. 5.47A). As in the penis, it has an attached part (root) and a free part (body).

- Unlike the root of penis, the **root of clitoris** technically consists only of the two crura. (Although the bulbs of the vestibule are attached to the glans clitoris by thin bands of erectile tissue, they are not included in the attached part of the clitoris.)
- The **body of clitoris,** which is formed only by the unattached parts of the two corpora cavernosa, angles posteriorly and is embedded in the connective tissues of the perineum.

The body of clitoris is supported by a suspensory ligament that attaches superiorly to the pubic symphysis (Fig. 5.48A). The glans clitoris is attached to the distal end of the body and is connected to the bulbs of the vestibule by small bands of erectile tissue. The glans clitoris is exposed in the perineum, and the body of the clitoris can be palpated through skin.

Penis

The penis is composed mainly of the two corpora cavernosa and the single corpus spongiosum, which contains the urethra (Fig. 5.47B) As in the clitoris, it has an attached part (root) and a free part (body):

- The **root of penis** consists of the two crura, which are proximal parts of the corpora cavernosa attached to the pubic arch, and the **bulb of penis,** which is the proximal part of the corpus spongiosum anchored to the perineal membrane.
- The **body of penis,** which is covered entirely by skin, is formed by the tethering of the two proximal free parts of the corpora cavernosa and the related free part of the corpus spongiosum.

The base of the body of penis is supported by two ligaments: the **suspensory ligament of penis** (attached superiorly to the pubic symphysis), and the more superficially positioned **fundiform ligament of penis** (attached above to the linea alba of the anterior abdominal wall and splits below into two bands that pass on each side of the penis and unite inferiorly) (Fig. 5.48B).

Because the anatomical position of the penis is erect, the paired corpora are defined as dorsal in the body of the penis and the single corpus spongiosum as ventral, even though the positions are reversed in the nonerect (flaccid) penis.

Table 5.6 Muscles of the superficial perineal pouch

Muscles of pelvic wall	Origin	Insertion	Innervation	Function
Ischiocavernosus	Ischial tuberosity and ramus	Crus of penis and clitoris	Pudendal nerve (S2 to S4)	Move blood from crura into the body of the erect penis and clitoris
Bulbospongiosus	In women: perineal body In men: perineal body, midline raphe	In women: bulb of vestibule, perineal membrane, body of clitoris, and corpus cavernosum In men: bulbospongiosus, perineal membrane, corpus cavernosum	Pudendal nerve (S2 to S4)	Move blood from attached parts of the clitoris and penis into the glans In men: removal of residual urine from urethra after urination; pulsatile emission of semen during ejaculation
Superficial transverse perineal	Ischial tuberosity and ramus	Perineal body	Pudendal nerve (S2 to S4)	Stabilize the perineal body

The corpus spongiosum expands to form the head of penis **(glans penis)** over the distal ends of the corpora cavernosa (Fig. 5.47B).

Erection

Erection of the penis and clitoris is a vascular event generated by parasympathetic fibers carried in pelvic splanchnic nerves from the anterior rami of S2 to S4, which enter the inferior hypogastric part of the prevertebral plexus and ultimately pass through the deep perineal pouch and perineal membrane to innervate the erectile tissues. Stimulation of these nerves causes specific arteries in the erectile tissues to relax. This allows blood to fill the tissues, causing the penis and clitoris to become erect.

Greater vestibular glands

The greater vestibular glands (Bartholin's glands) are seen in women. They are small, pea-shaped mucous glands that lie posterior to the bulbs of the vestibule on each side of the vaginal opening and are the female homologues of the bulbourethral glands in men (see Fig. 5.47). However, the bulbourethral glands are located within the deep perineal pouch, whereas the greater vestibular glands are in the superficial perineal pouch.

The duct of each greater vestibular gland opens into the vestibule of the perineum along the posterolateral margin of the vaginal opening.

Like the bulbourethral glands in men, the greater vestibular glands produce secretion during sexual arousal.

Muscles

The superficial perineal pouch contains three pairs of muscles: the **ischiocavernosus, bulbospongiosus, and superficial transverse perineal muscles** (Table 5.6, Fig. 5.48). Two of these three pairs of muscles are associated with the roots of the penis and clitoris; the other pair is associated with the perineal body.

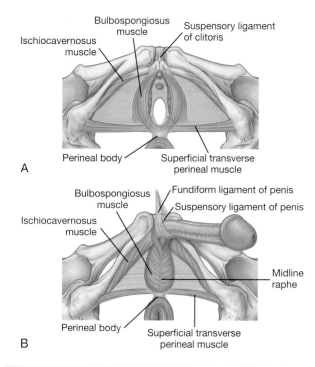

A

B

Fig. 5.48 Muscles in the superficial perineal pouch. A. In women. B. In men.

Surface anatomy

Superficial features of the external genitalia in women
In women, the clitoris and vestibular apparatus, together with a number of skin and tissue folds, form the **vulva** (Fig. 5.49A). On either side of the midline are two thin folds of skin termed the **labia minora**. The region enclosed between them, and into which the urethra and vagina open, is the **vestibule.** Anteriorly, the labia minora each bifurcate, forming a medial and a lateral fold. The medial folds unite to form the **frenulum of clitoris** that joins the glans clitoris (Fig. 5.49B). The lateral folds unite ventrally over the glans clitoris and the body of clitoris to form the **prepuce of clitoris** (hood) (Fig. 5.49B). The body of the clitoris extends anteriorly from the glans clitoris and is palpable deep to the prepuce and related skin. Posterior to the vestibule, the labia minora unite, forming a small transverse fold, the **frenulum of labia minora** (the **fourchette**) (Fig. 5.49C).

Within the vestibule, the vaginal orifice is surrounded to varying degrees by a ring-like fold of membrane, the **hymen,** which may have a small central perforation or may

Continued

completely close the vaginal opening. Following rupture of the hymen (resulting from first sexual intercourse or injury), irregular remnants of the hymen fringe the vaginal opening (Fig. 5.49C).

The orifices of the urethra and the vagina are associated with the openings of glands. The ducts of the para-urethral glands **(Skene's glands)** open into the vestibule, one on each side of the lateral margin of the urethra (Fig. 5.49D). The ducts of the greater vestibular glands **(Bartholin's glands)** open adjacent to the posterolateral margin of the vaginal opening in the crease between the vaginal orifice and remnants of the hymen (Fig. 5.49D).

Lateral to the labia minora are two broad folds, the **labia majora,** which unite anteriorly to form the mons pubis (Fig. 5.49A). The **mons pubis** overlies the inferior aspect of the pubic symphysis and is anterior to the vestibule and the clitoris. Posteriorly, the labia majora do not unite and are separated by a depression termed the **posterior commissure,** which overlies the position of the perineal body (Fig. 5.49A).

The cervix is visible when the vaginal canal is opened with a speculum (Fig. 5.49E). The external cervical os opens onto the surface

of the dome-shaped cervix. A recess or gutter, termed the *fornix,* occurs between the cervix and the vaginal wall and is further subdivided, based on location, into anterior, posterior, and lateral fornices.

The roots of the clitoris occur deep to surface features of the perineum and are attached to the ischiopubic rami and the perineal membrane.

The bulbs of the vestibule (Fig. 5.49F), composed of erectile tissues, lie deep to the labia minora on either side of the vestibule. These erectile masses are continuous, via thin bands of erectile tissues, with the glans clitoris, which is visible under the clitoral hood. The greater vestibular glands occur posterior to the bulbs of the vestibule on either side of the vaginal orifice.

The crura of clitoris are attached, one on each side, to the ischiopubic rami. Each crus is formed by the attached part of the corpus cavernosum. Anteriorly, these erectile corpora detach from bone, curve posteroinferiorly, and unite to form the body of the clitoris.

The body of clitoris underlies the ridge of skin immediately anterior to the clitoral hood (prepuce). The glans clitoris is positioned at the end of the body of clitoris.

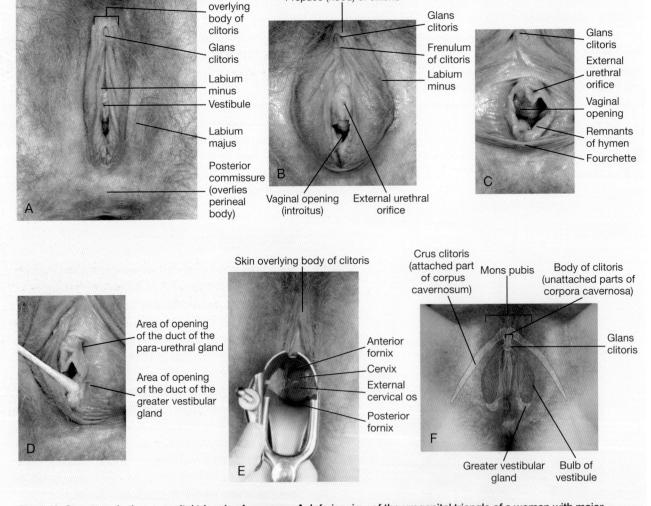

Fig. 5.49 Structures in the urogenital triangle of a woman. **A.** Inferior view of the urogenital triangle of a woman with major features indicated. **B.** Inferior view of the vestibule. The labia minora have been pulled apart to open the vestibule. Also indicated are the glans clitoris, the clitoral hood, and the frenulum of the clitoris. **C.** Inferior view of the vestibule showing the urethral and vaginal orifices and the hymen. The labia minora have been pulled further apart than in Fig. 5.49B. **D.** Inferior view of the vestibule with the left labium minus pulled to the side to show the regions of the vestibule into which the greater vestibular and para-urethral glands open. **E.** View through the vaginal canal of the cervix. **F.** Inferior view of the urogenital triangle of a woman with the erectile tissues of the clitoris and vestibule and the greater vestibular glands indicated with overlays.

Surface anatomy

Superficial features of the external genitalia in men

Superficial components of the genital organs in men consist of the scrotum and the penis (Fig. 5.50A). The urogenital triangle itself contains the root of the penis; however, the testes and associated structures, although they migrate into the scrotum from the abdomen, are generally evaluated with the penis during a physical examination.

The scrotum in men is homologous to the labia majora in women. Each oval testis is readily palpable through the skin of the scrotum (Fig. 5.50A). Posterolateral to the testis is an elongated mass of tissue, often visible as a raised ridge that contains lymphatics and blood vessels of the testis, and the epididymis and ductus deferens. A midline raphe (Fig. 5.50B) is visible on the skin, separating left and right sides of the scrotum. In some individuals, this raphe is prominent and extends from the anal aperture, over the scrotum, and along the ventral surface of the body of the penis to the frenulum of the glans.

The external urethral orifice is a sagittal slit, normally positioned at the tip of the glans (Fig. 5.50C). The inferior margin of the urethral orifice is continuous with a midline **raphe of penis,** which represents a line of fusion formed in the glans as the urethra develops in the fetus. The base of this raphe is continuous

with the **frenulum** of the glans, which is a median fold of skin that attaches the glans to more loosely attached skin proximal to the glans. The base of the glans is expanded to form a raised circular margin (the **corona of glans**) (Fig. 5.50D); the two lateral ends of the corona join inferiorly at the midline raphe of the glans. The depression posterior to the corona is the neck of the glans. Normally, a fold of skin at the neck of the glans is continuous anteriorly with thin skin that tightly adheres to the glans and posteriorly with thicker skin loosely attached to the body. This fold, known as the **prepuce,** extends forward to cover the glans. The prepuce is removed during male circumcision, leaving the glans exposed.

The root of the penis is formed by the attached parts of the corpus spongiosum and the corpora cavernosa. The corpus spongiosum is attached to the perineal membrane and can be easily palpated as a large mass anterior to the perineal body. This mass, which is covered by the bulbospongiosus muscles, is the bulb of penis (Fig. 5.50E).

The corpus spongiosum detaches from the perineal membrane anteriorly, becomes the ventral part of the body of penis (shaft of penis), and eventually terminates as the expanded glans penis.

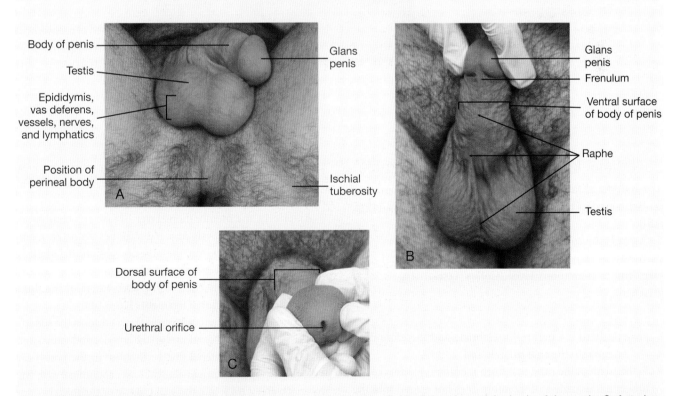

Fig. 5.50 Structures in the urogenital triangle of a man. **A.** Inferior view. **B.** Ventral surface of the body of the penis. **C.** Anterior view of the glans penis showing the urethral opening.

The crura of the penis, one crus on each side, are the attached parts of the corpora cavernosa and are anchored to the ischiopubic rami (Fig. 5.50E). The corpora cavernosa are unattached anteriorly and become the paired erectile masses that form the dorsal part of the body of the penis. The glans penis caps the anterior ends of the corpora cavernosa.

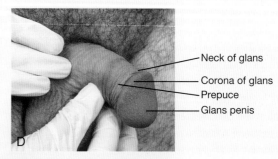

Neck of glans
Corona of glans
Prepuce
Glans penis

Fig. 5.50, cont'd D. Lateral view of the body of the penis and glans. **E.** Inferior view of the urogenital triangle of a man with the erectile tissues of the penis indicated with overlays.

Body of penis (unattached parts of corpus spongiosum and corpora cavernosa)

Crus of penis (attached part of corpus cavernosum)

Bulb of penis (attached part of corpus spongiosum)

Glans penis

Position of perineal body

Superficial fascia of the urogenital triangle

The superficial fascia of the urogenital triangle is continuous with similar fascia on the anterior abdominal wall (Fig. 5.51).

As with the superficial fascia of the abdominal wall, the perineal fascia has a membranous layer on its deep surface. This membranous layer **(Colles' fascia)** (Fig. 5.51) is attached:

- posteriorly to the perineal membrane and therefore does not extend into the anal triangle and
- to the ischiopubic rami that form the lateral borders of the urogenital triangle and therefore does not extend into the thigh.

It defines the external limits of the superficial perineal pouch, lines the scrotum or labia, and extends around the body of the penis and clitoris (Fig. 5.51A).

Anteriorly, the membranous layer of fascia is continuous over the pubic symphysis and pubic bones with the membranous layer of fascia on the anterior abdominal wall. In the lower lateral abdominal wall, the membranous layer of abdominal fascia is attached to the deep fascia of the thigh just inferior to the inguinal ligament (Fig. 5.51).

Because the membranous layer of fascia encloses the superficial perineal pouch and continues up the anterior abdominal wall, fluids or infectious material that accumulate in the pouch can track out of the perineum and onto the lower abdominal wall. This material will not track into the anal triangle or the thigh because the fascia fuses with deep tissues at the borders of these regions.

Clinical app

Urethral rupture

Urethral rupture may occur at a series of well-defined anatomical points.

The most common injury is a rupture of the proximal spongy urethra below the perineal membrane. The urethra is usually torn when structures of the perineum are caught between a hard object (e.g., a steel beam or cross bar of a bicycle) and the inferior pubic arch. Urine escapes through the rupture into the superficial perineal pouch and descends into the scrotum and onto the anterior abdominal wall deep to the superficial fascia.

In association with severe pelvic fractures, urethral rupture may occur at the prostatomembranous junction above the deep perineal pouch. The urine will extravasate into the true pelvis.

The worst and most serious urethral rupture is related to serious pelvic injuries where there is complete disruption of the puboprostatic ligaments. The prostate is dislocated superiorly not only by the ligamentous disruption but also by the extensive hematoma formed within the true pelvis. The diagnosis can be made by palpating the elevated prostate during a digital rectal examination.

Fig. 5.51 Superficial fascia. **A.** Lateral view. **B.** Anterior view.

Somatic nerves

Pudendal nerve

The major somatic nerve of the perineum is the pudendal nerve (see p. 236 and Fig. 5.52A). As it enters and courses through the perineum, it travels along the lateral wall of the ischio-anal fossa in the **pudendal canal,** which is a tubular compartment formed in the fascia that covers the obturator internus muscle. This pudendal canal also contains the internal pudendal artery and accompanying veins (Fig. 5.52A).

The pudendal nerve has three major terminal branches—the inferior rectal, perineal nerves, and the dorsal nerve of penis or clitoris—which are accompanied by branches of the internal pudendal artery (Fig. 5.52B).

- The **inferior rectal nerve** is often multiple, penetrates through the fascia of the pudendal canal, and courses medially across the ischio-anal fossa to innervate the external anal sphincter and related regions of the levator ani muscles. The nerve is also general sensory for the skin of the anal triangle.

- The **perineal nerve** passes into the urogenital triangle and gives rise to motor and cutaneous branches. The motor branches supply skeletal muscles in the superficial and deep perineal pouches. The largest of the sensory branches is the posterior scrotal nerve in men and the posterior labial nerve in women.

- The **dorsal nerve of penis** and **clitoris** enters the deep perineal pouch (Fig. 5.52). It passes along the lateral margin of the pouch and then exits by passing inferiorly through the perineal membrane in a position just inferior to the pubic symphysis where it meets the body of the clitoris or the penis. It courses along the dorsal surface of the body to reach the glans. The dorsal nerve is sensory to the penis and clitoris, particularly to the glans.

Other somatic nerves

Other somatic nerves that enter the perineum are mainly sensory and include branches of the ilio–inguinal, genitofemoral, posterior femoral cutaneous, and anococcygeal nerves.

Visceral nerves

Visceral nerves enter the perineum by two routes:

- Those to the skin, which consist mainly of postganglionic sympathetics, are delivered into the region along the

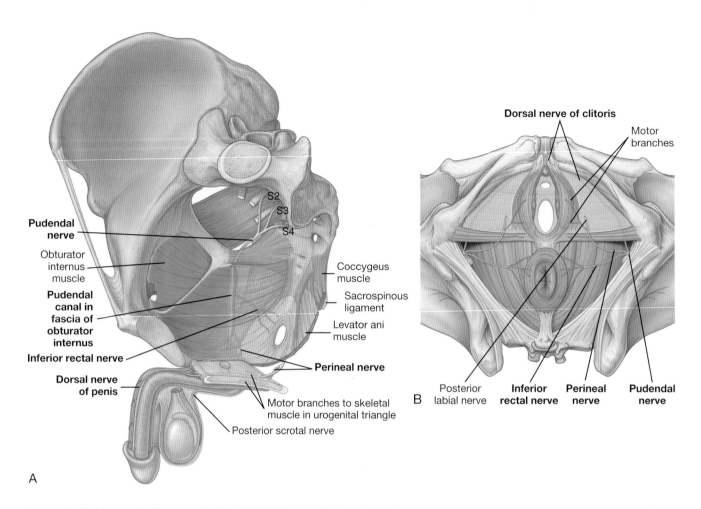

Dorsal nerve of clitoris

Motor branches

Pudendal nerve

Obturator internus muscle

Pudendal canal in fascia of obturator internus

Inferior rectal nerve

Dorsal nerve of penis

S2
S3
S4

Coccygeus muscle

Sacrospinous ligament

Levator ani muscle

Perineal nerve

Motor branches to skeletal muscle in urogenital triangle

Posterior scrotal nerve

A

Posterior labial nerve · **Inferior rectal nerve** · **Perineal nerve** · **Pudendal nerve**

B

Fig. 5.52 Pudendal nerve. **A.** In men. **B.** In women.

pudendal nerve (see Fig. 5.35). These fibers join the pudendal nerve from gray rami communicantes that connect pelvic parts of the sympathetic trunks to the anterior rami of the sacral spinal nerves.

■ Those to erectile tissues enter the region mainly by passing through the deep perineal pouch from the inferior hypogastric plexus in the pelvic cavity (see Fig. 5.38). The fibers that stimulate erection are parasympathetic fibers, which enter the inferior hypogastric plexus via pelvic splanchnic nerves from spinal cord levels of S2 to S4.

Blood vessels

Arteries

The most significant artery of the perineum is the internal pudendal artery (Fig. 5.53). Other arteries entering the area include the external pudendal, the testicular, and the cremasteric arteries.

Internal pudendal artery

The **internal pudendal artery** originates as a branch of the anterior trunk of the internal iliac artery in the pelvis (Fig. 5.53) and accompanies the pudendal nerve in the pudendal canal on the lateral wall of the ischio-anal fossa.

The branches of the internal pudendal artery are similar to those of the pudendal nerve in the perineum and include the inferior rectal and perineal arteries and branches to the erectile tissues of the penis and clitoris (Fig. 5.53).

Inferior rectal arteries

One or more **inferior rectal arteries** originate from the internal pudendal artery in the anal triangle and cross the ischio-anal fossa medially to branch and supply muscle and related skin (Fig. 5.53). They anastomose with middle and superior rectal arteries from the internal iliac artery and the inferior mesenteric artery, respectively,

Internal iliac artery

Internal pudendal artery

Inferior rectal artery

Internal pudendal artery
in fascia of obturator internus

Artery to bulb

Urethral artery

Deep artery of penis
(deep artery of clitoris in women)

Dorsal artery of penis
(dorsal artery of clitoris in women)

Perineal artery

Artery of bulb of penis
(artery of vestibular bulb in women)

Posterior scrotal artery
(posterior labial artery in women)

Fig. 5.53 Arteries in the perineum.

to form a network of vessels that supply the rectum and anal canal.

Perineal artery

The **perineal artery** originates near the anterior end of the pudendal canal and gives off a transverse perineal branch and a posterior scrotal or labial artery to surrounding tissues and skin (see Fig. 5.53).

Terminal part of the internal pudendal artery

The terminal part of the internal pudendal artery accompanies the dorsal nerve of the penis or clitoris into the deep perineal pouch and supplies branches to the tissues in the deep perineal pouch and erectile tissues.

Branches that supply the erectile tissues in men include the artery to the bulb of the penis, the urethral artery, the deep artery of the penis, and the dorsal artery of the penis (see Fig. 5.53).

- The **artery of bulb of penis** has a branch that supplies the bulbourethral gland and then penetrates the perineal membrane to supply the corpus spongiosum.

- A **urethral artery** also penetrates the perineal membrane and supplies the penile urethra and surrounding erectile tissue to the glans.

- Near the anterior margin of the deep perineal pouch, the internal pudendal artery bifurcates into two terminal branches. A **deep artery of penis** penetrates the perineal membrane to enter the crus and supply the crus and corpus cavernosum of the body. The **dorsal artery of penis** penetrates the anterior margin of the perineal membrane to meet the dorsal surface of the body of the penis. The vessel courses along the dorsal surface of the penis, medial to the dorsal nerve, and supplies the glans penis and superficial tissues of the penis; it also anastomoses with branches of the deep artery of penis and the urethral artery.

Branches that supply the erectile tissues in women are similar to those in men.

- **Arteries of the bulb of vestibule** supply the bulb of the vestibule and related vagina.

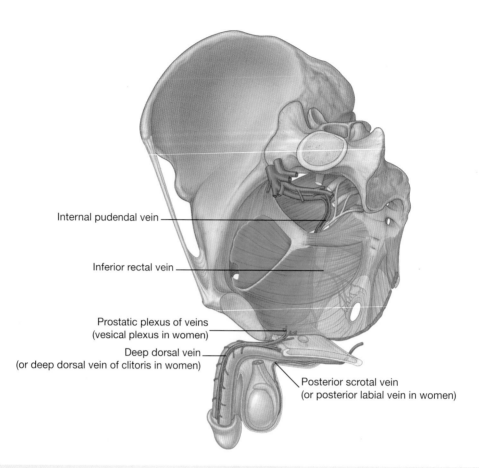

Internal pudendal vein

Inferior rectal vein

Prostatic plexus of veins
(vesical plexus in women)

Deep dorsal vein
(or deep dorsal vein of clitoris in women)

Posterior scrotal vein
(or posterior labial vein in women)

Fig. 5.54 Perineal veins.

- **Deep arteries of the clitoris** supply the crura and corpus cavernosum of the body.
- **Dorsal arteries of the clitoris** supply surrounding tissues and the glans.

External pudendal arteries

The **external pudendal arteries** consist of a superficial vessel and a deep vessel, which originate from the femoral artery in the thigh. They course medially to enter the perineum anteriorly and supply related skin of the penis and scrotum or the clitoris and labia majora.

Testicular and cremasteric arteries

In men, the **testicular arteries** originate from the abdominal aorta and descend into the scrotum through the inguinal canal to supply the testes. Also, **cremasteric arteries,** which originate from the inferior epigastric branch of the external iliac artery, accompany the spermatic cord into the scrotum.

In women, small cremasteric arteries follow the round ligament of the uterus through the inguinal canal.

Veins

Veins in the perineum generally accompany the arteries and join the **internal pudendal veins** that connect with the **internal iliac vein** in the pelvis (Fig. 5.54). The exception is the **deep dorsal vein of penis** or **clitoris** that drains mainly the glans and the corpora cavernosa. The deep dorsal vein courses along the midline between the dorsal arteries on each side of the body of penis or clitoris, passes though the gap between the inferior pubic ligament and the deep perineal pouch, and connects with the plexus of veins surrounding the prostate in men or bladder in women.

External pudendal veins, which drain anterior parts of the labia majora or the scrotum and overlap with the area of drainage of the internal pudendal veins, connect with the femoral vein in the thigh. Superficial dorsal veins of the penis or clitoris that drain skin are tributaries of the external pudendal veins.

Lymphatics

Lymphatic vessels from deep parts of the perineum accompany the internal pudendal blood vessels and drain mainly into **internal iliac nodes** in the pelvis.

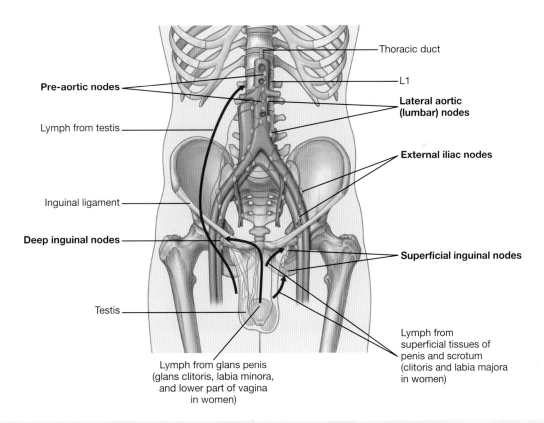

Pre-aortic nodes

Lymph from testis

Inguinal ligament

Deep inguinal nodes

Testis

Thoracic duct

L1

Lateral aortic (lumbar) nodes

External iliac nodes

Superficial inguinal nodes

Lymph from superficial tissues of penis and scrotum (clitoris and labia majora in women)

Lymph from glans penis (glans clitoris, labia minora, and lower part of vagina in women)

Fig. 5.55 Lymphatic drainage of the perineum.

Lymphatic channels from superficial tissues of the penis or the clitoris accompany the superficial external pudendal blood vessels and drain mainly into **superficial inguinal nodes,** as do lymphatic channels from the scrotum or labia majora (Fig. 5.55). The glans penis, the glans clitoris, labia minora, and the terminal inferior end of the vagina drain into **deep inguinal nodes** and **external iliac nodes.**

Lymphatics from the testes drain via channels that ascend in the spermatic cord, pass through the inguinal canal, and course up the posterior abdominal wall to connect directly with lateral aortic or lumbar nodes and pre-aortic nodes around the aorta at approximately vertebral levels LI and LII. Therefore disease from the testes tracks superiorly to nodes high in the posterior abdominal wall and not to inguinal or iliac nodes.

Imaging app

Visualizing the male pelvic cavity and perineum in the axial plane

Corpora cavernosa

Corpus spongiosum

Femur

Corpora cavernosa

Corpus spongiosum

Femur

Corpora cavernosa and crura of penis

Corpus spongiosum and bulb of penis

Femur

Anus

Fig. 5.56 A to C. Series of axial images that pass through the pelvic cavity and perineum from inferior to superior showing the various structures and their relationships to each other (T2-weighted MR images in axial plane).

Imaging app—cont'd

Corpora cavernosa

Spongy urethra

Ischiopubic ramus

Anal canal

Crus of penis
Bulb of penis
Femur

D

Ischiopubic ramus

Femur

Anal canal

Urethra
Bulb of penis

E

Pubic symphysis

Urethra

Femur

Ischiopubic ramus

Gluteus maximus

Anal canal

Puborectalis
(part of levator ani)

F

Fig. 5.56, cont'd D to **F.**

Continued

Imaging app—cont'd

Pubic symphysis

Prostate

Femur

Ischial tuberosity

Ischio-anal fossa

Obturator internus

Anal canal

Pudendal canal

Gluteus maximus

G

Prostate

Femur

Ischial tuberosity

Obturator internus

Anal canal

Ischio-anal fossa

Gluteus maximus

H

Femur   Bladder   Prostate

Ischium   Rectum

Femur   Bladder

Ischium   Rectum

I

J

Fig. 5.56, cont'd G to J.

Imaging app

Visualizing the female pelvic cavity and perineum in the sagittal plane

Fig. 5.57 A to **C**. Series of sagittal images that pass through the female pelvic cavity and perineum showing the various structures and their relationships to each other (T2-weighted MR images in sagittal plane).

Continued

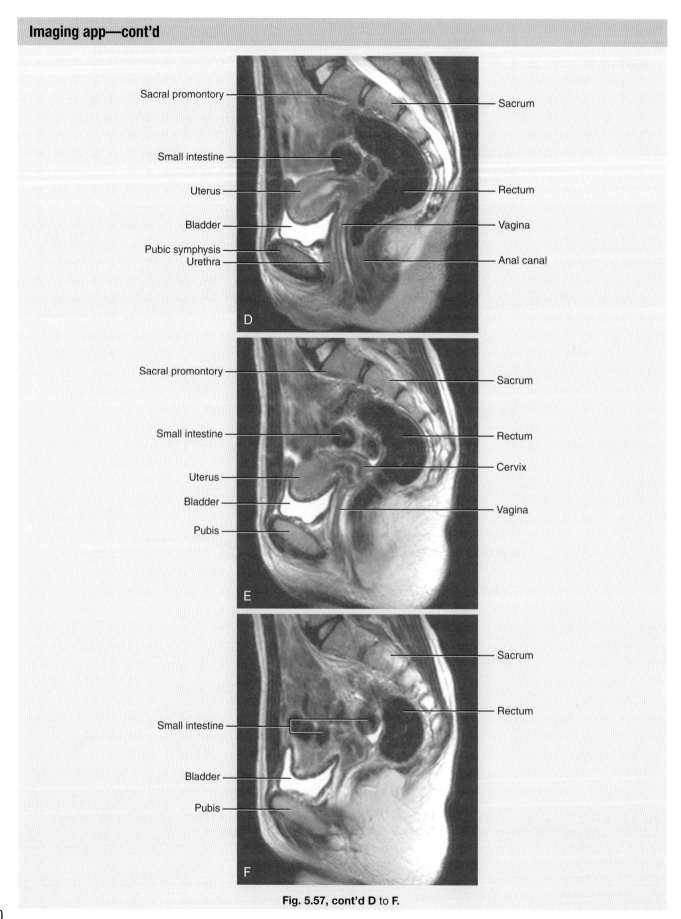

Fig. 5.57, cont'd D to **F.**

Imaging app

Visualizing the female pelvic cavity and perineum in the coronal plane

Fig. 5.58 A to **D.** Series of coronal images that pass through the pelvic cavity and perineum from anterior to posterior showing the various structures and their relationships to each other (T2-weighted MR images in coronal plane).

Imaging app

Visualizing the female pelvic cavity and perineum in the axial plane

Fig. 5.59 **A** to **D**. Series of axial images that pass through the pelvic cavity and perineum from inferior to superior showing the various structures and their relationships with each other (T2-weighted MR images in axial plane).

Imaging app—cont'd

Fig. 5.59, cont'd **E** to **H.**

6

Lower Limb

ADDITIONAL LEARNING RESOURCES
FOR CHAPTER 6, *LOWER LIMB*,
CAN BE FOUND ON THE ACCOMPANYING
EBOOK:

- Self-Assessment (scored) — National Board style
  multiple-choice questions, Chapter 6
- Short Questions (not scored) — these are
  questions requiring short responses, Chapter 6
- PT Case Studies
  Plantar fasciitis
  Achilles tendinitis and tendinosis
  Eversion ankle sprain
  High ankle sprain
  Patellofemoral pain syndrome
  Anterior lateral shin splints
  See more PT Case Studies online
- Clinical Cases
  Femoral hernia
  Groin injury
  Iliopsoas tendinitis
  Iliotibial band syndrome
  Nerve entrapment syndrome
  Pes cavus
  Varicose veins
  Knee joint injury
  Fracture of neck of femur
  Deep vein thrombosis
  See more Clinical Cases online

Regional anatomy **286**

The hip **287**
  Bony pelvis 287
  Proximal femur 290
  Hip joint 292
  Gateways to the lower
    limb 295
  Nerves 297
  Arteries 297
  Veins 298
  Lymphatics 299
  Deep fascia and
    the saphenous
    opening 300
  Femoral triangle 301

Gluteal region **303**
  Muscles 303
  Nerves 305
  Arteries 308
  Veins 308
  Lymphatics 308

Thigh **309**
  Bones 309
  Muscles 313
  Arteries 317
  Veins 321
  Nerves 321
  Knee joint 323
  Tibiofibular joint 329
  Popliteal fossa 329

Leg **331**
  Bones 331
  Joints 333
  Posterior compartment
    of leg 333
  Lateral compartment of
    leg 337
  Anterior compartment
    of the leg 338

Foot **340**
  Bones 340
  Joints 344
  Tarsal tunnel,
    retinacula, and
    arrangement of
    major structures at
    the ankle 351
  Arches of the
    foot 352
  Plantar
    aponeurosis 353
  Fibrous sheaths of
    toes 353
  Extensor hoods 354
  Intrinsic muscles 355
  Arteries 357
  Veins 359
  Nerves 359

Regional anatomy

The lower limb is divided into the gluteal region, thigh, leg, and foot on the basis of major joints, component bones, and superficial landmarks (Figs. 6.1, 6.2):

- The **gluteal region** is posterolateral and between the iliac crest and the fold of skin (gluteal fold) that defines the lower limit of the buttocks. The major bone of the gluteal region is the pelvic bone.
- Anteriorly, the **thigh** is between the inguinal ligament and the knee joint—the hip joint is just inferior to the middle third of the inguinal ligament, and the posterior thigh is between the gluteal fold and the knee. The bone of the thigh is the femur.
- The **leg** is between the knee and ankle joints. The bones of the leg are the tibia and fibula.
- The **foot** is distal to the ankle joint. Bones of the foot are the tarsals, metatarsals, and phalanges.

The major functions of the lower limb are:

- to support the weight of the body when standing, and
- to move the body through space.

When standing erect, the line of the center of gravity is slightly posterior to the hip joints, anterior to the knee and ankle joints, and directly over the almost circular support base formed by the feet on the ground. The organization of ligaments at the hip and knee joints, together with the shape of the articular surfaces particularly at the knee, facilitates "locking" of these joints into position, thereby reducing the muscular energy required to maintain a standing position.

When walking, integration of movements at all joints in the lower limb positions the foot on the ground and moves the body smoothly over the foot with minimal changes in the position of the body's center of gravity.

The lower limb is directly anchored to the axial skeleton by a sacro-iliac joint and by strong ligaments, which link the pelvic bone to the sacrum. This design serves to transmit the weight of the body above to the lower limb below.

Movements at the hip joint are flexion, extension, abduction, adduction, medial and lateral rotation, and circumduction (Fig. 6.3).

The knee and ankle joints are primarily hinge joints. Movements at the knee are mainly flexion and extension (Fig. 6.4A). Movements at the ankle are dorsiflexion

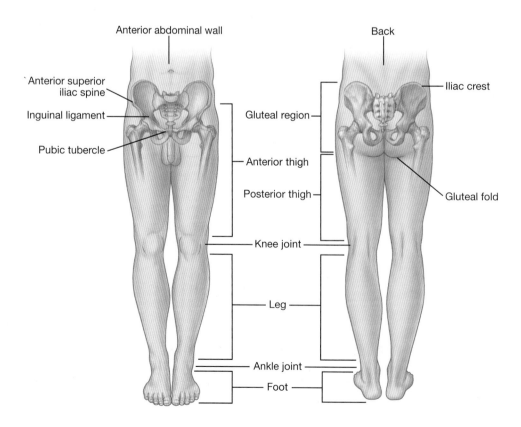

Fig. 6.1 Regions of the lower limb.

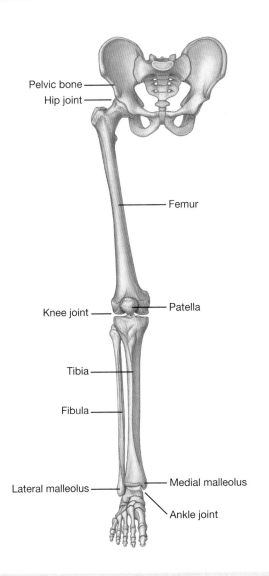

Fig. 6.2 Bones and joints of the lower limb.

(movement of the dorsal side of foot toward the leg) and plantarflexion (Fig. 6.4B).

THE HIP

Bony pelvis

The external surfaces of the pelvic bones, sacrum, and coccyx are predominantly the regions of the pelvis associated with the lower limb, although some muscles do originate from the deep or internal surfaces of these bones and from the deep surfaces of the lumbar vertebrae above.

Each pelvic bone is formed by three bones (**ilium, ischium,** and **pubis**), which fuse during childhood. The ilium is superior and the pubis and ischium are anteroinferior and posteroinferior, respectively (Fig. 6.5).

Ilium

The upper fan-shaped part of the ilium is associated on its inner side with the abdomen and on its outer side with the lower limb. The top of this region is the **iliac crest,** which ends anteriorly as the **anterior superior iliac spine** and posteriorly as the **posterior superior iliac spine** (Fig. 6.5). A prominent lateral expansion of the crest just posterior to the anterior superior iliac spine is the **tuberculum of iliac crest.**

The anterior inferior iliac spine is on the anterior margin of the ilium, and below this, where the ilium fuses with the pubis, is a raised area of bone (the **iliopubic eminence** [Fig. 6.5]).

The gluteal surface of the ilium faces posterolaterally, lies below the iliac crest, and provides attachment for the gluteal muscles. It is marked by three curved lines (inferior, anterior, and posterior gluteal lines (Fig. 6.5):

- The **inferior gluteal line** originates just superior to the anterior inferior iliac spine and curves inferiorly across the bone to end near the posterior margin of the acetabulum.
- The **anterior gluteal line** originates from the lateral margin of the iliac crest between the anterior superior iliac spine and the tuberculum of iliac crest and arches inferiorly across the ilium to disappear just superior to the upper margin of the greater sciatic foramen.
- The **posterior gluteal line** descends almost vertically from the iliac crest to a position near the posterior inferior iliac spine.

Ischial tuberosity

The **ischial tuberosity** is posteroinferior to the acetabulum and is associated mainly with the hamstring muscles of the posterior thigh (Fig. 6.6). It is divided into upper and lower areas by a transverse line.

The upper area of the ischial tuberosity is oriented vertically and is further subdivided into two parts by an oblique line that descends from medial to lateral across the surface.

The lower area of the ischial tuberosity is oriented horizontally and is divided into medial and lateral regions by a ridge of bone.

When sitting, this medial part supports the body weight.

The sacrotuberous ligament is attached to a sharp ridge on the medial margin of the ischial tuberosity.

Fig. 6.3 Movements of the hip joint. **A.** Flexion and extension. **B.** Abduction and adduction. **C.** External and internal rotation. **D.** Circumduction.

Fig. 6.4 Movements of the knee and ankle. **A.** Knee flexion and extension. **B.** Ankle dorsiflexion and plantarflexion.

Ischiopubic ramus and pubic bone

The external surfaces of the ischiopubic ramus anterior to the ischial tuberosity and the body of the pubis provide attachment for muscles of the medial compartment of thigh (Fig. 6.6).

Acetabulum

The large cup-shaped **acetabulum** for articulation with the head of the femur is on the lateral surface of the pelvic bone in the region where the ilium, pubis, and ischium fuse (Fig. 6.7).

The margin of the acetabulum is marked inferiorly by a prominent notch (**acetabular notch**).

The wall of the acetabulum consists of nonarticular and articular parts:

- The nonarticular part is rough and forms a shallow circular depression (the **acetabular fossa**) in central and inferior parts of the acetabular floor; the acetabular notch is continuous with the acetabular fossa (Fig. 6.7).

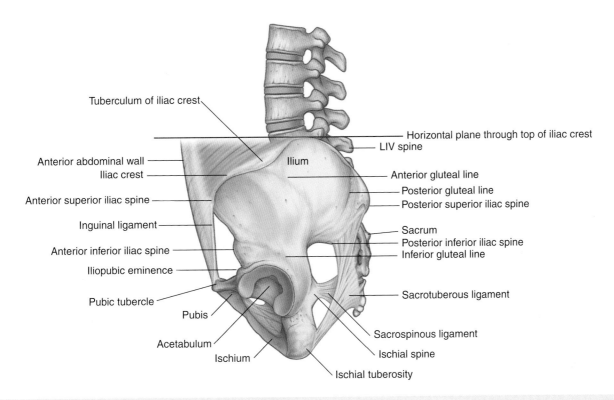

Fig. 6.5 External surface of the bony pelvis. Lateral view.

Tuberculum of iliac crest

Horizontal plane through top of iliac crest

LIV spine

Ilium

Anterior abdominal wall

Iliac crest

Anterior gluteal line

Posterior gluteal line

Posterior superior iliac spine

Anterior superior iliac spine

Inguinal ligament

Sacrum

Posterior inferior iliac spine

Anterior inferior iliac spine

Inferior gluteal line

Iliopubic eminence

Pubic tubercle

Sacrotuberous ligament

Pubis

Sacrospinous ligament

Acetabulum

Ischium

Ischial spine

Ischial tuberosity

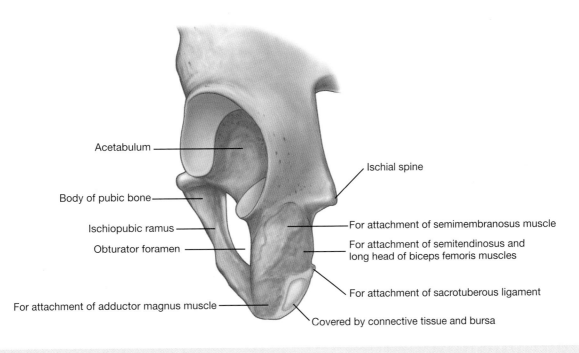

Fig. 6.6 Ischial tuberosity. Posterolateral view.

Acetabulum

Ischial spine

Body of pubic bone

For attachment of semimembranosus muscle

Ischiopubic ramus

For attachment of semitendinosus and long head of biceps femoris muscles

Obturator foramen

For attachment of sacrotuberous ligament

For attachment of adductor magnus muscle

Covered by connective tissue and bursa

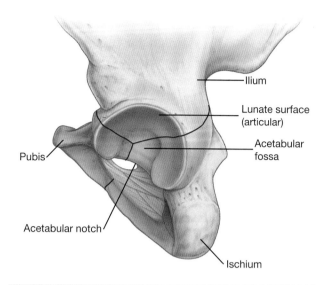

Fig. 6.7 Acetabulum.

- The articular **(lunate) surface** is broad and surrounds the anterior, superior, and posterior margins of the acetabular fossa (Fig. 6.7).

The smooth, crescent-shaped, articular surface (the lunate surface) is broadest superiorly where most of the body's weight is transmitted through the pelvis to the femur. The lunate surface is deficient inferiorly at the acetabular notch (Fig. 6.7).

The acetabular fossa provides attachment for the ligament of the head of the femur, whereas blood vessels and nerves pass through the acetabular notch.

Clinical app

Pelvic fractures

There are many ways of classifying pelvic fractures that enable a surgeon to determine the appropriate treatment and the patient's prognosis. The pelvic bones, sacrum, and associated joints form a bony ring surrounding the pelvic cavity.

Pelvic fractures are generally of four types.

- Type 1 injuries occur without disruption of the bony pelvic ring (e.g., a fracture of the iliac crest). These types of injuries are unlikely to represent significant trauma, though in the case of a fracture of the iliac crest, blood loss needs to be assessed.
- Type 2 injuries occur with a single break in the bony pelvic ring. An example of this would be a single fracture with diastasis (separation) of the pubic symphysis.

- Type 3 injuries occur with double breaks in the bony pelvic ring. These include bilateral fractures of the pubic rami, which may produce urethral damage.
- Type 4 injuries occur at and around the acetabulum.

Other types of pelvic ring injuries include disruption of the sacro-iliac joint with or without dislocation. This may involve significant visceral pelvic trauma and hemorrhage.

Other general pelvic injuries include stress fractures and insufficiency fractures, as seen in athletes and in elderly patients with osteoporosis, respectively.

Proximal femur

The femur is the bone of the thigh and the longest bone in the body. Its proximal end is characterized by a head and neck and two large projections (the greater and lesser trochanters) on the upper part of the shaft (Fig. 6.8).

The **head** of the femur is spherical and articulates with the acetabulum of the pelvic bone. It is characterized by a nonarticular pit **(fovea)** on its medial surface for the attachment of the ligament of the head.

The **neck** of the femur is a cylindrical strut of bone that connects the head to the shaft of the femur. It projects superomedially from the shaft at an angle of approximately 125° and projects slightly forward. The orientation of the neck relative to the shaft increases the range of movement of the hip joint.

The upper part of the **shaft** of the femur bears a greater and lesser trochanter, which are attachment sites for muscles that move the hip joint.

Greater and lesser trochanters

The **greater trochanter** extends superiorly from the shaft of the femur just lateral to the region where the shaft joins the neck of the femur (Fig. 6.8). It continues posteriorly where its medial surface is deeply grooved to form the **trochanteric fossa.** The lateral wall of this fossa bears a distinct oval depression for attachment of the obturator externus muscle.

The greater trochanter has an elongate ridge on its anterolateral surface for attachment of the gluteus minimus and a similar ridge more posteriorly on its lateral surface for attachment of the gluteus medius. Between these two points, the greater trochanter is palpable.

On the medial side of the superior aspect of the greater trochanter and just above the trochanteric fossa is a small impression for attachment of the obturator internus and its associated gemelli muscles, and immediately

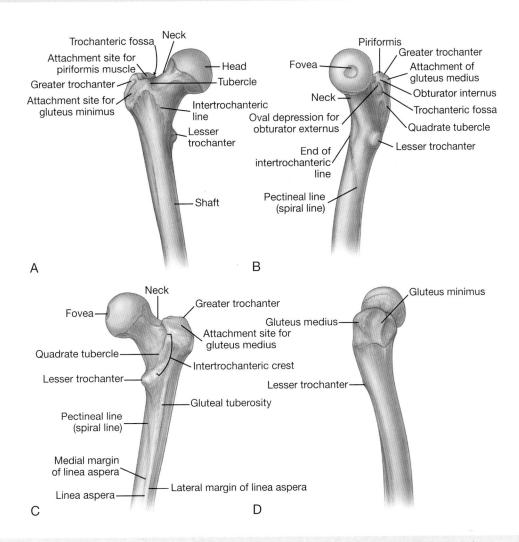

Fig. 6.8 Proximal end of the right femur. **A.** Anterior view. **B.** Medial view. **C.** Posterior view. **D.** Lateral view.

above and behind this feature is an impression on the margin of the trochanter for attachment of the piriformis muscle.

The **lesser trochanter** is smaller than the greater trochanter and has a blunt conical shape. It projects posteromedially from the shaft of femur just inferior to the junction with the neck (Fig. 6.8). It is the attachment site for the combined tendons of psoas major and iliacus muscles.

Extending between the two trochanters and separating the shaft from the neck of the femur are the intertrochanteric line and intertrochanteric crest.

Intertrochanteric line

The **intertrochanteric line** is a ridge of bone on the anterior surface of the upper margin of the shaft that descends medially from a tubercle on the anterior surface of the base of the greater trochanter to a position just anterior to the base of the lesser trochanter (Fig. 6.8). It is continuous with the **pectineal line** (spiral line), which curves medially under the lesser trochanter and around the shaft of the femur to merge with the medial margin of the **linea aspera** on the posterior aspect of the femur.

Intertrochanteric crest

The **intertrochanteric crest** is on the posterior surface of the femur and descends medially across the bone from the posterior margin of the greater trochanter to the base of the lesser trochanter (Fig. 6.8). It is a broad smooth ridge of bone with a prominent tubercle (the **quadrate tubercle**) on its upper half, which provides attachment for the quadratus femoris muscle.

Shaft of the femur

The shaft of the femur descends from lateral to medial in the coronal plane at an angle of 7° from the vertical axis (Fig. 6.9).

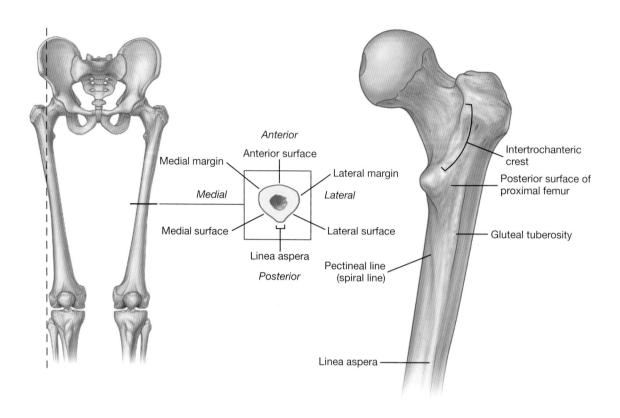

Fig. 6.9 Shaft of the femur. On the right is a posterior view of proximal shaft of right femur.

The distal end of the femur is therefore closer to the midline than the upper end of the shaft.

The middle third of the shaft of the femur is triangular in shape with smooth lateral and medial margins between anterior, lateral (posterolateral), and medial (posteromedial) surfaces. The posterior margin is broad and forms a prominent raised crest (the linea aspera) (Fig. 6.9).

The linea aspera is a major site of muscle attachment in the thigh. In the proximal third of the femur, the medial and lateral margins of the linea aspera diverge and continue superiorly as the pectineal line and gluteal tuberosity, respectively (Fig. 6.9):

- The pectineal line curves anteriorly under the lesser trochanter and joins the intertrochanteric line.
- The gluteal tuberosity is a broad linear roughening that curves laterally to the base of the greater trochanter.

The gluteus maximus muscle is attached to the gluteal tuberosity.

The triangular area enclosed by the pectineal line, the gluteal tuberosity, and the intertrochanteric crest is

the posterior surface of the proximal end of the femur (Fig. 6.9).

Hip joint

The hip joint is a synovial articulation between the head of the femur and the acetabulum of the pelvic bone (Fig. 6.11A; also see Fig. 6.16). The joint is a multiaxial ball-and-socket

Clinical app

Femoral neck fractures

Femoral neck fractures (Fig. 6.10) can interrupt blood supply to the femoral head. Blood supply to the head and neck is primarily from an arterial ring formed by the branches of the medial and lateral circumflex femoral arteries around the base of the femoral neck. From here, vessels course along the neck, penetrate the capsule, and supply the femoral head. Blood supply to the femoral head and femoral neck is further enhanced by the artery of the ligament of head of femur, a branch of the obturator artery, which is generally small and variable. Femoral neck fractures may disrupt associated vessels and lead to necrosis of the femoral head.

Fig. 6.10 This radiograph of the pelvis, anteroposterior view, demonstrates a fracture of the neck of the femur.

Fractured neck of femur

Clinical app

Femoral shaft fractures

An appreciable amount of energy is needed to fracture the femoral shaft. This type of injury is therefore accompanied by damage to the surrounding soft tissues, which include the muscle compartments and the structures they contain.

joint designed for stability and weightbearing at the expense of mobility.

When considering the effects of muscle action on the hip joint, the long neck of the femur and the angulation of the neck on the shaft of the femur must be kept in mind. For example, medial and lateral rotation of the femur involves muscles that move the greater trochanter forward and backward, respectively, relative to the acetabulum (Fig. 6.11B).

The articular surfaces of the hip joint are:

- the spherical head of the femur, and
- the lunate surface of the acetabulum of the pelvic bone (Fig. 6.12A).

The acetabulum almost entirely encompasses the hemispherical head of the femur and contributes substantially to joint stability. The nonarticular acetabular fossa contains loose connective tissue. The lunate surface is covered by hyaline cartilage and is broadest superiorly (Fig. 6.12).

Except for the fovea, the head of the femur is also covered by hyaline cartilage.

The rim of the acetabulum is raised slightly by a fibrocartilaginous collar (the **acetabular labrum**). Inferiorly, the labrum bridges across the acetabular notch as the **transverse acetabular ligament** and converts the notch into a foramen (Fig. 6.12A).

The **ligament of head of femur** is a flat band of delicate connective tissue that attaches at one end to the fovea on the head of the femur and at the other end to the acetabular fossa, transverse acetabular ligament, and margins of the acetabular notch

Clinical app

Intertrochanteric fractures

In these fractures, the break usually runs from the greater trochanter through to the lesser trochanter and does not involve the femoral neck. Intertrochanteric fractures preserve the femoral neck blood supply and do not render the femoral head ischemic.

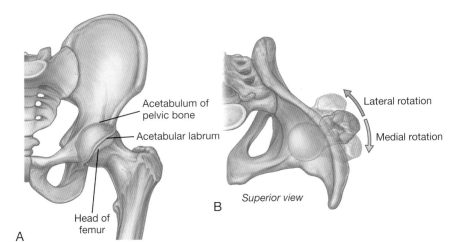

Acetabulum of pelvic bone

Acetabular labrum

Head of femur

A

Superior view

B

Lateral rotation

Medial rotation

Fig. 6.11 Hip joint. **A.** Articular surfaces. Anterior view. **B.** Movement of the neck of the femur during medial and lateral rotation. Superior view.

Fig. 6.12 Hip joint. **A.** Transverse acetabular ligament. **B.** Ligament of the head of the femur. The head of the femur has been laterally rotated out of the acetabulum to show the ligament.

Labels for A:
Acetabular labrum
Acetabular fossa
Lunate surface
Acetabular foramen
Transverse acetabular ligament
Obturator foramen

Labels for B:
Cut synovial membrane
Synovial sleeve around ligament
Obturator artery
Pubic tubercle
Pubis
Acetabular branch of obturator artery
Artery of ligament of head
Ligament of head of femur
Obturator membrane
Ischial tuberosity

Fig. 6.13 Synovial membrane of the hip joint.

Labels:
Synovial membrane
Line of attachment around head of femur
Membrane reflects back to attach to margin of acetabulum

(Fig. 6.12B). It carries a small branch of the obturator artery, which contributes to the blood supply of the head of the femur.

The synovial membrane attaches to the margins of the articular surfaces of the femur and acetabulum, forms a tubular covering around the ligament of head of femur, and lines the fibrous membrane of the joint (Figs. 6.12B, 6.13). From its attachment to the margin of the head of the femur, the synovial membrane covers the neck of the femur before reflecting onto the fibrous membrane (Fig. 6.13).

The fibrous membrane that encloses the hip joint is strong and generally thick. Medially, it is attached to the margin of the acetabulum, the transverse acetabular ligament, and the adjacent margin of the obturator foramen (Fig. 6.14A). Laterally, it is attached to the intertrochanteric line on the anterior aspect of the femur and to the neck of the femur just proximal to the intertrochanteric crest on the posterior surface.

Ligaments

Three ligaments reinforce the external surface of the fibrous membrane and stabilize the joint: the iliofemoral, pubofemoral, and ischiofemoral ligaments.

- The **iliofemoral ligament** is anterior to the hip joint and is triangular-shaped (Fig. 6.14B). Its apex is attached to the ilium between the anterior inferior iliac spine and the margin of the acetabulum and its base is attached along the intertrochanteric line of the femur. Parts of the ligament attached above and below the intertrochanteric line are thicker than those attached to the central part of the line. This results in the ligament having a Y appearance.
- The **pubofemoral ligament** is anteroinferior to the hip joint (Fig. 6.14B). It is also triangular in shape, with its base attached medially to the iliopubic eminence, adjacent bone, and obturator membrane. Laterally, it blends with the fibrous membrane and with the deep surface of the iliofemoral ligament.
- The **ischiofemoral ligament** reinforces the posterior aspect of the fibrous membrane (Fig. 6.14C). It is attached medially to the ischium just posteroinferior to the acetabulum and laterally to the greater trochanter deep to the iliofemoral ligament.

The fibers of all three ligaments are oriented in a spiral fashion around the hip joint so that they become taut when the joint is extended. This stabilizes the joint and reduces the amount of muscle energy required to maintain a standing position.

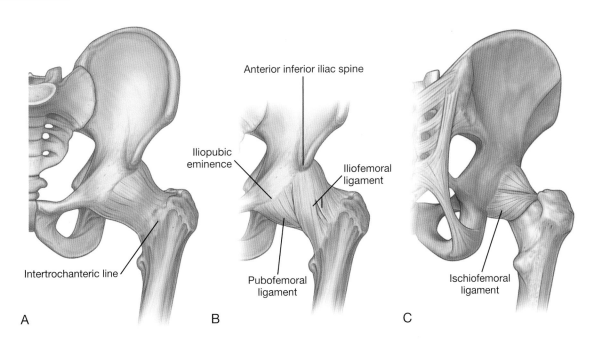

Fig. 6.14 Fibrous membrane and ligaments of the hip joint. **A.** Fibrous membrane of the joint capsule. Anterior view. **B.** Iliofemoral and pubofemoral ligaments. Anterior view. **C.** Ischiofemoral ligament. Posterior view.

Fig. 6.15 Blood supply of the hip joint.

Blood supply and innervation

Vascular supply to the hip joint is predominantly through branches of the **obturator artery, medial** and **lateral circumflex femoral arteries, superior** and **inferior gluteal arteries,** and the **first perforating branch** of the deep artery of the thigh. The articular branches of these vessels form a network around the joint (Fig. 6.15).

The hip joint is innervated by articular branches from the femoral, obturator, and superior gluteal nerves and the nerve to the quadratus femoris.

Gateways to the lower limb

There are four major routes by which structures pass from the abdomen and pelvis into and out of the lower limb (Fig. 6.17):

- **Obturator canal** — an almost vertically oriented passageway at the anterosuperior edge of the obturator foramen. The obturator canal connects the abdominopelvic region with the medial compartment of thigh.
- **Greater sciatic foramen** — formed on the posterolateral pelvic wall and is the major route for structures to pass between the pelvis and the gluteal region of the lower limb (Fig. 6.17). The piriformis muscle passes out of the pelvis into the gluteal region through the greater sciatic foramen and separates the foramen into two parts, a part above the muscle and a part below.
- **Lesser sciatic foramen** — inferior to the greater sciatic foramen on the posterolateral pelvic wall (Fig. 6.17). It is also inferior to the lateral attachment of the pelvic

Imaging app

Visualizing the hip joint

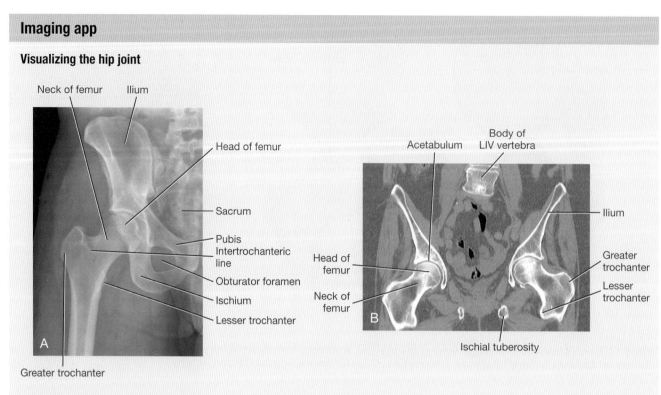

Neck of femur   Ilium

Head of femur

Sacrum

Pubis
Intertrochanteric
line

Obturator foramen

Ischium

Lesser trochanter

A

Greater trochanter

Body of
LIV vertebra

Acetabulum

Ilium

Head of
femur

Greater
trochanter

Neck of
femur

Lesser
trochanter

B

Ischial tuberosity

Fig. 6.16 Hip joint. **A.** Normal hip joint. Radiograph, anterior–posterior view. **B.** Hip joints. Computed tomography image in coronal plane.

Piriformis muscle   **Abdominal cavity**

Greater sciatic foramen above piriformis muscle:
• Superior gluteal nerve, artery, vein

Lesser sciatic foramen:
• Obturator internus muscle tendon
• Pudendal nerve and internal pudendal vessels pass into perineum from gluteal region

Greater sciatic foramen below piriformis muscle:
• Sciatic nerve
• Inferior gluteal nerve, artery, vein
• Pudendal nerve
• Internal pudendal artery and vein
• Posterior femoral cutaneous nerve
• Nerve to obturator internus and gemellus superior muscles
• Nerve to quadratus femoris and gemellus inferior muscles

Pelvic cavity

Sacrotuberous
ligament

Sacrospinous
ligament

Ilio-inguinal nerve

Obturator canal:
• Obturator nerve
• Obturator vessels

Gap between inguinal ligament and pelvic bone:
• Psoas major, iliacus, pectineus muscles
• Femoral artery
• Femoral vein
• Lymphatics
• Femoral branch of genitofemoral nerve
• Lateral cutaneous nerve of thigh
• Femoral nerve

   Fig. 6.17 Gateways to the lower limb.

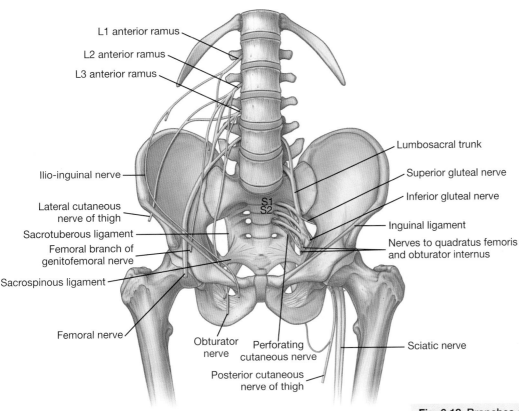

L1 anterior ramus
L2 anterior ramus
L3 anterior ramus

Ilio-inguinal nerve

Lateral cutaneous
nerve of thigh

Sacrotuberous ligament

Femoral branch of
genitofemoral nerve

Sacrospinous ligament

Femoral nerve

Obturator
nerve

Perforating
cutaneous nerve

Posterior cutaneous
nerve of thigh

Lumbosacral trunk

Superior gluteal nerve

Inferior gluteal nerve

Inguinal ligament

Nerves to quadratus femoris
and obturator internus

Sciatic nerve

S1
S2

Fig. 6.18 Branches of the lumbosacral plexus.

floor (levator ani and coccygeus muscles) to the pelvic wall and therefore connects the gluteal region with the perineum.

- Gap between the inguinal ligament and pelvic bone — a large crescent-shaped gap between the inguinal ligament above and the anterosuperior margin of the pelvic bone below is the major route of communication between the abdomen and the anteromedial aspect of the thigh (Fig. 6.17).

Nerves

Nerves that enter the lower limb from the abdomen and pelvis are terminal branches of the lumbosacral plexus on the posterior wall of the abdomen and the posterolateral walls of the pelvis (Fig. 6.18).

The **lumbar plexus** is formed by the anterior rami of spinal nerves L1 to L3 and part of L4. The rest of the anterior ramus of L4 and the anterior ramus of L5 combine to form the **lumbosacral trunk,** which enters the pelvic cavity and joins with the anterior rami of S1 to S3 and part of S4 to form the **sacral plexus.**

Nerves that originate from the lumbosacral plexus and that leave the abdomen and pelvis to enter the lower limb are indicated in Fig. 6.18 and described in Table 6.1, p. 278.

Arteries

Femoral artery

The major artery supplying the lower limb is the **femoral artery** (Fig. 6.19), which is the continuation of the external iliac artery in the abdomen. The external iliac artery becomes the femoral artery as the vessel passes under the inguinal ligament to enter the femoral triangle in the anterior aspect of the thigh. Branches supply most of the thigh and all of the leg and foot.

Superior and inferior gluteal arteries and the obturator artery

The **superior and inferior gluteal arteries** originate in the pelvic cavity as branches of the internal iliac artery (Fig. 6.19, see pp. 240–241) and supply the gluteal region. The superior gluteal artery leaves the pelvis through the greater sciatic foramen above the piriformis muscle, and the inferior gluteal artery leaves through the same foramen but below the piriformis muscle.

The **obturator artery** is also a branch of the internal iliac artery in the pelvic cavity (p. 241) and passes through the obturator canal to enter and supply the medial compartment of thigh (Fig. 6.19).

LI

LII

LIII

Aorta

Superior gluteal artery

Piriformis muscle

Inferior gluteal artery

Sacrotuberous ligament

Obturator foramen and membrane

Obturator canal

Sacrospinous ligament

Common iliac artery

Internal iliac artery

External iliac artery

Superior gluteal artery

Obturator artery

Inferior gluteal artery

Femoral vein

Femoral artery

Fig. 6.19 Arteries of the lower limb.

Branches of the femoral, inferior gluteal, superior gluteal, and obturator arteries, together with branches from the internal pudendal artery of the perineum, interconnect to form an anastomotic network in the upper thigh and gluteal region. The presence of these anastomotic channels may provide collateral circulation when one of the vessels is interrupted.

Veins

Veins draining the lower limb form superficial and deep groups (Fig. 6.20).

The deep veins generally follow the arteries (femoral, superior gluteal, inferior gluteal, and obturator). The major deep vein draining the limb is the **femoral vein** (Fig. 6.20). It becomes the external iliac vein when it passes under the inguinal ligament to enter the abdomen.

The superficial veins are in the subcutaneous connective tissue and are interconnected with and ultimately drain into the deep veins. The superficial veins form two major channels—the **great saphenous vein** and the **small saphenous vein.** Both veins originate from a dorsal venous arch in the foot (Fig. 6.20):

- The **great saphenous vein** originates from the medial side of the dorsal venous arch and then ascends up the medial side of the leg, knee, and thigh to connect with the femoral vein just inferior to the inguinal ligament.
- The **small saphenous vein** originates from the lateral side of the dorsal venous arch, ascends up the posterior surface

of the leg, and then penetrates deep fascia to join the popliteal vein posterior to the knee; proximal to the knee, the popliteal vein becomes the femoral vein.

Clinical app

Varicose veins

The normal flow of blood in the venous system depends on the presence of competent valves, which prevent reflux. Venous return is supplemented with contraction of the muscles in the lower limb, which pump the blood toward the heart. When venous valves become incompetent they tend to place extra pressure on more distal valves, which may also become incompetent. This condition produces dilated tortuous superficial veins (varicose veins) in the distribution of the great (long) and small (short) saphenous venous systems.

Clinical app

Deep vein thrombosis

Thrombosis resulting from venous stasis, injury to the vessel wall, or hypercoagulable states may occur in the deep veins of the lower limb and within the pelvic veins.

In some patients a deep vein thrombosis (DVT) in the veins of the leg may propagate into the femoral veins. This clot may break off and pass through the heart to enter the pulmonary circulation, resulting in occlusion of the pulmonary artery (pulmonary embolism), cardiopulmonary arrest, and death.

Inferior vena cava

Common
iliac vein

Internal iliac vein

External iliac vein

Inguinal ligament

Inferior and superior
gluteal veins

Obturator vein

Femoral vein

Popliteal vein

Anterior and posterior
tibial veins

Small
saphenous
vein

Superficial
veins

Great
saphenous
vein

Dorsal venous arch

Fig. 6.20 Veins of the lower limb.

Clinical app

Harvesting veins for grafts
Vein grafts have long been used for vascular conduits. Superficial veins of the arms and legs are harvested and used to bypass areas of arterial occlusion and stenoses. Typically vein bypass grafts are used for coronary artery bypass surgery and to bypass areas of vascular occlusion in the lower limb.

Clinical app—cont'd

The commonest vein used for bypass grafting is the great saphenous vein, but the radial artery is also used and, occasionally, the small saphenous vein. Historically, a long incision was required to obtain access to the vein, but now a small incision (approximately 2 inches) is made either above or below the knee and the vein is removed laparoscopically.

It is important to remember that veins contain valves and to use the vein as an appropriate conduit, it must either be reversed or, using special surgical techniques, the valves can be obliterated.

In coronary artery bypass grafting the vein is anastomosed to the ascending arch of the aorta and then anastomosed distal to the regions of occlusion on the coronary vessels. Similarly, in lower limb ischemic disease the vein can be used to bypass the regions of stenosis and occlusion within the femoral artery and the distal branches.

Lymphatics

Most lymphatic vessels in the lower limb drain into superficial and deep inguinal nodes located in the fascia just inferior to the inguinal ligament (Fig. 6.21).

Superficial inguinal nodes

The **superficial inguinal nodes,** of which there are approximately 10, are in the superficial fascia and parallel the course of the inguinal ligament in the upper thigh (Fig. 6.21). Medially, they extend inferiorly along the terminal part of the great saphenous vein.

Superficial inguinal nodes receive lymph from the gluteal region, lower abdominal wall, perineum, and superficial regions of the lower limb. They drain via vessels that accompany the femoral vessels into external iliac nodes associated with the external iliac artery in the abdomen.

Deep inguinal nodes

The **deep inguinal nodes,** of which there are up to three, are medial to the femoral vein (Fig. 6.21).

The deep inguinal nodes receive lymph from deep lymphatics associated with the femoral vessels and from the glans penis (or clitoris) in the perineum. They interconnect with the superficial inguinal nodes and drain into the external iliac nodes via vessels that pass along the medial side of the femoral vein as it passes under the inguinal ligament. The space through which the lymphatic vessels pass under the inguinal ligament is the femoral canal.

299

Table 6.1 Branches of the lumbosacral plexus associated with the lower limb

Branch	Spinal segments	Function: motor	Function: sensory (cutaneous)
Ilio-inguinal	L1	No motor function in lower limb but innervates muscles of the abdominal wall	Skin over anteromedial part of upper thigh and adjacent skin of perineum
Genitofemoral	L1, L2	No motor function in lower limb, but genital branch innervates cremaster muscle in the wall of the spermatic cord in men	Femoral branch innervates skin on anterior central part of upper thigh; the genital branch innervates skin in anterior part of perineum (anterior scrotum in men and mons pubis and anterior labia majora in women)
Femoral	L2 to L4	All muscles in the anterior compartment of thigh; in the abdomen, also gives rise to branches that supply iliacus and pectineus	Skin over the anterior thigh, anteromedial knee, medial side of the leg, and the medial side of the foot
Obturator	L2 to L4	All muscles in the medial compartment of thigh (except pectineus and the part of adductor magnus attached to the ischium); also innervates obturator externus	Skin over upper medial aspect of thigh
Sciatic	L4 to S3	All muscles in the posterior compartment of thigh and the part of adductor magnus attached to the ischium; all muscles in the leg and foot	Skin over lateral side of leg and foot and over the sole and dorsal surface of foot
Superior gluteal	L4 to S1	Muscles of the gluteal region (gluteus medius, gluteus minimus, tensor fasciae latae)	
Inferior gluteal	L5 to S2	Muscle of the gluteal region (gluteus maximus)	
Lateral cutaneous nerve of thigh	L2, L3		Parietal peritoneum in iliac fossa; skin over anterolateral thigh
Posterior cutaneous nerve of thigh	S1 to S3		Skin over gluteal fold and upper medial aspect of thigh and adjacent perineum, posterior aspect of thigh and upper posterior leg
Nerve to quadratus femoris	L4 to S1	Muscles of gluteal region (quadratus femoris and gemellus inferior)	
Nerve to obturator internus	L5 to S2	Muscles of gluteal region (obturator internus and gemellus superior)	
Perforating cutaneous nerve	S2, S3		Skin over medial aspect of gluteal fold

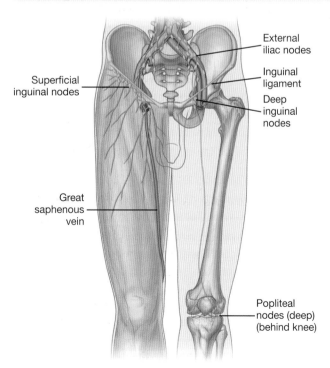

Fig. 6.21 Lymphatic drainage of the lower limb.

Popliteal nodes

In addition to the inguinal nodes, there is a small collection of deep nodes posterior to the knee close to the popliteal vessels (Fig. 6.21). These **popliteal nodes** receive lymph from superficial vessels, which accompany the small saphenous vein, and from deep areas of the leg and foot. They ultimately drain into the deep and superficial inguinal nodes.

Deep fascia and the saphenous opening

Fascia lata

The outer layer of deep fascia in the lower limb forms a thick "stocking-like" membrane, which covers the limb and lies beneath the superficial fascia (Fig. 6.22A). This deep fascia is particularly thick in the thigh and gluteal region and is termed the **fascia lata.**

The fascia lata is anchored superiorly to bone and soft tissues along a line of attachment that defines the upper margin of the lower limb.

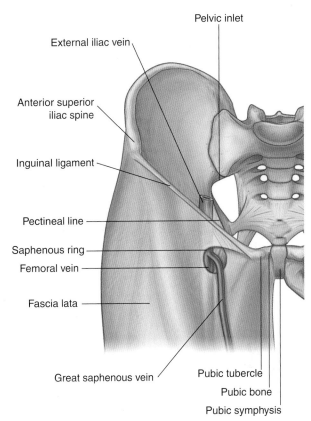

Fig. 6.23 Saphenous opening. Anterior view.

Fig. 6.22 Fascia lata. **A.** Right limb. Anterior view. **B.** Left limb. Lateral view.

Inferiorly, the fascia lata is continuous with the deep fascia of the leg.

Iliotibial tract

The fascia lata is thickened laterally into a longitudinal band (the **iliotibial tract**), which descends along the lateral margin of the limb from the tuberculum of iliac crest to a bony attachment just below the knee (Fig. 6.22B).

The superior aspect of the fascia lata in the gluteal region splits anteriorly to enclose the tensor fasciae latae muscle and posteriorly to enclose the gluteus maximus muscle:

- The tensor fasciae latae muscle is partially enclosed by and inserts into the superior and anterior aspects of the iliotibial tract.
- Most of the gluteus maximus muscle inserts into the posterior aspect of the iliotibial tract.

The tensor fasciae latae and gluteus maximus muscles, working through their attachments to the iliotibial tract, hold the leg in extension once other muscles have extended the leg at the knee joint. The iliotibial tract and its two associated muscles also stabilize the hip joint by preventing lateral displacement of the proximal end of the femur away from the acetabulum.

Saphenous opening

The fascia lata has one prominent aperture on the anterior aspect of the thigh just inferior to the medial end of the inguinal ligament (the **saphenous opening**), which allows the great saphenous vein to pass from superficial fascia through the deep fascia to connect with the femoral vein (Fig. 6.23).

Femoral triangle

The femoral triangle is a wedge-shaped depression formed by muscles in the upper thigh at the junction between the anterior abdominal wall and the lower limb (Fig. 6.24):

- The base of the triangle is the inguinal ligament.

Fig. 6.24 Boundaries of the femoral triangle.

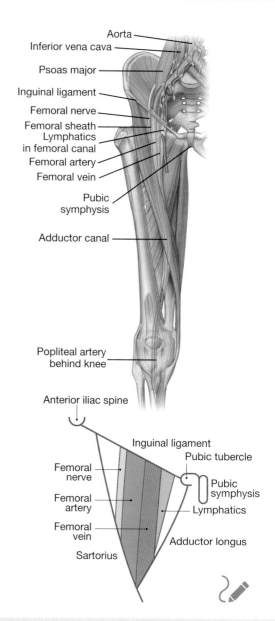

Fig. 6.25 Contents of the femoral triangle.

- The medial border is the medial margin of the adductor longus muscle in the medial compartment of thigh.
- The lateral margin is the medial margin of the sartorius muscle in the anterior compartment of thigh.
- The floor of the triangle is formed medially by the pectineus and adductor longus muscles in the medial compartment of thigh and laterally by the iliopsoas muscle descending from the abdomen.
- The apex of the femoral triangle points inferiorly and is continuous with a fascial canal (**adductor canal**), which descends medially down the thigh and posteriorly through an aperture in the lower end of one of the largest of the adductor muscles in the thigh (the adductor magnus muscle) to open into the popliteal fossa behind the knee.

The femoral nerve, artery, and vein, and lymphatics pass between the abdomen and lower limb under the inguinal ligament and in the femoral triangle (Fig. 6.25). The femoral artery and vein pass inferiorly through the adductor canal and become the popliteal vessels behind the knee where they meet and are distributed with branches of the sciatic nerve, which descends through the posterior thigh from the gluteal region.

From lateral to medial, major structures in the femoral triangle are the femoral nerve, the femoral artery, the femoral vein, and lymphatic vessels (Fig. 6.25).

Femoral sheath

In the femoral triangle, the femoral artery and vein and the associated lymphatic vessels are surrounded by a funnel-shaped sleeve of fascia (the **femoral sheath**) (Fig. 6.25). The sheath is continuous superiorly with the transversalis fascia and iliacus fascia of the abdomen and merges inferiorly with connective tissue associated with the vessels. Each of the three structures surrounded by the sheath is contained within a separate fascial compartment within the sheath. The most medial compartment (the **femoral canal**) contains the lymphatic vessels and is conical in shape. The opening of this canal superiorly is potentially a weak point in the lower abdomen and is the site for femoral hernias. The femoral nerve is lateral to and not contained within the femoral sheath.

Surface anatomy

Finding the femoral artery in the femoral triangle
The femoral artery descends into the thigh from the abdomen by passing under the inguinal ligament and into the femoral triangle (Fig. 6.26). In the femoral triangle, its pulse is easily felt just inferior to the inguinal ligament midway between the pubic symphysis and the anterior superior iliac spine. Medial to the artery is the femoral vein, and medial to the vein is the femoral canal, which contains lymphatics and lies immediately lateral to the pubic tubercle. The femoral nerve lies lateral to the femoral artery.

Anterior superior iliac spine
Inguinal ligament
Femoral nerve
Femoral artery
Femoral vein
Lymphatics passing through femoral canal
Pubic tubercle
Medial margin of sartorius muscle
Pubic symphysis

Medial margin of adductor longus muscle

Fig. 6.26 Position of the femoral artery in the femoral triangle.

GLUTEAL REGION

The gluteal region lies posterolateral to the bony pelvis and the proximal end of the femur (Fig. 6.27). Muscles in the region mainly abduct, extend, and laterally rotate the femur relative to the pelvic bone.

The gluteal region communicates anteromedially with the pelvic cavity and perineum through the greater and lesser sciatic foramina, respectively (Fig. 6.27). Inferiorly, it is continuous with the posterior thigh.

Muscles

Muscles of the gluteal region (Table 6.2, Fig. 6.28) compose mainly two groups:

- a deep group of small muscles that are mainly lateral rotators of the femur at the hip joint and include the **piriformis, obturator internus, gemellus superior, gemellus inferior,** and **quadratus femoris,** and
- a more superficial group of larger muscles that mainly abduct and extend the hip and include the **gluteus minimus, gluteus medius,** and **gluteus maximus.** An additional muscle in this group, the **tensor fasciae latae,** stabilizes the knee in extension by acting on a specialized longitudinal band of deep fascia (the iliotibial tract) that passes down the lateral side of the thigh to attach to the proximal end of the tibia in the leg.

The **piriformis** muscle is the most superior of the deep group of muscles (Fig. 6.28A) and is a muscle of the pelvic wall and of the gluteal region. It originates from between the anterior sacral foramina on the anterolateral surface of the sacrum and passes laterally and inferiorly

Sacrotuberous ligament

Greater sciatic foramen

Sacrospinous ligament

Quadrate tubercle

Gluteal tuberosity

Lesser sciatic foramen

Fig. 6.27 Gluteal region. Posterior view.

through the greater sciatic foramen. Piriformis is an important landmark because it divides the greater sciatic foramen into two regions, one above and one below the piriformis.

The obturator internus muscle, like the piriformis muscle, is a muscle of the pelvic wall and of the gluteal region (Fig. 6.28A). The muscle fibers of the obturator internus converge to form a tendon, which bends 90° around the ischium between the ischial spine and ischial tuberosity, and passes through the lesser sciatic foramen to enter the gluteal region. Gemellus superior and inferior (gemelli is Latin for "twins") are a pair of triangular muscles associated with the upper and lower margins of the obturator internus tendon (Fig. 6.28A).

The **gluteus medius** and **minimus** muscles abduct the pelvis over the stance limb at the hip joint and reduce pelvic drop over the opposite swing limb during walking (Fig. 6.28B).

Gluteus maximus is the largest muscle in the gluteal region and overlies most of the other gluteal muscles (Fig. 6.29). It is quadrangular and has a broad origin from the bony pelvis and associated ligaments and fascia. It is often described as being enclosed within two layers of the fascia lata, which covers the thigh and gluteal region. Laterally, the upper and superficial lower parts of the gluteus maximus insert into the

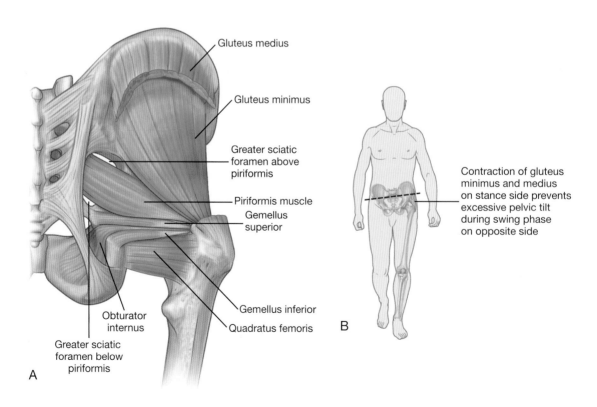

Gluteus medius

Gluteus minimus

Greater sciatic foramen above piriformis

Piriformis muscle

Gemellus superior

Contraction of gluteus minimus and medius on stance side prevents excessive pelvic tilt during swing phase on opposite side

Gemellus inferior

Obturator internus

Quadratus femoris

B

Greater sciatic foramen below piriformis

A

Fig. 6.28 Deep muscles in the gluteal region. **A.** Posterior view. **B.** Function.

iliotibial tract, which passes over the lateral surface of the greater trochanter and descends down the thigh and into the upper leg. Deep distal parts of the muscle attach to the elongate gluteal tuberosity of the proximal femur.

Clinical app

Trendelenburg's sign

Trendelenburg's sign occurs in people with weak or paralyzed abductor muscles (gluteus medius and gluteus minimus) of the hip. The sign is demonstrated by asking the patient to stand on one limb. When standing on the affected limb, the pelvis severely drops over the swing limb.

Positive findings are typically found in patients with damage to the superior gluteal nerve. Damage to this nerve may occur with associated pelvic fractures, space occupying lesions within the pelvis extending into the greater sciatic foramen and in some cases relating to hip surgery where there has been atrophy and disruption of the insertion of the gluteus medius and gluteus minimus tendons on the greater trochanter.

In patients with a positive Trendelenburg's sign, gait also is abnormal. Typically during the stance phase of the affected limb, the weakened abductor muscles allow the pelvis to tilt inferiorly over the swing limb. The patient compensates for the pelvic drop by lurching the trunk to the affected side in order to maintain the level of the pelvis throughout the gait cycle.

Nerves

Superior gluteal nerve

Of all the nerves that pass through the greater sciatic foramen, the **superior gluteal nerve** is the only one that passes above the piriformis muscle (Fig. 6.30A). After entering the gluteal region, the nerve loops up over the inferior margin of gluteus minimus and travels anteriorly and laterally in the plane between the gluteus minimus and medius muscles.

The superior gluteal nerve supplies branches to the gluteus minimus and medius muscles and terminates by innervating the tensor fasciae latae muscle.

Sciatic nerve

The **sciatic nerve** enters the gluteal region through the greater sciatic foramen inferior to the piriformis muscle (Fig. 6.30). It descends in the plane between the superficial and deep group of gluteal region muscles, crossing the posterior surfaces of first the obturator internus and associated gemellus muscles and then the quadratus femoris muscle. It lies just deep to the gluteus maximus at the midpoint between the ischial tuberosity and the greater trochanter. At

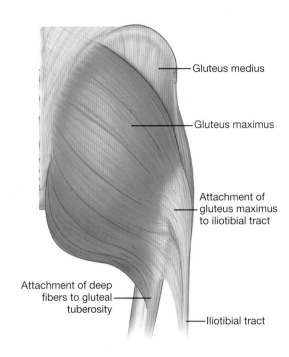

Fig. 6.29 Gluteus maximus muscle. Posterior view.

- Gluteus medius
- Gluteus maximus
- Attachment of gluteus maximus to iliotibial tract
- Attachment of deep fibers to gluteal tuberosity
- Iliotibial tract

the lower margin of the quadratus femoris muscle, the sciatic nerve enters the posterior thigh.

The sciatic nerve is the largest nerve in the body and innervates all muscles in the posterior compartment of thigh that flex the knee and all muscles that work the ankle and foot. It also innervates a large area of skin in the lower limb.

Nerve to quadratus femoris

The **nerve to the quadratus femoris** enters the gluteal region through the greater sciatic foramen inferior to the piriformis muscle and deep to the sciatic nerve (Fig. 6.30). Unlike other nerves in the gluteal region, the nerve to the quadratus femoris lies anterior to the plane of the deep muscles.

The nerve to the quadratus femoris descends along the ischium deep to the tendon of the obturator internus muscle and associated gemellus muscles to penetrate and innervate the quadratus femoris. It supplies a small branch to the gemellus inferior.

Nerve to obturator internus

The nerve to the **obturator internus** enters the gluteal region through the greater sciatic foramen inferior to the piriformis muscle and between the posterior cutaneous nerve of the thigh and the pudendal nerve (Fig. 6.30). It supplies a small branch to the gemellus superior and then passes over the ischial spine and through the lesser sciatic foramen to innervate the obturator internus muscle from the medial surface of the muscle in the perineum.

Table 6.2   Muscles of the gluteal region (spinal segments in **bold** are the major segments innervating the muscle)

Muscle	Origin	Insertion	Innervation	Function
Piriformis	Anterior surface of sacrum between anterior sacral foramina	Medial side of superior border of greater trochanter of femur	Branches from S1, **S2**	Laterally rotates the extended femur at hip joint; abducts flexed femur at hip joint
Obturator internus	Anterolateral wall of true pelvis; deep surface of obturator membrane and surrounding bone	Medial side of greater trochanter of femur	Nerve to obturator internus (L5, **S1**)	Laterally rotates the extended femur at hip joint; abducts flexed femur at hip joint
Gemellus superior	External surface of ischial spine	Along length of superior surface of the obturator internus tendon and into the medial side of greater trochanter of femur with obturator internus tendon	Nerve to obturator internus (**L5**, **S1**)	Laterally rotates the extended femur at hip joint; abducts flexed femur at hip joint
Gemellus inferior	Upper aspect of ischial tuberosity	Along length of inferior surface of the obturator internus tendon and into the medial side of greater trochanter of femur with obturator internus tendon	Nerve to quadratus femoris (**L5**, **S1**)	Laterally rotates the extended femur at hip joint; abducts flexed femur at hip joint
Quadratus femoris	Lateral aspect of the ischium just anterior to the ischial tuberosity	Quadrate tubercle on the intertrochanteric crest of the proximal femur	Nerve to quadratus femoris (**L5**, **S1**)	Laterally rotates femur at hip joint
Gluteus minimus	External surface of ilium between inferior and anterior gluteal lines	Linear facet on the anterolateral aspect of the greater trochanter	Superior gluteal nerve (L4, **L5**, S1)	Abducts femur at hip joint; holds pelvis secure over stance leg and prevents pelvic drop on the opposite swing side during walking; medially rotates thigh
Gluteus medius	External surface of ilium between anterior and posterior gluteal lines	Elongate facet on the lateral surface of the greater trochanter	Superior gluteal nerve (L4, **L5**, S1)	Abducts femur at hip joint; holds pelvis secure over stance leg and prevents pelvic drop on the opposite swing side during walking; medially rotates thigh
Gluteus maximus	Fascia covering gluteus medius, external surface of ilium behind posterior gluteal line, fascia of erector spinae, dorsal surface of lower sacrum, lateral margin of coccyx, external surface of sacrotuberous ligament	Posterior aspect of iliotibial tract of fascia lata and gluteal tuberosity of proximal femur	Inferior gluteal nerve (**L5**, **S1**, S2)	Powerful extensor of flexed femur at hip joint; lateral stabilizer of hip joint and knee joint; laterally rotates and abducts thigh
Tensor fasciae latae	Lateral aspect of crest of ilium between anterior superior iliac spine and tubercle of the crest	Iliotibial tract of fascia lata	Superior gluteal nerve (L4, **L5**, S1)	Stabilizes the knee in extension

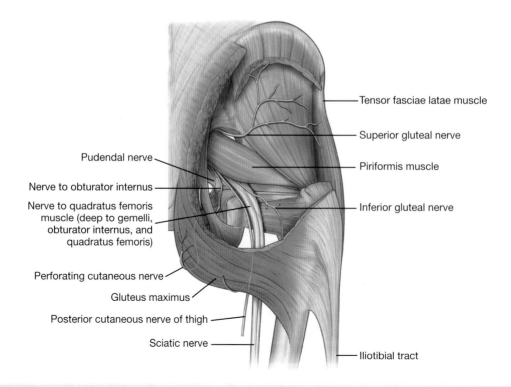

Pudendal nerve

Nerve to obturator internus

Nerve to quadratus femoris muscle (deep to gemelli, obturator internus, and quadratus femoris)

Perforating cutaneous nerve

Gluteus maximus

Posterior cutaneous nerve of thigh

Sciatic nerve

Tensor fasciae latae muscle

Superior gluteal nerve

Piriformis muscle

Inferior gluteal nerve

Iliotibial tract

Fig. 6.30 Nerves of the gluteal region.

Posterior cutaneous nerve of the thigh

The **posterior cutaneous nerve of the thigh** enters the gluteal region through the greater sciatic foramen inferior to the piriformis muscle and immediately medial to the sciatic nerve (Fig. 6.30). It descends through the gluteal region just deep to the gluteus maximus and enters the posterior thigh.

The posterior cutaneous nerve of the thigh has a number of gluteal branches, which loop around the lower margin of the gluteus maximus muscle to innervate skin over the gluteal fold. A small perineal branch passes medially to contribute to the innervation of skin of the scrotum or labia majora in the perineum. The main trunk of the posterior cutaneous nerve of the thigh passes inferiorly, giving rise to branches that innervate skin on the posterior thigh and leg.

Pudendal nerve

The **pudendal nerve** enters the gluteal region through the greater sciatic foramen inferior to the piriformis muscle and medial to the sciatic nerve (Fig. 6.30). It passes over the sacrospinous ligament and immediately passes through the lesser sciatic foramen to enter the perineum. The course of the pudendal nerve in the gluteal region is short and the nerve is often hidden by the overlying upper margin of the sacrotuberous ligament.

The pudendal nerve is the major somatic nerve of the perineum and has no branches in the gluteal region.

Inferior gluteal nerve

The **inferior gluteal nerve** enters the gluteal region through the greater sciatic foramen inferior to the piriformis muscle and along the posterior surface of the sciatic nerve (Fig. 6.30). It penetrates and supplies the gluteus maximus muscle.

Perforating cutaneous nerve

The **perforating cutaneous nerve** is the only nerve in the gluteal region that does not enter the area through the greater sciatic foramen. It is a small nerve that leaves the sacral plexus in the pelvic cavity by piercing the sacrotuberous ligament. It then loops around the lower border of the gluteus maximus to supply skin over the medial aspect of the gluteus maximus (Fig. 6.30).

Clinical app

Intramuscular injection in the gluteal region: avoiding the sciatic nerve
From time to time it is necessary to administer drugs intramuscularly; that is, by direct injection into muscles. This procedure must be carried out without injuring neurovascular structures. A typical site for an intramuscular injection is the gluteal region. The sciatic nerve passes through this region

Clinical app—cont'd

and needs to be avoided. The safest place to inject is the upper outer quadrant of either gluteal region.

The gluteal region can be divided into quadrants by two imaginary lines positioned using palpable bony landmarks (Fig. 6.31).

One line descends vertically from the highest point of the iliac crest.

The other line passes horizontally through the first line midway between the highest point of the iliac crest and the horizontal plane through the ischial tuberosity.

It is important to remember that the gluteal region extends as far forward as the anterior superior iliac spine. The sciatic nerve curves through the upper lateral corner of the lower medial quadrant and descends along the medial margin of the lower lateral quadrant.

Occasionally, the sciatic nerve bifurcates into its tibial and common fibular branches in the pelvis, in which case the common fibular nerve passes into the gluteal region through, or even above, the piriformis muscle.

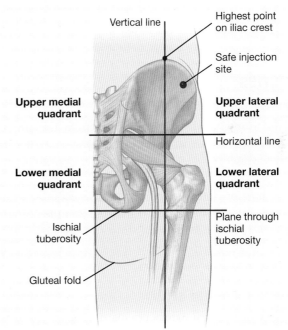

Fig. 6.31 Site for intramuscular injections.

The superior gluteal nerve and vessels normally enter the gluteal region above the piriformis and pass superiorly and forward.

The anterior corner of the upper lateral quadrant is normally used for injections to avoid injuring any part of the sciatic nerve or other nerves and vessels in the gluteal region. A needle placed in this region enters the gluteus medius anterosuperior to the margin of the gluteus maximus.

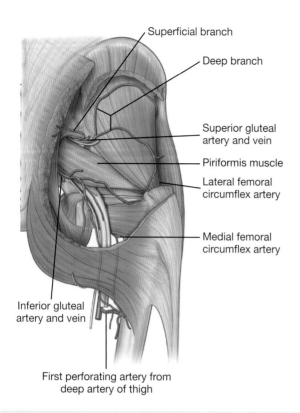

Fig. 6.32 Arteries of the gluteal region.

Fig. 6.33 Anastomoses between gluteal arteries and vessels originating from the femoral artery in the thigh. Posterior view.

Arteries

Inferior gluteal artery

The **inferior gluteal artery** originates from the anterior trunk of the internal iliac artery in the pelvic cavity. It leaves the pelvic cavity through the greater sciatic foramen inferior to the piriformis muscle (Fig. 6.32).

The inferior gluteal artery supplies adjacent muscles and descends through the gluteal region and into the posterior thigh where it supplies adjacent structures and anastomoses with perforating branches of the femoral artery. It also supplies a branch to the sciatic nerve.

Superior gluteal artery

The **superior gluteal artery** originates from the posterior trunk of the internal iliac artery in the pelvic cavity. It leaves the pelvic cavity through the greater sciatic foramen above the piriformis muscle (Fig. 6.32). In the gluteal region, it divides into a superficial branch and a deep branch:

- The superficial branch passes onto the deep surface of the gluteus maximus muscle.
- The deep branch passes between the gluteus medius and minimus muscles.

In addition to adjacent muscles, the superior gluteal artery contributes to the supply of the hip joint. Branches

of the artery also anastomose with the lateral and medial femoral circumflex arteries from the deep femoral artery in the thigh and with the inferior gluteal artery (Fig. 6.33).

Veins

Inferior and superior gluteal veins follow the inferior and superior gluteal arteries into the pelvis where they join the pelvic plexus of veins. Peripherally, the veins anastomose with superficial gluteal veins, which ultimately drain anteriorly into the femoral vein.

Lymphatics

Deep lymphatic vessels of the gluteal region accompany the blood vessels into the pelvic cavity and connect with internal iliac nodes.

Superficial lymphatics drain into the superficial inguinal nodes on the anterior aspect of the thigh.

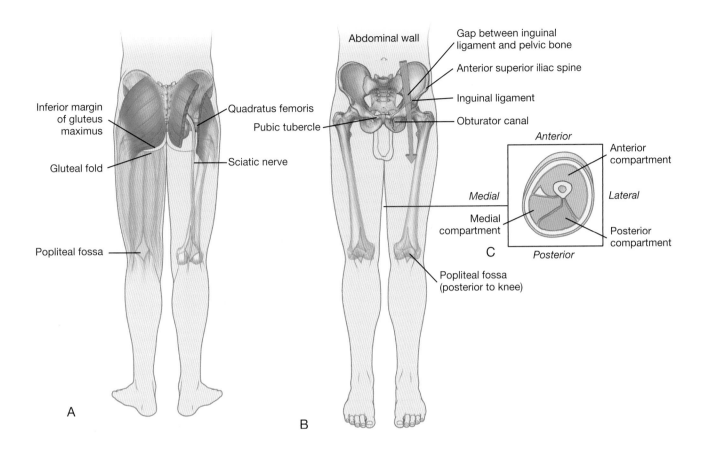

Fig. 6.34 Thigh. **A.** Posterior view. **B.** Anterior view. **C.** Cross-section through the mid-thigh.

THIGH

The thigh is the region of the lower limb that is approximately between the hip and knee joints (Fig. 6.34):

- Anteriorly, it is separated from the abdominal wall by the inguinal ligament.
- Posteriorly, it is separated from the gluteal region by the gluteal fold superficially and by the inferior margins of the gluteus maximus and quadratus femoris on deeper planes.

Structures enter and leave the top of the thigh by three routes:

- Posteriorly, the thigh is continuous with the gluteal region, and the major structure passing between the two regions is the sciatic nerve (Fig. 6.34A).
- Anteriorly, the thigh communicates with the abdominal cavity through the aperture between the inguinal ligament and pelvic bone (Fig. 6.34B), and major structures passing through this aperture are the iliopsoas and pectineus muscles, the femoral nerve, artery and vein, and lymphatic vessels.
- Medially, structures (including the obturator nerve and associated vessels) pass between the thigh and pelvic cavity through the obturator canal (Fig. 6.34B).

The thigh is divided into three compartments (anterior, medial, and posterior) by intermuscular septa between the posterior aspect of the femur and the fascia lata (the thick layer of deep fascia that completely surrounds or invests the thigh; Fig. 6.34C).

Bones

The skeletal support for the thigh is the femur (Fig. 6.35). Most of the large muscles in the thigh insert into the proximal ends of the two bones of the leg (tibia and fibula) and flex and extend the leg at the knee joint. The distal end of the femur provides origin for the gastrocnemius muscles, which are predominantly in the posterior compartment of leg and plantarflex the foot.

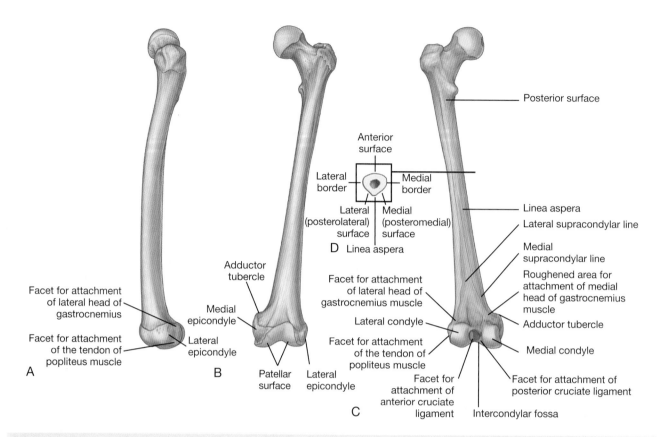

Fig. 6.35 Shaft and distal end of femur. **A.** Lateral view. **B.** Anterior view. **C.** Posterior view. **D.** Cross-section through shaft of femur.

Shaft and distal end of femur

The shaft of femur is bowed forward and has an oblique course from the neck of the femur to the distal end (Fig. 6.35A,B). As a consequence of this oblique orientation, the knee is close to the midline under the body's center of gravity.

The middle part of the shaft of the femur is triangular in cross-section (Fig. 6.35D). In the middle part of the shaft, the femur has smooth medial (posteromedial), lateral (posterolateral), and anterior surfaces and medial, lateral, and posterior borders. The medial and lateral borders are rounded, whereas the posterior border forms a broad roughened crest—the **linea aspera** (Fig. 6.35C).

In proximal and distal regions of the femur, the linea aspera widens to form an additional posterior surface. At the distal end of the femur, this posterior surface forms the floor of the popliteal fossa and its margins, which are continuous with the linea aspera above, form the **medial** and **lateral supracondylar lines.** The medial supracondylar line terminates at a prominent tubercle (the **adductor tubercle**) on the superior aspect of the **medial condyle** of the distal end. Just lateral to the lower end of the medial supracondylar line is an elongate roughened area of bone for the proximal attachment of the medial head of the gastrocnemius muscle (Fig. 6.35).

The distal end of the femur is characterized by two large condyles that articulate with the proximal head of the tibia (Fig. 6.35). The condyles are separated posteriorly by an **intercondylar fossa** and are joined anteriorly where they articulate with the patella.

The surfaces of the condyles that articulate with the tibia are rounded posteriorly and become flatter inferiorly. On each condyle, a shallow oblique groove separates the surface that articulates with the tibia from the more anterior surface that articulates with the patella. The surfaces of the medial and lateral condyles that articulate with the patella form a V-shaped trench, which faces anteriorly. The lateral surface of the trench is larger and steeper than the medial surface.

The walls of the intercondylar fossa bear two facets for the superior attachment of the cruciate ligaments, which stabilize the knee joint (Fig. 6.35C).

Epicondyles, for the attachment of collateral ligaments of the knee joint, are bony elevations on the nonarticular outer surfaces of the condyles (Fig. 6.35).

Additionally, just posterosuperior to the **medial epicondyle** is the adductor tubercle, and just posterior to the **lateral epicondyle** are facets for the attachment of the lateral head of the gastrocnemius and the popliteus muscles (Fig. 6.35C).

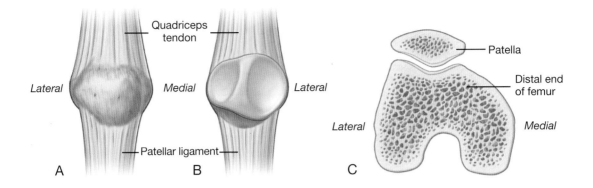

Fig. 6.36 Patella. **A.** Anterior view. **B.** Posterior view. **C.** Superior view.

Patella

The patella (knee cap) is the largest sesamoid bone (a bone formed within the tendon of a muscle) in the body and is formed within the tendon of the quadriceps femoris muscle as it crosses anterior to the knee joint to insert on the tibia.

The patella is triangular (Fig. 6.36):

- Its apex is pointed inferiorly for attachment to the patellar ligament, which connects the patella to the tibia.
- Its base is broad and thick for the attachment of the quadriceps tendon from above.
- Its posterior surface articulates with the femur and has medial and lateral facets (Fig. 6.36B) that slope away from a raised smooth ridge—the lateral facet is larger than the medial facet for articulation with the larger corresponding surface on the lateral condyle of the femur.

Proximal end of tibia

The tibia is the medial and larger of the two bones in the leg, and is the only one that articulates with the femur at the knee joint.

The proximal end of the tibia is expanded in the transverse plane for weight bearing and consists of a **medial condyle** and a **lateral condyle,** which are both flattened in the horizontal plane and overhang the shaft (Fig. 6.37).

The superior surfaces of the medial and lateral condyles are articular and separated by an intercondylar region, which contains sites of attachment for the cruciate ligaments and interarticular cartilages (menisci) of the knee joint (Fig. 6.37A).

The articular surfaces of the medial and lateral condyles and the intercondylar region together form a "tibial plateau," which articulates with and is anchored to the distal end of the femur. Inferior to the condyles on the proximal part of

the shaft is a large **tibial tuberosity** and the roughening for muscle and ligament attachments.

Tibial condyles and intercondylar areas

The tibial condyles are thick horizontal discs of bone attached to the top of the tibial shaft (Fig. 6.37).

The medial condyle is larger than the lateral condyle and is better supported over the shaft of the tibia. Its superior surface is oval for articulation with the medial condyle of the femur (Fig. 6.37A). The articular surface extends laterally onto the side of the raised **medial intercondylar tubercle.**

The superior surface of the lateral condyle is circular and articulates above with the lateral condyle of the femur (Fig. 6.37A). The medial edge of this surface extends onto the side of the **lateral intercondylar tubercle.**

The superior articular surfaces of both the lateral and medial condyles are concave, particularly centrally. The outer margins of the surfaces are flatter and are the regions in contact with the interarticular discs (menisci) of fibrocartilage in the knee joint.

The nonarticular posterior surface of the medial condyle bears a distinct horizontal groove for part of the attachment of the semimembranosus muscle, and the undersurface of the lateral condyle bears a distinct circular facet for articulation with the proximal head of the fibula.

The intercondylar region of the tibial plateau lies between the articular surfaces of the medial and lateral condyles (Fig. 6.37). It is narrow centrally where it is raised to form the **intercondylar eminence,** the sides of which are elevated further to form medial and lateral intercondylar tubercles.

The intercondylar region bears six distinct facets (Fig. 6.37A) for the attachment of menisci and cruciate ligaments. In addition to these facets, a large anterolateral region of the anterior intercondylar area is roughened and perforated by

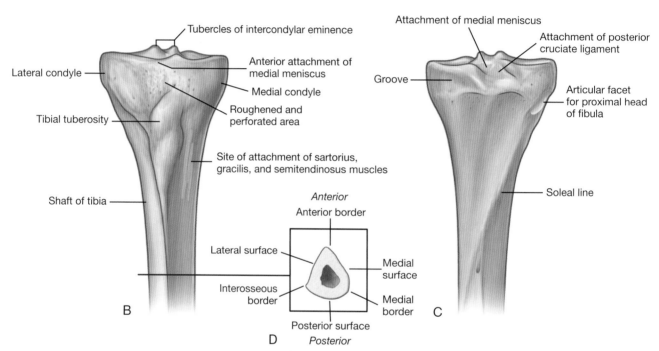

Fig. 6.37 Proximal end of the tibia. **A.** Superior view, tibial plateau. **B.** Anterior view. **C.** Posterior view. **D.** Cross-section through the shaft of tibia.

numerous small nutrient foramina for blood vessels. This region is continuous with a similar surface on the front of the tibia above the tuberosity and lies against infrapatellar connective tissue.

Tibial tuberosity

The tibial tuberosity is a palpable inverted triangular area on the anterior aspect of the tibia below the site of junction between the two condyles (Fig. 6.37A,B). It is the site of attachment for the **patellar ligament,** which is a continuation of the quadriceps femoris tendon below the patella.

Shaft of tibia

The shaft of the tibia is triangular in cross-section and has three surfaces (posterior, medial, and lateral) and three borders (anterior, interosseous, and medial) (Fig. 6.37D):

- The **anterior border** is sharp and descends from the tibial tuberosity where it is continuous superiorly with a ridge that passes along the lateral margin of the tuberosity and onto the lateral condyle.
- The **interosseous border** is a subtle vertical ridge that descends along the lateral aspect of the tibia from the region of bone anterior and inferior to the articular facet for the head of the fibula.
- The medial border is indistinct superiorly where it begins at the anterior end of the groove on the posterior surface of the medial tibial condyle but is sharp in the mid-shaft.

The large **medial surface** of the shaft of the tibia between the anterior and medial borders is smooth and subcutaneous and is palpable along almost its entire extent. Medial and somewhat inferior to the tibial tuberosity, this medial surface bears a subtle, slightly roughened elongate elevation. This elevation is the site of the combined attachment of three muscles (sartorius, gracilis, and semitendinosus), which descend from the thigh (Fig. 6.37B).

The **posterior surface** of the shaft of the tibia between the interosseous and medial borders is widest superiorly where it is crossed by a roughened oblique line (the soleal line) (Fig. 6.37C).

The **lateral surface** between the anterior and interosseous borders is smooth and unremarkable.

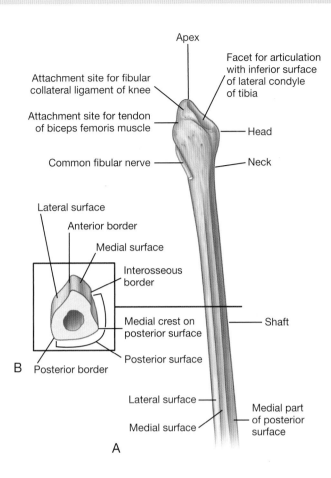

Fig. 6.38 Proximal end of the fibula. **A.** Anterior view. **B.** Cross-section through the shaft of fibula.

Clinical app

Shin splints

Shin splints are a generic term applied to patients with pain and discomfort in the midtibial region. The commonest causes of shin splints include tendinosis, tibial periostitis, medial tibial stress syndrome, compartment syndrome, and stress fractures. Most patients with shin splints present with pain during or after exercise usually related to high impact training, excessive training, or other biomechanical factors.

The cause of medial tibial stress syndrome is not entirely clear; however, it may be excessive periosteal tension relating to the muscle attachments in the midmedial tibial region. A resulting inflammatory response causes pain. In addition, the bone itself may become weakened and susceptible to small linear stress fractures.

Proximal end of fibula

The fibula is the lateral bone of the leg and does not take part in formation of the knee joint or in weight bearing. It is much smaller than the tibia and has a small proximal head, a narrow neck, and a delicate shaft, which ends as the lateral malleolus at the ankle.

The **head** of the fibula is a globe-shaped expansion at the proximal end of the fibula (Fig. 6.38). A circular facet on the superomedial surface is for articulation above with a similar facet on the inferior aspect of the lateral condyle of the tibia. Just posterolateral to this facet, the bone projects superiorly as a blunt apex (styloid process).

The **neck** of the fibula separates the expanded head from the **shaft.** The common fibular nerve lies against the posterolateral aspect of the neck (Fig. 6.38A).

Like the tibia, the shaft of the fibula has three borders (anterior, posterior, and interosseous) and three surfaces (lateral, posterior, and medial) that lie between the borders (Fig. 6.38B):

■ The **anterior border** is sharp mid-shaft and begins superiorly from the anterior aspect of the head.

■ The **posterior border** is rounded and descends from the region of the styloid process of the head.
■ The **interosseous border** is medial in position.

The three surfaces of the fibula are associated with the three muscular compartments (lateral, posterior, and anterior) of the leg.

Muscles

Muscles of the thigh are arranged in three compartments (anterior, medial, and posterior) separated by intermuscular septa (Fig. 6.39).

Anterior compartment (Table 6.3, Fig. 6.40)

The **anterior compartment of thigh** contains the **sartorius** and the four large **quadriceps femoris muscles (rectus femoris, vastus lateralis, vastus medialis,** and **vastus intermedius).** All are innervated by the femoral nerve. A tiny muscle **(articularis genus),** which is often part of the vastus intermedius muscle, originates from the femur just inferior to the origin of the vastus intermedius and inserts into the suprapatellar bursa associated with the knee joint. This articular muscle pulls the bursa away from the knee joint during extension. In addition to these muscles, the terminal ends of the psoas major and iliacus

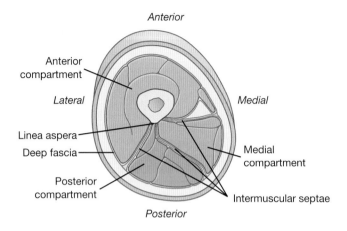

Fig. 6.39 Transverse section through the mid-thigh.

muscles pass into the upper part of the anterior compartment from sites of origin on the posterior abdominal wall (Fig. 6.41). These muscles are innervated by branches directly from the anterior rami of L1 to L3 (psoas major) or from the femoral nerve (iliacus) as it passes down the abdominal wall.

The sartorius muscle together with gracilis, and semitendinosus muscles from the medial and posterior compartments, respectively, attach to the tibia as part of a three-pronged pattern on the tibia. These combined tendons of insertion are often termed the **pes anserinus** (Latin for "goose foot")(Fig. 6.40).

Muscles in the anterior compartment act on the hip and knee joints:

- Psoas major and iliacus act on the hip joint.
- Sartorius and rectus femoris act on both the hip and knee joints.
- The vastus muscles act on the knee joint.

Fig. 6.40 Muscles of the anterior compartment of thigh.

Table 6.3　Muscles of the anterior compartment of thigh (spinal segments in **bold** are the major segments innervating the muscle)

Muscle	Origin	Insertion	Innervation	Function
Psoas major	Posterior abdominal wall (lumbar transverse processes, intervertebral discs, and adjacent bodies from TXII to LV and tendinous arches between these points)	Lesser trochanter of femur	Anterior rami (**L1**, **L2**, L3)	Flexes the thigh at the hip joint
Iliacus	Posterior abdominal wall (iliac fossa)	Lesser trochanter of femur	Femoral nerve (**L2**, L3)	Flexes the thigh at the hip joint
Vastus medialis	Femur—medial part of intertrochanteric line, pectineal line, medial lip of the linea aspera, medial supracondylar line	Quadriceps femoris tendon and medial border of patella	Femoral nerve (L2, **L3**, **L4**)	Extends the leg at the knee joint
Vastus intermedius	Femur—upper two-thirds of anterior and lateral surfaces	Quadriceps femoris tendon and lateral margin of patella	Femoral nerve (L2, **L3**, **L4**)	Extends the leg at the knee joint
Vastus lateralis	Femur—lateral part of intertrochanteric line, margin of greater trochanter, lateral margin of gluteal tuberosity, lateral lip of the linea aspera	Quadriceps femoris tendon and lateral margin of patella	Femoral nerve (L2, **L3**, **L4**)	Extends the leg at the knee joint
Rectus femoris	Straight head originates from the anterior inferior iliac spine; reflected head originates from the ilium just superior to the acetabulum	Quadriceps femoris tendon	Femoral nerve (L2, **L3**, **L4**)	Flexes the thigh at the hip joint and extends the leg at the knee joint
Sartorius	Anterior superior iliac spine	Medial surface of tibia just inferomedial to tibial tuberosity	Femoral nerve (**L2**, **L3**)	Flexes the thigh at the hip joint and flexes the leg at the knee joint

Clinical app

Quadriceps injury

Quadriceps muscle injuries include avulsion of the straight and reflected head of the rectus femoris muscles, proximal musculotendinous muscle tears, and quadriceps tendon disruption. Proximal injuries of the straight and reflected heads of the rectus femoris are uncommon. However, in adolescents it is possible to avulse these origins with a small fragment of bone. This can cause considerable pain and may result in the growth of a prominent bony tubercle.

Proximal injuries of the rectus femoris muscle occur very frequently in professional athletes and are the second most common thigh injury.

Quadriceps tendon disruption is a devastating injury. A typical history is "miss-kicking" a ball and hitting the ground, producing an abrupt deceleration and resulting in tearing the quadriceps tendon. Examination demonstrates that the patient is unable to extend the knee against resistance and in most cases a gap in the tendon can be palpated. In most instances, surgery is required to reattach the tendon to the patella.

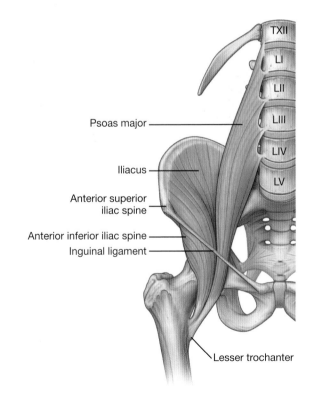

Fig. 6.41 Psoas major and iliacus muscles.

Patellar ligament

The patellar ligament is functionally the continuation of the quadriceps femoris tendon below the patella and is attached above to the apex and margins of the patella and below to the tibial tuberosity (Fig. 6.40). The more superficial fibers of the quadriceps femoris tendon and the patellar ligament are continuous over the anterior surface of the patella, and lateral and medial fibers are continuous with the ligament beside the margins of the patella.

315

Fig. 6.42 Muscles of the medial compartment of thigh. Anterior view.

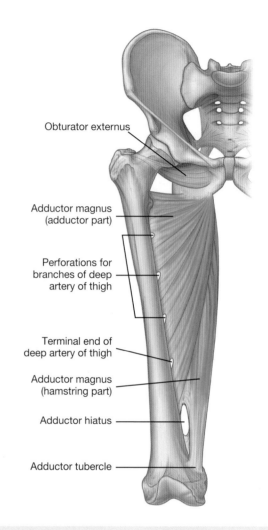

Fig. 6.43 Adductor magnus and obturator externus muscles. Anterior view.

Medial compartment (Table 6.4, Fig. 6.42)

The **medial compartment of thigh** contains six muscles (**gracilis, pectineus, adductor longus, adductor brevis, adductor magnus,** and **obturator externus**). All except the pectineus, which is innervated by the femoral nerve, and part of the adductor magnus, which is innervated by the sciatic nerve, are innervated by the obturator nerve. Collectively, all these muscles except the obturator externus mainly adduct the thigh at the hip joint; the adductor longus and magnus may also medially rotate the thigh. Obturator externus is a lateral rotator of the thigh at the hip joint, and the gracilis also flexes the leg at the knee joint.

The **adductor magnus** is the largest and deepest of the muscles in the medial compartment of thigh (Fig. 6.43). The muscle forms the distal posterior wall of the adductor canal. It is a triangular or fan-shaped muscle anchored by its apex to the pelvis and attached by its expanded base to the femur. The medial part of the adductor magnus, often called the *hamstring part,* originates from the ischial tuberosity of the pelvic bone and descends almost vertically along the thigh to insert via a rounded tendon into the adductor tubercle on the medial condyle of the distal head of the femur. The lateral or adductor part of the muscle inserts via an aponeurosis up onto the medial supracondylar line. A large circular gap inferiorly between the hamstring and adductor parts of the muscle is the **adductor hiatus** (Fig. 6.43), which allows the femoral artery and associated veins to pass between the adductor canal on the anteromedial aspect of the thigh and the popliteal fossa posterior to the knee. The adductor part of the muscle is innervated by the obturator nerve, and the hamstring part is innervated by the tibial division of the sciatic nerve.

Posterior compartment (Table 6.5, Fig. 6.44)

There are three long muscles in the posterior compartment of thigh: **biceps femoris, semitendinosus,** and **semimembranosus**—and they are collectively known as the hamstrings. All except the short head of biceps femoris cross both the hip and knee joints. As a group, the hamstrings flex the leg at the knee joint and extend the thigh at the hip joint.

They are also rotators at both joints. All are innervated by the sciatic nerve.

Arteries

Three arteries enter the thigh: the femoral artery, the obturator artery, and the inferior gluteal artery. Of these, the femoral artery is the largest and supplies most of the lower limb. The three arteries contribute to an anastomotic network of vessels around the hip joint.

Femoral artery

The femoral artery (Fig. 6.45) is the continuation of the external iliac artery and begins as the external iliac artery passes under the inguinal ligament to enter the femoral triangle on the anterior aspect of the upper thigh (Fig. 6.45).

The femoral artery passes vertically through the femoral triangle and then continues down the thigh in the adductor canal. It leaves the canal by passing through the adductor hiatus in the adductor magnus muscle and becomes the popliteal artery behind the knee (Fig. 6.45).

A cluster of four small branches—**superficial epigastric artery**, **superficial circumflex iliac artery**, **superficial external pudendal artery**, and **deep external pudendal artery**—originate from the femoral artery in the femoral triangle and supply cutaneous regions of the upper thigh, lower abdomen, and perineum (Fig. 6.45).

Deep artery of thigh

The largest branch of the femoral artery in the thigh is the **deep artery of thigh (profunda femoris artery)**, which

Table 6.4 Muscles of the medial compartment of thigh (spinal segments in **bold** are the major segments innervating the muscle)

Muscle	Origin	Insertion	Innervation	Function
Gracilis	A line on the external surfaces of the body of the pubis, the inferior pubic ramus, and the ramus of the ischium	Medial surface of proximal shaft of tibia	Obturator nerve (**L2**, L3)	Adducts thigh at hip joint and flexes leg at knee joint
Pectineus	Pectineal line (pecten pubis) and adjacent bone of pelvis	Oblique line extending from base of lesser trochanter to linea aspera on posterior surface of proximal femur	Femoral nerve (**L2**, L3)	Adducts and flexes thigh at hip joint
Adductor longus	External surface of body of pubis (triangular depression inferior to pubic crest and lateral to pubic symphysis)	Linea aspera on middle one-third of shaft of femur	Obturator nerve (anterior division) (**L2**, **L3**, L4)	Adducts and medially rotates thigh at hip joint
Adductor brevis	External surface of body of pubis and inferior pubic ramus	Posterior surface of proximal femur and upper one-third of linea aspera	Obturator nerve (**L2**, L3)	Adducts thigh at hip joint
Adductor magnus	Adductor part—ischiopubic ramus	Posterior surface of proximal femur, linea aspera, medial supracondylar line	Obturator nerve (**L2**, **L3**, L4)	Adducts and medially rotates thigh at hip joint
	Hamstring part—ischial tuberosity	Adductor tubercle and supracondylar line	Sciatic nerve (tibial division) (**L2**, **L3**, L4)	
Obturator externus	External surface of obturator membrane and adjacent bone	Trochanteric fossa	Obturator nerve (posterior division) (L3, **L4**)	Laterally rotates thigh at hip joint

originates from the lateral side of the femoral artery in the femoral triangle and is the major source of blood supply to the thigh (Fig. 6.46). The deep artery of thigh immediately passes:

- posteriorly between the pectineus and adductor longus muscles and then between the adductor longus and adductor brevis muscles; and
- then travels inferiorly between the adductor longus and adductor magnus, eventually penetrating through the

adductor magnus to connect with branches of the popliteal artery behind the knee.

The deep artery of thigh has lateral and medial circumflex femoral branches and three perforating branches.

Lateral circumflex femoral artery

The **lateral circumflex femoral artery** normally originates proximally from the lateral side of the deep artery of thigh but may arise directly from the femoral artery (Fig. 6.46).

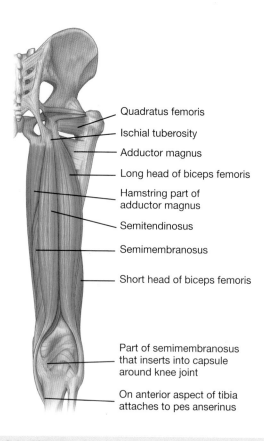

Quadratus femoris

Ischial tuberosity

Adductor magnus

Long head of biceps femoris

Hamstring part of adductor magnus

Semitendinosus

Semimembranosus

Short head of biceps femoris

Part of semimembranosus that inserts into capsule around knee joint

On anterior aspect of tibia attaches to pes anserinus

Fig. 6.44 Muscles of the posterior compartment of thigh. Posterior view.

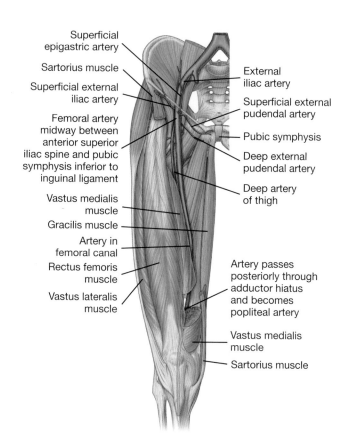

Superficial epigastric artery

Sartorius muscle

Superficial external iliac artery

Femoral artery midway between anterior superior iliac spine and pubic symphysis inferior to inguinal ligament

Vastus medialis muscle

Gracilis muscle

Artery in femoral canal

Rectus femoris muscle

Vastus lateralis muscle

External iliac artery

Superficial external pudendal artery

Pubic symphysis

Deep external pudendal artery

Deep artery of thigh

Artery passes posteriorly through adductor hiatus and becomes popliteal artery

Vastus medialis muscle

Sartorius muscle

Fig. 6.45 Femoral artery.

Table 6.5 Muscles of the posterior compartment of thigh (spinal segments in **bold** are the major segments innervating the muscle)

Muscle	Origin	Insertion	Innervation	Function
Biceps femoris	Long head—inferomedial part of the upper area of the ischial tuberosity; short head—lateral lip of linea aspera	Head of fibula	Sciatic nerve (L5, **S1**, S2)	Flexes leg at knee joint; extends and laterally rotates thigh at hip joint and laterally rotates leg at knee joint
Semitendinosus	Inferomedial part of the upper area of the ischial tuberosity	Medial surface of proximal tibia	Sciatic nerve (L5, **S1**, S2)	Flexes leg at knee joint and extends thigh at hip joint; medially rotates thigh at hip joint and leg at knee joint
Semimembranosus	Superolateral impression on the ischial tuberosity	Groove and adjacent bone on medial and posterior surface of medial tibial condyle	Sciatic nerve (L5, **S1**, S2)	Flexes leg at knee joint and extends thigh at hip joint; medially rotates thigh at hip joint and leg at knee joint

Fig. 6.46 Deep artery of thigh. **A.** Anterior view. **B.** Posterior view.

It passes deep to the sartorius and rectus femoris and divides into three terminal branches:

- One vessel (**ascending branch**) ascends laterally deep to the tensor fasciae latae muscle and connects with a branch of the medial circumflex femoral artery to form a channel, which circles the neck of the femur and supplies the neck and head of the femur.
- One vessel (**descending branch**) descends deep to the rectus femoris, penetrates the vastus lateralis muscle, and connects with a branch of the popliteal artery near the knee.
- One vessel (**transverse branch**) passes laterally to pierce the vastus lateralis and then circles around the proximal shaft of femur to anastomose with branches from the medial femoral circumflex artery, the inferior gluteal artery, and the first perforating artery to form the cruciate anastomosis around the hip (Fig. 6.46).

Medial circumflex femoral artery

The **medial circumflex femoral artery** normally originates proximally from the posteromedial aspect of the deep artery of thigh but may originate from the femoral artery (Fig. 6.46). It passes medially around the shaft of femur, first between the pectineus and iliopsoas and then between the obturator externus and adductor brevis muscles. Near the margin of the adductor brevis, the vessel gives off a small branch, which enters the hip joint through the acetabular notch and anastomoses with the acetabular branch of the obturator artery.

The main trunk of the medial circumflex femoral artery passes over the superior margin of the adductor magnus and divides into two major branches deep to the quadratus femoris muscle:

- One branch ascends to the trochanteric fossa and connects with branches of the gluteal and lateral circumflex femoral arteries.

319

Obturator artery

Acetabular branch

Artery of ligament of head of femur

Ligament of head of femur

Obturator externus muscle

Anterior branch

Posterior branch

Fig. 6.47 Obturator artery.

■ The other branch passes laterally to participate with branches from the lateral femoral circumflex artery, the inferior gluteal artery, and the first perforating artery in forming an anastomotic network of vessels around the hip.

Perforating arteries

The three **perforating arteries** branch from the deep artery of thigh (Fig. 6.46) as it descends anterior to the adductor brevis muscle—the first originates above the muscle, the second originates anterior to the muscle, and the third originates below the muscle. All three penetrate through the adductor magnus near its attachment to the linea aspera to enter and supply the posterior compartment of thigh. Here, the vessels have ascending and descending branches that interconnect to form a longitudinal channel, which participates above in forming an anastomotic network of vessels around the hip and inferiorly anastomoses with branches of the popliteal artery behind the knee.

Obturator artery

The **obturator artery** originates as a branch of the internal iliac artery in the pelvic cavity and enters the medial compartment of thigh through the obturator canal (Fig. 6.47). As it passes through the canal, it bifurcates into an **anterior branch** and a **posterior branch,** which, together, form a channel that circles the margin of the obturator membrane and lies within the attachment of the obturator externus muscle.

Vessels arising from the anterior and posterior branches supply adjacent muscles and anastomose with the inferior gluteal and medial circumflex femoral arteries. In addition, an acetabular vessel originates from the posterior branch, enters the hip joint through the acetabular notch, and contributes to the supply of the head of the femur.

Clinical app

Peripheral vascular disease
Peripheral vascular disease is often characterized by reduced blood flow to the legs. This disorder may be due to stenoses (narrowing) and/or occlusions (blockages) in the lower aorta, iliac, femoral, tibial, and fibular vessels. Patients typically have chronic leg ischemia and "acute on chronic" leg ischemia.

Chronic leg ischemia
Chronic leg ischemia is a disorder in which vessels have undergone atheromatous change, and often there is significant luminal narrowing (usually over 50%). Most patients with peripheral arterial disease have widespread arterial disease (including cardiovascular and cerebrovascular disease), which may be clinically asymptomatic. Some of these patients develop such severe ischemia that the viability of the limb is threatened **(critical limb ischemia).**

The commonest symptom of chronic leg ischemia is **intermittent claudication.** Patients typically have a history of pain that develops in the calf muscles (usually associated with occlusions or narrowing in the femoral artery) or the buttocks (usually associated with occlusion or narrowing in the aorto-iliac segments). The pain experienced in these muscles is often cramp-like and occurs with walking. The patient rests and is able to continue walking up to the same distance until the pain recurs and stops walking as before.

Acute on chronic ischemia
In some patients with chronic limb ischemia, an acute event blocks the vessels or reduces the blood supply to such a degree that the viability of the limb is threatened.

Occasionally a leg may become acutely ischemic with no evidence of underlying atheromatous disease. In these instances a blood clot is likely to have embolized from the heart. Patients with mitral valve disease and atrial fibrillation are prone to embolic disease.

Critical limb ischemia
Critical limb ischemia occurs when the blood supply to the limb is so poor that the viability of the limb is severely threatened, and in this case many patients develop gangrene, ulceration, and severe rest pain in the foot. These patients require urgent treatment, which may be in the form of surgical reconstruction, radiological angioplasty, or even amputation.

Veins

Veins in the thigh consist of superficial and deep veins. Deep veins generally follow the arteries and have similar names. Superficial veins are in the superficial fascia, interconnect with deep veins, and do not generally accompany arteries. The largest of the superficial veins in the thigh is the great saphenous vein.

Great saphenous vein

The great saphenous vein originates from a venous arch on the dorsal aspect of the foot and ascends along the medial side of the lower limb to the proximal thigh (see Fig. 6.20). Here it passes through the saphenous opening in the deep fascia covering the anterior thigh to connect with the femoral vein in the femoral triangle (see Fig. 6.23).

Nerves

There are three major nerves in the thigh, each associated with one of the three compartments. The **femoral nerve** is associated with the anterior compartment of thigh, the **obturator nerve** is associated with the medial compartment of thigh, and the **sciatic nerve** is associated with the posterior compartment of thigh.

Femoral nerve

The femoral nerve originates from the lumbar plexus (spinal cord segments L2 to L4) on the posterior abdominal wall and enters the femoral triangle of the thigh by passing under the inguinal ligament (Fig. 6.48). In the femoral triangle, the femoral nerve lies on the lateral side of the femoral artery and is outside the femoral sheath, which surrounds the vessels.

Before entering the thigh, the femoral nerve supplies branches to the iliacus and pectineus muscles.

Immediately after passing under the inguinal ligament, the femoral nerve divides into anterior and posterior branches, which supply muscles of the anterior compartment of thigh and skin on the anterior and medial aspects of the thigh and on the medial sides of the leg and foot.

Branches of the femoral nerve (Fig. 6.48) include:

- anterior cutaneous branches, which penetrate deep fascia to supply skin on the front of the thigh and knee;
- numerous motor nerves, which supply the quadriceps femoris muscle (rectus femoris, vastus lateralis, vastus intermedius, and vastus medialis muscles) and the sartorius muscle; and
- one long cutaneous nerve, the saphenous nerve, which supplies skin as far distally as the medial side of the foot.

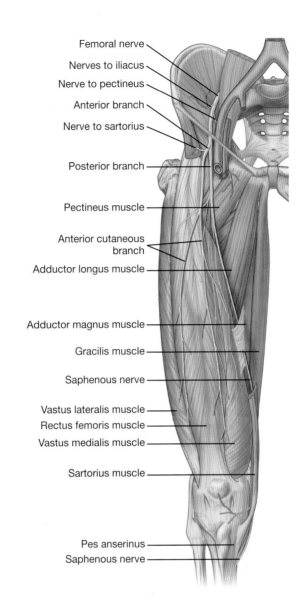

Fig. 6.48 Femoral nerve.

The **saphenous nerve** accompanies the femoral artery through the adductor canal but does not pass through the adductor hiatus with the femoral artery (Fig. 6.48). Rather, the saphenous nerve penetrates directly through connective tissues near the end of the canal to appear between the sartorius and gracilis muscles on the medial side of the knee. Here the saphenous nerve penetrates deep fascia and continues down the medial side of the leg to the foot, supplying skin on the medial side of the knee, leg, and foot.

Obturator nerve

The obturator nerve is a branch of the lumbar plexus (spinal cord segments L2 to L4) on the posterior abdominal

321

Fig. 6.49 Obturator nerve.

Fig. 6.50 Sciatic nerve.

wall. It descends in the psoas muscle and then passes out of the medial margin of the psoas muscle to enter the pelvis (Fig. 6.49). The obturator nerve continues along the lateral pelvic wall and then enters the medial compartment of thigh by passing through the obturator canal. It supplies most of the adductor muscles and skin on the medial aspect of the thigh. As the obturator nerve enters the thigh, it divides into two branches: an anterior branch and a posterior branch, which are separated by the adductor brevis muscle:

- The **posterior branch** descends behind the adductor brevis muscle and on the anterior surface of the adductor magnus muscle and supplies the obturator externus and adductor brevis muscles and the part of adductor magnus that attaches to the linea aspera.

- The **anterior branch** descends on the anterior surface of the adductor brevis muscle and is behind the pectineus and adductor longus muscles. It supplies branches to the adductor longus, gracilis, and adductor brevis muscles and often contributes to the supply of the pectineus muscle. Cutaneous branches innervate the skin on the medial side of the thigh.

Sciatic nerve

The sciatic nerve is a branch of the lumbosacral plexus (spinal cord segments L4 to S3) and descends into the posterior compartment of thigh from the gluteal region (Fig. 6.50). It innervates all muscles in the posterior compartment of thigh, and then its branches continue into the leg and foot.

In the posterior compartment of thigh, the sciatic nerve lies on the adductor magnus muscle and is crossed by the long head of biceps femoris muscle.

Proximal to the knee, and sometimes within the pelvis, the sciatic nerve divides into its two terminal branches: the **tibial nerve** and the **common fibular nerve** (Fig. 6.50). These nerves travel vertically down the thigh and enter the popliteal fossa posterior to the knee. Here, they meet the popliteal artery and vein.

The tibial nerve supplies branches to all muscles in the posterior compartment of thigh (long head of biceps femoris, semimembranosus, semitendinosus) except the short head of the biceps femoris, which is innervated by the common fibular part (Fig. 6.50).

The tibial nerve descends through the popliteal fossa, enters the posterior compartment of leg, and continues into the sole of the foot.

The tibial nerve innervates:

- all muscles in the posterior compartment of leg,
- all intrinsic muscles in the sole of the foot except for the first two dorsal interossei muscles, which are innervated by the deep fibular nerve, and
- skin on the posterolateral side of the lower half of the leg; lateral side of the ankle, foot, and little toe; and on the sole of the foot and toes.

The common fibular nerve supplies the short head of the biceps femoris in the posterior compartment of thigh and then continues into the lateral and anterior compartments of leg and onto the foot (Fig. 6.50).

The common fibular nerve innervates:

- all muscles in the anterior and lateral compartments of the leg,
- one muscle (extensor digitorum brevis) on the dorsal aspect of the foot,
- the first two dorsal interossei muscles in the sole of the foot, and
- skin over the lateral aspect of the leg and ankle and over the dorsal aspect of the foot and toes.

Knee joint

The knee joint is the largest synovial joint in the body (Fig. 6.51; also see Fig. 6.59). The detailed movements of the knee joint are complex, but basically the joint is a hinge joint that allows mainly flexion and extension. The joint consists of:

- the articulation between the femur and tibia, which is weight bearing, and
- the articulation between the patella and the femur, which allows the pull of the quadriceps femoris muscle to be directed anteriorly over the knee to the tibia without tendon wear.

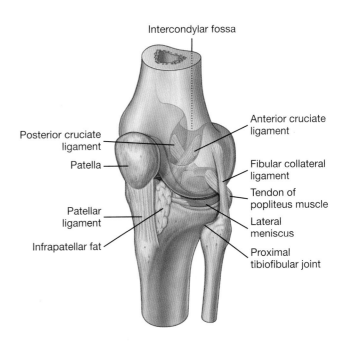

Fig. 6.51 Knee joint. Joint capsule is not shown.

Articular surfaces

The articular surfaces of the bones that contribute to the knee joint are covered by hyaline cartilage. The major surfaces involved include:

- the two femoral condyles, and
- the adjacent surfaces of the superior aspect of the tibial condyles.

The surfaces of the femoral condyles that articulate with the tibia in flexion of the knee are curved or round, whereas the surfaces that articulate in full extension are flat (Fig. 6.52A,B).

The articular surfaces between the femur and patella are the V-shaped trench on the anterior surface of the distal end of the femur where the two condyles join and the adjacent surfaces on the posterior aspect of the patella. The joint surfaces are all enclosed within a single articular cavity, as are the intra-articular menisci between the femoral and tibial condyles (Fig. 6.52C).

Menisci

There are two menisci, which are fibrocartilaginous C-shaped cartilages in the knee joint, one medial (**medial meniscus**) and the other lateral (**lateral meniscus**) (Fig. 6.53). Both are attached at each end to facets in the intercondylar region of the tibial plateau.

The medial meniscus is attached around its margin to the capsule of the joint and to the tibial collateral ligament,

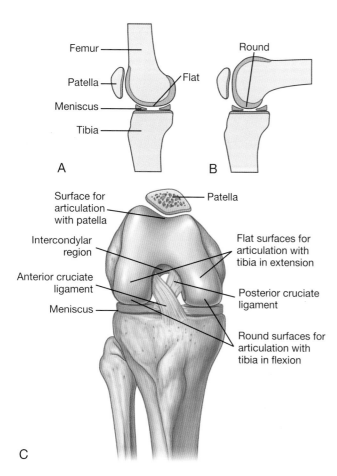

Fig. 6.52 Articular surfaces of the knee joint. **A.** Extended. **B.** Flexed. **C.** Anterior view (flexed).

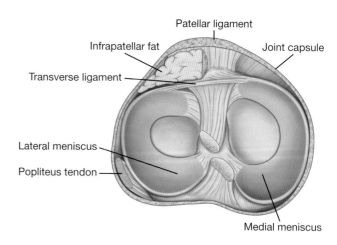

Fig. 6.53 Menisci of the knee joint. Superior view.

whereas the lateral meniscus is unattached to the capsule. Therefore the lateral meniscus is more mobile than the medial meniscus.

The menisci are interconnected anteriorly by a transverse ligament of the knee (Fig. 6.53). The lateral meniscus is also connected to the tendon of the popliteus muscle, which passes superolaterally between this meniscus and the capsule to insert on the femur (Fig. 6.53).

The menisci improve congruency between the femoral and tibial condyles during joint movements where the surfaces of the femoral condyles articulating with the tibial plateau change from small curved surfaces in flexion to large flat surfaces in extension (Fig. 6.52).

Synovial membrane

The synovial membrane of the knee joint attaches to the margins of the articular surfaces and to the superior and inferior outer margins of the menisci (Fig. 6.54A). The two cruciate ligaments, which attach in the intercondylar region of the tibia below and the intercondylar fossa of the femur

above, are outside the articular cavity but enclosed within the fibrous membrane of the knee joint.

Anteriorly, the synovial membrane is separated from the patellar ligament by an **infrapatellar fat pad** (Fig. 6.54). On each side of the pad, the synovial membrane forms a fringed margin (an **alar fold**), which projects into the articular cavity. In addition, the synovial membrane covering the lower part of the infrapatellar fat pad is raised into a sharp midline fold directed posteriorly (the **infrapatellar synovial fold**), which attaches to the margin of the intercondylar fossa of the femur.

The synovial membrane of the knee joint forms pouches in two locations to provide low friction surfaces for the movement of tendons associated with the joint:

- the small **subpopliteal recess** (Fig. 6.54A) extends between the lateral meniscus and the tendon of the popliteus muscle, and
- the large **suprapatellar bursa** (Fig. 6.54B) is a continuation of the articular cavity superiorly between the distal end of the shaft of the femur and the quadriceps femoris muscle and tendon. The apex of this bursa is attached to the small articularis genus muscle, which pulls the bursa away from the joint during extension of the knee.

Other bursae associated with the knee, but not normally communicating with the articular cavity, include the subcutaneous prepatellar bursa, deep and subcutaneous infrapatellar bursae, and numerous other bursae associated with tendons and ligaments around the joint (Fig. 6.54B).

The prepatellar bursa is subcutaneous and anterior to the patella. The deep and subcutaneous infrapatellar bursae are on the deep and subcutaneous sides of the patellar ligament, respectively.

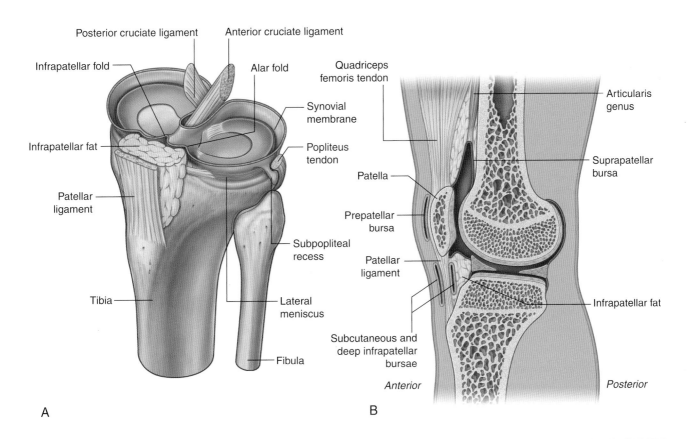

Fig. 6.54 Synovial membrane of the knee joint and associated bursae. **A.** Superolateral view; patella and femur not shown. **B.** Paramedial sagittal section through the knee.

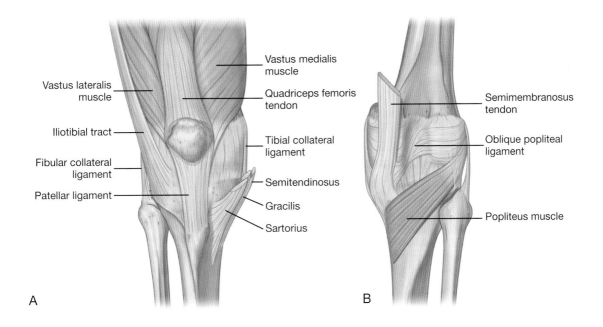

Fig. 6.55 Fibrous membrane of the knee joint capsule. **A.** Anterior view. **B.** Posterior view.

Fibular collateral ligament

Tendon of popliteus muscle

Biceps femoris

Iliotibial tract

Patellar ligament

A

Attaches to medial meniscus

Gracilis

Sartorius

Tibial collateral ligament

Attaches to capsule

Semitendinosus

B

Fig. 6.56 Collateral ligaments of the knee joint. **A.** Lateral view. **B.** Medial view.

Fibrous membrane

The fibrous membrane of the knee joint is extensive and is partly formed and reinforced by extensions from tendons of the surrounding muscles (Fig. 6.55). In general, the fibrous membrane encloses the articular cavity and the intercondylar region (Fig. 6.55):

- On the medial side of the knee joint, the fibrous membrane blends with the tibial collateral ligament and is attached on its internal surface to the medial meniscus.
- Laterally, the external surface of the fibrous membrane is separated by a space from the fibular collateral ligament, and the internal surface of the fibrous membrane is not attached to the lateral meniscus.
- Anteriorly, the fibrous membrane is attached to the margins of the patella where it is reinforced with tendinous expansions from the vastus lateralis and vastus medialis muscles, which also merge above with the quadriceps femoris tendon and below with the patellar ligament.

The fibrous membrane is reinforced anterolaterally by a fibrous extension from the iliotibial tract and posteromedially by an extension from the tendon of semimembranosus (the **oblique popliteal ligament**), which reflects superiorly across the back of the fibrous membrane from medial to lateral (Fig. 6.55B).

The upper end of the popliteus muscle passes through an aperture in the posterolateral aspect of the fibrous membrane of the knee and is enclosed by the fibrous membrane as its tendon travels around the joint to insert into the lateral aspect of the lateral femoral condyle (Fig. 6.55B).

Ligaments

The major ligaments associated with the knee joint are the patellar ligament, the tibial (medial) and fibular (lateral) collateral ligaments, and the anterior and posterior cruciate ligaments.

Patellar ligament

The **patellar ligament** is basically the continuation of the quadriceps femoris tendon inferior to the patella (Fig. 6.55A). It is attached above to the margins and apex of the patella and below to the tibial tuberosity.

Collateral ligaments

The collateral ligaments, one on each side of the joint, stabilize the hinge-like motion of the knee (Fig. 6.56).

The cord-like **fibular collateral ligament** is attached superiorly to the lateral femoral epicondyle just above the groove for the popliteus tendon (Fig. 6.56A). Inferiorly, it is attached to a depression on the lateral surface of the fibular head. It is separated from the fibrous membrane by a bursa.

The broad and flat **tibial collateral ligament** (Fig. 6.56B) is attached by much of its deep surface to the underlying fibrous membrane. It is anchored superiorly to the medial femoral epicondyle just inferior to the adductor tubercle and descends

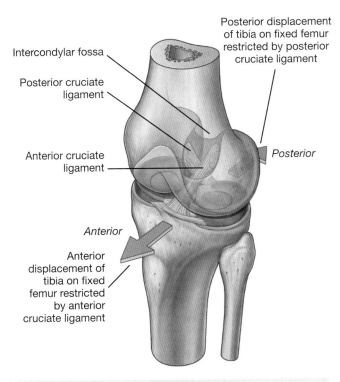

Fig. 6.57 Cruciate ligaments of the knee joint. Superolateral view.

Fig. 6.58 Knee "locking" mechanism.

anteriorly to attach to the medial margin and medial surface of the tibia above and behind the attachment of sartorius, gracilis, and semitendinosus tendons (Fig. 6.56B).

Cruciate ligaments

The two cruciate ligaments are in the intercondylar region of the knee and interconnect the femur and tibia (Fig. 6.57). They are termed *cruciate* (Latin for "shaped like a cross") because they cross each other in the sagittal plane between their femoral and tibial attachments:

- The **anterior cruciate ligament** attaches to a facet on the anterior part of the intercondylar area of the tibia and ascends posteriorly to attach to a facet at the back of the lateral wall of the intercondylar fossa of the femur (Fig. 6.57).
- The **posterior cruciate ligament** attaches to the posterior aspect of the intercondylar area of the tibia and ascends anteriorly to attach to the medial wall of the intercondylar fossa of the femur (Fig. 6.57).

The anterior cruciate ligament crosses lateral to the posterior cruciate ligament as they pass through the intercondylar region.

The anterior cruciate ligament prevents anterior displacement of the tibia relative to the femur and the posterior cruciate ligament restricts posterior displacement (Fig. 6.57).

Locking mechanism

When standing, the knee joint is locked into position, thereby reducing the amount of muscle work needed to maintain the standing position (Fig. 6.58).

One component of the locking mechanism is a change in the shape and size of the femoral surfaces that articulate with the tibia (see Fig. 6.52A,B):

- In flexion, the surfaces are the curved and rounded areas on the posterior aspects of the femoral condyles.
- As the knee is extended, the surfaces move to the broad and flat areas on the inferior aspects of the femoral condyles.

Consequently the joint surfaces become larger and more stable in extension.

Another component of the locking mechanism is medial rotation of the femur on the tibia during extension. Medial

Visualizing the knee joint

Fig. 6.59 Normal knee joint. **A.** Normal knee joint showing the tibial collateral ligament, the medial and lateral menisci, and the anterior and posterior cruciate ligaments. T1-weighted magnetic resonance image in the coronal plane. **B.** Radiograph, anterior–posterior view. **C.** Radiograph, lateral view.

rotation and full extension tightens all the associated ligaments.

Another feature that keeps the knee extended when standing is that the body's center of gravity is positioned along a vertical line that passes anterior to the knee joint.

The popliteus muscle unlocks the knee by initiating lateral rotation of the femur on the tibia.

Vascular supply and innervation

Vascular supply to the knee joint is predominantly through descending and genicular branches from the femoral, popliteal, and lateral circumflex femoral arteries in the thigh and the circumflex fibular artery and recurrent branches from the anterior tibial artery in the leg. These vessels form an anastomotic network around the joint (Fig. 6.60).

The knee joint is innervated by branches from the obturator, femoral, tibial, and common fibular nerves.

Soft tissue injuries to the knee

Soft tissue injuries are common at and around the knee joint.

The typical injuries include tears of the anterior and posterior cruciate ligaments, meniscal tears, and trauma to the collateral ligaments. Isolated soft tissue injuries may occur, but it is not uncommon for certain types of injuries to occur together, for example, anterior cruciate ligament disruption, tibial collateral ligament disruption, and tears of the medial or lateral menisci.

Clinical tests for tears in the cruciate ligaments:

- **Anterior drawer test**—a positive anterior drawer test is when the proximal head of a supine patient's tibia can be pulled anteriorly on the femur. The patient lies supine on a couch. The knee is flexed to 90° and the heel and sole of the foot are placed on the couch. If the tibia moves forward, the anterior cruciate ligament is torn.
- **Posterior drawer test**—a positive posterior drawer test occurs when the proximal head of a supine patient's tibia can be pushed posteriorly on the femur. The patient is placed in a supine position and the knee is flexed to approximately 90° with the foot in the neutral position. If the tibial plateau moves posteriorly, the posterior cruciate ligament is torn.

Arthroscopy

An arthroscope is a small camera that is placed into the knee joint through the anterolateral or anteromedial aspect of the knee joint. The joint is filled with a saline solution and the camera is manipulated around the knee joint to assess the cruciate ligaments, menisci, and cartilaginous surfaces. Any damage observed can be repaired or trimmed.

Femoral artery

Adductor magnus

Adductor hiatus

Descending branch of lateral circumflex femoral artery

Descending genicular artery

Saphenous branch

Superior medial genicular artery

Superior lateral genicular artery

Popliteal artery

Inferior lateral genicular artery

Inferior medial genicular artery

Circumflex fibular artery

Recurrent branch of anterior tibial

Posterior tibial artery

Interosseous membrane

Anterior tibial artery

Fig. 6.60 Anastomoses of arteries around the knee. Anterior view.

Tibiofibular joint

The small proximal tibiofibular joint is synovial in type and allows very little movement (Fig. 6.61). The opposing joint surfaces on the undersurface of the lateral condyle of the tibia and on the superomedial surface of the head of the fibula are flat and circular. The capsule is reinforced by anterior and posterior ligaments.

Popliteal fossa

The **popliteal fossa** is an important area of transition between the thigh and leg and is the major route by which structures pass from one region to the other.

The popliteal fossa is a diamond-shaped space behind the knee joint formed between muscles in the posterior compartments of thigh and leg (Fig. 6.62A):

- The margins of the upper part of the diamond are formed medially by the distal ends of the semitendinosus and semimembranosus muscles and laterally by the distal end of the biceps femoris muscle.
- The margins of the smaller lower part of the space are formed medially by the medial head of the gastrocnemius

Fibular collateral ligament

Proximal tibiofibular joint

Anterior ligament of joint

Interosseous membrane

Fig. 6.61 Tibiofibular joint.

muscle and laterally by the plantaris muscle and the lateral head of the gastrocnemius muscle.
- The floor of the fossa is formed by the capsule of the knee joint and adjacent surfaces of the femur and tibia, and, more inferiorly, by the popliteus muscle.
- The roof is formed by deep fascia, which is continuous above with the fascia lata of the thigh and below with deep fascia of the leg.

Contents

The major contents of the popliteal fossa are the popliteal artery, the popliteal vein, and the tibial and common fibular nerves (Fig. 6.62B).

The tibial and common fibular nerves originate proximal to the popliteal fossa as the two major branches of the sciatic nerve (Fig. 6.62B). They are the most superficial of the neurovascular structures in the popliteal fossa and enter the region directly from above under the margin of the biceps femoris muscle (Fig. 6.62B):

- The tibial nerve descends vertically through the popliteal fossa and exits deep to the margin of plantaris muscle to enter the posterior compartment of leg.
- The common fibular nerve exits by following the biceps femoris tendon over the lower lateral margin of the popliteal fossa and continues to the lateral side of the leg where it swings around the neck of the fibula and enters the lateral compartment of leg.

The popliteal artery is the continuation of the femoral artery in the anterior compartment of thigh, and begins as

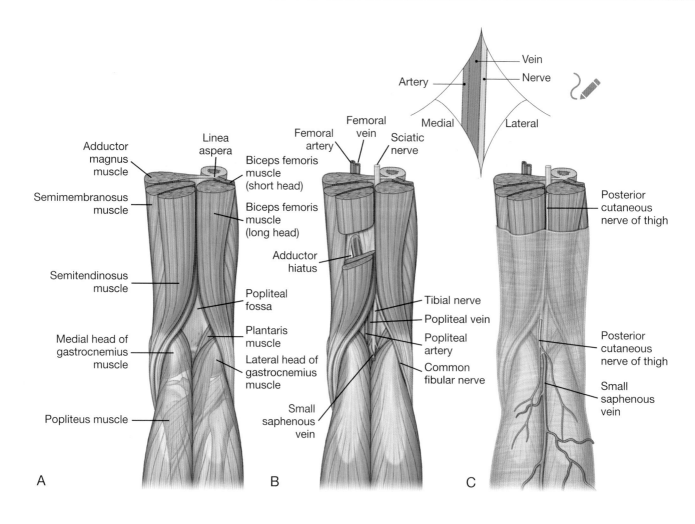

Fig. 6.62 Popliteal fossa. **A.** Boundaries. **B.** Nerves and vessels. **C.** Superficial structures.

the femoral artery passes posteriorly through the adductor hiatus in the adductor magnus muscle (Fig. 6.62B).

The popliteal artery appears deep in the popliteal fossa on the upper medial side under the margin of the semimembranosus muscle. It descends obliquely through the fossa with the tibial nerve and enters the posterior compartment of leg where it ends just lateral to the midline of the leg by dividing into the anterior and posterior tibial arteries.

In the popliteal fossa, the popliteal artery gives rise to branches, which supply adjacent muscles, and to a series of geniculate arteries, which contribute to vascular anastomoses around the knee (see Fig. 6.60).

The popliteal vein is superficial to and travels with the popliteal artery (Fig. 6.62B). It exits the popliteal fossa superiorly to become the femoral vein by passing through the adductor hiatus.

Roof of popliteal fossa

The roof of the popliteal fossa is covered by superficial fascia and skin (Fig. 6.62C). The most important structure in the superficial fascia is the small saphenous vein. This vessel ascends vertically in the superficial fascia on the back of the leg from the lateral side of the dorsal venous arch in the foot. It ascends to the back of the knee where it penetrates deep fascia, which forms the roof of the popliteal fossa and joins with the popliteal vein.

One other structure that passes through the roof of the fossa is the posterior cutaneous nerve of thigh, which descends through the thigh superficial to the hamstring muscles, passes through the roof of the popliteal fossa, and then continues inferiorly with the small saphenous vein to innervate skin on the upper half of the back of the leg.

Surface anatomy

Visualizing the contents of the popliteal fossa

The popliteal fossa is a diamond-shaped depression formed between the hamstrings and gastrocnemius muscle posterior to the knee. The tendons of the biceps femoris muscle and the semitendinosus muscle are palpable and often visible.

The head of the fibula is palpable on the lateral side of the knee and can be used as a landmark for identifying the biceps femoris tendon and the common fibular nerve, which curves laterally out of the popliteal fossa and crosses the neck of the fibula just inferior to the head.

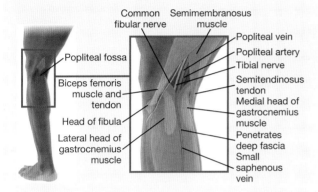

Fig. 6.63 Visualizing the contents of the popliteal fossa. Posterior view of the left knee.

The popliteal fossa contains the popliteal artery, the popliteal vein, the tibial nerve, and the common fibular nerve (Fig. 6.63). The popliteal artery is the deepest of the structures in the fossa and descends through the region from the upper medial side. As a consequence of its position, the popliteal artery pulse is difficult to find, but usually can be detected on deep palpation just medial to the midline of the fossa.

The small saphenous vein penetrates deep fascia in the upper part of the posterior leg and joins the popliteal vein.

LEG

The leg is that part of the lower limb between the knee joint and ankle joint (Fig. 6.64).

The bones of the leg are the lateral **fibula** and the medial **tibia.** The tibia is the weight-bearing bone of the leg and is therefore much larger than the fibula.

The leg is divided into anterior (extensor), posterior (flexor), and lateral (fibular) compartments (Fig. 6.64) by:

- an interosseous membrane, and
- two intermuscular septa, which pass between the fibula and deep fascia surrounding the limb.

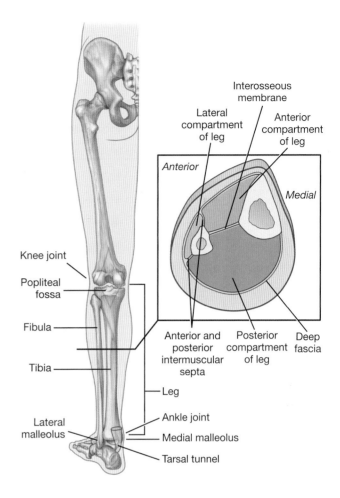

Fig. 6.64 Posterior view of leg; cross-section through the left leg (inset).

Muscles in the anterior compartment of leg dorsiflex the ankle, extend the toes, and invert the foot. Muscles in the posterior compartment plantarflex the ankle, flex the toes, and invert the foot. Muscles in the lateral compartment evert the foot. Major nerves and vessels supply or pass through each compartment.

Bones

Shaft and distal end of tibia

The shaft of tibia (Fig. 6.65A,B) is triangular in cross-section and has anterior, interosseous, and medial borders and medial, lateral, and posterior surfaces (Fig. 6.65C):

- The anterior and medial borders and the entire medial surface are subcutaneous and easily palpable.
- The interosseous border of the tibia is connected by the interosseous membrane along its length to the interosseous border of the fibula.
- The posterior surface is marked by an oblique line (the soleal line).

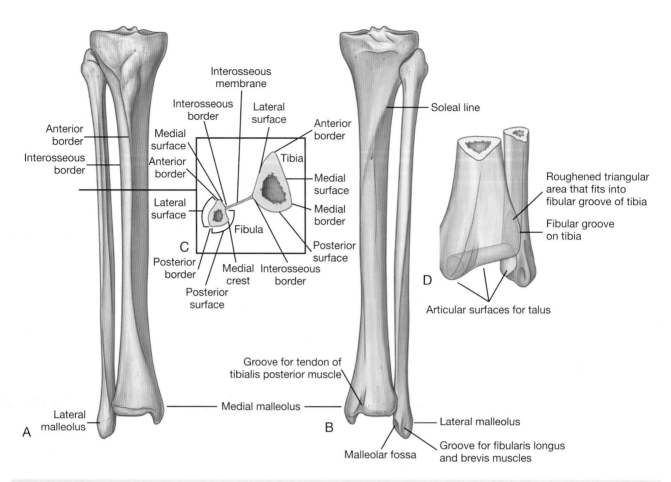

Fig. 6.65 Tibia and fibula. **A.** Anterior view. **B.** Posterior view. **C.** Cross-section through shafts. **D.** Posteromedial view of distal ends.

The soleal line descends across the bone from the lateral side to the medial side where it merges with the medial border. In addition, a vertical line descends down the upper part of the posterior surface from the midpoint of the soleal line. It disappears in the lower one-third of the tibia.

The shaft of the tibia expands at both the upper and lower ends to support the body's weight at the knee and ankle joints.

The distal end of the tibia is shaped like a rectangular box with a bony protuberance on the medial side (the **medial malleolus;** Fig. 6.65). The upper part of the box is continuous with the shaft of the tibia, whereas the lower surface and the medial malleolus articulate with one of the tarsal bones (talus) to form a large part of the ankle joint.

The posterior surface of the box-like distal end of the tibia is marked by a vertical groove, which continues inferiorly and medially onto the posterior surface of the medial malleolus. The groove is for the tendon of the tibialis posterior muscle.

The lateral surface of the distal end of the tibia is occupied by a deep triangular notch (the **fibular notch**) (Fig. 6.65D) to which the distal head of the fibula is anchored by a thickened part of the interosseous membrane.

Shaft and distal end of fibula

The fibula is not involved in weight bearing. The fibular shaft is therefore much narrower than the shaft of the tibia (Fig. 6.65A,B). Also, and except for the ends, the fibula is enclosed by muscles.

Like the tibia, the shaft of the fibula is triangular in cross-section and has three borders and three surfaces for the attachment of muscles, intermuscular septa, and ligaments (Fig. 6.65C). The interosseous border of the fibula faces and is attached to the interosseous border of the tibia by the interosseous membrane. Intermuscular septa attach to the anterior and posterior borders. Muscles attach to the three surfaces.

The narrow **medial surface** faces the anterior compartment of leg, the **lateral surface** faces the lateral compartment

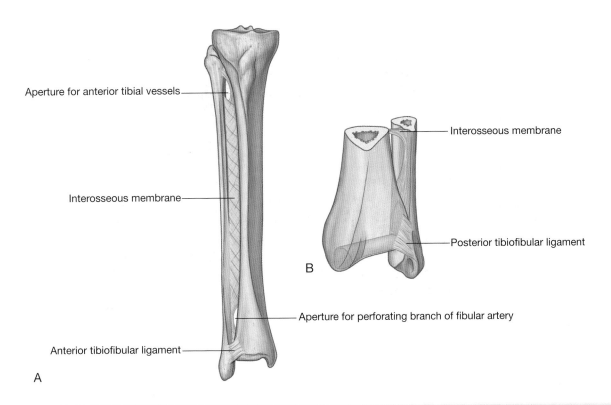

Aperture for anterior tibial vessels

Interosseous membrane

Interosseous membrane

Posterior tibiofibular ligament

B

Aperture for perforating branch of fibular artery

Anterior tibiofibular ligament

A

Fig. 6.66 Interosseous membrane. **A.** Anterior view. **B.** Posteromedial view.

of leg, and the **posterior surface** faces the posterior compartment of leg.

The posterior surface is marked by a vertical crest (**medial crest**), which divides the posterior surface into two parts, each attached to a different deep flexor muscle.

The distal end of the fibula expands to form the spade-shaped **lateral malleolus** (Fig. 6.65).

The medial surface of the lateral malleolus bears a facet for articulation with the lateral surface of talus, thereby forming the lateral part of the ankle joint. Just superior to this articular facet is a triangular area, which fits into the fibular notch on the distal end of the tibia (Fig. 6.65D). Here the tibia and fibula are joined together by the distal end of the interosseous membrane. Posteroinferior to the facet for articulation with the talus is a pit or fossa (the **malleolar fossa**) for the attachment of the posterior talofibular ligament associated with the ankle joint.

The posterior surface of the lateral malleolus is marked by a shallow groove for the tendons of the fibularis longus and fibularis brevis muscles.

Joints

Interosseous membrane of leg

The interosseous membrane of leg is a tough fibrous sheet of connective tissue that spans the distance between facing interosseous borders of the tibial and fibular shafts (Fig. 6.66A).

There are two apertures in the interosseous membrane, one at the top and the other at the bottom, for vessels to pass between the anterior and posterior compartments of the leg (Fig. 6.66A).

The interosseous membrane not only links the tibia and fibula together, but it also provides an increased surface area for muscle attachment.

The distal ends of the fibula and tibia are held together by the inferior aspect of the interosseous membrane, which spans the narrow space between the fibular notch on the lateral surface of the distal end of the tibia and the corresponding surface on the distal end of the fibula (Fig. 6.66A,B). This expanded end of the interosseous membrane is reinforced by anterior and posterior tibiofibular ligaments. This firm linking together of the distal ends of the tibia and fibula is essential to produce the skeletal framework for articulation with the foot at the ankle joint.

Posterior compartment of leg

Muscles

Muscles in the posterior (flexor) compartment of leg are organized into two groups, superficial and deep, separated by a layer of deep fascia. Generally, the muscles mainly plantarflex and invert the foot and flex the toes. All are innervated by the tibial nerve.

Table 6.6 Superficial group of muscles in the posterior compartment of leg (spinal segments in **bold** are the major segments innervating the muscle)

Muscle	Origin	Insertion	Innervation	Function
Gastrocnemius	Medial head—posterior surface of distal femur just superior to medial condyle; lateral head—upper posterolateral surface of lateral femoral condyle	Via calcaneal tendon, to posterior surface of calcaneus	Tibial nerve (**S1, S2**)	Plantarflexes foot and flexes knee
Plantaris	Inferior part of lateral supracondylar line of femur and oblique popliteal ligament of knee	Via calcaneal tendon, to posterior surface of calcaneus	Tibial nerve (**S1, S2**)	Plantarflexes foot and flexes knee
Soleus	Soleal line and medial border of tibia; posterior aspect of fibular head and adjacent surfaces of neck and proximal shaft; tendinous arch between tibial and fibular attachments	Via calcaneal tendon to posterior surface of calcaneus	Tibial nerve (**S1, S2**)	Plantarflexes the foot

Fig. 6.67 Superficial group of muscles in the posterior compartment of leg. **A.** Posterior view. **B.** Lateral view.

Superficial group

The superficial group of muscles in the posterior compartment of leg comprises three muscles—the **gastrocnemius**, **plantaris,** and **soleus** (Table 6.6, Fig. 6.67)—all of which insert onto the heel (calcaneus) of the foot and plantarflex the foot at the ankle joint (Fig. 6.67). As a unit, these muscles are large and powerful because they propel the body forward off the planted foot during walking and can elevate the body upward onto the toes when standing. Two of the muscles (gastrocnemius and plantaris) originate on the distal end of the femur and can also flex the knee.

Deep group

There are four muscles in the deep posterior compartment of leg (Table 6.7, Fig. 6.68)—the **popliteus, flexor hallucis** longus, **flexor digitorum longus,** and **tibialis posterior.** The popliteus muscle acts on the knee, whereas the other three muscles act mainly on the foot.

Fig. 6.68 Deep group of muscles in the posterior compartment of leg.

Arteries

Popliteal artery

The **popliteal artery** is the major blood supply to the leg and foot and enters the posterior compartment of leg from the popliteal fossa behind the knee (Fig. 6.69).

The popliteal artery passes into the posterior compartment of leg between the gastrocnemius and popliteus muscles. As it continues inferiorly it passes under the tendinous arch formed between the fibular and tibial heads of the soleus muscle and enters the deep region of the posterior compartment of leg where it immediately divides into an anterior tibial artery and a posterior tibial artery.

There are two large sural arteries, one on each side, that branch from the popliteal artery to supply the gastrocnemius, soleus, and plantaris muscles (Fig. 6.69). In addition, the popliteal artery gives rise to branches that contribute to a collateral network of vessels around the knee joint (see Fig. 6.60).

Anterior tibial artery

The **anterior tibial artery** passes forward through the aperture in the upper part of the interosseous membrane and enters and supplies the anterior compartment of leg (Fig. 6.69). It continues inferiorly onto the dorsal aspect of the foot.

Posterior tibial artery

The **posterior tibial artery** supplies the posterior and lateral compartments of the leg and continues into the sole of the foot (Fig. 6.69).

The posterior tibial artery descends through the deep region of the posterior compartment of leg on the superficial surfaces of the tibialis posterior and flexor digitorum longus muscles. It passes through the tarsal tunnel behind the medial malleolus and into the sole of the foot.

Table 6.7 Deep group of muscles in the posterior compartment of leg (spinal segments in **bold** are the major segments innervating the muscle)

Muscle	Origin	Insertion	Innervation	Function
Popliteus	Lateral femoral condyle	Posterior surface of proximal tibia	Tibial nerve (L4 to S1)	Stabilizes knee joint (resists lateral rotation of tibia on femur) Unlocks knee joint (laterally rotates femur on fixed tibia)
Flexor hallucis longus	Posterior surface of fibula and adjacent interosseous membrane	Plantar surface of distal phalanx of great toe	Tibial nerve (**S2**, S3)	Flexes great toe; particularly active during the toe-off phase of walking when the body is propelled forward off the stance leg and the great toe is the last part of the foot to leave the ground
Flexor digitorum longus	Medial side of posterior surface of the tibia	Plantar surfaces of bases of distal phalanges of the lateral four toes	Tibial nerve (**S2**, S3)	Flexes lateral four toes
Tibialis posterior	Posterior surfaces of interosseous membrane and adjacent regions of tibia and fibula	Mainly to tuberosity of navicular and adjacent region of medial cuneiform	Tibial nerve (L4, L5)	Inversion and plantarflexion of foot; support of medial arch of foot during walking

In the leg, the posterior tibial artery supplies adjacent muscles and bone and has two major branches, the circumflex fibular artery and the fibular artery:

- The **circumflex fibular artery** passes laterally through the soleus muscle and around the neck of the fibula to connect with the anastomotic network of vessels surrounding the knee (Fig. 6.69; see also Fig. 6.60).
- The **fibular artery** parallels the course of the tibial artery but descends along the lateral side of the posterior compartment adjacent to the medial crest on the posterior surface of the fibula, which separates the attachments of the tibialis posterior and flexor hallucis longus muscles (Fig. 6.69).

The fibular artery supplies adjacent muscles and bone in the posterior compartment of leg and also has branches that pass laterally through the intermuscular septum to supply the fibularis muscles in the lateral compartment of leg.

A **perforating branch** that originates from the fibular artery distally in the leg passes anteriorly through the inferior aperture in the interosseous membrane to anastomose with a branch of the anterior tibial artery.

The fibular artery passes behind the attachment between the distal ends of the tibia and fibula and terminates in a network of vessels over the lateral surface of the calcaneus.

Veins

Deep veins in the posterior compartment generally follow the arteries.

Nerves

Tibial nerve

The nerve associated with the posterior compartment of leg is the tibial nerve (Fig. 6.70A), a major branch of the sciatic nerve that descends into the posterior compartment from the popliteal fossa.

The tibial nerve passes under the tendinous arch formed between the fibular and tibial heads of the soleus muscle and passes vertically through the deep region of the posterior compartment of leg on the surface of the tibialis posterior muscle with the posterior tibial vessels.

The tibial nerve leaves the posterior compartment of leg at the ankle by passing through the tarsal tunnel behind the medial malleolus. It enters the foot to supply most intrinsic muscles and skin.

In the leg, the tibial nerve gives rise to:

- branches that supply all the muscles in the posterior compartment of leg, and
- two cutaneous branches, the **sural nerve** and **medial calcaneal nerve** (Fig. 6.70A,B).

Fig. 6.69 Arteries in the posterior compartment of leg.

Branches of the tibial nerve that innervate the superficial group of muscles of the posterior compartment and popliteus muscle of the deep group originate high in the leg between the two heads of the gastrocnemius muscle in the distal region of the popliteal fossa. Branches innervate the gastrocnemius, plantaris, and soleus muscles, and pass more deeply into the popliteus muscle.

Branches to the deep muscles of the posterior compartment originate from the tibial nerve deep to the soleus muscle in the upper half of the leg and innervate the tibialis posterior, flexor hallucis longus, and flexor digitorum longus muscles.

Sural nerve

The sural nerve originates high in the leg between the two heads of the gastrocnemius muscle (Fig. 6.70B). It

Fig. 6.70 Tibial nerve. **A.** Posterior view. **B.** Sural nerve.

descends superficial to the belly of the gastrocnemius muscle and penetrates through the deep fascia approximately in the middle of the leg where it is joined by a sural communicating branch from the common fibular nerve. It passes down the leg, around the lateral malleolus, and into the foot.

The sural nerve supplies skin on the lower posterolateral surface of the leg and the lateral side of the foot and little toe.

Medial calcaneal nerve

The medial calcaneal nerve is often multiple and originates from the tibial nerve low in the leg near the ankle and descends onto the medial side of the heel.

The medial calcaneal nerve innervates skin on the medial surface and sole of the heel (Fig. 6.70A).

Lateral compartment of leg
Muscles

There are two muscles in the lateral compartment of leg— **fibularis longus** and **fibularis brevis** (Table 6.8, Fig. 6.71). Both evert the foot (turn the sole outward) and are innervated by the superficial fibular nerve, which is a branch of the common fibular nerve.

Arteries

No major artery passes vertically through the lateral compartment of leg. It is supplied by branches (mainly from the fibular artery in the posterior compartment of leg) that penetrate into the lateral compartment (Fig. 6.72).

Veins

Deep veins generally follow the arteries.

Nerves
Superficial fibular nerve

The nerve associated with the lateral compartment of leg is the **superficial fibular nerve.** This nerve originates as one of the two major branches of the common fibular nerve, which enters the lateral compartment of leg from the popliteal fossa (Fig. 6.72B).

The common fibular nerve courses around the neck of the fibula (Fig. 6.72A) and enters the lateral compartment by passing between the attachments of the fibularis longus muscle to the head and shaft of fibula. Here the common fibular nerve divides into its two terminal branches (Fig. 6.72B):

- the superficial fibular nerve, and
- the deep fibular nerve.

The superficial fibular nerve descends in the lateral compartment deep to the fibularis longus and innervates the fibularis longus and fibularis brevis (Fig. 6.72B). It then penetrates deep fascia in the lower leg and enters the foot where it divides into medial and lateral branches, which supply dorsal areas of the foot and toes except for:

- the web space between the great and second toes, which is supplied by the deep fibular nerve, and
- the lateral side of the little toe, which is supplied by the sural branch of the tibial nerve.

The deep fibular nerve passes anteromedially through the intermuscular septum into the anterior compartment of leg, which it supplies.

Anterior compartment of leg
Muscles

There are four muscles in the anterior compartment of leg—the **tibialis anterior, extensor hallucis longus, extensor digitorum longus,** and **fibularis tertius** (Table 6.9, Fig. 6.73).

Collectively they dorsiflex the foot at the ankle joint, extend the toes, and invert the foot. All are innervated by the deep fibular nerve, which is a branch of the common fibular nerve.

Arteries

The artery associated with the anterior compartment of leg is the **anterior tibial artery,** which originates from the popliteal artery in the posterior compartment of leg and passes forward into the anterior compartment of leg through an aperture in the interosseous membrane.

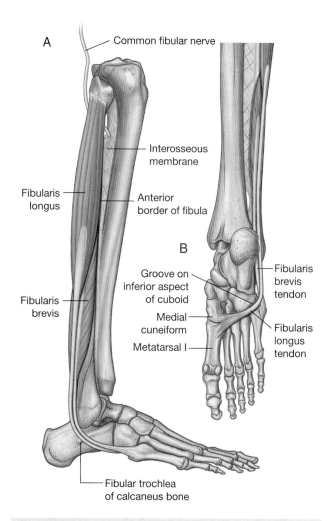

Fig. 6.71 Muscles in the lateral compartment of leg. **A.** Lateral view. **B.** Inferior view of the right foot, with the foot plantarflexed at the ankle.

Fig. 6.72 Common fibular nerve, and nerves and arteries of the lateral compartment of leg. **A.** Posterior view, right leg. **B.** Lateral view, right leg.

Table 6.8 Muscles of the lateral compartment of leg (spinal segments in **bold** are the major segments innervating the muscle)

Muscle	Origin	Insertion	Innervation	Function
Fibularis longus	Upper lateral surface of fibula, head of fibula, and occasionally the lateral tibial condyle	Undersurface of lateral sides of distal end of medial cuneiform and base of metatarsal I	Superficial fibular nerve (**L5, S1**, S2)	Eversion and plantarflexion of foot; supports mainly lateral and transverse arches of foot
Fibularis brevis	Lower two-thirds of lateral surface of shaft of fibula	Tuberosity at base of metatarsal V	Superficial fibular nerve (**L5, S1**, S2)	Eversion of foot

Table 6.9 Muscles of the anterior compartment of leg (spinal segments in **bold** are the major segments innervating the muscle)

Muscle	Origin	Insertion	Innervation	Function
Tibialis anterior	Lateral surface of tibia and adjacent interosseous membrane	Medial and inferior surfaces of medial cuneiform and adjacent surfaces on base of metatarsal I	Deep fibular nerve (**L4**, **L5**)	Dorsiflexion of foot at ankle joint; inversion of foot; dynamic support of medial arch of foot
Extensor hallucis longus	Middle one-half of medial surface of fibula and adjacent surface of interosseous membrane	Dorsal surface of base of distal phalanx of great toe	Deep fibular nerve (**L5**, **S1**)	Extension of great toe and dorsiflexion of foot
Extensor digitorum longus	Proximal one-half of medial surface of fibula and related surface of lateral tibial condyle	Via dorsal digital expansions into bases of distal and middle phalanges of lateral four toes	Deep fibular nerve (**L5**, **S1**)	Extension of lateral four toes and dorsiflexion of foot
Fibularis tertius	Distal part of medial surface of fibula	Dorsomedial surface of base of metatarsal V	Deep fibular nerve (**L5**, **S1**)	Dorsiflexion and eversion of foot

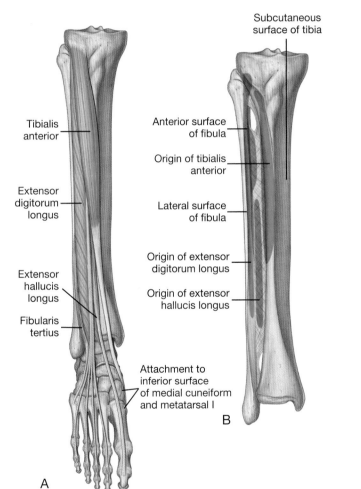

Fig. 6.73 Muscles of the anterior compartment of leg. **A.** Muscles. **B.** Proximal attachments.

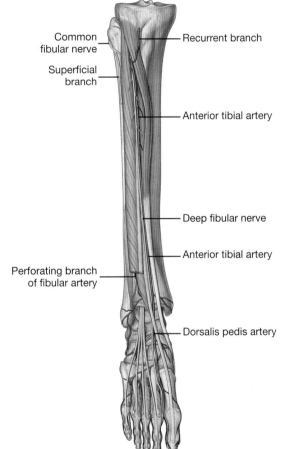

Fig. 6.74 Anterior tibial artery and deep fibular nerve.

The anterior tibial artery descends through the anterior compartment on the interosseous membrane (Fig. 6.74). In the distal leg, it lies between the tendons of the tibialis anterior and extensor hallucis longus muscles. It leaves the leg by passing anterior to the distal end of the tibia and ankle joint and continues onto the dorsal aspect of the foot as the dorsalis pedis artery.

In the proximal leg, the anterior tibial artery has a recurrent branch, which connects with the anastomotic network of vessels around the knee joint (see Fig. 6.60).

Along its course, the anterior tibial artery supplies numerous branches to adjacent muscles and is joined by the perforating branch of the fibular artery, which passes forward through the lower aspect of the interosseous membrane from the posterior compartment of leg.

Distally, the anterior tibial artery gives rise to an **anterior medial malleolar artery** and an **anterior lateral malleolar artery,** which pass posteriorly around the distal ends of the tibia and fibula, respectively, and connect with vessels from the posterior tibial and fibular arteries to form an anastomotic network around the ankle.

Veins

Deep veins follow the arteries and have similar names.

Nerves

Deep fibular nerve

The nerve associated with the anterior compartment of leg is the deep fibular nerve (Fig. 6.74). This nerve originates in the lateral compartment of leg as one of the two divisions of the common fibular nerve.

The deep fibular nerve passes through the intermuscular septum that separates the lateral from the anterior compartments of leg and then passes deep to the extensor digitorum longus. It reaches the anterior interosseous membrane where it meets and descends with the anterior tibial artery.

The deep fibular nerve:

- innervates all muscles in the anterior compartment; and
- then continues into the dorsal aspect of the foot where it innervates the extensor digitorum brevis, contributes to the innervation of the first two dorsal interossei muscles, and supplies the skin between the great and second toes.

Fig. 6.75 Foot. A. Dorsal aspect, right foot. **B.** Plantar aspect, right foot, showing the surface in contact with the ground when standing.

Clinical app

Foot drop

Foot drop is an inability to dorsiflex the foot. Patients with foot drop have a characteristic "steppage" gait. As the patient walks, the knee of the affected limb is elevated to an abnormal height during the swing phase to prevent the foot from dragging. At the end of the swing phase, the foot "slaps" the ground. Also, the unaffected limb often acquires a characteristic tiptoe pattern of gait during the stance phase. A typical cause of foot drop is damage to the common fibular nerve, which may occur with fractures of the fibular neck. Other causes include disc protrusion compressing the L5 nerve root, disorders of the sciatic nerve and the lumbosacral plexus, and pathologies of the spinal cord and brain.

FOOT

The foot is the region of the lower limb distal to the ankle joint. It is subdivided into the ankle, the metatarsus, and the digits.

There are five digits consisting of the medially positioned great toe (digit I) and four more laterally placed digits, ending laterally with the little toe (digit V) (Fig. 6.75).

The foot has a superior surface (**dorsum of foot)** and an inferior surface (**sole;** Fig. 6.75).

Abduction and adduction of the toes are defined with respect to the long axis of the second digit. Unlike in the hand where the thumb is oriented 90° to the other fingers, the great toe is oriented in the same position as the other toes. The foot is the body's point of contact with the ground and provides a stable platform for upright stance. It also levers the body forward during walking.

Bones

There are three groups of bones in the foot (Fig. 6.76):

- the seven **tarsal bones,** which form the skeletal framework for the ankle,
- **metatarsals (I to V),** which are the bones of the metatarsus, and
- the **phalanges,** which are the bones of the toes—each toe has three phalanges, except for the great toe, which has two.

Tarsal bones

The tarsal bones are arranged in a proximal group and a distal group with an intermediate bone between the two groups on the medial side of the foot (Fig. 6.76A).

Proximal group

The proximal group consists of two large bones, the talus (Latin for "ankle") and the calcaneus (Latin for "heel"):

■ The **talus** is the most superior bone of the foot and sits on top of and is supported by the calcaneus (Fig. 6.76B). It articulates above with the tibia and fibula to form the ankle joint and also projects forward to articulate with the intermediate tarsal bone (navicular) on the medial side of the foot.

■ The **calcaneus** is the largest of the tarsal bones (Fig. 6.76A,B)—posteriorly it forms the bony framework of the heel and anteriorly projects forward to articulate with one of the distal group of tarsal bones (cuboid) on the lateral side of the foot.

Talus

The talus, when viewed from the medial or lateral sides, is snail-shaped (Fig. 6.77A). It has a rounded **head,** which is projected forward and medially at the end of a short broad **neck,** which is connected posteriorly to an expanded body.

Anteriorly, the head of the talus is domed for articulation with a corresponding circular depression on the posterior surface of the navicular bone. Inferiorly, this domed articular surface is continuous with an additional three articular facets separated by smooth ridges (Fig. 6.76B):

■ The anterior and middle facets articulate with adjacent surfaces on the calcaneus bone.

■ The other facet, medial to the facets for articulation with the calcaneus, articulates with a ligament—the plantar calcaneonavicular ligament (spring ligament)—which connects the calcaneus to the navicular under the head of the talus.

The neck of the talus is marked inferiorly by a deep groove (the **sulcus tali**), which passes obliquely forward across the inferior surface from medial to lateral, and expands dramatically on the lateral side. Posterior to the sulcus tali is a large facet (posterior calcaneal articular facet) for articulation with the calcaneus.

The superior aspect of the body of the talus is elevated to fit into the socket formed by the distal ends of the tibia and fibula to form the ankle joint:

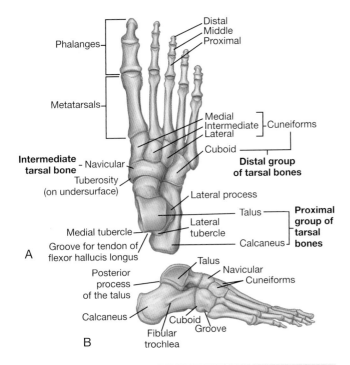

Fig. 6.76 Bones of the foot. **A.** Dorsal view, right foot. **B.** Lateral view, right foot.

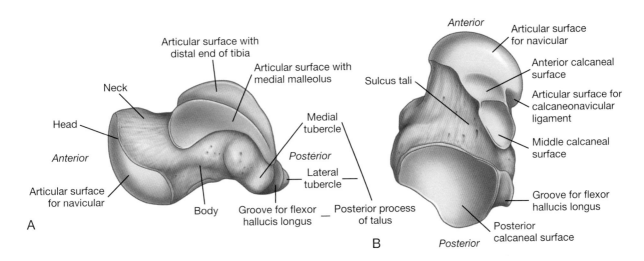

Fig. 6.77 Talus, right foot. **A.** Medial view. **B.** Inferior view.

- The upper (trochlear) surface of this elevated region articulates with the inferior end of the tibia.
- The medial surface articulates with the medial malleolus of the tibia.
- The lateral surface articulates with the lateral malleolus of the fibula.

Because the lateral malleolus is larger and projects more inferiorly than the medial malleolus at the ankle joint, the corresponding lateral articular surface on the talus is larger and projects more inferiorly than the medial surface.

The lower part of the lateral surface of the body of the talus, which supports the lower part of the facet for articulation with the fibula, forms a bony projection (the **lateral process**) (Fig. 6.76A).

The inferior surface of the body of the talus has a large oval concave facet (the **posterior calcaneal articular facet**) for articulation with the calcaneus (Fig. 6.77B).

The posterior aspect of the body of the talus consists of a backward and medially facing projection (the **posterior process**). The posterior process is marked on its surface by a lateral tubercle and a medial tubercle, which bracket between them the **groove for tendon of the flexor hallucis longus** as it passes from the leg into the foot.

Calcaneus

The calcaneus sits under and supports the talus. It is an elongate, irregular, box-shaped bone with its long axis generally oriented along the midline of the foot but deviating lateral to the midline anteriorly (Fig. 6.78).

The calcaneus projects behind the ankle joint to form the skeletal framework of the heel. The posterior surface of this heel region is circular and divided into upper, middle, and lower parts. The calcaneal tendon (Achilles tendon) attaches to the middle part:

- The upper part is separated from the calcaneal tendon by a bursa.
- The lower part curves forward, is covered by subcutaneous tissue, is the weight-bearing region of the heel, and is continuous onto the plantar surface of the bone as the **calcaneal tuberosity.**

The calcaneal tuberosity projects forward on the plantar surface as a large medial process and a small lateral process separated from each other by a V-shaped notch (Fig. 6.78B). At the anterior end of the plantar surface is a tubercle (the **calcaneal tubercle**) for the posterior attachment of the short plantar ligament of the sole of the foot.

The lateral surface of the calcaneus has a smooth contour except for two slightly raised regions (Fig. 6.78C). One of these raised areas—the **fibular trochlea** (peroneal tubercle)—is anterior to the middle of the surface and often has two shallow grooves, which pass, one above the other, obliquely across its surface. The tendons of the fibularis brevis and longus muscles are bound to the trochlea as they pass over the lateral side of the calcaneus.

Superior and posterior to the fibular trochlea is a second raised area or tubercle for attachment of the calcaneofibular part of the lateral collateral ligament of the ankle joint.

The medial surface of the calcaneus is concave and has one prominent feature associated with its upper margin (the **sustentaculum tali;** Fig. 6.78A), which is a shelf of bone projecting medially and supporting the more posterior part of the head of the talus.

The underside of the sustentaculum tali has a distinct groove running from posterior to anterior and along which the tendon of the flexor hallucis longus muscle travels into the sole of the foot (Fig. 6.78B).

The superior surface of the sustentaculum tali has a facet (**middle talar articular surface**) for articulation with the corresponding middle facet on the head of the talus (Fig. 6.78A,C).

Anterior and **posterior talar articular surfaces** are on the superior surface of the calcaneus itself (Fig. 6.78A):

- The anterior talar articular surface is small and articulates with the corresponding anterior facet on the head of the talus.
- The posterior talar articular surface is large and is approximately near the middle of the superior surface of the calcaneus.

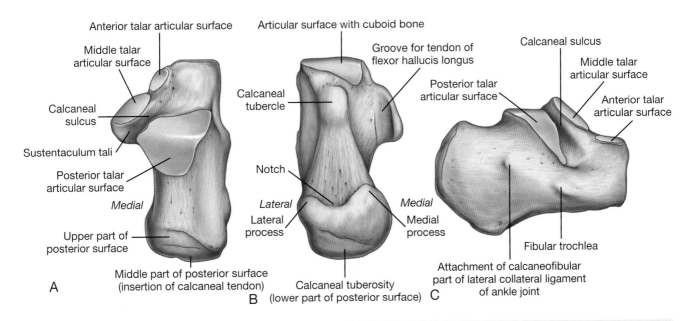

Fig. 6.78 Calcaneus, right foot. **A.** Superior view. **B.** Inferior view. **C.** Lateral view.

Between the posterior talar articular surface, which articulates with the body of the talus, and the other two articular surfaces, which articulate with the head of the talus, is a deep groove (the **calcaneal sulcus**; Fig. 6.78A,C).

The calcaneal sulcus on the superior surface of the calcaneus and the sulcus tali on the inferior surface of the talus together form the **tarsal sinus**, which is a large gap between the anterior ends of the calcaneus and talus that is visible when the skeleton of the foot is viewed from its lateral aspect (Fig. 6.79).

Intermediate tarsal bone

The intermediate tarsal bone on the medial side of the foot is the **navicular** (boat shaped) (see Fig. 6.76). This bone articulates behind with the talus and articulates in front and on the lateral side with the distal group of tarsal bones.

One distinctive feature of the navicular is a prominent rounded tuberosity for the attachment of the tibialis posterior tendon, which projects inferiorly on the medial side of the plantar surface of the bone.

Distal group

From lateral to medial, the distal group of tarsal bones consists of (see Fig. 6.76):

- The **cuboid** (Greek for "cube"), which articulates posteriorly with the calcaneus, medially with the lateral cuneiform, and anteriorly with the bases of the lateral two metatarsals—the tendon of the fibularis longus muscle lies in a prominent groove on the anterior plantar surface, which passes obliquely forward across the bone from lateral to medial.
- Three **cuneiforms** (Latin for "wedge")—the **lateral, intermediate,** and **medial** cuneiform bones, in addition to articulating with each other, articulate posteriorly with the navicular bone and anteriorly with the bases of the medial three metatarsals (see Fig. 6.76).

Metatarsals

There are five metatarsals in the foot, numbered I to V from medial to lateral (Fig. 6.80; also see Fig. 6.81). Metatarsal I, associated with the great toe, is shortest and thickest. The second is the longest.

Each metatarsal has a **head** at the distal end, an elongate **shaft** in the middle, and a proximal **base.**

The head of each metatarsal articulates with the proximal phalanx of a toe and the base articulates with one or more of the distal group of tarsal bones. The plantar surface of

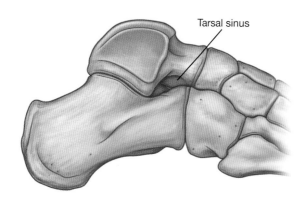

Fig. 6.79 Tarsal sinus. Lateral view, right foot.

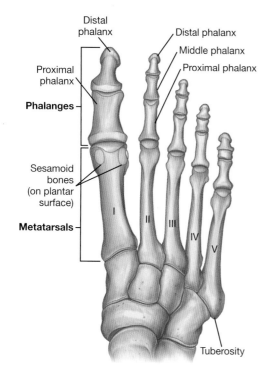

Fig. 6.80 Metatarsals and phalanges. Dorsal view, right foot.

the head of metatarsal I also articulates with two sesamoid bones.

The sides of the bases of metatarsals II to V also articulate with each other. The lateral side of the base of metatarsal V has a prominent **tuberosity**, which projects posteriorly and is the attachment site for the tendon of the fibularis brevis muscle (Fig. 6.80).

Phalanges

The phalanges are the bones of the toes (Figs. 6.80 and 6.81). Each toe has three phalanges (**proximal, middle,** and **distal**), except for the great toe, which has only two (proximal and distal).

Each phalanx consists of a **base,** a **shaft,** and a distal **head:**

- The base of each proximal phalanx articulates with the head of the related metatarsal.
- The head of each distal phalanx is nonarticular and flattened into a crescent-shaped plantar tuberosity under the plantar pad at the end of the digit.

In each toe, the total length of the phalanges combined is much shorter than the length of the associated metatarsal.

Imaging app

Visualizing the bones of the foot

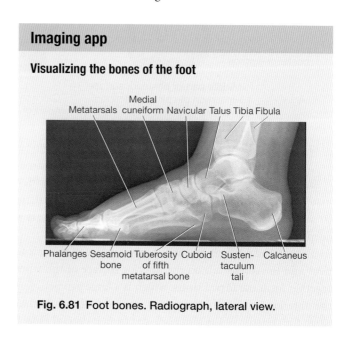

Fig. 6.81 Foot bones. Radiograph, lateral view.

Joints
Ankle joint

The ankle joint is synovial in type and involves the talus of the foot and the tibia and fibula of the leg (Fig. 6.82; also see Fig. 6.86).

The ankle joint mainly allows hinge-like dorsiflexion and plantarflexion of the foot on the leg.

The distal end of the fibula is firmly anchored to the larger distal end of the tibia by strong ligaments. Together, the fibula and tibia create a deep bracket-shaped socket for the upper expanded part of the body of the talus:

- The roof of the socket is formed by the inferior surface of the distal end of the tibia.
- The medial side of the socket is formed by the medial malleolus of the tibia.
- The longer lateral side of the socket is formed by the lateral malleolus of the fibula.

The articular surfaces are covered by hyaline cartilage.

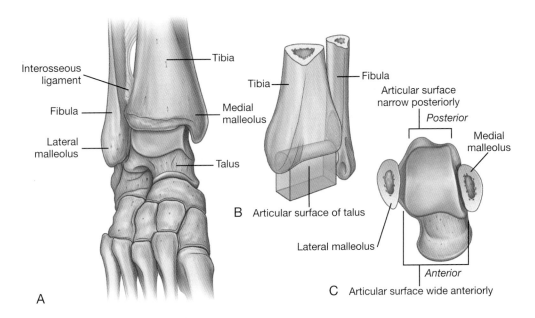

Fig. 6.82 Ankle joint. **A.** Anterior view with foot plantarflexed, right foot. **B.** Schematic of joint. **C.** Superior view of the talus to show the shape of the articular surface.

The articular part of the talus is shaped like a short half cylinder tipped onto its flat side with one end facing lateral and the other end facing medial. The curved upper surface of the half cylinder and the two ends are covered by hyaline cartilage and fit into the bracket-shaped socket formed by the distal ends of the tibia and fibula (Fig. 6.82C).

When viewed from above, the articular surface of the talus is much wider anteriorly than it is posteriorly. As a result, the bone fits tighter into its socket when the foot is dorsiflexed, and the wider surface of the talus moves into the ankle joint than when the foot is plantarflexed and the narrower part of the talus is in the joint. The joint is therefore most stable when the foot is dorsiflexed.

The articular cavity is enclosed by a synovial membrane, which attaches around the margins of the articular surfaces, and by a fibrous membrane, which covers the synovial membrane and is also attached to the adjacent bones.

The ankle joint is stabilized by **medial** (deltoid) and **lateral ligaments** (Figs. 6.83 and 6.84).

Medial ligament (deltoid ligament)

The medial (deltoid) ligament is large, strong (Fig. 6.83), and triangular in shape. Its apex is attached above to the medial malleolus and its broad base is attached below to a line that extends from the tuberosity of the navicular bone in front to the medial tubercle of the talus behind.

The medial ligament is subdivided into four parts based on the inferior points of attachment (Fig. 6.83):

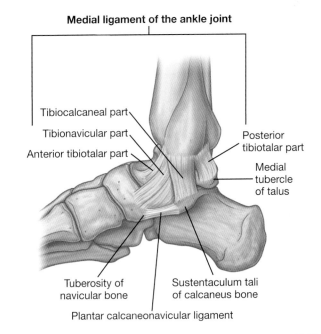

Fig. 6.83 Medial ligament of the ankle joint, right foot.

- The part that attaches in front to the tuberosity of the navicular and the associated margin of the plantar calcaneonavicular ligament (spring ligament), which connects the navicular bone to the sustentaculum tali of the calcaneus bone behind, is the **tibionavicular part** of the medial ligament.
- The **tibiocalcaneal part,** which is more central, attaches to the sustentaculum tali of the calcaneus bone.

Lower Limb

- The **posterior tibiotalar part** attaches to the medial side and medial tubercle of the talus.
- The fourth part (the **anterior tibiotalar part**) is deep to the tibionavicular and tibiocalcaneal parts of the medial ligament and attaches to the medial surface of the talus.

Lateral ligament

The lateral ligament of the ankle is composed of three separate ligaments: the anterior talofibular ligament, the posterior talofibular ligament, and the calcaneofibular ligament (Fig. 6.84).

- The **anterior talofibular ligament** is a short ligament and attaches the anterior margin of the lateral malleolus to the adjacent region of the talus.
- The **posterior talofibular ligament** runs horizontally backward and medially from the malleolar fossa on the medial side of the lateral malleolus to the posterior process of the talus.

- The **calcaneofibular ligament** is attached above to the malleolar fossa on the posteromedial side of the lateral malleolus and passes posteroinferiorly to attach below to a tubercle on the lateral surface of the calcaneus.

Intertarsal joints

The numerous synovial joints between the individual tarsal bones mainly invert, evert, supinate, and pronate the foot (Fig. 6.85):

- Inversion and eversion is turning the whole sole of the foot inward and outward, respectively.
- Pronation is rotating the front of the foot laterally relative to the back of the foot, and supination is the reverse movement.

Pronation and supination allow the foot to maintain normal contact with the ground when in different stances or when standing on irregular surfaces.

The major joints at which movements occur include the subtalar, talocalcaneonavicular, and calcaneocuboid joints (see Fig. 6.85). The talocalcaneonavicular and calcaneocuboid joints together form what is often referred to as the **transverse tarsal joint.**

Intertarsal joints between the cuneiforms and between the cuneiforms and the navicular allow only limited movement.

The joint between the cuboid and navicular is normally fibrous.

Fig. 6.84 Lateral ligament of the ankle joint, right foot. **A.** Lateral view. **B.** Posterior view.

346

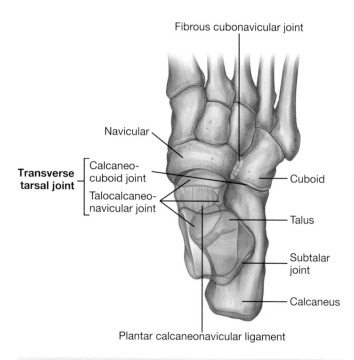

Fig. 6.85 Intertarsal joints, right foot.

Imaging app

Visualizing the ankle joint

Fig. 6.86 Normal ankle joint. **A.** Radiograph, lateral view. **B.** Radiograph, anterior–posterior view. **C.** Coronal view of the ankle joint showing the medial ligament (deltoid ligament). T2-weighted magnetic resonance (MR) image in coronal plane. **D.** Coronal view of ankle joint showing posterior talofibular and calcaneofibular ligaments. T2-weighted MR image in coronal plane.

Ankle injuries

The anatomy of the ankle joint is complex. However, from a clinical perspective it may be regarded as a fibro-osseous ring oriented in the coronal plane.

- The upper part of the ring is formed by the joint between the distal ends of the fibula and tibia and by the ankle joint itself.
- The sides of the ring are formed by the ligaments that connect the medial malleolus and lateral malleolus to the adjacent tarsal bones.
- The bottom of the ring is not part of the ankle joint but consists of the subtalar joint and the associated ligaments.

Injuries may occur as fractures or ligament disruptions. Typically, two parts of this fibro-osseous ring are disrupted. Inversion injuries of the ankle joint are common. In this injury, the anterior talofibular and calcaneofibular parts of the lateral ligament are disrupted. These structures, once disrupted, allow the ankle to invert, often producing a fracture of the medial malleolus or a partial tear to the medial (deltoid) ligament.

Subtalar joint

The subtalar joint is between (Fig. 6.87):

- the large posterior calcaneal facet on the inferior surface of the talus, and
- the corresponding posterior talar facet on the superior surface of the calcaneus.

The articular cavity is enclosed by synovial membrane, which is covered by a fibrous membrane.

The subtalar joint allows gliding and rotation, which are involved in inversion and eversion of the foot. **Lateral, medial, posterior,** and **interosseous talocalcaneal ligaments** stabilize the joint. The interosseous talocalcaneal ligament lies in the tarsal sinus (Fig. 6.87).

Talocalcaneonavicular joint

The **talocalcaneonavicular joint** (Fig. 6.88) is a complex joint in which the head of the talus articulates with the calcaneus and plantar calcaneonavicular ligament (spring ligament) below and the navicular in front (Fig. 6.88A).

The talocalcaneonavicular joint allows gliding and rotation movements, which, together with similar movements of the subtalar joint, are involved with inversion

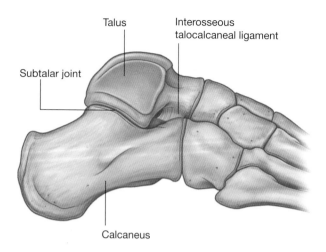

Fig. 6.87 Interosseous talocalcaneal ligament. Lateral view, right foot.

and eversion of the foot. It also participates in pronation and supination.

The parts of the talocalcaneonavicular joint between the talus and calcaneus are:

- the anterior and middle calcaneal facets on the inferior surface of the talar head, and
- the corresponding anterior and middle talar facets on the superior surface and sustentaculum tali, respectively, of the calcaneus (Fig. 6.88B).

The part of the joint between the talus and the plantar calcaneonavicular ligament (spring ligament) is between the ligament and a facet on the inferior surface of the talar head.

The joint between the navicular and talus is the largest part of the talocalcaneonavicular joint and is between the ovoid anterior end of the talar head and the corresponding concave posterior surface of the navicular.

Ligaments

The capsule of the talocalcaneonavicular joint, which is a synovial joint, is reinforced (Fig. 6.88A,B,C):

- posteriorly by the interosseous talocalcaneal ligament,
- superiorly by the **talonavicular ligament,** which passes between the neck of the talus and adjacent regions of the navicular, and
- inferiorly by the plantar calcaneonavicular ligament (spring ligament).

The lateral part of the talocalcaneonavicular joint is reinforced by the calcaneonavicular part of the **bifurcate ligament,** which is a Y-shaped ligament superior to the joint

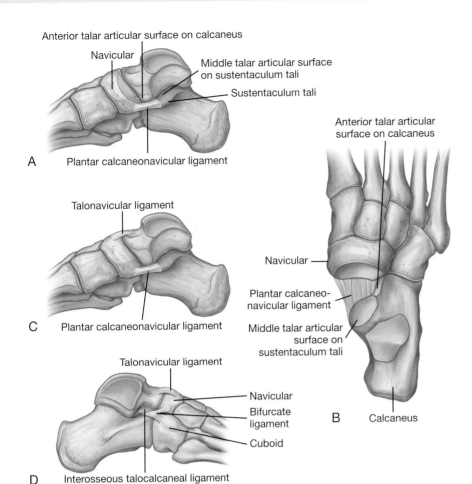

A — Anterior talar articular surface on calcaneus / Navicular / Middle talar articular surface on sustentaculum tali / Sustentaculum tali / Plantar calcaneonavicular ligament

C — Talonavicular ligament / Plantar calcaneonavicular ligament

D — Talonavicular ligament / Navicular / Bifurcate ligament / Cuboid / Interosseous talocalcaneal ligament

B — Anterior talar articular surface on calcaneus / Navicular / Plantar calcaneo-navicular ligament / Middle talar articular surface on sustentaculum tali / Calcaneus

Fig. 6.88 Talocalcaneonavicular joint. **A.** Medial view, right foot. **B.** Superior view, right foot, talus removed. **C.** Ligaments, medial view, right foot. **D.** Ligaments, lateral view, right foot.

(Fig. 6.88D). The base of the bifurcate ligament is attached to the anterior aspect of the superior surface of the calcaneus and its arms are attached to:

- the dorsomedial surface of the cuboid (**calcaneocuboid ligament**), and
- the dorsolateral part of the navicular (**calcaneonavicular ligament**).

The **plantar calcaneonavicular ligament** (spring ligament) is a broad thick ligament that spans the space between the sustentaculum tali behind and the navicular bone in front (Fig. 6.88B,C). It supports the head of the talus, takes part in the talocalcaneonavicular joint, and resists depression of the medial arch of the foot.

Calcaneocuboid joint

The **calcaneocuboid joint** is a synovial joint between:

- the facet on the anterior surface of the calcaneus, and
- the corresponding facet on the posterior surface of the cuboid.

The calcaneocuboid joint allows sliding and rotating movements involved with inversion and eversion of the foot, and also contributes to pronation and supination of the forefoot on the hindfoot.

Ligaments

The calcaneocuboid joint is reinforced by the bifurcate ligament (see previous discussion) and by the long plantar ligament and the plantar calcaneocuboid ligament (short plantar ligament) (Fig. 6.89).

The **plantar calcaneocuboid ligament** (short plantar ligament) is short, wide, and very strong and connects the calcaneal tubercle to the inferior surface of the cuboid (Fig. 6.89A). It not only supports the calcaneocuboid joint, but it also assists the long plantar ligament in resisting depression of the lateral arch of the foot.

The **long plantar ligament** is the longest ligament in the sole of the foot and lies inferior to the plantar calcaneocuboid ligament (Fig. 6.89B):

- Posteriorly, it attaches to the inferior surface of the calcaneus between the tuberosity and the calcaneal tubercle.

Fibularis longus tendon

Plantar calcaneocuboid ligament (short plantar ligament)

Plantar calcaneonavicular ligament

Calcaneocuboid joint

Calcaneal tubercle

Long plantar ligament

A

B

Fig. 6.89 Plantar ligaments, right foot. **A.** Plantar calcaneocuboid ligament (short plantar ligament). **B.** Long plantar ligament.

Interphalangeal joints

Collateral ligaments

Interphalangeal joint

Collateral ligaments

Metatarso-phalangeal joints

Plantar ligaments

Deep transverse metatarsal ligament

Tarsometatarsal joints

Fig. 6.90 Tarsometatarsal, metatarsophalangeal, and interphalangeal joints and the deep transverse metatarsal ligaments, right foot.

■ Anteriorly, it attaches to a broad ridge and a tubercle on the inferior surface of the cuboid bone behind the groove for the fibularis longus tendon.

More superficial fibers of the long plantar ligament extend to the bases of the metatarsal bones.

The long plantar ligament supports the calcaneocuboid joint and is the strongest ligament, resisting depression of the lateral arch of the foot.

Tarsometatarsal joints

The **tarsometatarsal joints** between the metatarsal bones and adjacent tarsal bones are plane joints and allow limited sliding movements (Fig. 6.90).

The range of movement of the tarsometatarsal joint between the metatarsal of the great toe and the medial cuneiform is greater than that of the other tarsometatarsal joints and allows flexion, extension, and rotation. The tarsometatarsal joints, with the transverse tarsal joint, take part in pronation and supination of the foot.

Metatarsophalangeal joints

The metatarsophalangeal joints are ellipsoid synovial joints between the sphere-shaped heads of the metatarsals and the corresponding bases of the proximal phalanges of the digits.

The metatarsophalangeal joints allow extension and flexion and limited abduction, adduction, rotation, and circumduction.

The joint capsules are reinforced by medial and lateral **collateral ligaments** and by **plantar ligaments,** which have grooves on their plantar surfaces for the long tendons of the digits (Fig. 6.90).

Clinical app

Bunions

Clinically, a bunion is a significant protuberance of bone that may include soft tissue around the medial aspect of the first metatarsophalangeal joint. This area is an extremely important region of the foot because it is crossed by tendons and ligaments that transmit and distribute the body's weight during movement. It is postulated that abnormal stresses in this region of the joint may actually produce the bunion deformity. As the bunion progresses, the great toe appears to move toward the smaller toes, producing crowding of the digits. Typically the patient's symptoms are pain, swelling, and inflammation.

The metatarsal of the great toe is oriented in the same plane as the metatarsals of the other toes and is linked to the metatarsal of the second toe by a deep transverse metatarsal ligament. In addition, the joint between the metatarsal of the great toe and medial cuneiform has a limited range of motion. The great toe therefore has a very restricted independent function.

Interphalangeal joints

The interphalangeal joints are hinge joints that allow mainly flexion and extension. They are reinforced by medial and lateral **collateral ligaments** and by **plantar ligaments** (Fig. 6.90).

Tarsal tunnel, retinacula, and arrangement of major structures at the ankle

The tarsal tunnel is formed on the posteromedial side of the ankle by (Fig. 6.91):

- a depression formed by the medial malleolus of the tibia, the medial and posterior surfaces of the talus, the medial surface of the calcaneus, and the inferior surface of the sustentaculum tali of the calcaneus; and
- an overlying flexor retinaculum.

Flexor retinaculum

The flexor retinaculum is a strap-like layer of connective tissue that spans the bony depression formed by the medial malleolus, the medial and posterior surfaces of the talus, the medial surface of calcaneus, and the inferior surface of the sustentaculum tali (Fig. 6.91). It attaches above to the medial malleolus and below and behind to the inferomedial margin of the calcaneus.

The retinaculum is continuous above with the deep fascia of the leg and below with deep fascia (plantar aponeurosis) of the foot.

Septa from the flexor retinaculum convert grooves on the bones into tubular connective tissue channels for the tendons of the flexor muscles as they pass into the sole of the foot from the posterior compartment of leg (Fig. 6.91). Free movement of the tendons in the channels is facilitated by synovial sheaths, which surround the tendons.

Two compartments on the posterior surface of the medial malleolus are for the tendons of the tibialis posterior and flexor digitorum longus muscles. The tendon of the tibialis posterior is medial to the tendon of the flexor digitorum longus.

Immediately lateral to the tendons of the tibialis posterior and flexor digitorum longus, the posterior tibial artery with its associated veins and the tibial nerve pass through the tarsal tunnel into the sole of the foot.

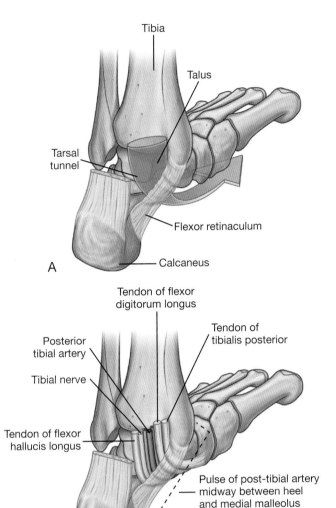

Tibia

Talus

Tarsal tunnel

Flexor retinaculum

Calcaneus

A

Tendon of flexor digitorum longus

Tendon of tibialis posterior

Posterior tibial artery

Tibial nerve

Tendon of flexor hallucis longus

Pulse of post-tibial artery midway between heel and medial malleolus

B

Tibialis posterior

Flexor digitorum longus

Tibial artery

Tibial vein

Tibial nerve

Flexor hallucis longus

Fig. 6.91 Tarsal tunnel and flexor retinaculum. Posteromedial view, left foot. **A.** Bones. **B.** Tarsal tunnel and flexor retinaculum.

Deep transverse metatarsal ligaments

Four **deep transverse metatarsal ligaments** link the heads of the metatarsals together and enable the metatarsals to act as a single unified structure (Fig. 6.90). The ligaments blend with the plantar ligaments of the adjacent metatarsophalangeal joints.

Lower Limb

Lateral to the tibial nerve is the compartment on the posterior surface of the talus and the undersurface of the sustentaculum tali for the tendon of the flexor hallucis longus muscle.

Surface anatomy

Finding the tarsal tunnel—the gateway to the foot

The tarsal tunnel (Fig. 6.92) is formed on the medial side of the foot in the groove between the medial malleolus and the heel (calcaneal tuberosity) and by the overlying flexor retinaculum.

The posterior tibial artery and tibial nerve enter the foot through the tarsal tunnel. The tendons of the tibialis posterior, flexor digitorum longus, and flexor hallucis longus also pass through the tarsal tunnel in compartments formed by septa of the flexor retinaculum.

The order of structures passing through the tunnel from the anteromedial to posterolateral are the tendon of the tibialis posterior, the tendon of the flexor digitorum longus, the posterior tibial artery and associated veins, the tibial nerve, and the tendon of the flexor hallucis longus ("Tom, Dick, and a very nervous Harry").

The tibial artery is palpable just posteroinferior to the medial malleolus on the anterior face of the visible groove between the heel and medial malleolus.

Fig. 6.92 Finding the tarsal tunnel—the gateway to the foot.

Extensor retinacula

Two extensor retinacula strap the tendons of the extensor muscles to the ankle region and prevent tendon bowing during extension of the foot and toes (Fig. 6.93):

- A **superior extensor retinaculum** is a thickening of deep fascia in the distal leg just superior to the ankle joint and attached to the anterior borders of the fibula and tibia.
- An **inferior retinaculum** is Y-shaped, attached by its base to the lateral side of the upper surface of the calcaneus, and crosses medially over the foot to attach by one of its arms to the medial malleolus, whereas the other arm wraps medially around the foot and attaches to the medial side of the plantar aponeurosis.

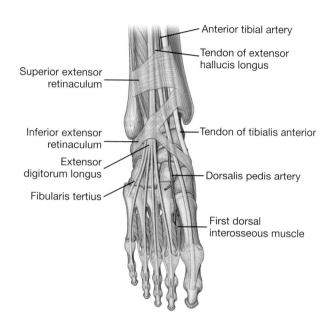

Fig. 6.93 Extensor retinacula, right foot.

The tendons of the extensor digitorum longus and fibularis tertius pass through a compartment on the lateral side of the proximal foot. Medial to these tendons, the dorsalis pedis artery (terminal branch of the anterior tibial artery), the tendon of the extensor hallucis longus muscle, and finally the tendon of the tibialis anterior muscle pass under the extensor retinacula.

Fibular retinacula

Fibular (peroneal) retinacula bind the tendons of the fibularis longus and fibularis brevis muscles to the lateral side of the foot (Fig. 6.94):

- A **superior fibular retinaculum** extends between the lateral malleolus and the calcaneus.
- An **inferior fibular retinaculum** attaches to the lateral surface of the calcaneus around the fibular trochlea and blends above with the fibers of the inferior extensor retinaculum.

At the fibular trochlea, a septum separates the compartment for the tendon of the fibularis brevis muscle above from that for the fibularis longus below.

Arches of the foot

The bones of the foot do not lie in a horizontal plane. Instead, they form longitudinal and transverse arches relative to the ground (Fig. 6.95), which absorb and distribute downward

Tendons of fibularis longus
and brevis muscles

Superior fibular
retinaculum

Inferior fibular retinaculum
(at fibular trochlea on calcaneus)

Fig. 6.94 Fibular retinacula. Lateral view, right foot.

Medial longitudinal arch

A

Lateral longitudinal arch

B

Transverse arch

Fig. 6.95 Arches of the foot. **A.** Longitudinal arches, right foot. **B.** Transverse arch, left foot.

forces from the body during standing and moving on different surfaces.

Longitudinal arch

The longitudinal arch of the foot is formed between the posterior end of the calcaneus and the heads of the metatarsals (Fig. 6.95A). It is highest on the medial side where it forms the medial part of the longitudinal arch and lowest on the lateral side where it forms the lateral part.

Transverse arch

The transverse arch of the foot is highest in a coronal plane that cuts through the head of the talus and disappears near the heads of the metatarsals where these bones are held together by the deep transverse metatarsal ligaments (Fig. 6.95B).

Ligaments and muscles support the arches of the foot (Fig. 6.96):

- Ligaments that support the arches include the plantar calcaneonavicular (spring ligament), plantar calcaneocuboid (short plantar ligament), long plantar ligament, and the plantar aponeurosis.
- Muscles that provide dynamic support for the arches during walking include the tibialis anterior and posterior, and the fibularis longus.

Plantar aponeurosis

The plantar aponeurosis is a thickening of deep fascia in the sole of the foot (Fig. 6.97). It is firmly anchored to the medial

process of the calcaneal tuberosity and extends forward as a thick band of longitudinally arranged connective tissue fibers. The fibers diverge as they pass anteriorly and form digital bands, which enter the toes and connect with bones, ligaments, and dermis of the skin.

Distal to the metatarsophalangeal joints, the digital bands of the plantar aponeurosis are interconnected by transverse fibers that form superficial transverse metatarsal ligaments.

The plantar aponeurosis supports the longitudinal arch of the foot and protects deeper structures in the sole.

Fibrous sheaths of toes

The tendons of the flexor digitorum longus, flexor digitorum brevis, and flexor hallucis longus muscles enter fibrous digital sheaths or tunnels on the plantar aspect of the digits (Fig. 6.98). These fibrous sheaths begin anterior to the metacarpophalangeal joints and extend to the distal phalanges. They are formed by fibrous arches and cruciate (cross-shaped) ligaments attached posteriorly to the margins of the phalanges and to the plantar ligaments associated with the metatarsophalangeal and interphalangeal joints.

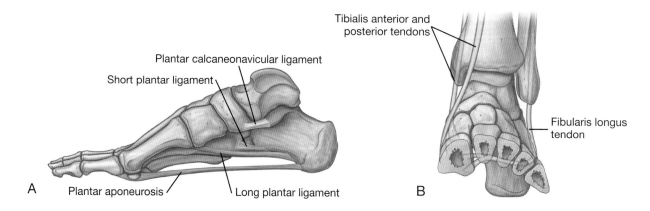

Fig. 6.96 Support for arches of the foot. **A.** Ligaments. Medial view, right foot. **B.** Cross-section through the foot to show tendons of muscles supporting the arches, left foot.

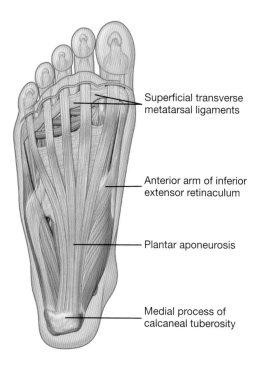

Fig. 6.97 Plantar aponeurosis, right foot.

Fig. 6.98 Fibrous digital sheaths, right foot.

These fibrous tunnels hold the tendons to the bony plane and prevent tendon bowing when the toes are flexed. Within each tunnel, the tendons are surrounded by a synovial sheath.

Extensor hoods

The tendons of the extensor digitorum longus, extensor digitorum brevis, and extensor hallucis longus pass into the dorsal aspect of the digits and expand over the proximal phalanges to form complex dorsal digital expansions ("extensor hoods") (Fig. 6.99).

Each extensor hood is triangular with the apex attached to the distal phalanx, the central region attached to the middle (toes II to V) or proximal (toe I) phalanx, and each corner of the base wrapped around the sides of the metatarsophalangeal joint. The corners of the hoods attach mainly to the deep transverse metatarsal ligaments.

Many of the intrinsic muscles of the foot insert into the free margin of the hood on each side. The attachment of these muscles into the extensor hoods allows the forces from these muscles to be distributed over the toes to cause flexion of the metatarsophalangeal joints while extending the interphalangeal joints (Fig. 6.99). The function of these movements in the foot is uncertain, but they may prevent overextension of the metatarsophalangeal joints and flexion of the interphalangeal joints when the heel is elevated off the ground and the toes grip the ground during walking.

Intrinsic muscles

Intrinsic muscles of the foot originate and insert in the foot:

- the **extensor digitorum brevis** and **extensor hallucis brevis** on the dorsal aspect of the foot (Table 6.10, Fig. 6.100);
- all other intrinsic muscles are on the plantar side of the foot where they are organized into four layers.

Intrinsic muscles mainly modify the actions of the long tendons and generate fine movements of the toes.

All intrinsic muscles of the foot are innervated by the medial and lateral plantar branches of the tibial nerve except for the extensor digitorum brevis, which is innervated by the deep fibular nerve. The first two dorsal interossei also may receive part of their innervation from the deep fibular nerve.

First layer

There are three components in the first layer of muscles, which is the most superficial of the four layers in the sole of the foot and is immediately deep to the plantar aponeurosis (Table 6.11, Fig. 6.101). From medial to lateral, these muscles are the **abductor hallucis, flexor digitorum brevis,** and **abductor digiti minimi.**

Second layer

The second muscle layer in the sole of the foot is associated with the tendons of the flexor digitorum longus muscle, which pass through this layer, and consists of the **quadratus plantae** and **four lumbrical muscles** (Table 6.12, Fig. 6.102).

Third layer

There are three muscles in the third layer in the sole of the foot (Table 6.13, Fig. 6.103):

Fig. 6.99 Extensor hoods, right foot.

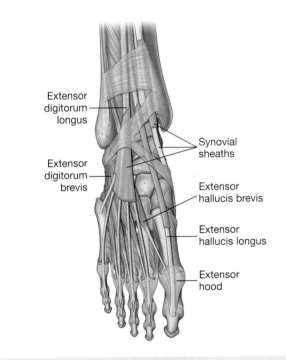

Fig. 6.100 Extensor digitorum brevis muscle, right foot.

Table 6.10 Muscle of the dorsal aspect of the foot (spinal segments in **bold** are the major segments innervating the muscle)

Muscle	Origin	Insertion	Innervation	Function
Extensor hallucis brevis and extensor digitorum brevis	Superolateral surface of the calcaneus	Base of proximal phalanx of great toe and lateral sides of the tendons of extensor digitorum longus of toes II to IV	Deep fibular nerve (**S1, S2**)	Extension of metatarsophalangeal joint of great toe and extension of toes II to IV

Table 6.11   First layer of muscles in the sole of the foot (spinal segments in **bold** are the major segments innervating the muscle)

Muscle	Origin	Insertion	Innervation	Function
Abductor hallucis	Medial process of calcaneal tuberosity	Medial side of base of proximal phalanx of great toe	Medial plantar nerve from the tibial nerve (**S1**, **S2**, **S3**)	Abducts and flexes great toe at metatarsophalangeal joint
Flexor digitorum brevis	Medial process of calcaneal tuberosity and plantar aponeurosis	Sides of plantar surface of middle phalanges of lateral four toes	Medial plantar nerve from the tibial nerve (**S1**, **S2**, **S3**)	Flexes lateral four toes at proximal interphalangeal joint
Abductor digiti minimi	Lateral and medial processes of calcaneal tuberosity and band of connective tissue connecting calcaneus with base of metatarsal V	Lateral side of base of proximal phalanx of little toe	Lateral plantar nerve from the tibial nerve (**S1**, **S2**, **S3**)	Abducts little toe at the metatarsophalangeal joint

Table 6.12   Second layer of muscles in the sole of the foot (spinal segments in **bold** are the major segments innervating the muscle)

Muscle	Origin	Insertion	Innervation	Function
Quadratus plantae	Medial surface of calcaneus and lateral process of calcaneal tuberosity	Lateral side of tendon of flexor digitorum longus in proximal sole of the foot	Lateral plantar nerve from tibial nerve (**S1**, **S2**, **S3**)	Assists flexor digitorum longus tendon in flexing toes II to V
Lumbricals	First lumbrical—medial side of tendon of flexor digitorum longus associated with toe II; second, third, and fourth lumbricals—adjacent surfaces of adjacent tendons of flexor digitorum longus	Medial free margins of extensor hoods of toes II to V	First lumbrical—medial plantar nerve from the tibial nerve; second, third, and fourth lumbricals—lateral plantar nerve from the tibial nerve (**S2**, **S3**)	Flexion of metatarsophalangeal joint and extension of interphalangeal joints; act through the extensor hoods to resist excessive extension of the metatarsophalangeal joints and flexion of the interphalangeal joints when the heel leaves the ground during walking

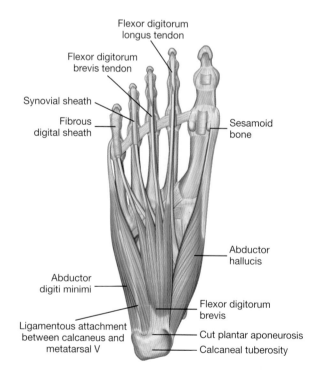

Fig. 6.101 First layer of muscles in the sole of the foot, right foot.

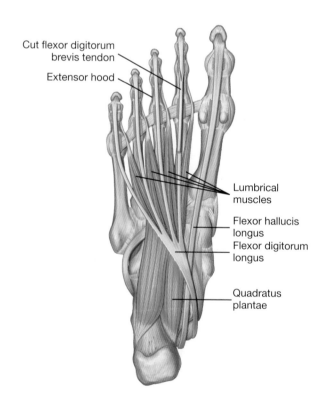

Fig. 6.102 Second layer of muscles in the sole of the foot, right foot.

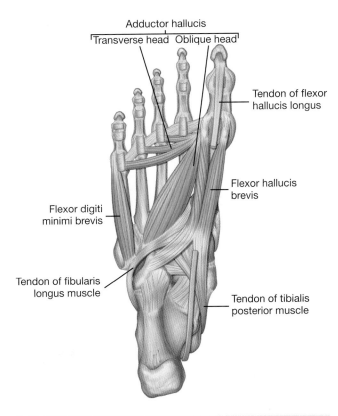

Adductor hallucis
Transverse head Oblique head
Tendon of flexor hallucis longus
Flexor hallucis brevis
Flexor digiti minimi brevis
Tendon of fibularis longus muscle
Tendon of tibialis posterior muscle

Fig. 6.103 Third layer of muscles in the sole of the foot, right foot.

Abduct (dorsal interossei)
Adduct (plantar interossei)
Deep transverse metatarsal ligaments
Plantar ligaments
Third plantar interosseus
First dorsal interosseous muscle

Fig. 6.104 Fourth layer of muscles in the sole of the foot, right foot.

- Two (the **flexor hallucis brevis** and **adductor hallucis**) are associated with the great toe.
- The third (the **flexor digiti minimi brevis**) is associated with the little toe.

Fourth layer

There are two muscle groups in the deepest muscle layer in the sole of the foot: the **dorsal** and **plantar interossei** (Table 6.14, Fig. 6.104).

Arteries

Blood supply to the foot is by branches of the posterior tibial and dorsalis pedis (dorsal artery of the foot) arteries.

Posterior tibial artery and plantar arch

The posterior tibial artery enters the foot through the tarsal tunnel on the medial side of the ankle and posterior to the medial malleolus. Here it bifurcates into a small medial plantar artery and a much larger lateral plantar artery (Fig. 6.105).

Lateral plantar artery

The **lateral plantar artery** passes anterolaterally into the sole of the foot, first deep to the proximal end of the abductor

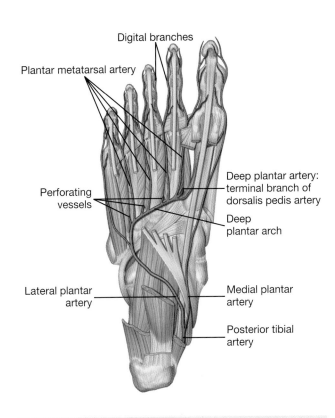

Digital branches
Plantar metatarsal artery
Perforating vessels
Deep plantar artery: terminal branch of dorsalis pedis artery
Deep plantar arch
Lateral plantar artery
Medial plantar artery
Posterior tibial artery

Fig. 6.105 Arteries in the sole of the foot, right foot.

357

Table 6.13 Third layer of muscles in the sole of the foot (spinal segments in **bold** are the major segments innervating the muscle)

Muscle	Origin	Insertion	Innervation	Function
Flexor hallucis brevis	Plantar surface of cuboid and lateral cuneiform; tendon of tibialis posterior	Lateral and medial sides of base of proximal phalanx of the great toe	Medial plantar nerve from tibial nerve (**S1**, S2)	Flexes metatarsophalangeal joint of the great toe
Adductor hallucis	Transverse head—ligaments associated with metatarsophalangeal joints of lateral three toes; oblique head—bases of metatarsals II to IV and from sheath covering fibularis longus	Lateral side of base of proximal phalanx of great toe	Lateral plantar nerve from tibial nerve (**S2, S3**)	Adducts great toe at metatarsophalangeal joint
Flexor digiti minimi brevis	Base of metatarsal V and related sheath of fibularis longus tendon	Lateral side of base of proximal phalanx of little toe	Lateral plantar nerve from tibial nerve (**S2, S3**)	Flexes little toe at metatarsophalangeal joint

Table 6.14 Fourth layer of muscles in the sole of the foot (spinal segments in **bold** are the major segments innervating the muscle)

Muscle	Origin	Insertion	Innervation	Function
Dorsal interossei	Sides of adjacent metatarsals	Extensor hoods and bases of proximal phalanges of toes II to IV	Lateral plantar nerve from tibial nerve; first and second dorsal interossei also innervated by deep fibular nerve (**S2, S3**)	Abduction of toes II to IV at metatarsophalangeal joints; act through the extensor hoods to resist extension of metatarsophalangeal joints and flexion of interphalangeal joints
Plantar interossei	Medial sides of metatarsals of toes III to V	Extensor hoods and bases of proximal phalanges of toes III to V	Lateral plantar nerve from tibial nerve (**S2, S3**)	Adduction of toes III to V at metatarsophalangeal joints; act through the extensor hoods to resist extension of the metatarsophalangeal joints and flexion of the interphalangeal joints

hallucis muscle and then between the quadratus plantae and flexor digitorum brevis muscles (Fig. 6.105). It reaches the base of metatarsal V where it lies in the groove between the flexor digitorum brevis and abductor digiti minimi muscles. From here, the lateral plantar artery curves medially to form the **deep plantar arch,** which crosses the deep plane of the sole on the metatarsal bases and the interossei muscles.

Between the bases of metatarsals I and II, the deep plantar arch joins with the terminal branch (deep plantar artery) of the dorsalis pedis artery, which enters the sole from the dorsal side of the foot.

Major branches of the deep plantar arch include:

- a digital branch to the lateral side of the little toe;
- four plantar metatarsal arteries, which supply digital branches to adjacent sides of toes I to V and the medial side of the great toe; and
- three perforating arteries, which pass between the bases of metatarsals II to V to anastomose with vessels on the dorsal aspect of the foot.

Medial plantar artery

The **medial plantar artery** passes into the sole of the foot by passing deep to the proximal end of the abductor hallucis muscle (Fig. 6.105). It supplies a deep branch to adjacent muscles and then passes forward in the groove between the

abductor hallucis and the flexor digitorum brevis muscles. It ends by joining the digital branch of the deep plantar arch, which supplies the medial side of the great toe.

Near the base of metatarsal I, the medial plantar artery gives rise to a superficial branch, which divides into three vessels that pass superficial to the flexor digitorum brevis muscle to join the plantar metatarsal arteries from the deep plantar arch.

Dorsalis pedis artery

The **dorsalis pedis artery** is the continuation of the anterior tibial artery and begins as the anterior tibial artery crosses the ankle joint (Fig. 6.106). It passes anteriorly over the dorsal aspect of the talus, navicular, and intermediate cuneiform bones and then passes inferiorly as the **deep plantar artery** between the two heads of the first dorsal interosseous muscle to join the deep plantar arch in the sole of the foot.

Branches of the dorsalis pedis artery include lateral and medial tarsal branches, an arcuate artery, and a first dorsal metatarsal artery (Fig. 6.106):

- The **tarsal arteries** pass medially and laterally over the tarsal bones, supplying adjacent structures and anastomosing with a network of vessels formed around the ankle.
- The **arcuate artery** passes laterally over the dorsal aspect of the metatarsals near their bases and gives rise to three

Fig. 6.106 Dorsalis pedis artery, right foot.

Labels (figure left):
- Anterior tibial artery
- Anterior medial malleolar artery
- Anterior lateral malleolar artery
- Medial and lateral tarsal branches
- Dorsalis pedis artery
- Arcuate artery
- Extensor hallucis longus
- First dorsal metatarsal artery
- Tendon of extensor digitorum longus to toe II
- Deep plantar artery
- First dorsal interosseous muscle
- Extensor hood
- Dorsal digital arteries

It is palpable in this position. The terminal branch of the dorsalis pedis artery passes into the plantar surface of the foot between the two heads of the first dorsal interosseous muscle.

Fig. 6.107 Finding the dorsalis pedis artery, right foot.

Labels (figure right):
- Extensor hallucis longus tendon
- Dorsalis pedis artery
- Extensor digitorum longus tendon to second toe

dorsal metatarsal arteries that supply **dorsal digital arteries** to adjacent sides of digits II to V and to a dorsal digital artery that supplies the lateral side of digit V.

- The **first dorsal metatarsal artery** (the last branch of the dorsalis pedis artery before the dorsalis pedis artery continues as the deep plantar artery into the sole of the foot) supplies dorsal digital branches to adjacent sides of the great and second toes.

The dorsal metatarsal arteries connect with perforating branches from the deep plantar arch and similar branches from the plantar metatarsal arteries.

Surface anatomy

Finding the dorsalis pedis artery

The nature of the dorsalis pedis pulse (Fig. 6.107) is important for assessing peripheral circulation because the dorsalis pedis artery is the farthest palpable vessel from the heart. Also, it is the lowest palpable artery in the body when a person is standing.

The dorsalis pedis artery passes onto the dorsal aspect of the foot and anteriorly over the tarsal bones where it lies between and is parallel to the tendon of the extensor hallucis longus and the tendon of the extensor digitorum longus to the second toe.

Veins

There are interconnected networks of deep and superficial veins in the foot. The deep veins follow the arteries. Superficial veins drain into a dorsal venous arch on the dorsal surface of the foot over the metatarsals (Fig. 6.108):

- The **great saphenous vein** originates from the medial side of the arch and passes anterior to the medial malleolus and onto the medial side of the leg.
- The **small saphenous vein** originates from the lateral side of the arch and passes posterior to the lateral malleolus and onto the back of the leg.

Nerves

The foot is supplied by the tibial, deep fibular, superficial fibular, sural, and saphenous nerves:

- All five nerves contribute to cutaneous or general sensory innervation.
- The tibial nerve innervates all intrinsic muscles of the foot except for the extensor digitorum brevis, which is innervated by the deep fibular nerve.

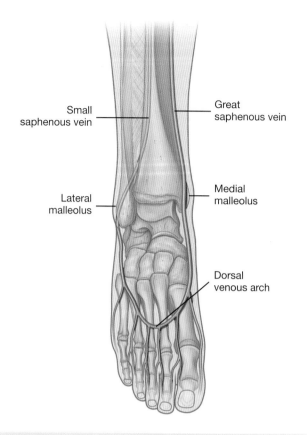

Small
saphenous vein

Great
saphenous vein

Lateral
malleolus

Medial
malleolus

Dorsal
venous arch

Fig. 6.108 Superficial veins of the foot, right foot.

- The deep fibular nerve often also contributes to the innervation of the first and second dorsal interossei.

Tibial nerve

The **tibial nerve** enters the foot through the tarsal tunnel posterior to the medial malleolus. In the tunnel, the nerve is lateral to the posterior tibial artery and gives origin to **medial calcaneal branches,** which penetrate the flexor retinaculum to supply the heel. Midway between the medial malleolus and the heel, the tibial nerve bifurcates with the posterior tibial artery into (Fig. 6.109):

- a large medial plantar nerve, and
- a smaller lateral plantar nerve.

The medial and lateral plantar nerves lie together between their corresponding arteries.

Medial plantar nerve

The **medial plantar nerve** is the major sensory nerve in the sole of the foot (Fig. 6.109B). It innervates skin on most of the anterior two-thirds of the sole and adjacent surfaces of the medial three and one-half toes, which includes the great toe. In addition to this large area of plantar skin, the nerve also innervates four intrinsic muscles—the abductor hallucis, flexor digitorum brevis, flexor hallucis brevis, and the first lumbrical.

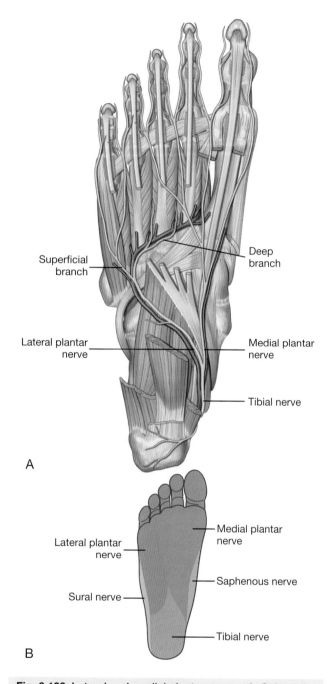

Superficial
branch

Deep
branch

Lateral plantar
nerve

Medial plantar
nerve

Tibial nerve

A

Medial plantar
nerve

Lateral plantar
nerve

Saphenous nerve

Sural nerve

Tibial nerve

B

Fig. 6.109 Lateral and medial plantar nerves. **A.** Sole of the right foot. **B.** Cutaneous distribution.

The medial plantar nerve passes into the sole of the foot deep to the abductor hallucis muscle and forward in the groove between the abductor hallucis and flexor digitorum brevis, supplying branches to both these muscles.

The medial plantar nerve supplies a digital branch (**proper plantar digital nerve**) to the medial side of the great toe and then divides into three nerves (**common plantar digital nerves**) on the plantar surface of the flexor digitorum brevis, which continue forward to supply proper plantar digital branches to adjacent surfaces of toes I to IV. The nerve to the first lumbrical originates from the first common plantar digital nerve.

Lateral plantar nerve

The **lateral plantar nerve** is an important motor nerve in the foot because it innervates all intrinsic muscles in the sole except for the muscles supplied by the medial plantar nerve (the abductor hallucis, flexor digitorum brevis, flexor hallucis brevis, and first lumbrical; Fig. 6.109). It also innervates a strip of skin on the lateral side of the anterior two-thirds of the sole and the adjacent plantar surfaces of the lateral one and one-half digits.

The lateral plantar nerve enters the sole of the foot by passing deep to the proximal attachment of the abductor hallucis muscle. It continues laterally and anteriorly across the sole between the flexor digitorum brevis and quadratus plantae muscles, supplying branches to both these muscles, and then divides near the head of metatarsal V into a deep and superficial branch (Fig. 6.109).

The **superficial branch** of the lateral plantar nerve gives rise to a **proper plantar digital nerve,** which supplies skin on the lateral side of the little toe and to a **common plantar digital nerve,** which divides to supply proper plantar digital nerves to skin on the adjacent sides of toes IV and V.

The proper plantar digital nerve to the lateral side of the little toe also innervates the flexor digiti minimi brevis and the dorsal and plantar interossei muscles between metatarsals IV and V.

The **deep branch** of the lateral plantar nerve is motor and accompanies the lateral plantar artery deep to the long flexor tendons and the adductor hallucis muscle. It supplies branches to the second to fourth lumbrical muscles, the adductor hallucis muscle, and all interossei except those between metatarsals IV and V, which are innervated by the superficial branch.

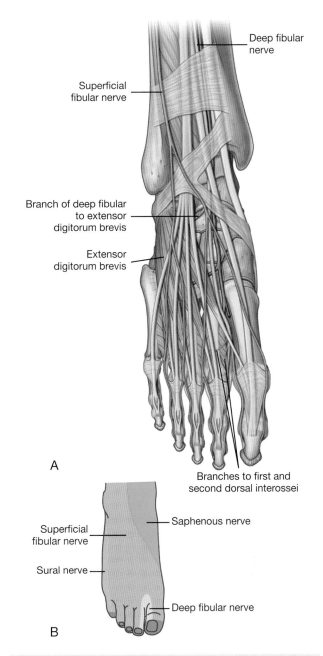

A

B

Fig. 6.110 A. Terminal branches of superficial and deep fibular nerves in the right foot. **B.** Cutaneous distribution.

Deep fibular nerve

The **deep fibular nerve** innervates the extensor digitorum brevis, contributes to the innervation of the first two dorsal interossei muscles, and supplies general sensory branches to the skin on the adjacent dorsal sides of the first and second toes and to the web space between them (Fig. 6.110).

The deep fibular nerve enters the dorsal aspect of the foot on the lateral side of the dorsalis pedis artery and is parallel with and lateral to the tendon of the extensor hallucis longus muscle. Just distal to the ankle joint, the nerve gives origin to a lateral branch, which innervates the extensor digitorum brevis from its deep surface.

The deep fibular nerve continues forward on the dorsal surface of the foot, penetrates deep fascia between metatarsals I and II near the metatarsophalangeal joints, and then divides into two **dorsal digital nerves,** which supply skin over adjacent surfaces of toes I and II down to the beginning of the nail beds (Fig. 6.110).

Small motor branches that contribute to the supply of the first two dorsal interossei muscles originate from the deep fibular nerve before it penetrates deep fascia.

Superficial fibular nerve

The **superficial fibular nerve** is sensory to most skin on the dorsal aspect of the foot and toes except for skin on adjacent sides of toes I and II (which is innervated by the deep fibular nerve) and skin on the lateral side of the foot and little toe (which is innervated by the sural nerve; Fig. 6.110).

The superficial fibular nerve penetrates deep fascia on the anterolateral side of the lower leg and enters the dorsal aspect of the foot in superficial fascia. It gives rise to cutaneous branches and **dorsal digital nerves** along its course.

Sural nerve

The sural nerve is a cutaneous branch of the tibial nerve that originates high in the leg. It enters the foot in superficial fascia posterior to the lateral malleolus close to the short saphenous vein. Terminal branches innervate skin on the lateral side of the foot and dorsolateral surface of the little toe (Fig. 6.110B).

Saphenous nerve

The saphenous nerve is a cutaneous branch of the femoral nerve that originates in the thigh. Terminal branches enter the foot in superficial fascia on the medial side of the ankle and supply skin on the medial side of the proximal foot (Fig. 6.110B).

Clinical app

Dermatomes and myotomes in the lower limb

General sensory and somatic motor innervation of the lower limb is by peripheral nerves emanating from the lumbar and sacral plexuses on the posterior abdominal and pelvic walls. These plexuses are formed by the anterior rami of L1 to L3 and most of L4 (lumbar plexus) and L4 to S5 (sacral plexus).

Nerves originating from the lumbar and sacral plexuses and entering the lower limb carry fibers from spinal cord levels L1 to S3. As a consequence of this innervation, lumbar and upper sacral nerves are tested clinically by examining the lower limb. In addition, clinical signs (such as pain, pins and needles, paresthesia, and fascicular muscle twitching) resulting from any disorder affecting these spinal nerves (e.g., herniated intervertebral disc in the lumbar region) appear in the lower limb.

Dermatomes

Dermatomes in the lower limb are shown in Fig. 6.111. Regions that can be tested for sensation and are reasonably autonomous (have minimal overlap) are:

- over the inguinal ligament—L1
- lateral side of the thigh—L2
- lower medial side of the thigh—L3
- medial side of the great toe (digit I)—L4
- medial side of digit II—L5
- little toe (digit V)—S1
- back of the thigh—S2
- skin over the gluteal fold—S3

Fig. 6.111 Dermatomes of the lower limb. Dots indicate autonomous zones (i.e., with minimal overlap).

Clinical app—cont'd

Myotomes

Selected joint movements are used to test myotomes (Fig. 6.112). For example:

- Flexion of the hip is controlled primarily by L1 and L2.
- Extension of the knee is controlled mainly by L3 and L4.
- Knee flexion is controlled mainly by L5 to S2.
- Plantarflexion of the foot is controlled predominantly by S1 and S2.
- Adduction of the digits is controlled by S2 and S3.

Fig. 6.112 Movements generated by myotomes.

Clinical app

Testing sensory innervation carried by major peripheral nerves in the lower limb

In addition to innervating major muscle groups, each of the major peripheral nerves originating from the lumbar and sacral plexuses carries general sensory information from patches of skin (Fig. 6.113). Sensation from these areas can be used to test for peripheral nerve lesions:

- The femoral nerve innervates skin on the anterior thigh, medial side of the leg, and medial side of the ankle.
- The obturator nerve innervates the medial side of the thigh.
- The tibial part of the sciatic nerve innervates the lateral side of the ankle and foot.
- The common fibular nerve innervates the lateral side of the leg and the dorsum of the foot.

Fig. 6.113 Regions of skin innervated by peripheral nerves.

363

Tendon taps in the lower limb

In an unconscious patient, both somatic sensory and somatic motor functions of spinal cord levels can be tested using tendon reflexes:

- A tap on the patellar ligament at the knee tests predominantly L3 and L4.
- A tendon tap on the calcaneal tendon posterior to the ankle (tendon of gastrocnemius and soleus) tests S1 and S2.

Gait and gait defects

The body's center of gravity lies just anterior to the anterior edge of the SII vertebra in the pelvis. During walking, many anatomical features of the lower limbs contribute to minimizing fluctuations in the body's center of gravity and thereby reduce the amount of energy needed to maintain locomotion and produce a smooth, efficient gait (Fig. 6.114). They include pelvic tilt in the coronal plane, pelvic rotation in the transverse plane, movement of the knees toward the midline, flexion of the knees, and complex interactions between the hip, knee, and ankle. As a result, during walking, the body's center of gravity normally fluctuates only 5 cm in both vertical and lateral directions.

Any pathology that alters the determinants of gait changes the gait pattern and increases the amount of energy required to walk.

Fig. 6.114 Some of the determinants of gait.

Surface anatomy

Pulse points

Peripheral pulses can be felt at four locations in the lower limb (Fig. 6.115):

- **femoral pulse** in the femoral triangle—femoral artery inferior to the inguinal ligament and midway between the anterior superior iliac spine and the pubic symphysis
- **popliteal pulse** in the popliteal fossa—popliteal artery deep in the popliteal fossa medial to the midline

- **posterior tibial pulse** in the tarsal tunnel—posterior tibial artery posteroinferior to the medial malleolus in the groove between the medial malleolus and the heel (calcaneal tuberosity)
- **dorsalis pedis pulse** on the dorsal aspect of the foot—dorsalis pedis artery as it passes distally over the tarsal bones between the tendon of the extensor hallucis longus and the tendon of the extensor digitorum longus to the second toe

Femoral pulse

Popliteal pulse

Posterior tibial pulse

Dorsalis pedis pulse

Fig. 6.115 Where to feel peripheral arterial pulses in the lower limb.

7
Upper Limb

Regional anatomy 368

Shoulder 370
Bones 370
Joints 372
Muscles 377
Posterior scapular region 379
Gateways to the posterior scapular region 379
Nerves 380
Arteries and veins 381

Axilla 381
Axillary inlet 382
Anterior wall 382
Medial wall 383
Lateral wall 384
Posterior wall 384
Gateways in the posterior wall 386
Floor 386
Contents of the axilla 386
Arm 398
Bones 398
Muscles 401
Nerves 401
Arteries and veins 403
Elbow joint 405
Cubital fossa 408
Forearm 410
Bones 410
Joints 412
Anterior compartment of the forearm 414
Muscles 414
Arteries and veins 414
Nerves 417
Posterior compartment of the forearm 418
Muscles 418
Arteries and veins 418
Nerves 421
Hand 422
Bones 423
Joints 425
Carpal tunnel and structures at the wrist 426
Palmar aponeurosis 427
Anatomical snuffbox 428
Fibrous digital sheaths 429
Extensor hoods 429
Muscles 430
Arteries and veins 432
Nerves 435

Regional anatomy

Based on the position of its major joints, the upper limb is divided into the shoulder, arm, forearm, and hand (Fig. 7.1):

- The shoulder is the area of upper limb attachment to the trunk. The bones of the shoulder include the scapula, clavicle, and proximal end of the humerus.
- The arm is between the shoulder and the elbow joint. the bone of the arm is the humerus.
- The forearm is between the elbow joint and the wrist joint. The bones of the forearm are the ulna and radius.
- The hand is distal to the wrist joint. Bones of the hand are the carpals, metacarpals, and phalanges.

The major function of the upper limb is to position the hand in space for use as a mechanical and sensory tool.

Unlike the lower limb, which is used for support, stability, and locomotion, the upper limb is designed to be flexible. The shoulder is suspended from the trunk predominantly by muscles and can therefore be moved relative to the body. Sliding (protraction and retraction) and rotating the scapula on the thoracic wall changes the position of the **glenohumeral joint (shoulder joint)** and extends the reach of the hand (Fig. 7.2). The glenohumeral joint allows the arm to move around three axes with a wide range of motion. Movements of the arm at this joint are flexion, extension, abduction, adduction, medial rotation (internal rotation), lateral rotation (external rotation), and circumduction (Fig. 7.3).

The major movements at the **elbow joint** are flexion and extension of the forearm (Fig. 7.4A). At the other end of the forearm, the distal end of the lateral bone, the radius, can be flipped over the adjacent head of the medial bone, the ulna. Because the hand is articulated with the radius, it can be efficiently moved from a palm-anterior position to a palm-posterior position simply by crossing the distal end of the radius over the ulna (Fig. 7.4B). This movement, termed *pronation,* occurs solely in the forearm. Supination returns the hand to the anatomical position.

At the **wrist joint,** the hand can be abducted, adducted, flexed, extended, and circumducted (Fig. 7.5). These movements, combined with those of the shoulder, arm, and forearm, enable the hand to be placed in a wide range of positions relative to the body.

The thumb is positioned at right angles to the orientation of the index, middle, ring, and little fingers (Fig. 7.6 As a result, movements of the thumb occur at right angles to those of the other digits. For example, flexion brings the thumb across the palm, whereas abduction moves it away from the fingers at right angles to the palm (Fig. 7.6A,B).

Importantly, with the thumb positioned at right angles to the palm. Only a slight rotation of the thumb brings it into a position directly facing the other fingers (Fig. 7.6C). This opposition of the thumb is essential for normal hand function.

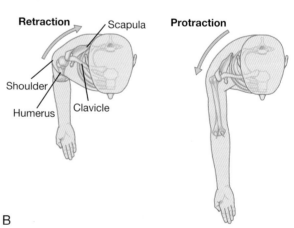

Fig. 7.2 Movements of the scapula. **A.** Rotation. **B.** Protraction and retraction.

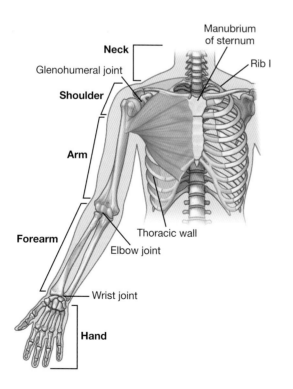

Fig. 7.1 Anterior view of the upper limb.

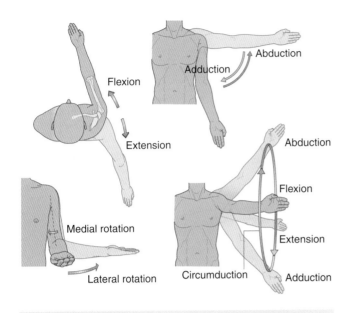

Fig. 7.3 Movements of the arm at the glenohumeral joint.

A

B **Palm anterior** **Palm posterior** **Palm anterior**

Fig. 7.4 Movements of the forearm. **A.** Flexion and extension at the elbow joint. **B.** Pronation and supination.

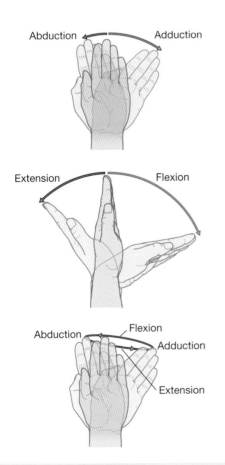

Fig. 7.5 Movements of the hand at the wrist joint.

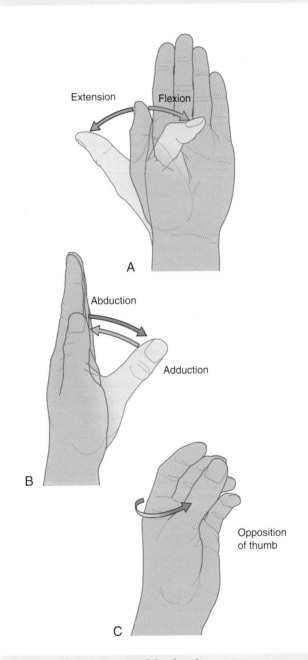

Fig. 7.6 A-C. Movements of the thumb.

SHOULDER

The bone framework of the shoulder consists of:

- the clavicle and scapula, which form the **pectoral girdle (shoulder girdle),** and
- the proximal end of the humerus.

The superficial muscles of the shoulder consist of the trapezius and deltoid muscles, which together form the smooth muscular contour over the lateral part of the shoulder. These muscles connect the scapula and clavicle to the trunk and to the arm, respectively.

Bones

Clavicle

The clavicle is the only bony attachment between the trunk and the upper limb. It is palpable along its entire length and has a gentle S-shaped contour with the forward-facing convex part medial and the forward-facing concave part lateral. The acromial (lateral) end of the clavicle is flat, whereas the sternal (medial) end is more robust and somewhat quadrangular (Fig. 7.7).

The acromial end of the clavicle has a small oval facet on its surface for articulation with a similar facet on the medial surface of the acromion of the scapula.

The sternal end has a much larger facet for articulation mainly with the manubrium of the sternum and, to a lesser extent, with the first costal cartilage.

The inferior surface of the lateral third of the clavicle possesses a distinct tuberosity consisting of a tubercle (the **conoid tubercle**) and lateral roughening (the **trapezoid line**) for attachment of the important coracoclavicular ligament.

In addition, the surfaces and margins of the clavicle are roughened by the attachment of muscles that connect the clavicle to the thorax, neck, and upper limb. The superior surface is smoother than the inferior surface.

Scapula

The scapula is a large, flat triangular bone with (Fig. 7.8):

- three angles (lateral, superior, and inferior);
- three borders (superior, lateral, and medial);
- two surfaces (costal and posterior); and
- three processes (acromion, spine, and coracoid process)

The **lateral angle** of the scapula is marked by a shallow, somewhat comma-shaped **glenoid cavity** that articulates with the head of the humerus to form the glenohumeral joint (Fig. 7.8B,C).

A large triangular-shaped roughening (the **infraglenoid tubercle**) inferior to the glenoid cavity is the site of attachment for the long head of the triceps brachii muscle (Fig. 7.8B,C).

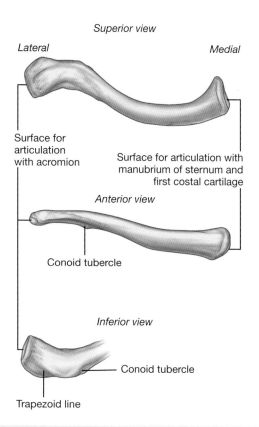

Superior view

Lateral   *Medial*

Surface for articulation with acromion

Surface for articulation with manubrium of sternum and first costal cartilage

Anterior view

Conoid tubercle

Inferior view

Conoid tubercle

Trapezoid line

Fig. 7.7 Right clavicle.

A less distinct **supraglenoid tubercle** is located superior to the glenoid cavity and is the site of attachment for the long head of the biceps brachii muscle (Fig. 7.8C).

A prominent spine subdivides the posterior surface of the scapula into a small, superior **supraspinous fossa** and a much larger, inferior **infraspinous fossa** (Fig. 7.8A).

The **acromion,** which is an anterolateral projection of the spine, arches over the glenohumeral joint and articulates, via a small oval facet on its distal end, with the clavicle (Fig. 7.8B).

The region between the lateral angle of the scapula and the attachment of the spine to the posterior surface of the scapula is the **greater scapular notch (spinoglenoid notch)** (Fig. 7.8A).

Unlike the posterior surface, the **costal surface** of the scapula is unremarkable, being characterized by a shallow concave **subscapular fossa** over much of its extent (Fig. 7.8B). The costal surface and margins provide for muscle attachment, and the costal surface, together with its related muscle **(subscapularis),** moves freely over the underlying thoracic wall.

The lateral border of the scapula is strong and thick for muscle attachment, whereas the medial border and much of the superior border is thin and sharp.

The superior border is marked on its lateral end by:

- the **coracoid process** (Fig. 7.8B,C), a hook-like structure that projects anterolaterally and is positioned directly inferior to the lateral part of the clavicle; and

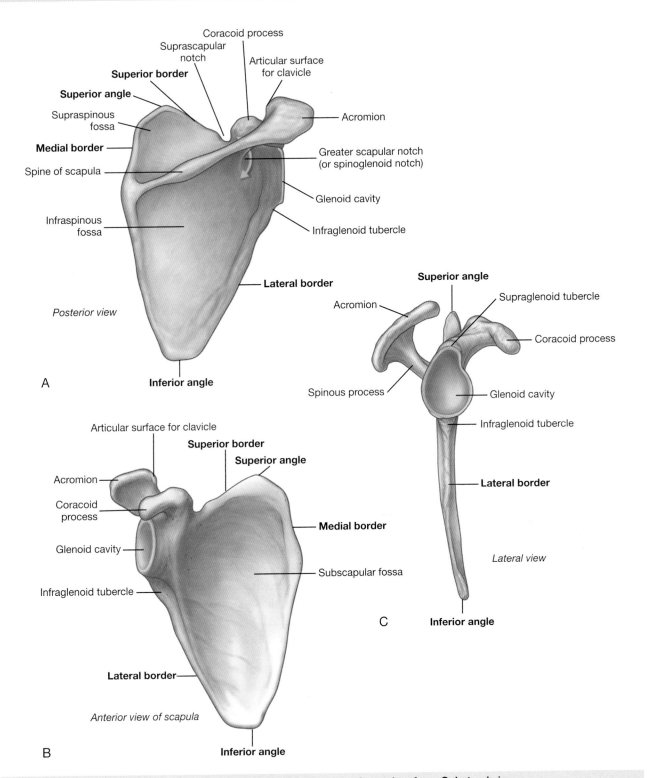

Fig. 7.8 Scapula. **A.** Posterior view of right scapula. **B.** Anterior view of costal surface. **C.** Lateral view.

- the small but distinct **suprascapular notch** (Fig. 7.8A), which lies immediately medial to the root of the coracoid process.

The spine and acromion can be readily palpated on a patient, as can the tip of the coracoid process, the inferior angle, and much of the medial border of the scapula.

Proximal humerus

The proximal end of the humerus consists of the head, the anatomical neck, the greater and lesser tubercles, the surgical neck, and the superior half of the shaft of humerus (Fig. 7.9).

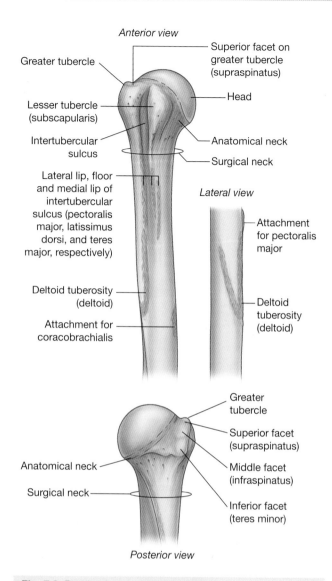

Anterior view

Greater tubercle

Superior facet on greater tubercle (supraspinatus)

Lesser tubercle (subscapularis)

Head

Intertubercular sulcus

Anatomical neck

Surgical neck

Lateral lip, floor and medial lip of intertubercular sulcus (pectoralis major, latissimus dorsi, and teres major, respectively)

Lateral view

Attachment for pectoralis major

Deltoid tuberosity (deltoid)

Deltoid tuberosity (deltoid)

Attachment for coracobrachialis

Greater tubercle

Superior facet (supraspinatus)

Anatomical neck

Middle facet (infraspinatus)

Surgical neck

Inferior facet (teres minor)

Posterior view

Fig. 7.9 Proximal end of right humerus.

The **head** is half-spherical and projects medially and somewhat superiorly to articulate with the much smaller glenoid cavity of the scapula.

The **anatomical neck** is very short and is formed by a narrow constriction immediately distal to the head. It lies between the head and the greater and lesser tubercles laterally and between the head and the shaft more medially.

Greater and lesser tubercles

The **greater** and **lesser tubercles** are prominent landmarks on the proximal end of the humerus and serve as attachment sites for the four rotator cuff muscles of the glenohumeral joint (Fig. 7.9).

The greater tubercle is lateral in position. Its superior surface and posterior surface are marked by three large smooth facets for muscle tendon attachment (Fig. 7.9):

- The superior facet is for attachment of the supraspinatus muscle.
- The middle facet is for attachment of infraspinatus.
- The inferior facet is for attachment of teres minor.

The lesser tubercle is anterior in position, and its surface is marked by a large smooth impression for attachment of the subscapularis muscle.

A deep **intertubercular sulcus (bicipital groove)** separates the lesser and greater tubercles and continues inferiorly onto the proximal shaft of the humerus (Fig. 7.9). The tendon of the long head of the biceps brachii passes through this sulcus.

Roughenings on the lateral and medial lips and on the floor of the intertubercular sulcus mark sites for the attachment of the pectoralis major, teres major, and latissimus dorsi muscles, respectively.

The lateral lip of the intertubercular sulcus is continuous inferiorly with a large V-shaped **deltoid tuberosity** on the lateral surface of the humerus midway along its length (Fig. 7.9), which is where the deltoid muscle inserts onto the humerus.

In approximately the same position but on the medial surface of the bone there is a thin vertical roughening for attachment of the coracobrachialis muscle.

Surgical neck

One of the most important features of the proximal end of the humerus is the **surgical neck** (Fig. 7.9). This region is oriented in the horizontal plane between the expanded proximal part of the humerus (head, anatomical neck, and tubercles) and the narrower shaft. The axillary nerve and the posterior circumflex humeral artery, which pass into the deltoid region from the axilla, do so immediately posterior to the surgical neck. Because the surgical neck is weaker than more proximal regions of the bone, it is one of the sites where the humerus commonly fractures.

Clinical app

Fracture of the proximal humerus

Typically, fractures occur around the surgical neck of the humerus. Although the axillary nerve and posterior circumflex humeral artery may be damaged with this type of fracture, this rarely happens. However, it is important that the axillary nerve is tested to be sure that the injury has not damaged the nerve and that the treatment itself does not cause a neurologic deficit.

Joints

The three joints in the shoulder complex are the sternoclavicular, acromioclavicular, and glenohumeral joints.

The sternoclavicular joint and the acromioclavicular joint link the two bones of the pectoral girdle to each other and to

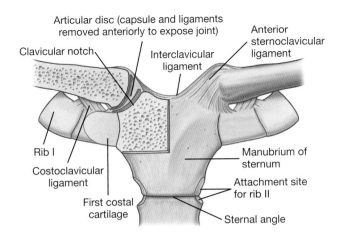

Articular disc (capsule and ligaments removed anteriorly to expose joint)

Anterior sternoclavicular ligament

Clavicular notch

Interclavicular ligament

Rib I

Costoclavicular ligament

First costal cartilage

Manubrium of sternum

Attachment site for rib II

Sternal angle

Fig. 7.10 Sternoclavicular joint.

the trunk. The combined movements at these two joints enable the scapula to be positioned over a wide range on the thoracic wall, substantially increasing "reach" by the upper limb.

The glenohumeral joint (shoulder joint) is the articulation between the humerus of the arm and the scapula.

Sternoclavicular joint

The **sternoclavicular joint** occurs between the proximal end of the clavicle and the **clavicular notch** of the **manubrium of sternum** together with a small part of the first costal cartilage (Figs. 7.10, 7.11). It is synovial and saddle-shaped. The articular cavity is completely separated into two compartments by an articular disc. The sternoclavicular joint allows movement of the clavicle, predominantly in the anteroposterior and vertical planes, although some rotation also occurs.

The sternoclavicular joint is surrounded by a joint capsule and is reinforced by four ligaments (Fig. 7.10):

- The **anterior and posterior sternoclavicular ligaments** are anterior and posterior, respectively, to the joint.
- An **interclavicular ligament** links the ends of the two clavicles to each other and to the superior surface of the manubrium of sternum.
- The **costoclavicular ligament** is positioned laterally to the joint and links the proximal end of the clavicle to the first rib and related costal cartilage.

Acromioclavicular joint

The **acromioclavicular joint** is a small synovial joint between an oval facet on the medial surface of the acromion and a similar facet on the acromial end of the clavicle (Figs. 7.12, 7.13). It allows movement in the anteroposterior and vertical planes together with some axial rotation.

The acromioclavicular joint is surrounded by a joint capsule and is reinforced by (Fig. 7.12):

- a small **acromioclavicular ligament** superior to the joint and passing between adjacent regions of the clavicle and acromion; and
- a much larger **coracoclavicular ligament,** which is not directly related to the joint but is an important strong accessory ligament, providing much of the weight-bearing support for the upper limb on the clavicle and maintaining the position of the clavicle on the acromion. It spans the distance between the coracoid process of the scapula and the inferior surface of the acromial end of the clavicle and comprises an anterior **trapezoid ligament** (which attaches to the trapezoid line on the clavicle) and a posterior **conoid ligament** (which attaches to the related conoid tubercle).

Glenohumeral joint

The **glenohumeral joint** is a synovial ball-and-socket articulation between the head of the humerus and the glenoid cavity of the scapula (Fig. 7.14; see Fig. 7.15). It is multiaxial with a wide range of movements provided at the cost of skeletal stability. Joint stability is provided instead by the rotator cuff muscles, the long head of the biceps brachii muscle, related bony processes, and extracapsular ligaments.

The articular surfaces of the glenohumeral joint are the large spherical head of the humerus and the small glenoid cavity of the scapula (Fig. 7.14).

The glenoid cavity is deepened and expanded peripherally by a fibrocartilaginous collar (the **glenoid labrum**), which attaches to the margin of the fossa (Fig. 7.14). Superiorly, this labrum is continuous with the tendon of the long head of the biceps brachii muscle, which attaches to the supraglenoid tubercle and passes through the articular cavity superior to the head of the humerus.

The synovial membrane attaches to the margins of the articular surfaces and lines the fibrous membrane of the

Imaging app

Visualizing the sternoclavicular joint

Vertebral body of TII   Left clavicle   Rib I

Sternal angle   Manubrium of sternum   Rib II

Fig. 7.11 Anterior view of normal sternoclavicular joints. Volume-rendered reconstruction using multidetector computed tomography.

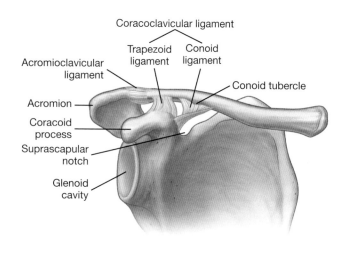

Fig. 7.12 Right acromioclavicular joint.

Imaging app

Visualizing the acromioclavicular joint

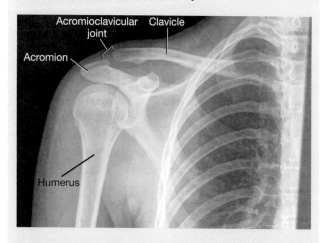

Fig. 7.13 Radiograph of a normal right acromioclavicular joint (anteroposterior view).

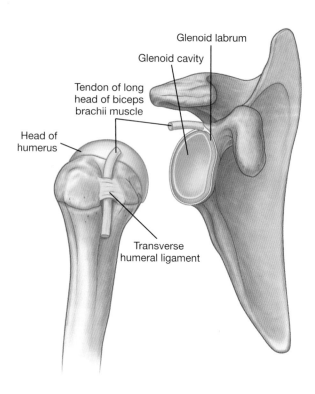

Fig. 7.14 Articular surfaces of right glenohumeral joint.

structures reduce friction between the tendons and adjacent joint capsule and bone.

In addition to bursae that communicate with the articular cavity through apertures in the fibrous membrane, other bursae are associated with the joint but are not connected to it. These occur:

- between the acromion (or deltoid muscle) and supraspinatus muscle (or joint capsule) (the **subacromial** or **subdeltoid bursa**) (Fig. 7.17);
- between the acromion and skin;
- between the coracoid process and the joint capsule; and
- in relationship to tendons of muscles around the joint (coracobrachialis, teres major, long head of triceps brachii, and latissimus dorsi muscles).

The fibrous membrane of the joint capsule attaches to the margin of the glenoid cavity outside the attachment of the glenoid labrum and the long head of the biceps brachii muscle and to the anatomical neck of the humerus (Fig. 7.18).

On the humerus, the medial attachment occurs more inferiorly than the neck and extends onto the shaft. In this region, the fibrous membrane is also loose or folded in the anatomical position. This redundant area of the fibrous membrane accommodates abduction of the arm.

Openings in the fibrous membrane provide continuity of the articular cavity with bursae that occur between the joint capsule and surrounding muscles and around the tendon of

joint capsule (Fig. 7.16). The synovial membrane is loose inferiorly. This redundant region of synovial membrane and related fibrous membrane accommodates abduction of the arm.

The synovial membrane protrudes through apertures in the fibrous membrane to form bursae, which lie between the tendons of surrounding muscles and the fibrous membrane. The most consistent of these is the **subtendinous bursa of the subscapularis** (Figs. 7.16, 7.17), which lies between the subscapularis muscle and the fibrous membrane. The synovial membrane also folds around the tendon of the long head of the biceps brachii muscle in the joint and extends along the tendon as it passes into the intertubercular sulcus (Figs. 7.16, 7.18). All these synovial

Imaging app

Visualizing the glenohumeral joint

Clavicle Glenoid cavity Acromion

Head of humerus

Fig. 7.15 Radiograph of a normal glenohumeral joint.

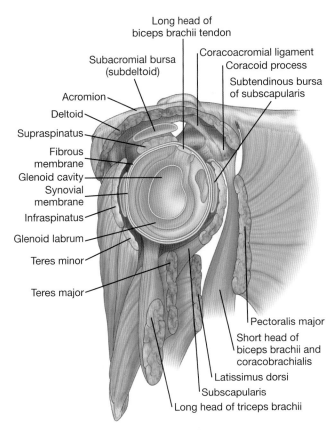

Long head of biceps brachii tendon
Subacromial bursa (subdeltoid)
Coracoacromial ligament
Coracoid process
Subtendinous bursa of subscapularis
Acromion
Deltoid
Supraspinatus
Fibrous membrane
Glenoid cavity
Synovial membrane
Infraspinatus
Glenoid labrum
Teres minor
Teres major
Pectoralis major
Short head of biceps brachii and coracobrachialis
Latissimus dorsi
Subscapularis
Long head of triceps brachii

Fig. 7.17 Lateral view of right glenohumeral joint and surrounding muscles with proximal end of humerus removed.

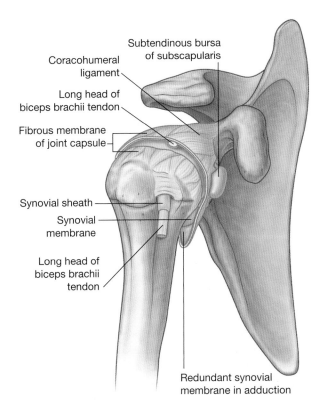

Coracohumeral ligament
Subtendinous bursa of subscapularis
Long head of biceps brachii tendon
Fibrous membrane of joint capsule
Synovial sheath
Synovial membrane
Long head of biceps brachii tendon
Redundant synovial membrane in adduction

Fig. 7.16 Synovial membrane and joint capsule of right glenohumeral joint.

the long head of the biceps brachii muscle in the intertubercular sulcus.

The fibrous membrane of the joint capsule is thickened (Fig. 7.18):

- anterosuperiorly in three locations to form **superior, middle, and inferior glenohumeral ligaments,** which pass from the superomedial margin of the glenoid cavity to the lesser tubercle and inferiorly related anatomical neck of the humerus;
- superiorly between the base of the coracoid process and the greater tubercle of the humerus (the **coracohumeral ligament;** and
- between the greater and lesser tubercles of the humerus **(transverse humeral ligament)**—this holds the tendon of the long head of the biceps brachii muscle in the intertubercular sulcus.

Joint stability is provided by surrounding muscle tendons and a skeletal arch formed superiorly by the coracoid process and acromion and the coracoacromial ligament (Figs. 7.17 and 7.19).

Tendons of the rotator cuff muscles (the supraspinatus, infraspinatus, teres minor, and subscapularis muscles) blend with the joint capsule and form a musculotendinous collar

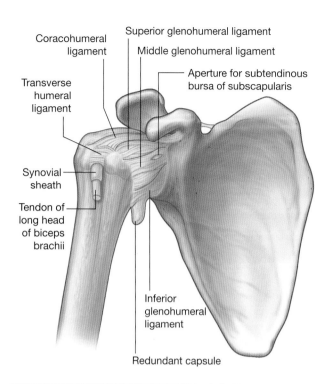

Coracohumeral ligament

Superior glenohumeral ligament

Middle glenohumeral ligament

Transverse humeral ligament

Aperture for subtendinous bursa of subscapularis

Synovial sheath

Tendon of long head of biceps brachii

Inferior glenohumeral ligament

Redundant capsule

Fig. 7.18 Capsule of right glenohumeral joint.

Imaging app

Visualizing the rotator cuff muscles

Infraspinatus

Supraspinatus

Acromion

Clavicle

Posterior

Anterior

Head of humerus

Coracoid process

Teres minor

Subscapularis

Fig. 7.19 Magnetic resonance image (T1-weighted) of a normal glenohumeral joint in the sagittal plane.

that surrounds the posterior, superior, and anterior aspects of the glenohumeral joint (see Figs. 7.17; 7.19). This cuff of muscles stabilizes and holds the head of the humerus in the glenoid cavity of the scapula without compromising the arm's flexibility and range of motion. The tendon of the long head of the biceps brachii muscle passes superiorly through the joint and restricts upward movement of the humeral head on the glenoid cavity.

Vascular supply to the glenohumeral joint is predominantly through branches of the anterior and posterior circumflex humeral and suprascapular arteries.

The glenohumeral joint is innervated by branches from the posterior cord of the brachial plexus and from the suprascapular, axillary, and lateral pectoral nerves.

Clinical app

Fractures of the clavicle and dislocations of the acromioclavicular and sternoclavicular joints

The clavicle is often fractured because of its small size and the large forces that it often transmits from the upper limb to the trunk. The typical site of fracture is the middle third (Fig. 7.20), proximal to the attachment of the coracoclavicular ligament.

The acromial end of the clavicle tends to dislocate at the acromioclavicular joint with trauma (Fig. 7.21). A minor injury tends to tear the fibrous joint capsule and ligaments of the

Fracture of clavicle

Acromioclavicular joint

Fig. 7.20 Radiograph showing an oblique fracture of the middle third of the right clavicle.

Acromion

Head of humerus

Clavicle

Fig. 7.21 Radiograph of dislocated right acromioclavicular joint (shoulder separation).

Clinical app—cont'd

acromioclavicular joint, resulting in acromioclavicular separation on a plain radiograph. More severe trauma will disrupt the conoid and trapezoid ligaments of the coracoclavicular ligament, which results in elevation and upward subluxation of the clavicle.

The typical injury at the medial end of the clavicle is an anterior or posterior dislocation of the sternoclavicular joint. Importantly, a posterior dislocation of the clavicle may impinge on the great vessels and compress or disrupt them.

Clinical app

Dislocations of the glenohumeral joint

The glenohumeral joint is extremely mobile, providing a wide range of movement at the expense of stability. The relatively small bony glenoid cavity, supplemented by the less robust fibrocartilaginous glenoid labrum and the ligamentous support, makes it susceptible to dislocation.

Anteroinferior dislocation (Fig. 7.22) occurs most frequently and is usually associated with an isolated traumatic incident (clinically, all anterior dislocations are anteroinferior). In some cases, the anteroinferior glenoid labrum is torn with or without a small bony fragment. Once the joint capsule and cartilage are disrupted, the joint is susceptible to further (recurrent) dislocations. When an anteroinferior dislocation occurs, the axillary nerve may be injured by direct compression of the humeral head on the nerve inferiorly as it passes through the quadrangular space. Furthermore, the "lengthening" effect of the humerus may stretch the radial nerve, which is tightly bound within the radial groove, and produce a radial nerve paralysis. Occasionally, an anteroinferior dislocation is associated with a fracture. Posterior dislocation is extremely rare.

Glenoid cavity

Acromion Clavicle

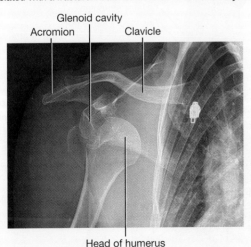

Head of humerus

Fig. 7.22 Radiograph showing an anteroinferior dislocation of the shoulder joint with an accompanying fracture of the greater tubercle and the glenoid rim.

Clinical app

Rotator cuff disorders

The two main disorders of the rotator cuff are impingement and tendinopathy. The muscle most commonly involved is supraspinatus as it passes beneath the acromion and the acromioclavicular ligament. This space, beneath which the supraspinatus tendon passes, is of fixed dimensions. Swelling of the supraspinatus muscle, excessive fluid within the subacromial/subdeltoid bursa, or subacromial bony spurs may produce significant impingement when the arm is abducted.

The blood supply to the supraspinatus tendon is relatively poor. Repeated trauma in certain circumstances makes the tendon susceptible to degenerative change, which may result in calcium deposition, producing extreme pain.

When the supraspinatus tendon has undergone significant degenerative change, it is further susceptible to trauma and partial- or full-thickness tears may develop (Fig. 7.23). These tears are most common in older patients and may result in considerable difficulty in carrying out normal activities of daily living such as combing hair. However, complete tears may be entirely asymptomatic.

Torn supraspinatus tendon

Humeral head

Fig. 7.23 Magnetic resonance image of a full-thickness tear of the supraspinatus tendon as it inserts onto the greater tubercle of the humerus.

Muscles

The two most superficial muscles of the shoulder are the **trapezius** and **deltoid** muscles (Table 7.1, Fig. 7.24). Together, they provide the characteristic contour of the shoulder:

- The trapezius attaches the scapula and clavicle to the trunk.
- The deltoid attaches the scapula and clavicle to the humerus.

Table 7.1 Muscles of the shoulder (spinal segments indicated in **bold** are the major segments innervating the muscle)

Muscle	Origin	Insertion	Innervation	Function
Trapezius	Superior nuchal line, external occipital protuberance, medial margin of the ligamentum nuchae, spinous processes of CVII to TXII and the related supraspinous ligaments	Superior edge of the crest of the spine of the scapula, acromion, posterior border of lateral one-third of clavicle	Motor accessory nerve Cranial nerve [XI]. Sensory (proprioception) anterior rami of C3 and C4	Powerful elevator of the scapula; rotates the scapula during abduction of humerus above horizontal; middle fibers retract scapula; lower fibers depress scapula
Deltoid	Inferior edge of the crest of the spine of the scapula, lateral margin of the acromion, anterior border of lateral one-third of clavicle	Deltoid tuberosity of humerus	Axillary nerve [**C5**, C6]	Major abductor of arm; clavicular fibers assist in flexing the arm; posterior fibers assist in extending the arm
Levator scapulae	Transverse processes of CI and CII vertebrae and posterior tubercles of transverse processes of CIII and CIV vertebrae	Posterior surface of medial border of scapula from superior angle to root of spine of the scapula	Branches directly from anterior rami of **C3** and **C4** spinal nerves and by branches [**C5**] from the dorsal scapular nerve	Elevates the scapula
Rhomboid minor	Lower end of ligamentum nuchae and spinous processes of CVII and TI vertebrae	Posterior surface of medial border of scapula at the root of the spine of the scapula	Dorsal scapular nerve [**C4, C5**]	Elevates and retracts the scapula
Rhomboid major	Spinous processes of TII–TV vertebrae and intervening supraspinous ligaments	Posterior surface of medial border of scapula from the root of the spine of the scapula to the inferior angle	Dorsal scapular nerve [**C4, C5**]	Elevates and retracts the scapula

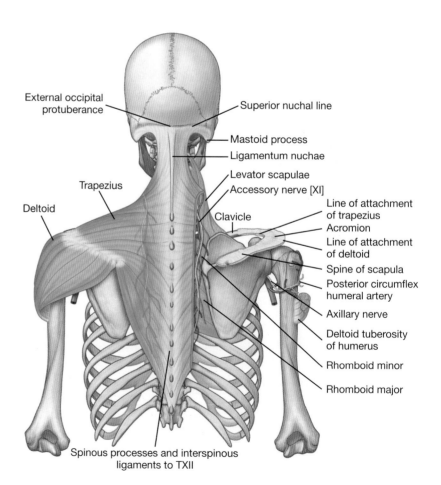

External occipital protuberance
Superior nuchal line
Mastoid process
Ligamentum nuchae
Levator scapulae
Accessory nerve [XI]
Trapezius
Deltoid
Clavicle
Line of attachment of trapezius
Acromion
Line of attachment of deltoid
Spine of scapula
Posterior circumflex humeral artery
Axillary nerve
Deltoid tuberosity of humerus
Rhomboid minor
Rhomboid major
Spinous processes and interspinous ligaments to TXII

Fig. 7.24 Attachment and neurovascular supply of the trapezius and deltoid muscles.

Table 7.2   Muscles of the posterior scapular region (spinal segments indicated in **bold** are the major segments innervating the muscle)

Muscle	Origin	Insertion	Innervation	Function
Supraspinatus	Medial two-thirds of the supraspinous fossa of the scapula and the deep fascia that covers the muscle	Most superior facet on the greater tubercle of the humerus	Suprascapular nerve [**C5**, C6]	**Rotator cuff muscle;** participates in abduction of the glenohumeral jont; stabilization of glenohumeral joint
Infraspinatus	Medial two-thirds of the infraspinous fossa of the scapula and the deep fascia that covers the muscle	Middle facet on posterior surface of the greater tubercle of the humerus	Suprascapular nerve [**C5**, C6]	**Rotator cuff muscle;** lateral rotation of arm at the glenohumeral joint; stabilization of glenohumeral joint
Teres minor	Upper two-thirds of a flattened strip of bone on the posterior surface of the scapula immediately adjacent to the lateral border of the scapula	Inferior facet on the posterior surface of the greater tubercle of the humerus	Axillary nerve [**C5**, C6]	**Rotator cuff muscle;** lateral rotation of arm at the glenohumeral joint; stabilization of glenohumeral joint
Teres major	Elongate oval area on the posterior surface of the inferior angle of the scapula	Medial lip of the intertubercular sulcus on the anterior surface of the humerus	Inferior subscapular nerve [**C5, C6, C7**]	Medial rotation and extension of the arm at the glenohumeral joint; stabilization of glenohumeral joint
Long head of triceps brachii	Infraglenoid tubercle on scapula	Common tendon of insertion with medial and lateral heads on the olecranon process of ulna	Radial nerve [C6, **C7, C8**]	Extension of the forearm at the elbow joint; accessory adductor and extensor of the arm at the glenohumeral joint

Both the trapezius and deltoid are attached to opposing surfaces and margins of the spine of the scapula, the acromion, and the clavicle, and these structures can be palpated between the attachments of trapezius and deltoid.

Deep to the trapezius the scapula is attached to the vertebral column by three muscles—the **levator scapulae, rhomboid minor,** and **rhomboid major** (Table 7.1, Fig. 7.24). These three muscles work with the trapezius (and with muscles found anteriorly) to position the scapula on the trunk.

POSTERIOR SCAPULAR REGION

The posterior scapular region occupies the posterior aspect of the scapula and is located deep to the trapezius and deltoid muscles. It contains four muscles that pass between the scapula and proximal end of the humerus: the **supraspinatus, infraspinatus, teres minor,** and **teres major** muscles (Table 7.2, Fig. 7.25).

The posterior scapular region also contains part of one additional muscle, the **long head of the triceps brachii,** which passes between the scapula and the proximal end of the forearm (Fig. 7.25). The importance of the triceps brachii in the posterior scapular region is that its vertical course between the teres minor and teres major together with these muscles and the humerus forms spaces through which nerves and vessels pass between regions.

The supraspinatus, infraspinatus, and teres minor muscles are three of the four components of the rotator cuff, which stabilizes the glenohumeral joint. The other component is **subscapularis** that is on the anterior aspect of the scapula.

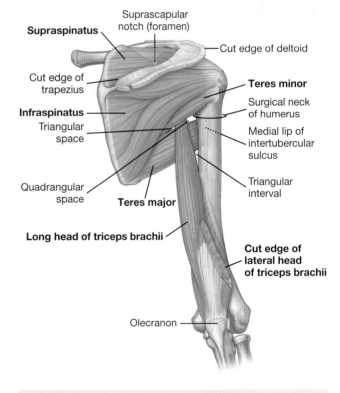

Fig. 7.25 Right posterior scapular region.

Gateways to the posterior scapular region

Suprascapular foramen

The **suprascapular foramen** is the route through which structures pass between the base of the neck and the posterior scapular region. It is formed by the suprascapular notch of the scapula and the **superior transverse scapular**

379

(suprascapular) ligament, which converts the notch into a foramen (Fig. 7.26).

The suprascapular nerve passes through the suprascapular foramen; the suprascapular artery and the suprascapular vein follow the same course as the nerve but normally pass immediately superior to the superior transverse scapular ligament and not through the foramen (Fig. 7.26).

Quadrangular space (from posterior)

The quadrangular space provides a passageway for nerves and vessels passing between more anterior regions (the axilla) and the posterior scapular region (Figs. 7.25, 7.26). In the posterior scapular region, its boundaries are formed by:

- the inferior margin of the teres minor,
- the surgical neck of the humerus,
- the superior margin of the teres major, and
- the lateral margin of the long head of triceps brachii.

The axillary nerve and the posterior circumflex humeral artery and vein pass through this space (Fig. 7.26).

Clinical app

Quadrangular space syndrome
Hypertrophy of the muscles around the quadrangular space or fibrosis of the muscle edges may impinge on the axillary nerve. This may produce weakness of the deltoid muscle. It may also produce atrophy of the teres minor muscle, which may affect the control that the rotator cuff muscles exert on shoulder movement.

Triangular space

The triangular space is an area of communication between the axilla and the posterior scapular region (see Fig. 7.25). When viewed from the posterior scapular region, the triangular space is formed by:

- the medial margin of the long head of triceps brachii,
- the superior margin of the teres major, and
- the inferior margin of the teres minor.

The circumflex scapular artery and vein pass through this gap (see Fig. 7.26).

Triangular interval

The triangular interval is formed by (see Fig. 7.25):

- the lateral margin of the long head of triceps brachii,
- the shaft of the humerus, and
- the inferior margin of the teres major.

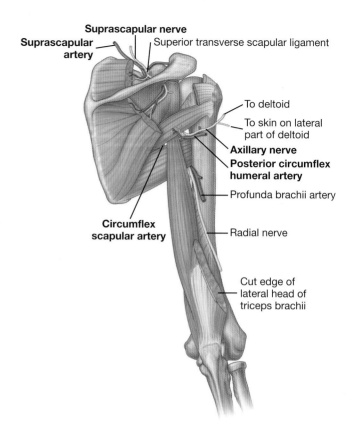

Fig. 7.26 Arteries and nerves associated with gateways in the posterior scapular region.

Because this space is below the inferior margin of the teres major, which defines the inferior boundary of the axilla, the triangular interval serves as a passageway between the anterior and posterior compartments of the arm and between the posterior compartment of the arm and the axilla. The radial nerve, the **profunda brachii artery (deep artery of arm),** and associated veins pass through it (see Fig. 7.26).

Nerves

The two major nerves of the posterior scapular region are the suprascapular and axillary nerves (see Fig. 7.25), both of which originate from the brachial plexus in the axilla.

Suprascapular nerve

The **suprascapular nerve** originates in the base of the neck from the superior trunk of the brachial plexus. It passes posterolaterally from its origin through the suprascapular foramen to reach the posterior scapular region where it lies in the plane between bone and muscle (see Fig. 7.26).

It innervates the supraspinatus muscle, then passes through the greater scapular (spinoglenoid) notch between the root of the spine of the scapula and the glenoid cavity to terminate in and innervate the infraspinatus muscle.

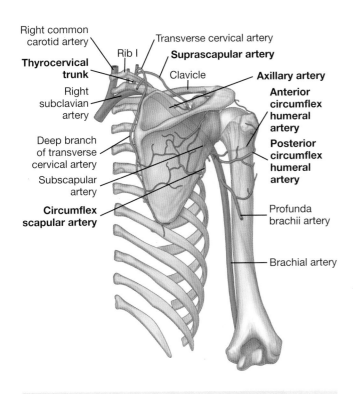

Right common carotid artery

Transverse cervical artery

Rib I

Suprascapular artery

Thyrocervical trunk

Clavicle

Axillary artery

Right subclavian artery

Anterior circumflex humeral artery

Deep branch of transverse cervical artery

Posterior circumflex humeral artery

Subscapular artery

Circumflex scapular artery

Profunda brachii artery

Brachial artery

Fig. 7.27 Arterial anastomoses around the shoulder.

Generally, the suprascapular nerve has no cutaneous branches.

Axillary nerve

The **axillary nerve** originates from the posterior cord of the brachial plexus. It exits the axilla by passing through the quadrangular space in the posterior wall of the axilla and enters the posterior scapular region (see Fig. 7.26). Together with the posterior circumflex humeral artery and vein, it is directly related to the posterior surface of the surgical neck of the humerus.

The axillary nerve innervates the deltoid and teres minor muscles. In addition, it has a cutaneous branch, the superior lateral cutaneous nerve of the arm, which carries general sensation from the skin over the inferior part of the deltoid muscle.

Arteries and veins

Three major arteries are found in the posterior scapular region: the suprascapular, posterior circumflex humeral, and circumflex scapular arteries. These arteries contribute to an interconnected vascular network around the scapula (Fig. 7.27).

Suprascapular artery

The **suprascapular artery** originates in the base of the neck as a branch of the thyrocervical trunk, which, in turn, is a

major branch of the subclavian artery (Fig. 7.27). The vessel may also originate directly from the third part of the subclavian artery.

The suprascapular artery normally enters the posterior scapular region superior to the suprascapular foramen, whereas the nerve passes through the foramen. In the posterior scapular region, the vessel runs with the suprascapular nerve (see Fig. 7.26).

In addition to supplying the supraspinatus and infraspinatus muscles, the suprascapular artery contributes branches to numerous structures along its course.

Posterior circumflex humeral artery

The **posterior circumflex humeral** artery originates from the third part of the axillary artery in the axilla (Figs. 7.26, 7.27).

The posterior circumflex humeral artery and axillary nerve leave the axilla through the quadrangular space in the posterior wall and enter the posterior scapular region. The vessel supplies the related muscles and the glenohumeral joint.

Circumflex scapular artery

The **circumflex scapular artery** is a branch of the subscapular artery that also originates from the third part of the axillary artery in the axilla (Fig. 7.27; also see Fig. 7.26). The circumflex scapular artery leaves the axilla through the triangular space and enters the posterior scapular region, passes through the origin of the teres minor muscle, and forms anastomotic connections with other arteries in the region.

Veins

Veins in the posterior scapular region generally follow the arteries and connect with vessels in the neck, back, arm, and axilla.

AXILLA

The axilla is the gateway to the upper limb, providing an area of transition between the neck and the arm (Fig. 7.28A). Formed by the clavicle, the scapula, the upper thoracic wall, the humerus, and related muscles, the axilla is an irregularly shaped pyramidal space with (Fig. 7.28A,B):

- four sides,
- an inlet, and
- a floor (base).

The axillary inlet is continuous superiorly with the neck, and the lateral part of the floor opens into the arm.

All major structures passing into and out of the upper limb pass through the axilla (Fig. 7.28C). Apertures formed

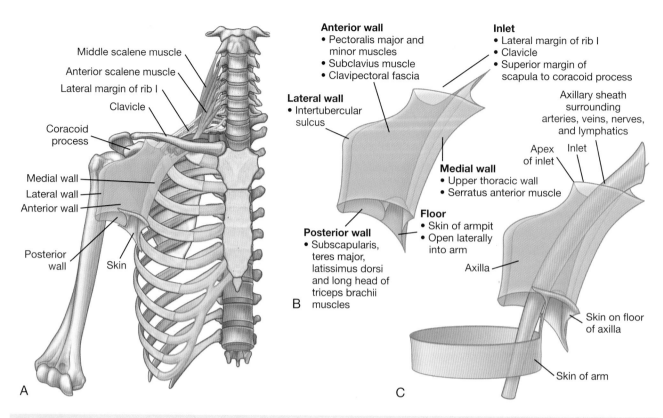

Fig. 7.28 Axilla. **A.** Walls and transition between neck and arm. **B.** Boundaries. **C.** Continuity with the arm.

between muscles in the anterior and posterior walls enable structures to pass between the axilla and immediately adjacent regions (the posterior scapular, pectoral, and deltoid regions).

Axillary inlet

The axillary inlet is oriented in the horizontal plane and is somewhat triangular with its apex directed laterally (Fig. 7.28). The margins of the inlet are completely formed by bone:

- The medial margin is the lateral border of rib I.
- The anterior margin is the posterior surface of the clavicle.
- The posterior margin is the superior border of the scapula up to the coracoid process.

The apex of the triangularly shaped axillary inlet is lateral in position and is formed by the medial aspect of the coracoid process.

Major vessels and nerves pass between the neck and the axilla by crossing over the lateral border of rib I and through the axillary inlet (Fig. 7.28A).

The subclavian artery, the major blood vessel supplying the upper limb, becomes the axillary artery as it crosses the lateral margin of rib I and enters the axilla. Similarly, the axillary vein becomes the subclavian vein as it passes over the lateral margin of rib I and leaves the axilla to enter the neck.

At the axillary inlet, the axillary vein is anterior to the axillary artery, which, in turn, is anterior to the trunks of the brachial plexus (Fig. 7.28A)

The inferior trunk (lower trunk) of the brachial plexus lies directly on rib I in the neck as does the subclavian artery and vein. As they pass over rib I, the vein and artery are separated by the insertion of the anterior scalene muscle (Fig. 7.28A).

Anterior wall

The anterior wall of the axilla is formed by the lateral part of the **pectoralis major muscle,** the underlying **pectoralis minor** and **subclavius muscles,** and the **clavipectoral fascia** (Table 7.3, Figs. 7.28B, 7.29).

Clavipectoral fascia

The clavipectoral fascia is a thick sheet of connective tissue that connects the clavicle to the floor of the axilla (Fig. 7.30). It encloses the subclavius and pectoralis minor muscles and spans the gap between them.

Structures travel between the axilla and the anterior wall of the axilla by passing through the clavipectoral fascia

Table 7.3 Muscles of the anterior wall of the axilla (spinal segments indicated in **bold** are the major segments innervating the muscle)

Muscle	Origin	Insertion	Innervation	Function
Pectoralis major	Clavicular head—anterior surface of medial half of clavicle; sternocostal head—anterior surface of sternum; first seven costal cartilages; sternal end of sixth rib; aponeurosis of external oblique	Lateral lip of intertubercular sulcus of humerus	Medial and lateral pectoral nerves; clavicular head [**C5**, C6]; sternocostal head [C6, **C7**, C8, T1]	Flexion, adduction, and medial rotation of arm at glenohumeral joint; clavicular head—flexion of extended arm; sternocostal head—extension of flexed arm
Subclavius	First rib at junction between rib and costal cartilage	Groove on inferior surface of middle one-third of clavicle	Nerve to subclavius [**C5, C6**]	Pulls tip of shoulder down; pulls clavicle medially to stabilize sternoclavicular joint
Pectoralis minor	Anterior surfaces and superior borders of ribs III to V; and from deep fascia overlying the related intercostal spaces	Coracoid process of scapula (medial border and upper surface)	Medial pectoral nerve (with a contribution from lateral pectoral nerve) [C5, C6, **C7, C8**, T1]	Pulls tip of shoulder down; protracts scapula

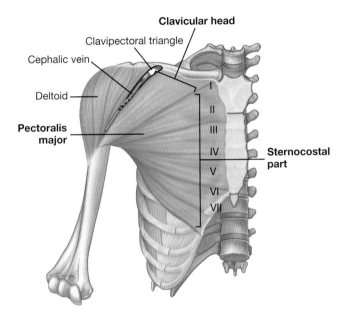

Fig. 7.29 Pectoralis major muscle.

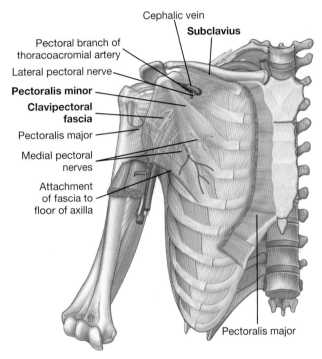

Fig. 7.30 Pectoralis minor and subclavius muscles and clavipectoral fascia.

either between the pectoralis minor and subclavius muscles or inferior to the pectoralis minor muscle.

Important structures that pass between the subclavius and pectoralis minor muscles include the cephalic vein, the thoracoacromial artery, and the lateral pectoral nerve.

The lateral thoracic artery leaves the axilla by passing through the fascia inferior to the pectoralis minor muscle.

The medial pectoral nerve leaves the axilla by penetrating directly through the pectoralis minor muscle to supply this muscle and to reach the pectoralis major muscle. Occasionally, branches of the medial pectoral nerve pass around the lower margin of the pectoralis minor to reach and innervate the overlying pectoralis major muscle.

Medial wall

The medial wall of the axilla consists of the upper thoracic wall (the ribs and related intercostal tissues) and the **serratus anterior muscle** (Table 7.4, Fig. 7.31; see Fig. 7.28B).

The only major structure that passes directly through the medial wall and into the axilla is the **intercostobrachial nerve** (Fig. 7.31C). This nerve is the lateral cutaneous branch of the second intercostal nerve (anterior ramus of T2). It communicates with a branch of the brachial plexus (the medial cutaneous nerve of the arm) in the axilla and supplies skin on the upper posteromedial side of the arm, which is part of the T2 dermatome.

Table 7.4 Muscles of the medial wall of the axilla (spinal segments indicated in **bold** are the major segments innervating the muscle)

Muscle	Origin	Insertion	Innervation	Function
Serratus anterior	Lateral surfaces of upper 8-9 ribs and deep fascia overlying the related intercostal spaces	Costal surface of medial border of scapula	Long thoracic nerve [**C5**, C6, C7]	Protraction and rotation of the scapula; keeps medial border and inferior angle of scapula opposed to thoracic wall

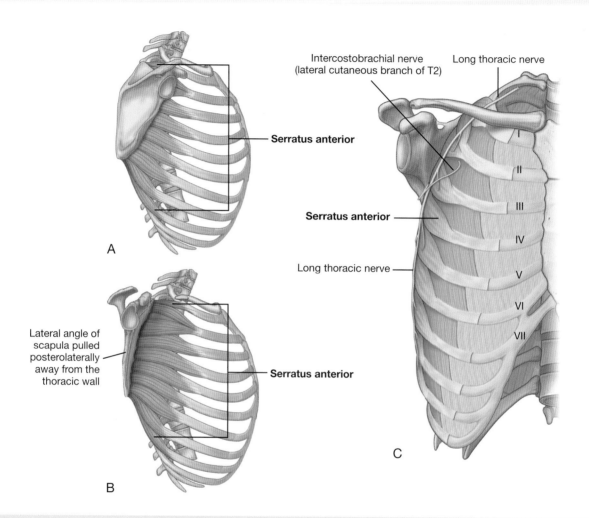

Fig. 7.31 Medial wall of the axilla. **A.** Lateral view. **B.** Lateral view with lateral angle of scapula retracted posteriorly. **C.** Anterior view.

Clinical app

"Winging" of the scapula

Because the long thoracic nerve passes down the lateral thoracic wall on the external surface of the serratus anterior muscle just deep to skin and subcutaneous fascia, it is vulnerable to damage (see Fig. 7.31C). Loss of function of this muscle causes the medial border and, particularly, the inferior angle of the scapula to elevate away from the thoracic wall, resulting in characteristic "winging" of the scapula on pushing forward with the arm. Furthermore, normal elevation of the arm is no longer possible.

Lateral wall

The lateral wall of the axilla is narrow and formed entirely by the **intertubercular sulcus** of the humerus (Fig. 7.32). The pectoralis major muscle of the anterior wall attaches to the lateral lip of the intertubercular sulcus. The latissimus dorsi and teres major muscles of the posterior wall attach to the floor and medial lip of the intertubercular sulcus, respectively (Table 7.5, Fig. 7.32).

Posterior wall

The posterior wall of the axilla is complex (Table 7.5, Figs. 7.28B, 7.33). Its bone framework is formed by the costal surface of the scapula. Muscles of the wall are:

Table 7.5 Muscles of the lateral and posterior wall of the axilla (spinal segments indicated in **bold** are the major segments innervating the muscle; spinal segments enclosed in parentheses do not consistently innervate the muscle)

Muscle	Origin	Insertion	Innervation	Function
Subscapularis	Medial two-thirds of subscapular fossa	Lesser tubercle of humerus	Upper and lower subscapular nerves [C5, **C6**, (C7)]	**Rotator cuff muscle;** medial rotation of the arm at the glenohumeral joint
Teres major	Elongate oval area on the posterior surface of the inferior angle of the scapula	Medial lip of the intertubercular sulcus on the anterior surface of the humerus	Lower subscapular nerve [**C5, C6, C7**]	Medial rotation and extension of the arm at the glenohumeral joint
Latissimus dorsi	Spinous processes of lower six thoracic vertebrae and related interspinous ligaments; via the thoracolumbar fascia to the spinous processes of the lumbar vertebrae, related interspinous ligaments, and iliac crest; lower 3-4 ribs	Floor of intertubercular sulcus	Thoracodorsal nerve [C6, **C7**, C8]	Adduction, medial rotation, and extension of the arm at the glenohumeral joint
Long head of triceps brachii	Infraglenoid tubercle on scapula	Common tendon of insertion with medial and lateral heads on the olecranon process of ulna	Radial nerve [C6, **C7**, C8]	Extension of the forearm at the elbow joint; accessory adductor and extensor of the arm at the glenohumeral joint

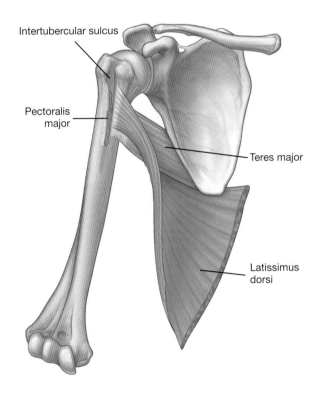

Fig. 7.32 Lateral wall of the axilla (anterior view).

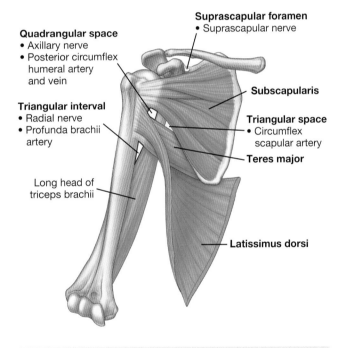

Fig. 7.33 Posterior wall of the axilla (anterior view).

- the **subscapularis** muscle (associated with the costal surface of the scapula),
- the distal parts of the **latissimus dorsi** and **teres major** muscles (which pass into the wall from the back and posterior scapular region), and
- the proximal part of the long head of the **triceps brachii** muscle (which passes vertically down the wall and into the arm).

Gaps between the muscles of the posterior wall form apertures through which structures pass between the axilla, posterior scapular region, and posterior compartment of the arm (Fig. 7.33).

Together with three muscles of the posterior scapular region (the supraspinatus, infraspinatus, and teres minor muscles), the subscapularis is a member of the rotator cuff muscles, which stabilize the glenohumeral joint.

The **long head of the triceps brachii** muscle passes vertically through the posterior wall of the axilla and, together with surrounding muscles and adjacent bones, results in the formation of three apertures through which major structures pass through the posterior wall (Fig. 7.33):

- the quadrangular space,
- the triangular space, and
- the triangular interval.

Gateways in the posterior wall

(See also "Gateways to the posterior scapular region," p. 379, and Fig. 7.25.)

Quadrangular space

The quadrangular space provides a passageway for nerves and vessels passing between the axilla and the more posterior scapular and deltoid regions (Fig. 7.33). When viewed anteriorly, its boundaries are formed by:

- the inferior margin of the subscapularis muscle;
- the surgical neck of the humerus;
- the superior margin of the teres major muscle; and
- the lateral margin of the long head of the triceps brachii muscle.

Passing through the quadrangular space are the axillary nerve and the posterior circumflex humeral artery and vein (see Fig. 7.26).

Triangular space

The **triangular space** is an area of communication between the axilla and the posterior scapular region (Fig. 7.33). When viewed anteriorly, it is formed by:

- the medial margin of the long head of the triceps brachii muscle,
- the superior margin of the teres major muscle. and
- the inferior margin of the subscapularis muscle.

The circumflex scapular artery and vein pass into this space (see Fig. 7.26).

Triangular interval

This triangular interval is formed by (Fig. 7.33):

- the lateral margin of the long head of the triceps brachii muscle,
- the shaft of the humerus, and
- the inferior margin of the teres major muscle.

The radial nerve passes out of the axilla traveling through this interval to reach the posterior compartment of the arm (see Fig. 7.26).

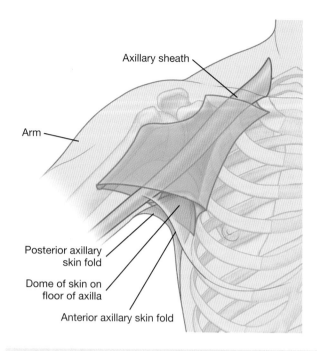

Fig. 7.34 Floor of the axilla.

Floor

The floor of the axilla (Fig. 7.34; also see Fig 7.28B) is formed by fascia and a dome of skin that spans the distance between the inferior margins of the walls. It is supported by the clavipectoral fascia.

Inferiorly, structures pass into and out of the axilla immediately lateral to the floor where the anterior and posterior walls of the axilla converge and where the axilla is continuous with the anterior compartment of the arm.

Contents of the axilla

Passing through the axilla are the major vessels, nerves, and lymphatics of the upper limb. The space also contains the proximal parts of two muscles (**biceps brachii** and **coracobrachialis muscles;** Table 7.6) of the arm, the axillary process of the breast, and collections of lymph nodes, which drain the upper limb and chest wall.

Axillary artery

The axillary artery supplies the walls of the axilla and related regions and continues as the major blood supply to the more distal parts of the upper limb (Fig. 7.35).

The subclavian artery in the neck becomes the axillary artery at the lateral margin of rib I and passes through the axilla, becoming the brachial artery at the inferior margin of the teres major muscle.

Table 7.6 Muscles having parts that pass through the axilla (spinal segments indicated in **bold** are the major segments innervating the muscle)

Muscle	Origin	Insertion	Innervation	Function
Biceps brachii	Long head—supraglenoid tubercle of scapula; short head—apex of coracoid process	Radial tuberosity	Musculocutaneous nerve **[C5, C6]**	Powerful flexor of the forearm at the elbow joint and supinator of the forearm; accessory flexor of the arm at the glenohumeral joint
Coracobrachialis	Apex of coracoid process	Linear roughening on mid-shaft of humerus on medial side	Musculocutaneous nerve **[C5, C6, C7]**	Flexor of the arm at the glenohumeral joint; adducts arm

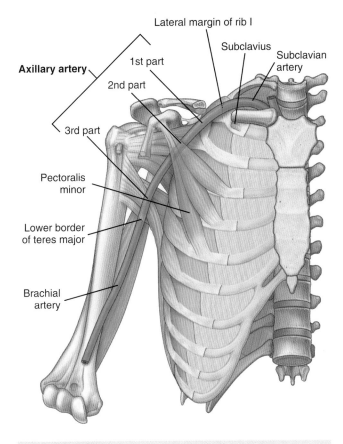

Fig. 7.35 Contents of the axilla: the axillary artery.

The axillary artery is separated into three parts by the pectoralis minor muscle, which crosses anteriorly to the vessel (Fig. 7.35):

- The first part is proximal to pectoralis minor.
- The second part is posterior to pectoralis minor.
- The third part is distal to pectoralis minor.

Generally, six branches arise from the axillary artery (Fig. 7.36):

- One branch, the **superior thoracic artery,** originates from the first part.

- Two branches, the **thoracoacromial artery** and the **lateral thoracic artery,** originate from the second part.
- Three branches, the **subscapular artery,** the **anterior circumflex humeral artery,** and the **posterior circumflex humeral artery,** originate from the third part.

Superior thoracic artery

The **superior thoracic artery** is small and originates from the anterior surface of the first part of the axillary artery (Fig. 7.36). It supplies upper regions of the medial and anterior axillary walls.

Thoracoacromial artery

The **thoracoacromial artery** is short and originates from the anterior surface of the second part of the axillary artery just posterior to the medial (superior) margin of the pectoralis minor muscle (Fig. 7.36). It curves around the superior margin of the muscle, penetrates the clavipectoral fascia, and immediately divides into four branches (the pectoral, deltoid, clavicular, and acromial branches), which supply the anterior axillary wall and related regions.

Additionally, the pectoral branch contributes vascular supply to the breast, and the deltoid branch passes into the clavipectoral triangle where it accompanies the cephalic vein and supplies adjacent structures (see Fig. 7.30).

Lateral thoracic artery

The **lateral thoracic artery** arises from the anterior surface of the second part of the axillary artery posterior to the lateral (inferior) margin of pectoralis minor (Fig. 7.36). It follows the margin of the muscle to the thoracic wall and supplies the medial and anterior walls of the axilla. In women, branches emerge from around the inferior margin of the pectoralis major muscle and contribute to the vascular supply of the breast.

Subscapular artery

The **subscapular artery** is the largest branch of the axillary artery and is the major blood supply to the posterior wall of

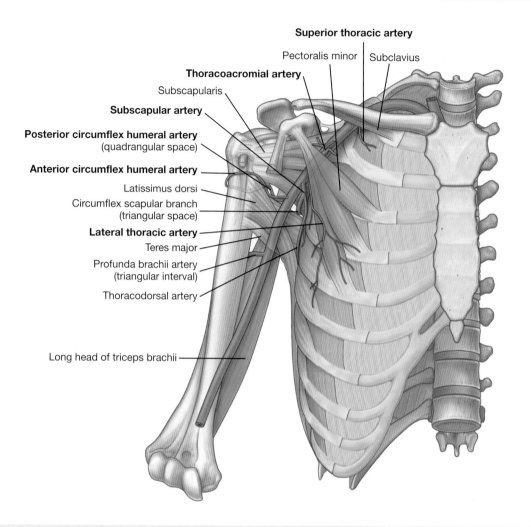

Fig. 7.36 Branches of the axillary artery.

the axilla (Fig. 7.36). It also contributes to the blood supply of the posterior scapular region.

The subscapular artery originates from the posterior surface of the third part of the axillary artery, follows the inferior margin of the subscapularis muscle for a short distance, then divides into its two terminal branches, the **circumflex scapular artery** and the **thoracodorsal artery** (Fig. 7.36).

The circumflex scapular artery passes through the triangular space between the subscapularis, teres major, and long head of the triceps muscles. Posteriorly, it passes inferior to, or pierces, the origin of the teres minor muscle to enter the infraspinous fossa. It anastomoses with the suprascapular artery and the **deep branch (dorsal scapular artery)** of the transverse cervical artery, thereby contributing to an anastomotic network of vessels around the scapula.

The thoracodorsal artery approximately follows the lateral border of the scapula to the inferior angle. It contributes to the vascular supply of the posterior and medial walls of the axilla.

Anterior circumflex humeral artery

The **anterior circumflex humeral artery** is small compared to the posterior circumflex humeral artery and originates from the lateral side of the third part of the axillary artery (Fig. 7.36). It passes anterior to the surgical neck of the humerus and anastomoses with the posterior circumflex humeral artery.

This anterior circumflex humeral artery supplies branches to surrounding tissues, which include the glenohumeral joint and the head of the humerus.

Posterior circumflex humeral artery

The **posterior circumflex humeral artery** originates from the lateral surface of the third part of the axillary artery immediately posterior to the origin of the anterior circumflex humeral artery (Fig. 7.36). With the axillary nerve, it leaves the axilla by passing through the quadrangular space between the teres major, teres minor, and the long head of the triceps brachii muscle and the surgical neck of the humerus (see Fig. 7.26).

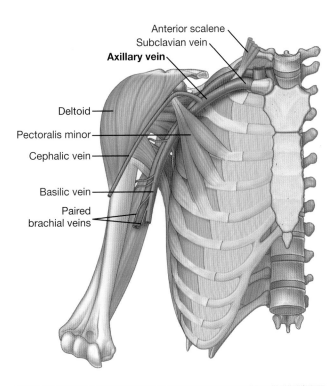

Anterior scalene
Subclavian vein
Axillary vein
Deltoid
Pectoralis minor
Cephalic vein
Basilic vein
Paired
brachial veins

Fig. 7.37 Axillary vein.

The posterior circumflex humeral artery curves around the surgical neck of the humerus and supplies the surrounding muscles and the glenohumeral joint. It anastomoses with the anterior circumflex humeral artery, and with branches from the profunda brachii, suprascapular, and thoracoacromial arteries.

Axillary vein

The axillary vein begins at the lower margin of the teres major muscle and is the continuation of the basilic vein (Fig. 7.37), which is a superficial vein that drains the posteromedial surface of the hand and forearm and penetrates the deep fascia in the middle of the arm.

The axillary vein passes through the axilla medial and anterior to the axillary artery and becomes the subclavian vein as the vessel crosses the lateral border of rib I at the axillary inlet. Tributaries of the axillary vein generally follow the branches of the axillary artery. Other tributaries include brachial veins that follow the brachial artery and the cephalic vein (Fig. 7.37).

The cephalic vein is a superficial vein that drains the lateral and posterior parts of the hand, the forearm, and the arm. In the area of the shoulder, it passes into an inverted triangular cleft (the **clavipectoral triangle**) between the deltoid muscle, pectoralis major muscle, and the clavicle. In the superior part of the clavipectoral triangle, the cephalic vein passes deep to the clavicular head of the pectoralis major muscle and pierces the clavipectoral fascia to join the axillary vein.

Brachial plexus

The brachial plexus is a somatic nerve plexus formed by the **anterior rami** of C5 to C8 and most of the anterior ramus of T1 (Fig. 7.38). It originates in the neck, passes laterally and inferiorly over rib I, and enters the axilla.

The parts of the brachial plexus, from medial to lateral, are roots, trunks, divisions, and cords. All major nerves that innervate the upper limb originate from the brachial plexus, mostly from the cords. Proximal parts of the brachial plexus are posterior to the subclavian artery in the neck, while more distal regions of the plexus surround the axillary artery.

Roots

The roots of the brachial plexus are the anterior rami of C5 to C8 and most of T1. Close to their origin, the roots receive **gray rami communicantes** from the sympathetic

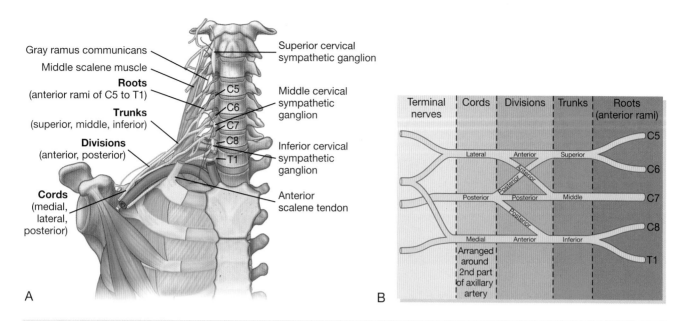

Fig. 7.38 Brachial plexus. **A.** Major components in the neck and axilla. **B.** Schematic showing parts of the brachial plexus.

trunk (Fig. 7.38). These carry postganglionic sympathetic fibers onto the roots for distribution to the periphery. The roots and trunks enter the **posterior triangle** of the neck by passing between the anterior scalene and middle scalene muscles and lie superior and posterior to the subclavian artery.

Trunks

The three trunks of the brachial plexus originate from the roots, pass laterally over rib I, and enter the axilla (Fig. 7.38):

- The **superior trunk** is formed by the union of C5 and C6 roots.
- The **middle trunk** is a continuation of the C7 root.
- The **inferior trunk** is formed by the union of the C8 and T1 roots.

The inferior trunk lies on rib I posterior to the subclavian artery; the middle and superior trunks are more superior in position.

Divisions

Each of the three trunks of the brachial plexus divides into an **anterior** and a **posterior division** (Fig. 7.38):

- The three anterior divisions form parts of the brachial plexus that ultimately give rise to peripheral nerves associated with the anterior compartments of the arm and forearm.
- The three posterior divisions combine to form parts of the brachial plexus that give rise to nerves associated with the posterior compartments.

Cords

The three cords of the brachial plexus originate from the divisions and are related to the second part of the axillary artery (Fig. 7.38):

- The **lateral cord** results from the union of the anterior divisions of the upper and middle trunks and therefore has contributions from C5 to C7; it is positioned lateral to the second part of the axillary artery;
- The **medial cord** is medial to the second part of the axillary artery and is the continuation of the anterior division of the inferior trunk; it contains contributions from C8 and T1.
- The **posterior cord** occurs posterior to the second part of the axillary artery and originates as the union of all three posterior divisions; it contains contributions from all roots of the brachial plexus (C5 to T1).

Most of the major peripheral nerves of the upper limb originate from the cords of the brachial plexus. Generally, nerves associated with the anterior compartments of the upper limb arise from the medial and lateral cords and nerves associated with the posterior compartments originate from the posterior cord.

Branches (Table 7.7)
Branches of the roots

In addition to small segmental branches from C5 to C8 to muscles of the neck and a contribution of C5 to the phrenic nerve, the roots of the brachial plexus give rise to the dorsal scapular and long thoracic nerves (Figs. 7.39, 7.40).

Table 7.7   Branches of brachial plexus ([brackets] indicate that a spinal segment is a minor component of the nerve or is inconsistently present in the nerve)

Branch

Dorsal scapular
  Origin: C5 root
  Spinal segment: C5

Function: motor
Rhomboid major, rhomboid minor

Long thoracic
  Origin: C5 to C7 roots
  Spinal segments:
  C5 to C7

Function: motor
Serratus anterior

Suprascapular
  Origin: Superior trunk
  Spinal segments: C5, C6

Function: motor
Supraspinatus, infraspinatus

Nerve to subclavius
  Origin: Superior trunk
  Spinal segments: C5, C6

Function: motor
Subclavius

Lateral pectoral
  Origin: Lateral cord
  Spinal segments:
  C5 to C7

Function: motor
Pectoralis major

Musculocutaneous
  Origin: Lateral cord
  Spinal segments:
  C5 to C7

Function: motor
All muscles in the anterior compartment of the arm
Function: sensory
Skin on lateral side of forearm

Medial pectoral
  Origin: Medial cord
  Spinal segments: C8, T1
  (also receives contributions from spinal
  segments C5 to C7 through a communication
  with the lateral pectoral nerve)

Function: motor
Pectoralis major, pectoralis minor

Medial cutaneous of arm
  Origin: Medial cord
  Spinal segments: C8, T1

Function: sensory
Skin on medial side of distal one-third of arm

Continued

Table 7.7　Branches of brachial plexus ([brackets] indicate that a spinal segment is a minor component of the nerve or is inconsistently present in the nerve)—cont'd

Medial cutaneous of forearm
　Origin: Medial cord
　Spinal segments: C8, T1

Function: sensory
Skin on medial side of forearm

Median
　Origin: Medial and lateral cords
　Spinal segments:
　　[C5], C6 to T1

Function: motor
All muscles in the anterior compartment of the forearm (except flexor carpi ulnaris and medial half of flexor digitorum profundus), three thenar muscles of the thumb, and two lateral lumbrical muscles
Function: sensory
Skin over the palmar surface of the lateral three and one-half digits and over the lateral side of the palm and middle of the wrist

Ulnar
　Origin: Medial cord
　Spinal segments:
　　[C7], C8, T1

Function: motor
All intrinsic muscles of the hand (except three thenar muscles and two lateral lumbricals); also flexor carpi ulnaris and the medial half of flexor digitorum profundus in the forearm
Function: sensory
Skin over the palmar surface of the medial one and one-half digits and associated palm and wrist and skin over the dorsal surface of the medial one and one-half digits

Superior subscapular
　Origin: Posterior cord
　Spinal segments: C5, C6

Function: motor
Subscapularis

Thoracodorsal
　Origin: Posterior cord
　Spinal segments:
　　C6 to C8

Function: motor
Latissimus dorsi

Inferior subscapular
　Origin: Posterior cord
　Spinal segments: C5, C6

Function: motor
Subscapularis, teres major

Axillary
　Origin: Posterior cord
　Spinal segments: C5, C6

Function: motor
Deltoid, teres minor
Function: sensory
Skin over upper lateral part of arm

Radial
　Origin: Posterior cord
　Spinal segments:
　　C5 to C8, [T1]

Function: motor
All muscles in the posterior compartments of arm and forearm
Function: sensory
Skin on the posterior aspects of the arm and forearm, the lower lateral surface of the arm, and the dorsal lateral surface of the hand

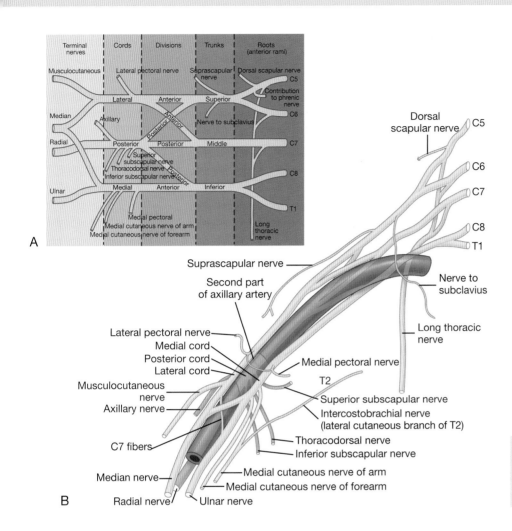

Fig. 7.39 Brachial plexus.
A. Schematic showing branches of the brachial plexus. **B.** Relationships to the axillary artery.

The **dorsal scapular nerve:**

■ originates from the C5 root of the brachial plexus,
■ passes posteriorly, often piercing the middle scalene muscle in the neck, to reach and travel along the medial border of the scapula, and
■ innervates the rhomboid major and minor muscles from their deep surfaces.

The **long thoracic nerve:**

■ originates from the anterior rami of C5 to C7,
■ passes vertically down the neck, through the axillary inlet, and down the medial wall of the axilla to supply the serratus anterior muscle, and
■ lies on the superficial aspect of the serratus anterior muscle.

Clinical app

Damage to long thoracic nerve

A mastectomy (surgical removal of the breast) involves excision of the breast tissue to the pectoralis major muscle and fascia. Within the axilla, the breast tissue must be removed from the medial

Clinical app—cont'd

axillary wall. Closely applied to the medial axillary wall is the long thoracic nerve. Damage to this nerve can result in paralysis of the serratus anterior muscle, producing a characteristic "winged" scapula. This nerve also can be injured during placement of chest tubes or by trauma to the lateral body wall.

Branches of the trunks

The only branches from the trunks of the brachial plexus are two nerves that originate from the superior trunk (upper trunk): the suprascapular nerve and the nerve to the subclavius muscle (Figs. 7.39, 7.40).

The **suprascapular nerve** (C5 and C6):

■ originates from the superior trunk of the brachial plexus,
■ passes laterally through the posterior triangle of the neck and through the suprascapular foramen to enter the posterior scapular region,
■ innervates the supraspinatus and infraspinatus muscles, and
■ is accompanied in the lateral parts of the neck and in the posterior scapular region by the suprascapular artery.

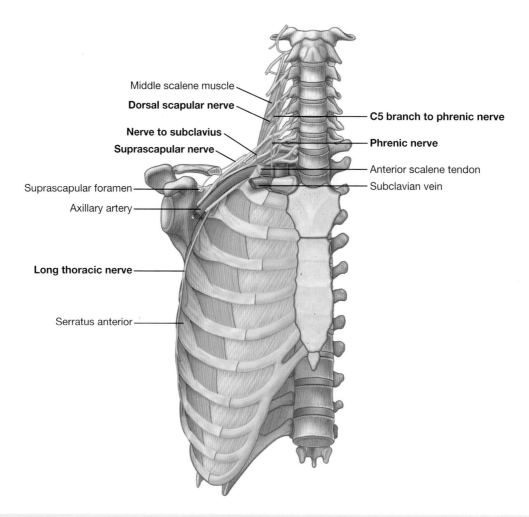

Middle scalene muscle

Dorsal scapular nerve

C5 branch to phrenic nerve

Nerve to subclavius

Suprascapular nerve

Phrenic nerve

Suprascapular foramen

Anterior scalene tendon

Subclavian vein

Axillary artery

Long thoracic nerve

Serratus anterior

Fig. 7.40 Branches of the roots and trunks of the brachial plexus.

The **nerve to subclavius muscle** (C5 and C6) is a small nerve that:

- originates from the superior trunk of the brachial plexus,
- passes anteroinferiorly over the subclavian artery and vein, and
- innervates the subclavius muscle.

Branches of the lateral cord

Three nerves originate entirely or partly from the lateral cord (Figs. 7.39, 7.41).

The **lateral pectoral nerve** is the most proximal of the branches from the lateral cord. It passes anteriorly together with the thoracoacromial artery to penetrate the clavipectoral fascia that spans the gap between the subclavius and pectoralis minor muscles and innervates the pectoralis major muscle.

The **musculocutaneous nerve** is a large terminal branch of the lateral cord. It passes laterally to penetrate the coracobrachialis muscle, passes between the biceps brachii and brachialis muscles in the arm, and innervates all three flexor

muscles in the anterior compartment of the arm, terminating as the **lateral cutaneous nerve of forearm.**

The **lateral root of median nerve** is the largest terminal branch of the lateral cord and passes medially to join a similar branch from the medial cord to form the median nerve.

Branches of the medial cord

The medial cord has five branches (Figs. 7.39, 7.41).

The **medial pectoral nerve** is the most proximal branch. It receives a communicating branch from the lateral pectoral nerve and then passes anteriorly between the axillary artery and axillary vein. Branches of the nerve penetrate and supply the pectoralis minor muscle. Some of these branches pass through the muscle to reach and supply the pectoralis major muscle. Other branches occasionally pass around the inferior or lateral margin of the pectoralis minor muscle to reach the pectoralis major muscle.

The **medial cutaneous nerve of arm (medial brachial cutaneous nerve)** passes through the axilla and into the arm where it penetrates deep fascia and supplies skin over the medial side of the distal third of the arm. In the axilla, the

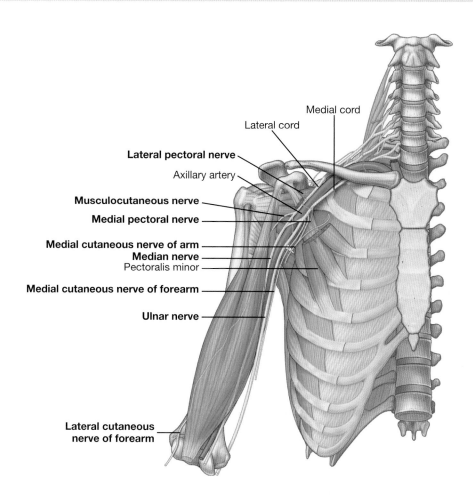

Fig. 7.41 Branches of the lateral and medial cords of the brachial plexus.

nerve communicates with the **intercostobrachial nerve** of T2. Fibers of the medial cutaneous nerve of arm innervate the upper part of the medial surface of the arm and floor of the axilla.

The **medial cutaneous nerve of forearm (medial antebrachial cutaneous nerve)** originates just distal to the origin of the medial cutaneous nerve of arm. It passes out of the axilla and into the arm where it gives off a branch to the skin over the biceps brachii muscle and then continues down the arm to penetrate the deep fascia with the basilic vein, continuing inferiorly to supply the skin over the anterior surface of the forearm. It innervates skin over the medial surface of the forearm down to the wrist.

The **medial root of median nerve** passes laterally to join with a similar root from the lateral cord to form the median nerve anterior to the third part of the axillary artery.

The **ulnar nerve** is a large terminal branch of the medial cord. However, near its origin, it often receives a communicating branch from the lateral root of the median nerve originating from the lateral cord and carrying fibers from C7 (see Fig. 7.39B). The ulnar nerve passes through the arm and forearm into the hand where it innervates all intrinsic

muscles of the hand (except for the three thenar muscles and the two lateral lumbrical muscles). On passing through the forearm, branches of the ulnar nerve innervate the flexor carpi ulnaris muscle and the medial half of the flexor digitorum profundus muscle. The ulnar nerve innervates skin over the palmar surface of the little finger, medial half of the ring finger, associated palm and wrist, and over the dorsal surface of the medial part of the hand.

Median nerve. The median nerve is formed anterior to the third part of the axillary artery by the union of lateral and medial roots originating from the lateral and medial cords of the brachial plexus (Figs. 7.39, 7.41). It passes into the arm anterior to the brachial artery and through the arm into the forearm where branches innervate most of the muscles in the anterior compartment of the forearm (except for the flexor carpi ulnaris muscle and the medial half of the flexor digitorum profundus muscle, which are innervated by the ulnar nerve).

The median nerve continues into the hand to innervate:

- the three thenar muscles associated with the thumb,
- the two lateral lumbrical muscles associated with movement of the index and middle fingers, and

■ the skin over the palmar surface of the lateral three and one-half digits and over the lateral side of the palm and middle of the wrist.

The musculocutaneous nerve, the lateral root of the median nerve, the median nerve, the medial root of the median nerve, and the ulnar nerve form an M over the third part of the axillary artery (Fig. 7.41). This feature, together with penetration of the coracobrachialis muscle by the musculocutaneous nerve, can be used to identify components of the brachial plexus in the axilla.

Branches of the posterior cord

Five nerves originate from the posterior cord of the brachial plexus (Figs. 7.39, 7.42):

■ the superior subscapular nerve,
■ the thoracodorsal nerve,
■ the inferior subscapular nerve,
■ the axillary nerve, and
■ the radial nerve.

All these nerves except the radial nerve innervate muscles associated with the shoulder region or the posterior wall of the axilla; the radial nerve passes into the arm and forearm.

The **superior subscapular nerve,** the thoracodorsal, and the **inferior subscapular nerves** originate sequentially from the posterior cord and pass directly into muscles associated with the posterior wall of the axilla (Fig. 7.42). The **superior subscapular nerve** is short and passes into and supplies the subscapularis muscle. The **thoracodorsal nerve** is the longest of these three nerves and passes vertically along the posterior axillary wall. It penetrates and innervates the latissimus dorsi muscle. The **inferior subscapular nerve** also passes inferiorly along the posterior axillary wall and innervates the subscapularis and teres major muscles.

The **axillary nerve** originates from the posterior cord and passes inferiorly and laterally along the posterior wall to exit the axilla through the quadrangular space (Fig. 7.42). It passes posteriorly around the surgical neck of the humerus and innervates both the deltoid and teres minor muscles. A **superior lateral cutaneous nerve** of arm originates from the axillary nerve after passing through the quadrangular space and loops around the posterior margin of the deltoid muscle to innervate skin in that region. The **axillary nerve** is accompanied by the posterior circumflex humeral artery.

The **radial nerve** is the largest terminal branch of the posterior cord (Fig. 7.42). It passes out of the axilla and into the posterior compartment of the arm by passing through the triangular interval between the inferior border of the

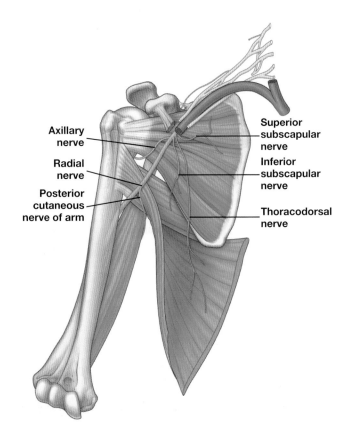

Fig. 7.42 Branches of the posterior cord of the brachial plexus.

teres major muscle, the long head of the triceps brachii muscle, and the shaft of the humerus. It is accompanied through the triangular interval by the profunda brachii artery, which originates from the brachial artery in the anterior compartment of the arm. The radial nerve and its branches innervate:

■ all muscles in the posterior compartments of the arm and forearm, and
■ the skin on the posterior aspect of the arm and forearm, the lower lateral surface of the arm, and the dorsolateral surface of the hand.

The **posterior cutaneous nerve of arm (posterior brachial cutaneous nerve)** originates from the radial nerve in the axilla and innervates skin on the posterior surface of the arm.

Lymphatics

All lymphatics from the upper limb drain into lymph nodes in the axilla (Fig. 7.43).

In addition, axillary nodes receive drainage from an extensive area on the adjacent trunk, which includes regions of the upper back and shoulder, the lower neck, the chest,

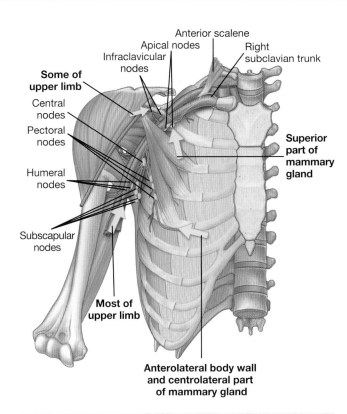

Fig. 7.43 Lymph nodes and vessels in the axilla.

Fig. 7.44 Axillary process of the breast.

and the upper anterolateral abdominal wall. Axillary nodes also receive drainage from approximately 75% of the mammary gland.

The 20 to 30 axillary nodes are generally divided into five groups on the basis of location (Fig. 7.43).

Humeral (lateral) nodes posteromedial to the axillary vein receive most of the lymphatic drainage from the upper limb.

Pectoral (anterior) nodes occur along the inferior margin of the pectoralis minor muscle and along the course of the lateral thoracic vessels. They receive drainage from the abdominal wall, the chest, and the mammary gland.

Subscapular (posterior) nodes on the posterior axillary wall in association with the subscapular vessels drain the posterior axillary wall and receive lymphatics from the back, the shoulder, and the neck.

Central nodes are embedded in axillary fat and receive tributaries from humeral, subscapular, and pectoral groups of nodes.

Apical nodes are the most superior group of nodes in the axilla and drain all other groups of nodes in the region. In addition, they receive lymphatic vessels that accompany the cephalic vein as well as vessels that drain the superior region of the mammary gland.

Efferent vessels from the apical group converge to form the subclavian trunk, which usually joins the venous system

at the junction between the right subclavian vein and the right internal jugular vein in the neck. On the left, the subclavian trunk usually joins the thoracic duct in the base of the neck.

Axillary process of the mammary gland

Although the mammary gland is in superficial fascia overlying the thoracic wall, its superolateral region extends along the inferior margin of the pectoralis major muscle toward the axilla. In some cases, this may pass around the margin of the muscle to penetrate deep fascia and enter the axilla (Fig. 7.44). This axillary process rarely reaches as high as the apex of the axilla.

Lymphatic drainage and breast cancer

Lymphatic drainage from the lateral part of the breast passes through nodes in the axilla. Significant disruption to the normal lymphatic drainage of the upper limb may occur if a mastectomy or a surgical axillary nodal clearance has been carried out for breast cancer. Furthermore, some patients have radiotherapy to the axilla to prevent the spread of metastatic disease, but a side effect of this is the destruction of the tiny lymphatics as well as the cancer cells. If the lymphatic drainage of the upper limb is damaged, the arm may swell (lymphedema).

ARM

The arm is the region of the upper limb between the shoulder and the elbow (Fig. 7.45A). The superior aspect of the arm communicates medially with the axilla. Inferiorly, a number of important structures pass between the arm and the forearm through the cubital fossa, which is positioned anterior to the elbow joint.

The arm is divided into two compartments by medial and lateral intermuscular septa, which pass from each side of the humerus to the outer sleeve of deep fascia that surrounds the limb (Fig. 7.45B).

The anterior compartment of the arm contains muscles that predominantly flex the elbow joint; the posterior compartment contains muscles that extend the joint. Major nerves and vessels supply and pass through each compartment.

Bones

The skeletal support for the arm is the humerus (Fig. 7.46). However, most of the large muscles of the arm insert into the proximal ends of the two bones of the forearm, the radius and the ulna, and flex and extend the forearm at the elbow joint. In addition, the muscles predominantly situated in the forearm that move the hand originate at the distal end of the humerus.

Shaft and distal end of the humerus

In cross-section, the shaft of the humerus is somewhat triangular with (Fig. 7.46):

- **anterior, lateral,** and **medial borders,** and
- **anterolateral, anteromedial,** and **posterior surfaces.**

The posterior surface of the humerus is marked on its superior aspect by a linear roughening for the attachment of the lateral head of the triceps brachii muscle, beginning just

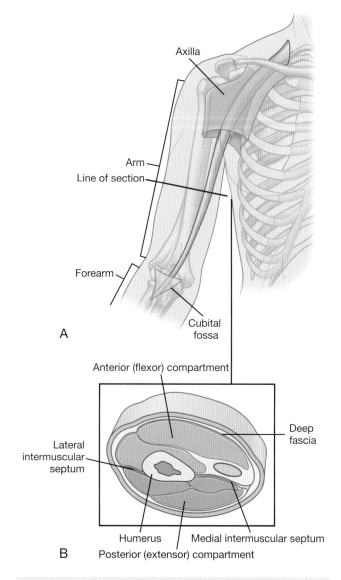

Fig. 7.45 Arm. A. Proximal and distal relationships. **B.** Transverse section through the middle of the arm.

inferior to the surgical neck and passing diagonally across the bone to the **deltoid tuberosity** (Fig. 7.46).

The middle part of the posterior surface and adjacent part of the anterolateral surface are marked by the shallow **radial groove,** which passes diagonally down the bone and parallel to the sloping posterior margin of the deltoid tuberosity (Fig. 7.46). The radial nerve and the profunda brachii artery lie in this groove.

Approximately in the middle of the shaft, the medial border is marked by a thin elongated roughening for the attachment of the coracobrachialis muscle (Fig. 7.46).

Intermuscular septa, which separate the anterior compartment from the posterior compartment, attach to the medial and lateral borders (Fig. 7.47A).

Distally, the humerus becomes flattened, and these borders expand as the **lateral supraepicondylar ridge (lateral**

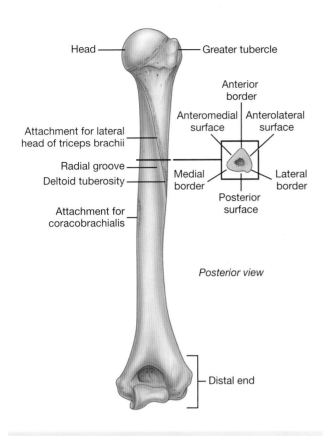

Fig. 7.46 Humerus. Posterior view.

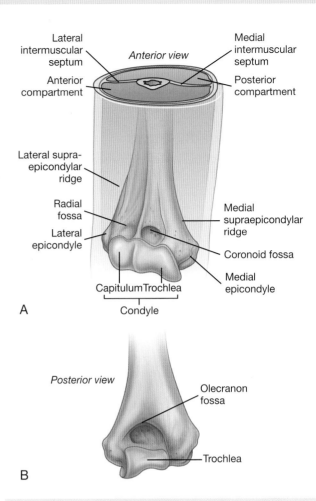

Fig. 7.47 Distal end of the humerus. **A.** Anterior view. **B.** Posterior view.

supracondylar ridge) and the **medial supraepicondylar ridge (medial supracondylar ridge)** (Fig. 7.47A). The lateral supraepicondylar ridge is more pronounced than the medial and is roughened for the attachment of muscles found in the posterior compartment of the forearm.

The distal end of the humerus, which is flattened in the anteroposterior plane, bears a condyle, two epicondyles, and three fossae, as follows.

The condyle

The two articular parts of the condyle, the **capitulum** and the **trochlea** (Fig. 7.47A), articulate with the two bones of the forearm.

The capitulum articulates with the radius of the forearm. Lateral in position and hemispherical in shape, it projects anteriorly and somewhat inferiorly and is not visible when the humerus is viewed from the posterior aspect.

The trochlea articulates with the ulna of the forearm. It is pulley shaped and lies medial to the capitulum. Its medial edge is more pronounced than its lateral edge and, unlike the capitulum, it extends onto the posterior surface of the bone.

The two epicondyles

The two epicondyles lie adjacent and somewhat superior to the trochlea and capitulum (Fig. 7.47A).

The **medial epicondyle,** a large bony protuberance, is the major palpable landmark on the medial side of the elbow and projects medially from the distal end of the humerus. On its surface, it bears a large oval impression for the attachment of muscles in the anterior compartment of the forearm (common flexor origin). The ulnar nerve passes from the arm into the forearm around the posterior surface of the medial epicondyle and can be palpated against the bone in this location.

The **lateral epicondyle** is much less pronounced than the medial epicondyle. It is lateral to the capitulum and has a large irregular impression for the attachment of muscles in the posterior compartment of the forearm (common extensor origin).

The three fossae

Three fossae occur superior to the trochlea and capitulum on the distal end of the humerus (Fig. 7.47).

The **radial fossa** is the least distinct of the fossae and occurs immediately superior to the capitulum on the anterior surface of the humerus.

The **coronoid fossa** is adjacent to the radial fossa and is superior to the trochlea.

The largest of the fossae, the **olecranon fossa,** occurs immediately superior to the trochlea on the posterior surface of the distal end of the humerus (Fig. 7.47B).

These three fossae accommodate projections from the bones in the forearm during movements of the elbow joint.

Proximal end of the radius

The proximal end of the radius consists of a head, a neck, and the radial tuberosity (Fig. 7.48).

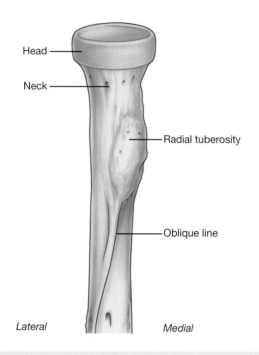

Fig. 7.48 Anterior view of the proximal end of the radius.

The **head** of the radius is a thick disc-shaped structure oriented in the horizontal plane. The circular superior surface is concave for articulation with the capitulum of the humerus. The thick margin of the disc is broad medially where it articulates with the radial notch on the proximal end of the ulna.

The **neck** of the radius is a short and narrow cylinder of bone between the expanded head and the radial tuberosity on the shaft.

The **radial tuberosity** is a large blunt projection medial to the distal part of the neck. Much of its surface is roughened for the attachment of the biceps brachii tendon. The oblique line of the radius continues diagonally across the shaft of the bone from the inferior margin of the radial tuberosity.

Proximal end of the ulna

The proximal end of the ulna is much larger than the proximal end of the radius and consists of the olecranon, the coronoid process, the trochlear notch, the radial notch, and the tuberosity of ulna (Fig. 7.49).

The **olecranon** is a large projection of bone that extends proximally from the ulna. Its anterolateral surface is articular and contributes to the formation of the trochlear notch, which articulates with the trochlea of the humerus. The superior surface is marked by a large roughened impression for the attachment of the triceps brachii muscle. The posterior surface is smooth, shaped somewhat triangularly, and can be palpated as the "tip of the elbow."

The **coronoid process** projects anteriorly from the proximal end of the ulna (Fig. 7.49). Its superolateral surface is articular and participates with the olecranon

Fig. 7.49 Lateral, anterior, medial, and posterior views of the proximal end of the ulna.

Table 7.8 Muscles of the anterior compartment of the arm (spinal segments indicated in **bold** are the major segments innervating the muscle)

Muscle	Origin	Insertion	Innervation	Function
Coracobrachialis	Apex of coracoid process	Linear roughening on mid-shaft of humerus on medial side	Musculocutaneous nerve [**C5, C6, C7**]	Flexor of the arm at the glenohumeral joint
Biceps brachii	Long head—supraglenoid tubercle of scapula; short head—apex of coracoid process	Radial tuberosity	Musculocutaneous nerve [**C5, C6**]	Powerful flexor of the forearm at the elbow joint and supinator of the forearm; accessory flexor of the arm at the glenohumeral joint
Brachialis	Anterior aspect of humerus (medial and lateral surfaces) and adjacent intermuscular septae	Tuberosity of the ulna	Musculocutaneous nerve [C5, **C6**]; (small contribution by the radial nerve [C7] to lateral part of muscle)	Powerful flexor of the forearm at the elbow joint

in forming the **trochlear notch.** The lateral surface is marked by the **radial notch** for articulation with the head of the radius.

Just inferior to the radial notch is a fossa that allows the radial tuberosity to change position during pronation and supination. The posterior margin of this fossa is broadened to form the **supinator crest.** The anterior surface of the coronoid process is triangular, with the apex directed distally, and has a number of roughenings for muscle attachment. The largest of these roughenings, the **tuberosity of ulna,** is at the apex of the anterior surface and is the attachment site for the brachialis muscle.

Clinical app

Rupture of biceps tendon

It is relatively unusual for muscles and their tendons to rupture in the upper limb; however, the tendon that most commonly ruptures is the tendon of the long head of the biceps brachii muscle. In isolation, this has relatively little effect on the upper limb, but it does produce a characteristic deformity—on flexing the elbow, there is an extremely prominent bulge of the muscle belly as its unrestrained fibers contract—the "Popeye" sign.

Muscles

The anterior compartment of the arm contains three muscles—the **coracobrachialis, brachialis,** and **biceps brachii** muscles (Table 7.8, Fig. 7.50)—which are innervated predominantly by the musculocutaneous nerve.

The posterior compartment contains one muscle—the **triceps brachii** muscle (Table 7.9, Fig. 7.51)—which is innervated by the radial nerve.

Nerves
Musculocutaneous nerve

The musculocutaneous nerve leaves the axilla and enters the arm by passing through the coracobrachialis muscle

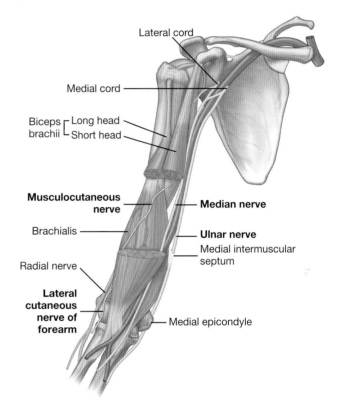

Fig. 7.50 Musculocutaneous, median, and ulnar nerves in the arm.

(Fig. 7.50). It passes diagonally down the arm in the plane between the biceps brachii and brachialis muscles. After giving rise to motor branches in the arm, it emerges laterally to the tendon of the biceps brachii muscle at the elbow, penetrates deep fascia, and continues as the **lateral cutaneous nerve** of forearm.

The musculocutaneous nerve provides:

- motor innervation to all muscles in the anterior compartment of the arm, and
- sensory innervation to skin on the lateral surface of the forearm.

Table 7.9 Muscle of the posterior compartment of the arm (spinal segments indicated in **bold** are the major segments innervating the muscle)

Muscle	Origin	Insertion	Innervation	Function
Triceps brachii	Long head—infraglenoid tubercle of scapula; medial head—posterior surface of humerus; lateral head—posterior surface of humerus	Olecranon	Radial nerve [C6, **C7**, C8]	Extension of the forearm at the elbow joint. Long head can also extend and adduct the arm at the shoulder joint

Fig. 7.51 Radial nerve in the arm.

Median nerve

The median nerve enters the arm from the axilla at the inferior margin of the teres major muscle (Fig. 7.50). It passes vertically down the medial side of the arm in the anterior compartment and is related to the brachial artery throughout its course:

- In proximal regions, the median nerve is immediately lateral to the brachial artery.
- In more distal regions, the median nerve crosses to the medial side of the brachial artery and lies anterior to the elbow joint.

The median nerve has no major branches in the arm, but a branch to one of the muscles of the forearm, the pronator teres muscle, may originate from the nerve immediately proximal to the elbow joint.

Clinical app

Median nerve injury in the arm

In the arm and forearm the median nerve is usually not injured by trauma because of its relatively deep position. On very rare occasions, a fibrous band may arise from the anterior aspect of the humerus beneath which the median nerve passes. This is an embryological remnant of the coracobrachialis muscle and is sometimes called the *ligament of Struthers;* occasionally, it may calcify. This band can compress the median nerve, resulting in weakness of the flexor muscles in the forearm and the thenar muscles in the hand. Nerve conduction studies can demonstrate the site of nerve compression.

Ulnar nerve

The ulnar nerve enters the arm with the median nerve and axillary artery (Fig. 7.50). It passes through proximal regions medial to the axillary artery. In the middle of the arm, the ulnar nerve penetrates the medial intermuscular septum and enters the posterior compartment where it lies anterior to the medial head of the triceps brachii muscle. It passes posterior to the medial epicondyle of the humerus and then into the anterior compartment of the forearm.

The ulnar nerve has no major branches in the arm.

Radial nerve

The radial nerve originates from the posterior cord of the brachial plexus and enters the arm by crossing the inferior margin of the teres major muscle (Fig. 7.51). As it enters the arm, it lies posterior to the brachial artery. Accompanied by the profunda brachii artery, the radial nerve enters the posterior compartment of the arm by passing through the triangular interval.

As the radial nerve passes diagonally from medial to lateral through the posterior compartment, it lies in the radial groove directly on bone. On the lateral side of the arm, it passes anteriorly through the lateral intermuscular septum and enters the anterior compartment where it lies between the brachialis muscle and a muscle of the posterior compartment of the forearm—the brachioradialis muscle, which attaches to the lateral supraepicondylar ridge of the humerus. The radial nerve enters the forearm anterior to the lateral epicondyle of the humerus just deep to the brachioradialis muscle.

In the arm, the radial nerve has muscular and cutaneous branches (Fig. 7.51).

Muscular branches include those to the triceps brachii, brachioradialis, and extensor carpi radialis longus muscles. In addition, the radial nerve contributes to the innervation of the lateral part of the brachialis muscle. One of the branches to the medial head of the triceps brachii muscle arises before the radial nerve's entrance into the posterior compartment and passes vertically down the arm in association with the ulnar nerve.

Cutaneous branches of the radial nerve that originate in the posterior compartment of the arm are the **inferior lateral cutaneous nerve** of arm and the **posterior cutaneous nerve of forearm,** both of which penetrate through the lateral head of the triceps brachii muscle and the overlying deep fascia to become subcutaneous.

Clinical app

Radial nerve injury in the arm
The radial nerve is tightly bound with the profunda brachii artery between the medial and lateral heads of the triceps brachii muscle in the radial groove. If the humerus is fractured (Fig. 7.52), the radial nerve may become stretched or transected in this region, leading to permanent damage and loss of function. The nerve should always be tested when a fracture of the mid-shaft of the humerus is suspected. The patient's symptoms usually include wrist drop (due to denervation of the extensor muscles) and sensory changes over the dorsum of the hand.

Fig. 7.52 Radiograph of the humerus demonstrating a mid-shaft fracture, which may disrupt the radial nerve.

A

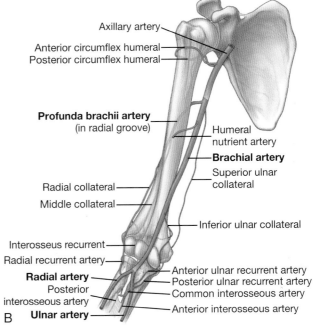

B

Fig. 7.53 Brachial artery. A. Brachial artery. B. Branches.

Arteries and veins
Brachial artery

The major artery of the arm, the **brachial artery,** is found in the anterior compartment (Fig. 7.53A). Beginning as a continuation of the axillary artery at the lower border of the teres major muscle, it terminates just distal to the elbow joint where it divides into the radial and ulnar arteries.

In the proximal arm, the brachial artery lies on the medial side. In the distal arm, it moves laterally to assume a position midway between the lateral epicondyle and the medial epicondyle of the humerus (Fig. 7.53A). It crosses anteriorly to the elbow joint where it lies immediately medial to the tendon of the biceps brachii muscle. The brachial artery is palpable along its length. In proximal regions, the brachial artery can be compressed against the medial side of the humerus.

Branches of the brachial artery in the arm include those to muscles and two ulnar collateral vessels, which contribute to a network of arteries around the elbow joint (Fig. 7.53B). Additional branches are the profunda brachii artery and nutrient arteries to the humerus, which pass through a foramen in the anteromedial surface of the humeral shaft.

Surface anatomy

Locating the brachial artery in the right arm

The brachial artery is on the medial side of the arm in the cleft between the biceps brachii and triceps brachii muscles (Fig. 7.54). The median nerve courses with the brachial artery, whereas the ulnar nerve deviates posteriorly from the vessel in distal regions.

Fig. 7.54 Locating the brachial artery in the right arm (medial view of arm with brachial artery, median nerve, and ulnar nerve).

Profunda brachii artery

The **profunda brachii artery,** the largest branch of the brachial artery, passes into and supplies the posterior compartment of the arm (Fig. 7.53B). It enters the posterior compartment with the radial nerve and together they pass

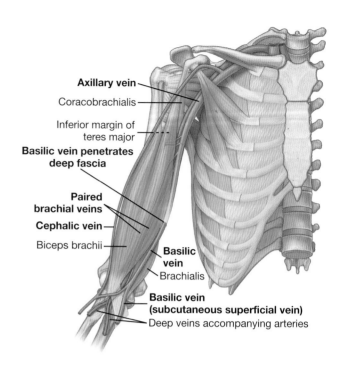

Fig. 7.55 Veins of the arm.

through the triangular interval, which is formed by the shaft of the humerus, the inferior margin of the teres major muscle, and the lateral margin of the long head of the triceps muscle. They then pass along the radial groove on the posterior surface of the humerus deep to the lateral head of the triceps brachii muscle.

Branches of the profunda brachii artery supply adjacent muscles and anastomose with the posterior circumflex humeral artery. The artery terminates as two collateral vessels, which contribute to an anastomotic network of arteries around the elbow joint.

Veins

Paired brachial veins pass along the medial and lateral sides of the brachial artery, receiving tributaries that accompany branches of the artery (Fig. 7.55).

In addition to these deep veins, two large subcutaneous veins, the basilic vein and the cephalic vein, are located in the arm (Fig. 7.55).

The basilic vein passes vertically in the distal half of the arm, penetrates deep fascia to assume a position medial to the brachial artery, and then becomes the axillary vein at the lower border of the teres major muscle. The brachial veins join the basilic, or axillary, vein.

The cephalic vein passes superiorly on the anterolateral aspect of the arm and through the anterior wall of the axilla to reach the axillary vein.

Fig. 7.57 Synovial membrane of elbow joint (anterior view).

Fig. 7.56 Components and movements of the elbow joint.
A. Bones and joint surfaces. **B.** Flexion and extension.
C. Pronation and supination.

ELBOW JOINT

The elbow joint is a complex joint involving three separate articulations that share a common synovial cavity (Fig. 7.56; also see Fig. 7.60).

The joints between the trochlear notch of the ulna and the trochlea of the humerus and between the head of the radius and the capitulum of the humerus are primarily involved with hinge-like flexion and extension of the forearm on the arm and, together, are the principal articulations of the elbow joint.

The joint between the head of the radius and the radial notch of the ulna, the proximal radioulnar joint, is involved with pronation and supination of the forearm.

The synovial membrane originates from the edges of the articular cartilage and lines the radial fossa, the coronoid fossa, the olecranon fossa, the deep surface of the joint capsule, and the medial surface of the trochlea (Fig. 7.57).

The synovial membrane is separated from the fibrous membrane of the joint capsule by pads of fat in regions overlying the coronoid fossa, the olecranon fossa, and the radial fossa (Fig. 7.57). These fat pads accommodate the related bony processes during extension and flexion of the elbow. Attachments of the brachialis and triceps brachii muscles to the joint capsule overlying these regions pull the attached fat pads out of the way when the adjacent bony processes are moved into the fossae.

The fibrous membrane of the joint capsule overlies the synovial membrane, encloses the joint, and attaches to the medial epicondyle and the margins of the olecranon, coronoid, and radial fossae of the humerus (Fig. 7.58). It also attaches to the coronoid process and olecranon of the ulna. On the lateral side, the free inferior margin of the joint capsule passes around the neck of the radius from an anterior attachment to the coronoid process of the ulna to a posterior attachment to the base of the olecranon.

The fibrous membrane of the joint capsule is thickened medially and laterally to form collateral ligaments, which support the flexion and extension movements of the elbow joint (Fig. 7.58).

405

Radial collateral ligament

Anular ligament of radius

Sacciform recess of synovial membrane

Ulnar collateral ligament

Fig. 7.58 Joint capsule and ligaments of the right elbow joint.

In addition, the external surface of the joint capsule is reinforced laterally where it cuffs the head of the radius with a strong **anular ligament of radius** (Fig. 7.58). Although this ligament blends with the fibrous membrane of the joint capsule in most regions, they are separate posteriorly. The anular ligament of radius also blends with the **radial collateral ligament** (Fig. 7.58).

The anular ligament of radius and related joint capsule allow the radial head to slide against the radial notch of the ulna and pivot on the capitulum during pronation and supination of the forearm.

The deep surface of the fibrous membrane of the joint capsule and the related anular ligament of radius that articulate with the sides of the radial head are lined by cartilage. A pocket of synovial membrane (sacciform recess) protrudes from the inferior free margin of the joint capsule and facilitates rotation of the radial head during pronation and supination (Fig. 7.58).

Vascular supply to the elbow joint is through an anastomotic network of vessels derived from collateral and recurrent branches of the brachial, profunda brachii, radial, and ulnar arteries.

The elbow joint is innervated predominantly by branches of the radial and musculocutaneous nerves, but there may be some innervation by branches of the ulnar and median nerves.

Imaging app

Developmental changes in the elbow joint

In an adult it is usually not difficult to interpret a radiograph, but in children developmental patterns have to be considered (Fig. 7.59).

As the elbow develops, numerous secondary ossification centers appear before and around puberty. It is easy to mistakenly interpret these as fractures. In addition, it is also possible for the epiphyses and apophyses to be "pulled off" or disrupted. Therefore when interpreting a child's radiograph of the elbow, the physician must know the child's age. Fusion occurs at around the time of puberty. The approximate ages of appearance of the secondary ossification centers around the elbow joint and are:

- capitulum—1 year,
- head (of radius)—5 years,
- medial epicondyle—5 years,
- trochlea—11 years,
- olecranon—12 years, and
- lateral epicondyle—13 years.

Fig. 7.59 Radiographs of elbow joint development. **A.** At age 2 years. **B.** At age 5 years. **C.** At age 5 or 6 years. **D.** At age 12 years.

Imaging app

Visualizing the elbow joint

Humerus

Lateral epicondyle

Medial epicondyle

Capitulum

Trochlea

Head of radius

Radius

Ulna

A

Radial tuberosity Capitulum Humerus

B

Coronoid process Trochlear notch Olecranon

Radial collateral ligament Humerus Medial epicondyle

C

Head of radius Ulna Ulnar collateral ligament

Fig. 7.60 Elbow joint **A.** Radiograph (anteroposterior view). **B.** Radiograph (lateral view). **C.** Magnetic resonance image (coronal plane).

Clinical app

Supracondylar fracture of the humerus

Elbow injuries in children may result in a transverse fracture of the distal end of the humerus above the level of the epicondyles. This fracture is termed a *supracondylar fracture.* The distal fragment and its soft tissues are pulled posteriorly by the triceps muscle. This posterior displacement effectively "bowstrings" the brachial artery over the irregular proximal fracture fragment. In children, this is a relatively devastating injury: the muscles of the anterior compartment of the forearm are rendered ischemic and form severe contractions, significantly reducing the function of the anterior compartment and flexor muscles (Volkmann's ischemic contracture).

Clinical app

Pulled elbow

Pulled elbow is a disorder that typically occurs in children younger than 5 years of age. It is commonly caused by a sharp pull of the child's hand, usually when the child is pulled up onto a curb. The not-yet-developed head of the radius and the laxity of the anular ligament of radius allow the head to sublux from this cuff of tissue.

Clinical app

Fracture of the head of radius

A fracture of the head of radius is a common injury and can cause appreciable morbidity. It is one of the typical injuries that occur with a fall on the outstretched hand. On falling, the force is transmitted to the radial head, which fractures. These fractures result in loss of full extension, and potential surgical reconstruction may require long periods of physiotherapy to obtain a full range of movement at the elbow joint.

Clinical app

"Tennis" and "golfer's" elbow (epicondylitis)

It is not uncommon for people who are involved in sports such as golf and tennis to develop an overuse strain of the origins of the flexor and extensor muscles of the forearm. The pain is typically around the epicondyles and usually resolves after rest. If pain and inflammation persist, surgical division of the extensor or flexor origin from the bone may be necessary. Typically, in tennis players this pain occurs on the lateral epicondyle and common extensor origin (tennis elbow), whereas in golfers it occurs on the medial epicondyle and common flexor origin (golfer's elbow).

Clinical app

Ulnar nerve injury at the elbow

Posterior to the medial epicondyle of the humerus, the ulnar nerve is bound in a fibro-osseous tunnel (the cubital tunnel) by a retinaculum. Older patients may develop degenerative changes within this tunnel, which compresses the ulnar nerve when the elbow joint is flexed. The repeated action of flexion and extension of the elbow joint may cause local nerve damage, resulting in impaired function of the ulnar nerve. Localized neuritis in this region secondary to direct trauma may also produce ulnar nerve damage.

CUBITAL FOSSA

The cubital fossa is an important area of transition between the arm and the forearm. It is located anterior to the elbow joint and appears as a triangular depression formed between two forearm muscles (Fig. 7.61A):

- the brachioradialis muscle originating from the lateral supraepicondylar ridge of the humerus, and
- the pronator teres muscle originating from the medial epicondyle of the humerus.

The base of the triangle is an imaginary horizontal line between the medial and lateral epicondyles. The bed or floor of the fossa is formed mainly by the brachialis muscle.

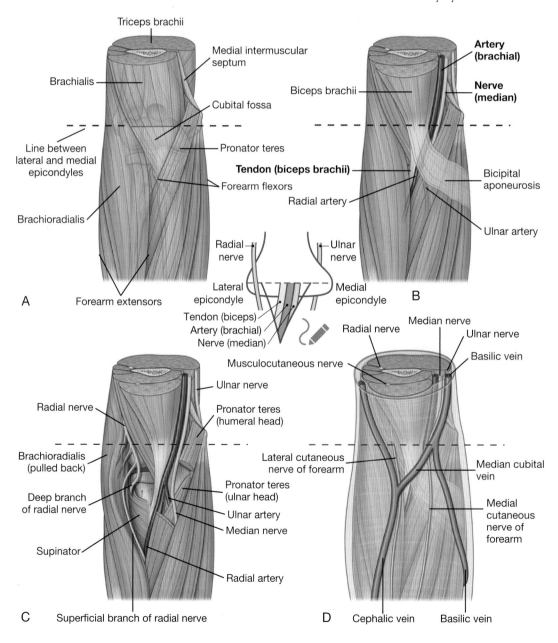

Fig. 7.61 Cubital fossa. A. Margins. B. Contents. C. Position of the radial nerve. D. Superficial structures.

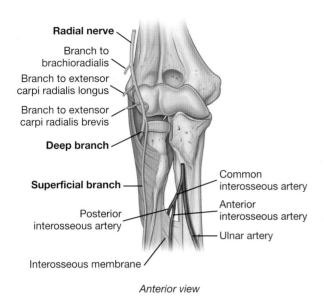

Radial nerve
Branch to brachioradialis
Branch to extensor carpi radialis longus
Branch to extensor carpi radialis brevis
Deep branch
Superficial branch
Posterior interosseous artery
Interosseous membrane
Common interosseous artery
Anterior interosseous artery
Ulnar artery

Anterior view

Fig. 7.62 Radial nerve in posterior compartment of forearm.

The major contents of the cubital fossa from lateral to medial are (Fig. 7.61B):

- the tendon of the biceps brachii muscle,
- the brachial artery, and
- the median nerve.

The brachial artery normally bifurcates into the radial and ulnar arteries in the apex of the fossa, although this bifurcation may occur much higher in the arm, even in the axilla (Fig. 7.61C). When taking a blood pressure reading from a patient, the clinician places the stethoscope over the brachial artery in the cubital fossa.

The median nerve lies immediately medial to the brachial artery and leaves the fossa by passing between the ulnar and humeral heads of the pronator teres muscle (Fig. 7.61C).

The brachial artery and the median nerve are covered and protected anteriorly in the distal part of the cubital fossa by the bicipital aponeurosis (Fig. 7.61B). This flat connective tissue membrane passes between the medial side of the tendon of the biceps brachii muscle and deep fascia of the forearm. The sharp medial margin of the bicipital aponeurosis can often be felt.

The radial nerve lies just under the lip of the brachioradialis muscle, which forms the lateral margin of the fossa (Fig. 7.61C). In this position, the radial nerve divides into superficial and deep branches:

- The superficial branch continues into the forearm just deep to the brachioradialis muscle.
- The deep branch passes between the two heads of the supinator muscle (Fig. 7.62) to access the posterior compartment of the forearm.

The ulnar nerve does not pass through the cubital fossa. Instead, it passes posterior to the medial epicondyle.

The roof of the cubital fossa is formed by superficial fascia and skin. The most important structure within the roof is the median cubital vein (Fig. 7.61D), which passes diagonally across the roof and connects the cephalic vein on the lateral side of the upper limb with the basilic vein on the medial side. The bicipital aponeurosis separates the median cubital vein from the brachial artery and median nerve. Other structures within the roof are cutaneous nerves—the medial cutaneous and lateral cutaneous nerves of the forearm.

Clinical app

Construction of a dialysis fistula

Many patients throughout the world require renal dialysis for kidney failure. The patient's blood is filtered and cleaned by the dialysis machine. Blood therefore has to be taken from patients into the filtering device and then returned to them. This process of dialysis occurs over many hours and requires flow rates of 250 to 500 mL/min. To enable such large volumes of blood to be removed from and returned to the body, the blood is taken from vessels that have a high flow. As no veins in the peripheral limbs have such high flow, a surgical procedure is necessary to create such a system. In most patients, the brachial artery is anastomosed (joined) to the cephalic vein at the elbow, or the radial artery is anastomosed to the cephalic vein at the wrist. Some surgeons place an arterial graft between these vessels. After 6 weeks, the veins increase in size in response to their arterial blood flow and are amenable to direct cannulation or dialysis.

Clinical app

Blood pressure measurement

Blood pressure measurement is an extremely important physiological parameter. High blood pressure (hypertension) requires treatment to prevent long-term complications such as stroke. Low blood pressure may be caused by extreme blood loss, widespread infection, or poor cardiac output (e.g., after myocardial infarction). Accurate measurement of blood pressure is essential.

Most clinicians use a sphygmomanometer and a stethoscope. The sphygmomanometer is a device that inflates a cuff around the midportion of the arm to compress the brachial artery against the humerus. The cuff is inflated so it exceeds the systolic blood pressure (greater than 120 mm Hg). The clinician places a stethoscope over the brachial artery in the cubital fossa and listens (auscultates) for the pulse. As the pressure in the arm cuff of the sphygmomanometer is reduced just below the level of the systolic blood pressure, the pulse becomes audible as a regular thumping sound. As the pressure in the sphygmomanometer continues to drop, the regular thumping sound becomes clearer. When the pressure in

Continued

Clinical app—cont'd

the sphygmomanometer is less than that of the diastolic blood pressure, the audible thumping sound becomes inaudible. Using the simple scale on the sphygmomanometer, the patient's blood pressure can be determined. The normal range is 90–120/60–80 mm Hg (systolic blood pressure/diastolic blood pressure).

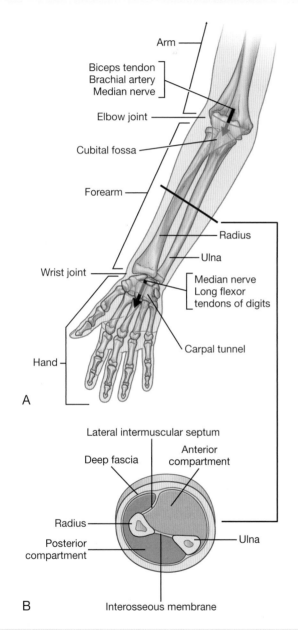

Fig. 7.63 Forearm. **A.** Proximal and distal relationships of the forearm. **B.** Transverse section through the middle of the forearm.

FOREARM

The forearm is the part of the upper limb that extends between the elbow joint and the wrist joint.

Structures pass between the forearm and the hand through, or anterior to, the carpal tunnel (Fig. 7.63A). The

major exception is the radial artery, which passes dorsally around the wrist to enter the hand posteriorly.

The bone framework of the forearm consists of two parallel bones, the radius and the ulna (Figs. 7.63A, 7.65). The radius is lateral in position and is small proximally where it articulates with the humerus and large distally where it forms the wrist joint with the carpal bones of the hand.

The ulna is medial in the forearm, and its proximal and distal dimensions are the reverse of those for the radius: the ulna is large proximally and small distally. Proximal and distal joints between the radius and the ulna allow the distal end of the radius to swing over the adjacent end of the ulna, resulting in pronation and supination of the hand.

As in the arm, the forearm is divided into anterior and posterior compartments (Fig. 7.63B). In the forearm, these compartments are separated by:

- a lateral intermuscular septum, which passes from the anterior border of the radius to deep fascia surrounding the limb;
- an interosseous membrane, which links adjacent borders of the radius and ulna along most of their length; and
- the attachment of deep fascia along the posterior border of the ulna.

Muscles in the anterior compartment of the forearm flex the wrist and digits and pronate the hand. Muscles in the posterior compartment extend the wrist and digits and supinate the hand. Major nerves and vessels supply or pass through each compartment.

Bones
Shaft and distal end of radius

The shaft of the radius is narrow proximally where it is continuous with the radial tuberosity and neck, and much broader distally where it expands to form the distal end (Fig. 7.64).

Throughout most of its length, the shaft of the radius is triangular in cross-section and has (Fig. 7.64):

- three borders (anterior, posterior, and interosseous), and
- three surfaces (anterior, posterior, and lateral).

The **anterior border** begins on the medial side of the bone as a continuation of the radial tuberosity. In the superior third of the bone, it crosses the shaft diagonally, from medial to lateral, as the oblique line of the radius. The **posterior border** is distinct only in the middle third of the bone. The **interosseous border** is sharp and is the attachment site for the interosseous membrane, which links the radius to the ulna.

The anterior and posterior surfaces of the radius are generally smooth, whereas an oval roughening for the attachment of pronator teres marks approximately the middle of the lateral surface of the radius.

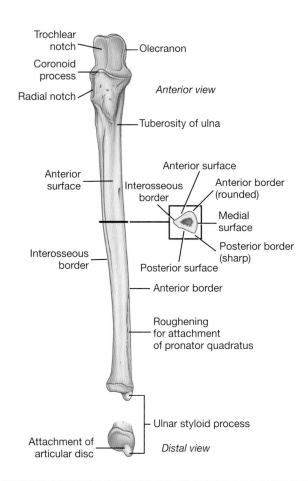

Fig. 7.64 Shaft and distal end of the right radius.

Imaging app

Visualizing the forearm

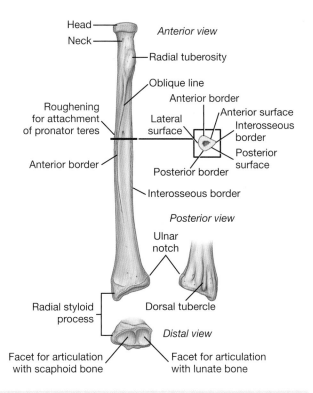

Fig. 7.65 Radiograph of the forearm (anteroposterior view).

Fig. 7.66 Shaft and distal end of right ulna.

Viewed anteriorly, the distal end of the radius is broad and somewhat flattened anteroposteriorly (Fig. 7.64). Consequently, the radius has expansive anterior and posterior parts and narrow medial and lateral parts. Its anterior surface is smooth and unremarkable, except for the prominent sharp ridge that forms its lateral margin.

The posterior part of the radius is characterized by the presence of a large **dorsal tubercle** (Fig. 7.64) that acts as a pulley for the tendon of one of the extensor muscles of the thumb (extensor pollicis longus). The medial part is marked by a prominent facet for articulation with the distal end of the ulna (Fig. 7.64). The lateral part of the distal end of the radius is diamond shaped and extends distally as a **radial styloid process** (Fig. 7.64).

The distal end of the bone is marked by two facets for articulation with two carpal bones (the scaphoid and lunate) (Fig. 7.64).

Shaft and distal end of ulna

The shaft of the ulna is broad superiorly where it is continuous with the large proximal end and narrow distally to form a small distal head (Fig. 7.66). Like the radius, the shaft of the ulna is triangular in cross-section and has:

411

- three borders (anterior, posterior, and interosseous), and
- three surfaces (anterior, posterior, and medial).

The **anterior border** is smooth and rounded. The **posterior border** is sharp and palpable along its entire length. The interosseous border is also sharp and is the attachment site for the interosseous membrane, which joins the ulna to the radius.

The **anterior surface** of the ulna is smooth, except distally where there is a prominent linear roughening for the attachment of the pronator quadratus muscle. The **medial surface** is smooth and unremarkable. The **posterior surface** is marked by lines that separate different regions of muscle attachments to bone.

The distal end of the ulna is small and characterized by a rounded head and the **ulnar styloid process** (Fig. 7.66). The anterolateral and distal part of the head is covered by articular cartilage. The ulnar styloid process originates from the posteromedial aspect of the ulna and projects distally.

Clinical app

Fractures of the radius and ulna
When a severe injury occurs to the forearm it usually involves both bones, resulting in either fracture of both bones or more commonly a fracture of one bone and a dislocation of the other. Commonly, the mechanism of injury and the age of the patient determine which of these are likely to occur. Whenever a fracture of the radius or ulna is demonstrated radiographically, further images of the elbow and wrist should be obtained to exclude dislocations.

Joints
Distal radioulnar joint

The distal radioulnar joint occurs between the articular surface of the head of the ulna with the ulnar notch on the end of the radius and with a fibrous articular disc, which separates the radioulnar joint from the wrist joint (Fig. 7.67).

The triangular-shaped articular disc is attached by its apex to a roughened depression on the ulna between the styloid process and the articular surface of the head and by its base to the angular margin of the radius between the ulnar notch and the articular surface for the carpal bones.

Synovial membrane is attached to the margins of the distal radioulnar joint and is covered on its external surface by a fibrous joint capsule.

The distal radioulnar joint allows the distal end of the radius to move anteromedially over the ulna.

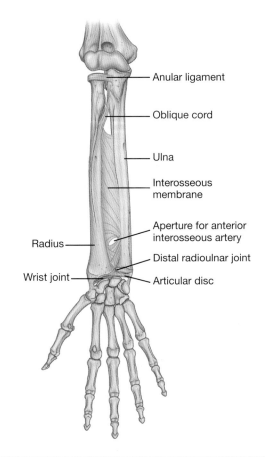

Fig. 7.67 Distal radioulnar joint and the interosseous membrane.

Interosseous membrane

The interosseous membrane is a thin fibrous sheet that connects the medial and lateral borders of the radius and ulna, respectively (Fig. 7.67). Collagen fibers within the sheet pass predominantly inferiorly from the radius to the ulna.

The interosseous membrane has a free upper margin that is situated just inferior to the radial tuberosity and a small circular aperture in its distal third. Vessels pass between the anterior and posterior compartments superior to the upper margin and through the inferior aperture.

The interosseous membrane connects the radius and ulna without restricting pronation and supination and provides attachment for muscles in the anterior and posterior compartments. The orientation of fibers in the membrane is also consistent with its role in transferring forces from the radius to the ulna and ultimately, therefore, from the hand to the humerus.

Pronation and supination

Pronation and supination of the hand occur entirely in the forearm and involve rotation of the radius at the elbow and movement of the distal end of the radius over the ulna (Fig. 7.68).

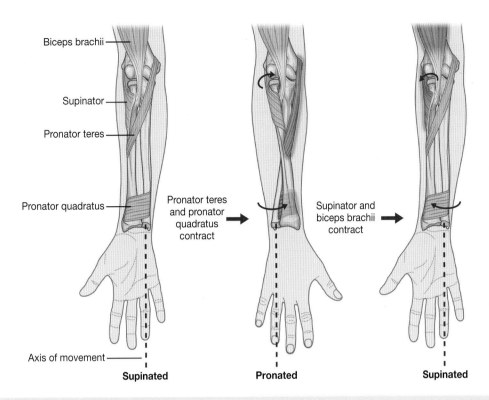

Biceps brachii

Supinator

Pronator teres

Pronator quadratus

Pronator teres
and pronator
quadratus
contract

Supinator and
biceps brachii
contract

Axis of movement

Supinated

Pronated

Supinated

Fig. 7.68 Pronation and supination.

At the elbow, the superior articular surface of the radial head spins on the capitulum while the articular surface on the side of the head slides against the radial notch of the ulna and adjacent areas of the joint capsule and anular ligament of radius. At the distal radioulnar joint, the ulnar notch of the radius slides anteriorly over the convex surface of the head of the ulna. During these movements, the bones are held together by:

- the anular ligament of radius at the proximal radioulnar joint,
- the interosseous membrane along the lengths of the radius and ulna, and
- the articular disc at the distal radioulnar joint.

Because the hand articulates predominantly with the radius, the translocation of the distal end of the radius medially over the ulna moves the hand from the palm-anterior (supinated) position to the palm-posterior (pronated) position.

Two muscles (biceps brachii and supinator) supinate and two muscles (pronator teres and pronator quadratus) pronate the hand (Fig. 7.68).

Abduction of the ulna during pronation

Abduction of the distal end of the ulna occurs during pronation to maintain the position of the palm of the hand over a central point (Fig. 7.69). The muscle involved in this

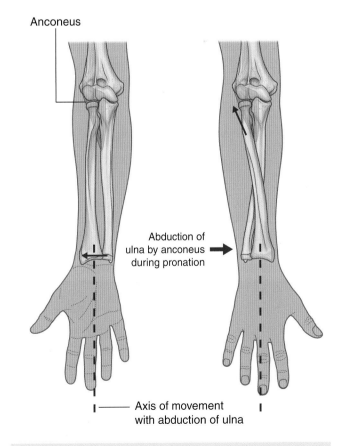

Anconeus

Abduction of
ulna by anconeus
during pronation

Axis of movement
with abduction of ulna

Fig. 7.69 Abduction of the distal end of the ulna by the anconeus muscle during pronation.

Table 7.10 Superficial layer of muscles in the anterior compartment of the forearm (spinal segments indicated in **bold** are the major segments innervating the muscle)

Muscle	Origin	Insertion	Innervation	Function
Flexor carpi ulnaris	Humeral head—medial epicondyle of humerus; ulnar head—olecranon and posterior border of ulna	Pisiform bone, and then via pisohamate and pisometacarpal ligaments into the hamate and base of metacarpal V	Ulnar nerve [C7, **C8**, T1]	Flexes and adducts the wrist joint
Palmaris longus (absent in 15% of the population)	Medial epicondyle of humerus	Palmar aponeurosis of hand	Median nerve [**C7, C8**]	Flexes wrist joint; because the palmar aponeurosis anchors skin of the hand, contraction of the muscle resists shearing forces when gripping
Flexor carpi radialis	Medial epicondyle of humerus	Base of metacarpals II and III	Median nerve [**C6, C7**]	Flexes and abducts the wrist
Pronator teres	Humeral head—medial epicondyle and adjacent supraepicondylar ridge; ulnar head—medial side of coronoid process	Roughening on lateral surface, mid-shaft of radius	Median nerve [**C6, C7**]	Pronation

movement is the anconeus muscle, which is a triangular muscle in the posterior compartment of the forearm that runs from the lateral epicondyle to the lateral surface of the proximal end of the ulna.

ANTERIOR COMPARTMENT OF THE FOREARM

Muscles

Muscles in the anterior (flexor) compartment of the forearm occur in three layers: superficial, intermediate, and deep. Generally, these muscles are associated with:

- movements of the wrist joint,
- flexion of the fingers including the thumb, and
- pronation.

All muscles in the anterior compartment of the forearm are innervated by the median nerve, except for the flexor carpi ulnaris muscle and the medial half of the flexor digitorum profundus muscle, which are innervated by the ulnar nerve.

Superficial layer

All four muscles in the superficial layer—the **flexor carpi ulnaris, palmaris longus, flexor carpi radialis, and pronator teres**—have a common origin from the medial epicondyle of the humerus and, except for the pronator teres, extend distally from the forearm into the hand (Table 7.10, Fig. 7.70).

Intermediate layer

The only muscle in the intermediate layer of the anterior compartment of the forearm is the **flexor digitorum superficialis** muscle (Table 7.11, Fig. 7.71).

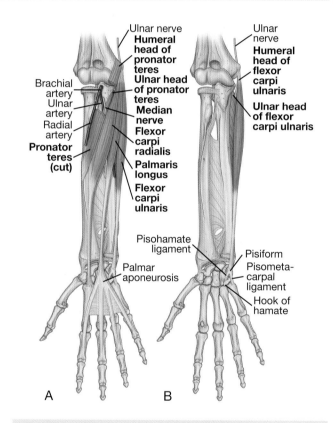

Fig. 7.70 Superficial layer of forearm muscles. A. Superficial muscles (flexor retinaculum not shown). B. Flexor carpi ulnaris muscle.

Deep layer

There are three deep muscles in the anterior compartment of the forearm: **the flexor digitorum profundus, flexor pollicis longus,** and **pronator quadratus** (Table 7.12, Fig. 7.72).

Arteries and veins

The largest arteries in the forearm are in the anterior compartment, pass distally to supply the hand, and give rise to vessels that supply the posterior compartment (Fig. 7.73).

414

Table 7.11 Intermediate layer of muscles in the anterior compartment of the forearm (spinal segments indicated in **bold** are the major segments innervating the muscle)

Muscle	Origin	Insertion	Innervation	Function
Flexor digitorum superficialis	Humeroulnar head—medial epicondyle of humerus and adjacent margin of coronoid process; radial head—oblique line of radius	Four tendons that attach to the palmar surfaces of the middle phalanges of the index, middle, ring, and little fingers	Median nerve [**C8**, T1]	Flexes proximal interphalangeal joints of the index, middle, ring, and little fingers; can also flex metacarpophalangeal joints of the same fingers and the wrist joint

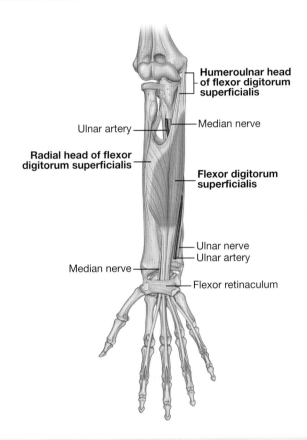

Fig. 7.71 Intermediate layer of forearm muscles.

The brachial artery enters the forearm from the arm by passing through the cubital fossa. At the apex of the cubital fossa, it divides into its two major branches, the radial and ulnar arteries.

Radial artery

The radial artery originates from the brachial artery at approximately the neck of the radius and passes along the lateral aspect of the forearm (Fig. 7.73). It is:

- just deep to the brachioradialis muscle in the proximal half of the forearm;
- related on its lateral side to the superficial branch of the radial nerve in the middle third of the forearm;
- medial to the tendon of the brachioradialis muscle and covered only by deep fascia, superficial fascia, and skin in the distal forearm.

In the distal forearm, the radial artery lies immediately lateral to the large tendon of the flexor carpi radialis muscle and directly anterior to the pronator quadratus muscle and the distal end of the radius (Fig. 7.73).

The radial artery leaves the forearm, passes around the lateral side of the wrist, and penetrates the posterolateral aspect of the hand between the bases of metacarpals I and II (Fig. 7.73). Branches of the radial artery in the hand often provide the major blood supply to the thumb and lateral side of the index finger.

Branches of the radial artery originating in the forearm include:

- a **radial recurrent artery,** which contributes to an anastomotic network around the elbow joint and to numerous vessels that supply muscles on the lateral side of the forearm (see Fig. 7.53B);
- a small **palmar carpal branch,** which contributes to an anastomotic network of vessels that supply the carpal bones and joints; and
- a somewhat larger branch, the **superficial palmar branch,** which enters the hand by passing through, or superficial to, the thenar muscles at the base of the thumb (Fig. 7.73), which anastomoses with the superficial palmar arch formed by the ulnar artery.

Ulnar artery

The ulnar artery is larger than the radial artery and passes down the medial side of the forearm (Fig. 7.73). It leaves the cubital fossa by passing deep to the pronator teres muscle and then passes through the forearm in the fascial plane between the flexor carpi ulnaris and flexor digitorum profundus muscles.

In the distal forearm, the ulnar artery often remains tucked under the lateral lip of the flexor carpi ulnaris tendon.

In distal regions of the forearm, the ulnar nerve is immediately medial to the ulnar artery.

The ulnar artery leaves the forearm, enters the hand by passing lateral to the pisiform bone and superficial to the flexor retinaculum of the wrist, and arches over the palm (Fig. 7.73). It is often the major blood supply to the medial three and one-half digits.

Table 7.12 Deep layer of muscles in the anterior compartment of the forearm (spinal segments indicated in **bold** are the major segments innervating the muscle)

Muscle	Origin	Insertion	Innervation	Function
Flexor digitorum profundus	Anterior and medial surfaces of ulna and anterior medial half of interosseous membrane	Four tendons, which attach to the palmar surfaces of the distal phalanges of the index, middle, ring, and little fingers	Lateral half by median nerve (anterior interosseous nerve); medial half by ulnar nerve [**C8**, T1]	Flexes distal interphalangeal joints of the index, middle, ring, and little fingers; can also flex metacarpophalangeal joints of the same fingers and the wrist joint
Flexor pollicis longus	Anterior surface of radius and radial half of interosseous membrane	Palmar surface of base of distal phalanx of thumb	Median nerve (anterior interosseous nerve) [C7, **C8**]	Flexes interphalangeal joint of the thumb; can also flex metacarpophalangeal joint of the thumb
Pronator quadratus	Linear ridge on distal anterior surface of ulna	Distal anterior surface of radius	Median nerve (anterior interosseous nerve) [C7, **C8**]	Pronation

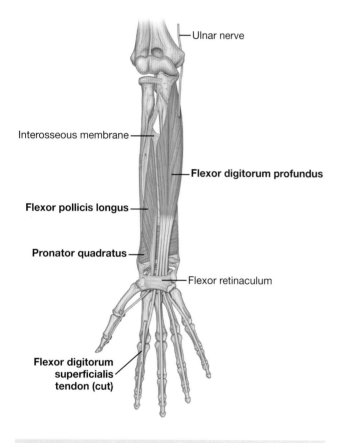

Fig. 7.72 Deep layer of forearm muscles.

Branches of the ulnar artery that arise in the forearm include:

- the **ulnar recurrent artery** with **anterior** and **posterior branches,** which contribute to an anastomotic network of vessels around the elbow joint (see Fig. 7.53B);
- numerous muscular arteries, which supply surrounding muscles;
- the **common interosseous artery,** which divides into **anterior** and **posterior interosseous arteries** (Fig. 7.73); and

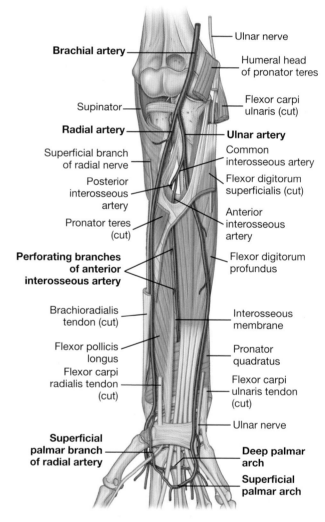

Fig. 7.73 Arteries of the anterior compartment of the forearm.

- two small carpal arteries (**dorsal carpal branch** and **palmar carpal branch**), which supply the wrist.

The **posterior interosseous artery** passes dorsally over the proximal margin of the interosseous membrane into the posterior compartment of the forearm.

The **anterior interosseous artery** passes distally along the anterior aspect of the interosseous membrane and supplies muscles of the deep compartment of the forearm and the radius and ulna (Fig. 7.73). It has numerous branches, which perforate the interosseous membrane to supply deep muscles of the posterior compartment; it also has a small branch, which contributes to the vascular network around the carpal bones and joints. Perforating the interosseous membrane in the distal forearm, the anterior interosseous artery terminates by joining the posterior interosseous artery.

Veins

Deep veins of the anterior compartment generally accompany the arteries and ultimately drain into brachial veins associated with the brachial artery in the cubital fossa.

Nerves

Nerves in the anterior compartment of the forearm are the median and ulnar nerves and the superficial branch of the radial nerve (Fig. 7.74).

Median nerve

The median nerve innervates the muscles in the anterior compartment of the forearm except for the flexor carpi ulnaris and the medial part of the flexor digitorum profundus (ring and little fingers). It leaves the cubital fossa by passing between the two heads of the pronator teres muscle and passing between the humeroulnar and radial heads of the flexor digitorum superficialis muscle (Fig. 7.74).

The median nerve continues a straight linear course distally down the forearm in the fascia on the deep surface of the flexor digitorum superficialis muscle. Just proximal to the wrist, it moves around the lateral side of the muscle and becomes more superficial in position, lying between the tendons of the palmaris longus and flexor carpi radialis muscles. It leaves the forearm and enters the palm of the hand by passing through the carpal tunnel deep to the flexor retinaculum (Fig. 7.74).

Most branches to the muscles in the superficial and intermediate layers of the forearm originate medially from the nerve just distal to the elbow joint (Fig. 7.74).

The largest branch of the median nerve in the forearm is the **anterior interosseous nerve,** which originates between the two heads of the pronator teres. It passes distally down the forearm with the anterior interosseous artery, innervates the muscles in the deep layer (the flexor pollicis longus, the lateral half of flexor digitorum profundus, and pronator quadratus), and terminates as articular branches to joints of the distal forearm and wrist.

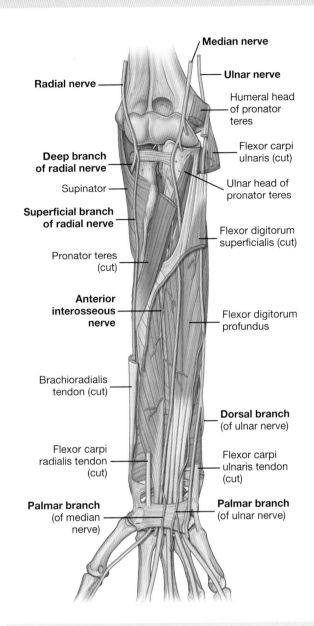

Fig. 7.74 Nerves of anterior forearm.

A small **palmar branch** originates from the median nerve in the distal forearm immediately proximal to the flexor retinaculum, passes superficial to the flexor retinaculum of the wrist into the hand, and innervates the skin over the base and central palm.

Ulnar nerve

The ulnar nerve passes through the forearm and into the hand where most of its major branches occur. In the forearm, the ulnar nerve innervates only the flexor carpi ulnaris muscle and the medial part (ring and little fingers) of the flexor digitorum profundus muscle (Fig. 7.74).

The ulnar nerve enters the anterior compartment of the forearm by passing posteriorly around the medial epicondyle of the humerus and between the humeral and ulnar heads of the flexor carpi ulnaris muscle. After passing down the medial side of the forearm in the plane between the flexor carpi ulnaris and the flexor digitorum profundus muscles, it lies under the lateral lip of the tendon of the flexor carpi ulnaris proximal to the wrist.

The ulnar artery is lateral to the ulnar nerve in the distal two-thirds of the forearm, and both the ulnar artery and nerve enter the hand by passing superficial to the flexor retinaculum and immediately lateral to the pisiform bone (Fig. 7.74).

In the forearm the ulnar nerve gives rise to:

- **muscular branches** to the flexor carpi ulnaris and to the medial half of the flexor digitorum profundus that arise soon after the ulnar nerve enters the forearm; and
- two small cutaneous branches—the **palmar branch** originates in the middle of the forearm and passes into the hand to supply skin on the medial side of the palm (Fig. 7.74), and the larger **dorsal branch** originates from the ulnar nerve in the distal forearm and passes posteriorly deep to the tendon of the flexor carpi ulnaris and innervates skin on the posteromedial side of the back of the hand and most skin on the posterior surfaces of the medial one and one-half digits (Fig. 7.74).

Radial nerve

The radial nerve bifurcates into deep and superficial branches under the margin of the brachioradialis muscle in the lateral border of the cubital fossa (Fig. 7.74).

The **deep branch** is predominantly motor and passes between the superficial and deep layers of the supinator muscle to access and supply muscles in the posterior compartment of the forearm.

The **superficial branch** of the radial nerve is sensory. It passes down the anterolateral aspect of the forearm deep to the brachioradialis muscle and in association with the radial artery. Approximately two-thirds of the way down the forearm, the superficial branch of the radial nerve passes laterally and posteriorly around the radial side of the forearm deep to the tendon of the brachioradialis. The nerve continues into the hand where it innervates skin on the posterolateral surface.

POSTERIOR COMPARTMENT OF THE FOREARM

Muscles

Muscles in the posterior compartment of the forearm occur in two layers: a superficial and a deep layer. The muscles are associated with:

- movement of the wrist joint,
- extension of the fingers and thumb, and
- supination.

All muscles in the posterior compartment of the forearm are innervated by the radial nerve.

Superficial layer

The seven muscles in the superficial layer are the **brachioradialis, extensor carpi radialis longus, extensor carpi radialis brevis, extensor digitorum, extensor digiti minimi, extensor carpi ulnaris,** and **anconeus** (Table 7.13, Fig. 7.75). All have a common origin from the supraepicondylar ridge and lateral epicondyle of the humerus and, except for the brachioradialis and anconeus, extend as tendons into the hand.

Deep layer

The deep layer of the posterior compartment of the forearm consists of five muscles: **supinator, abductor pollicis longus, extensor pollicis brevis, extensor pollicis longus, and extensor indicis** (Table 7.14, Fig. 7.76).

Except for the supinator muscle, all these deep layer muscles originate from the posterior surfaces of the radius, ulna, and interosseous membrane and pass into the thumb and fingers.

Three of these muscles—the abductor pollicis longus, extensor pollicis brevis, and extensor pollicis longus—emerge from between the extensor digitorum and the extensor carpi radialis brevis tendons of the superficial layer and pass into the thumb.

Two of these three "outcropping" muscles (the abductor pollicis longus and extensor pollicis brevis) form a distinct muscular bulge in the distal posterolateral surface of the forearm.

All muscles of the deep layer are innervated by the posterior interosseous nerve, the continuation of the deep branch of the radial nerve.

Arteries and veins

The blood supply to the posterior compartment of the forearm occurs predominantly through branches of the radial, posterior interosseous, and anterior interosseous arteries (Fig. 7.77; also see Fig. 7.73).

Posterior interosseous artery

The posterior interosseous artery originates in the anterior compartment from the common interosseous branch of the ulnar artery and passes posteriorly over the proximal margin of the interosseous membrane and into the posterior compartment of the forearm (see Fig. 7.73). It contributes a branch, the **recurrent**

Table 7.13 Superficial layer of muscles in the posterior compartment of the forearm (spinal segments indicated in **bold** are the major segments innervating the muscle)

Muscle	Origin	Insertion	Innervation	Function
Brachioradialis	Proximal part of lateral supraepicondylar ridge of humerus and adjacent intermuscular septum	Lateral surface of distal end of radius	Radial nerve [C5, **C6**] before division into superficial and deep branches	Accessory flexor of elbow joint when forearm is mid-pronated
Extensor carpi radialis longus	Distal part of lateral supraepicondylar ridge of humerus and adjacent intermuscular septum	Dorsal surface of base of metacarpal II	Radial nerve [**C6**, C7] before division into superficial and deep branches	Extends and abducts the wrist
Extensor carpi radialis brevis	Lateral epicondyle of humerus and adjacent intermuscular septum	Dorsal surface of base of metacarpals II and III	Deep branch of radial nerve [**C7**, C8] before penetrating supinator muscle	Extends and abducts the wrist
Extensor digitorum	Lateral epicondyle of humerus and adjacent intermuscular septum and deep fascia	Four tendons, which insert via extensor hoods into the dorsal aspects of the bases of the middle and distal phalanges of the index, middle, ring, and little fingers	Posterior interosseous nerve [**C7**, C8]	Extends the index, middle, ring, and little fingers; can also extend the wrist
Extensor digiti minimi	Lateral epicondyle of humerus and adjacent intermuscular septum together with extensor digitorum	Extensor hood of the little finger	Posterior interosseous nerve [**C7**, C8]	Extends the little finger
Extensor carpi ulnaris	Lateral epicondyle of humerus and posterior border of ulna	Tubercle on the base of the medial side of metacarpal V	Posterior interosseous nerve [**C7**, C8]	Extends and adducts the wrist
Anconeus	Lateral epicondyle of humerus	Olecranon and proximal posterior surface of ulna	Radial nerve [C6, C7, C8] (via branch to medial head of triceps brachii)	Abduction of the ulna in pronation; accessory extensor of the elbow joint

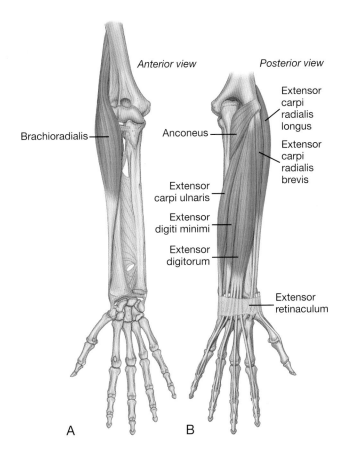

Anterior view　　*Posterior view*

Brachioradialis

Anconeus

Extensor carpi ulnaris

Extensor digiti minimi

Extensor digitorum

Extensor carpi radialis longus

Extensor carpi radialis brevis

Extensor retinaculum

A　　B

Fig. 7.75 Superficial layer of muscles in the posterior compartment of the forearm. A. Brachioradialis muscle (anterior view). B. Superficial muscles (posterior view).

interosseous artery (see Fig. 7.53B) to the vascular network around the elbow joint and then passes between the supinator and abductor pollicis longus muscles to supply the superficial extensors (Fig. 7.77). After receiving the terminal end of the anterior interosseous artery, the posterior interosseous artery terminates by joining the dorsal carpal arch of the wrist.

Anterior interosseous artery

The anterior interosseous artery, also a branch of the common interosseous branch of the ulnar artery (see Fig. 7.73), is situated in the anterior compartment of the forearm on the interosseous membrane. It has numerous perforating branches that pass directly through the interosseous membrane to supply deep muscles of the posterior compartment. The terminal end of the anterior interosseous artery passes posteriorly through an aperture in the interosseous membrane in distal regions of the forearm to join the posterior interosseous artery (Fig. 7.77).

Radial artery

The radial artery has muscular branches that contribute to the supply of the extensor muscles on the radial side of the forearm.

Veins

Deep veins of the posterior compartment generally accompany the arteries. They ultimately drain into brachial veins associated with the brachial artery in the cubital fossa.

Table 7.14 Deep layer of muscles in the posterior compartment of the forearm (spinal segments indicated in **bold** are the major segments innervating the muscle)

Muscle	Origin	Insertion	Innervation	Function
Supinator	Superficial layer—lateral epicondyle of humerus, radial collateral and anular ligaments; deep layer—supinator crest of the ulna	Lateral surface of radius superior to the anterior oblique line	Posterior interosseous nerve [**C6**, C7]	Supination
Abductor pollicis longus	Posterior surfaces of ulna and radius (distal to the attachments of supinator and anconeus), and intervening interosseous membrane	Lateral side of base of metacarpal I	Posterior interosseous nerve [**C7**, C8]	Abducts carpometacarpal joint of thumb; accessory extensor of the thumb
Extensor pollicis brevis	Posterior surface of radius (distal to abductor pollicis longus) and the adjacent interosseous membrane	Dorsal surface of base of proximal phalanx of the thumb	Posterior interosseous nerve [**C7**, C8]	Extends metacarpophalangeal joint of the thumb; can also extend the carpometacarpal joint of the thumb
Extensor pollicis longus	Posterior surface of ulna (distal to the abductor pollicis longus) and the adjacent interosseous membrane	Dorsal surface of base of distal phalanx of thumb	Posterior interosseous nerve [**C7**, C8]	Extends interphalangeal joint of the thumb; can also extend carpometacarpal and metacarpophalangeal joints of the thumb
Extensor indicis	Posterior surface of ulna (distal to extensor pollicis longus) and adjacent interosseous membrane	Extensor hood of index finger	Posterior interosseous nerve [**C7**, C8]	Extends index finger

Fig. 7.76 Deep layer of muscles in the posterior compartment of the forearm.

Fig 7.77 Arteries and radial nerve in the posterior compartment of the forearm.

Nerves
Radial nerve

The nerve of the posterior compartment of the forearm is the radial nerve (Fig. 7.77). Most of the muscles are innervated by the deep branch, which originates from the radial nerve in the lateral wall of the cubital fossa deep to the brachioradialis muscle and becomes **the posterior interosseous nerve** (Fig. 7.77), after emerging from between the two layers of the supinator muscle in the posterior compartment of the forearm (Fig. 7.77).

In the lateral wall of the cubital fossa and before dividing into **superficial** and **deep branches,** the radial nerve innervates the brachioradialis and extensor carpi radialis longus muscles.

The deep branch innervates the extensor carpi radialis brevis then passes between the two heads of the supinator muscle and follows the plane of separation between the two heads dorsally and laterally around the proximal shaft of the radius to the posterior aspect of the forearm. It supplies the supinator muscle and then emerges as the **posterior interosseous nerve** from the muscle to lie between the superficial and deep layers of muscles.

The posterior interosseous nerve supplies the remaining muscles in the posterior compartment and terminates as articular branches, which pass deep to the extensor pollicis longus muscle to reach the wrist.

Surface anatomy

Identifying tendons and locating major vessels and nerves in the distal forearm

Tendons that pass from the forearm into the hand are readily visible in the distal forearm and can be used as landmarks to locate major vessels and nerves.

In the anterior aspect of the distal forearm, the tendons of the flexor carpi radialis, flexor carpi ulnaris, and palmaris longus muscles can be easily located either by palpating or by asking a patient to flex the wrist against resistance (Fig. 7.78A).

The tendon of flexor carpi radialis is located approximately at the junction between the lateral and middle thirds of an imaginary line drawn transversely across the distal forearm. The radial artery is immediately lateral to this tendon, and this site is used for taking a radial pulse (Fig. 7.78A).

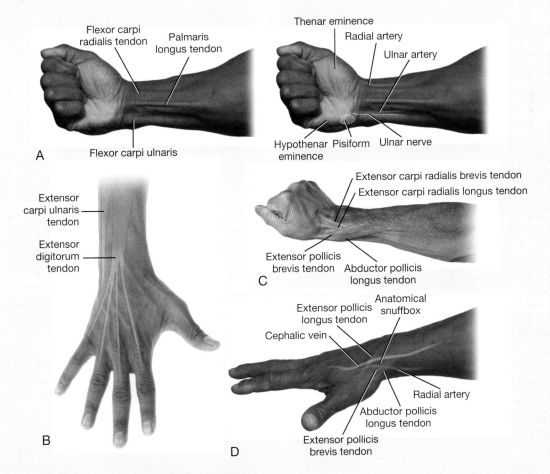

Fig. 7.78 Identifying tendons and locating major vessels and nerves in the distal right forearm. **A.** Anterior distal forearm and wrist. **B.** Posterior distal forearm and wrist. **C.** Lateral view of posterior wrist and forearm. **D.** Anatomical snuffbox.

Continued

Surface anatomy—cont'd

The tendon of the flexor carpi ulnaris is easily palpated along the medial margin of the forearm and inserts on the pisiform, which can also be palpated by following the tendon to the base of the hypothenar eminence of the hand (Fig. 7.78A). The ulnar artery and ulnar nerve travel through the distal forearm and into the hand under the lateral lip of the flexor carpi ulnaris tendon and lateral to the pisiform (Fig. 7.78A).

The palmaris longus tendon may be absent but, when present, lies medial to the flexor carpi radialis tendon and is particularly prominent when the wrist is flexed against resistance (Fig. 7.78A). The median nerve is also medial to the flexor carpi radialis tendon and lies under the palmaris longus tendon.

The long tendons of the digits of the hand are deep to the median nerve and between the long flexors of the wrist. Their position can be visualized by rapidly and repeatedly flexing and extending the fingers from medial to lateral.

In the posterior distal forearm and wrist, the tendons of the extensor digitorum (Fig. 7.78B) are in the midline and radiate into the index, middle, ring, and little fingers from the wrist.

The distal ends of the tendons of the extensor carpi radialis longus and brevis muscles are on the lateral side of the wrist (Fig. 7.78C) and can be accentuated by making a tight fist and extending the wrist against resistance.

The tendon of the extensor carpi ulnaris can be felt on the far medial side of the wrist between the distal end of the ulna and the wrist (Fig. 7.78B).

Hyperextension and abduction of the thumb reveals the anatomical snuffbox (Fig. 7.78D). The medial margin of this triangular area is the tendon of the extensor pollicis longus, which swings around the dorsal tubercle of the radius and then travels into the thumb. The lateral margin is formed by the tendons of the extensor pollicis brevis and abductor pollicis longus. The radial artery passes through the anatomical snuffbox when traveling laterally around the wrist to reach the back of the hand and penetrate the base of the first dorsal interosseous muscle to access the deep aspect of the palm of the hand. The pulse of the radial artery can be felt in the floor of the anatomical snuffbox in the relaxed wrist (Fig. 7.78D). The cephalic vein crosses the roof of the anatomical snuffbox, and cutaneous branches of the radial nerve can be felt by moving a finger back and forth along the tendon of the extensor pollicis longus muscle.

HAND

The hand (Fig. 7.79) is the region of the upper limb distal to the wrist joint and is a mechanical and sensory tool. It is subdivided into three parts:

- the wrist (carpus),
- the metacarpus, and
- the digits (five fingers including the thumb).

The five digits consist of the laterally positioned thumb; medial to the thumb are the remaining four fingers—the index, middle, ring, and little fingers.

In the normal resting position, the fingers form a flexed arcade, with the little finger flexed most and the index finger flexed least. In the anatomical position, the fingers are extended.

The hand has an anterior surface (**palm**) and a dorsal surface (**dorsum of hand**).

Abduction and adduction of the fingers are defined with respect to the long axis of the middle finger (Fig. 7.79). In the anatomical position, the long axis of the thumb is rotated 90° to the rest of the digits so that the pad of the thumb points medially; consequently, movements of the thumb are defined at right angles to the movements of the other digits of the hand.

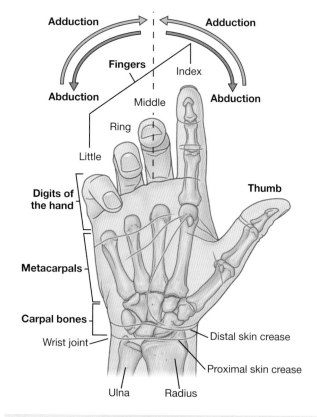

Fig. 7.79 Right hand. The fingers are shown in a normal resting arcade in which they are flexed. In the anatomical position, the digits are straight and adducted.

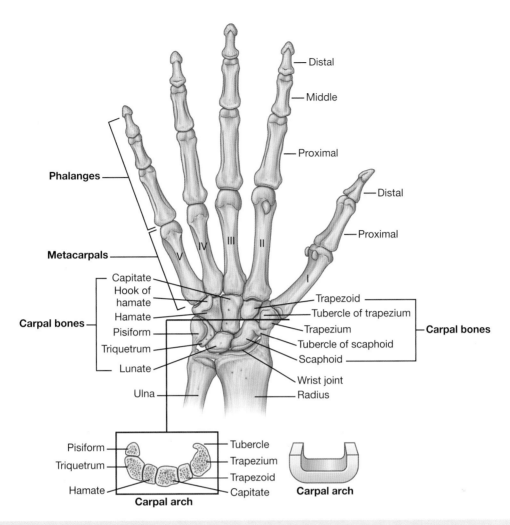

Fig 7.80 Bones of the right hand and wrist.

Bones

There are three groups of bones in the hand (Figs. 7.80; 7.81A):

- The eight **carpal bones** are the bones of the wrist.
- The five **metacarpals (I to V)** are the bones of the metacarpus.
- The **phalanges** are the bones of the digits—the thumb has only two, the rest of the digits have three (Fig. 7.80).

The carpal bones and metacarpals of the index, middle, ring, and little fingers (metacarpals II to V) tend to function as a unit and form much of the bony framework of the palm. The metacarpal bone of the thumb functions independently and has increased flexibility at the carpometacarpal joint to provide opposition of the thumb to the fingers.

Carpal bones

The small carpal bones of the wrist are arranged in two rows, a proximal and a distal row, each consisting of four bones (Fig. 7.80).

Proximal row

From lateral to medial and when viewed anteriorly, the proximal row of bones consists of (Fig. 7.80):

- the boat-shaped **scaphoid,**
- the **lunate,** which has a crescent shape,
- the three-sided **triquetrum,** and
- the pea-shaped **pisiform.**

The pisiform is a sesamoid bone in the tendon of the flexor carpi ulnaris and articulates with the anterior surface of the triquetrum.

The scaphoid has a prominent **tubercle** on its lateral palmar surface that is directed anteriorly.

Distal row

From lateral to medial and when viewed anteriorly, the distal row of carpal bones consists of (Fig. 7.80):

- the irregular four-sided **trapezium,**

423

- the four-sided **trapezoid,**
- the **capitate,** which has a head, and
- the **hamate,** which has a hook.

The trapezium articulates with the metacarpal bone of the thumb and has a distinct **tubercle** on its palmar surface that projects anteriorly.

The largest of the carpal bones, the capitate, articulates with the base of metacarpal III.

The hamate, which is positioned just lateral and distal to the pisiform, has a prominent hook **(hook of hamate)** on its palmar surface that projects anteriorly.

Articular surfaces

The carpal bones have numerous articular surfaces (Fig. 7.80). All of them articulate with each other, and the carpal bones in the distal row articulate with the metacarpals of the digits. With the exception of the metacarpal of the thumb, all movements of the metacarpal bones on the carpal bones are limited.

The expansive proximal surfaces of the scaphoid and lunate articulate with the radius to form the wrist joint (Figs. 7.80, 7.81B).

Carpal arch

The carpal bones do not lie in a flat plane; rather they form an arch whose base is directed anteriorly (Fig. 7.80). The lateral side of this base is formed by the tubercles of the scaphoid and trapezium. The medial side is formed by the pisiform and the hook of hamate.

The flexor retinaculum attaches to and spans the distance between the medial and lateral sides of the base to form the anterior wall of the so-called carpal tunnel. The sides and roof of the carpal tunnel are formed by the arch of the carpal bones.

Metacarpals

Each of the five metacarpal bones is related to one digit (Figs. 7.80, 7.81A):

- Metacarpal I is related to the thumb.
- Metacarpals II to V are related to the index, middle, ring, and little fingers, respectively.

Each metacarpal consists of a **base,** a **shaft (body),** and, distally, a **head.**

Imaging app

Visualizing the hand and wrist joint

Fig. 7.81 Hand and wrist joint. **A.** Radiograph of a normal hand and wrist joint (anteroposterior view). **B.** Magnetic resonance image of a normal wrist joint in the coronal plane.

All of the bases of the metacarpals articulate with the carpal bones; in addition, the bases of the metacarpal bones of the fingers articulate with each other.

All of the heads of the metacarpal bones articulate with the proximal phalanges of the digits. The heads form the knuckles on the dorsal surface of the hand when the fingers are flexed.

Phalanges

The phalanges are the bones of the digits (Figs. 7.80, 7.81A):

- The thumb has two—a **proximal** and a **distal phalanx.**
- The rest of the digits have three—a **proximal**, a **middle**, and a **distal phalanx.**

Each phalanx has a **base**, a **shaft (body)**, and, distally, a **head.**

The base of each proximal phalanx articulates with the head of the related metacarpal bone.

The head of each distal phalanx is nonarticular and flattened into a crescent-shaped palmar tuberosity, which lies under the palmar pad at the end of the digit.

Joints
Wrist joint

The wrist joint is a synovial joint between the distal end of the radius and the articular disc overlying the distal end of the ulna and the scaphoid, lunate, and triquetrum (Fig. 7.81B; also see Fig. 7.80). Together, the articular surfaces of the carpals form an oval shape with a convex contour that articulates with the corresponding concave surface of the radius and articular disc.

The wrist joint allows movement around two axes. The hand can be abducted, adducted, flexed, and extended at the wrist joint.

The capsule of the wrist joint is reinforced by **palmar radiocarpal, palmar ulnocarpal,** and **dorsal radiocarpal ligaments.** In addition, **radial and ulnar collateral ligaments of the wrist joint** span the distance between the styloid processes of the radius and ulna and the adjacent carpal bones. These ligaments reinforce the medial and lateral sides of the wrist joint and support them during flexion and extension.

Carpal joints

The synovial joints between the carpal bones share a common articular cavity. The joint capsule of the joints is reinforced by numerous ligaments.

Although movement at the **carpal joints (intercarpal joints)** is limited, they do contribute to the positioning of the hand in abduction, adduction, flexion, and, particularly, extension.

Carpometacarpal joints

There are five carpometacarpal joints between the metacarpals and the related distal row of carpal bones (Fig. 7.81B; also see Fig. 7.80).

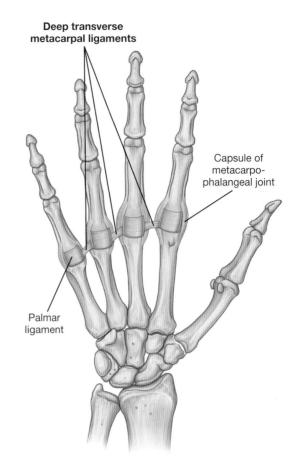

Fig. 7.82 Deep transverse metacarpal ligaments, right hand.

The saddle joint between metacarpal I and the trapezium imparts a wide range of mobility to the thumb that is not a feature of the rest of the digits. Movements at this carpometacarpal joint are flexion, extension, abduction, adduction, rotation, and circumduction.

The carpometacarpal joints between metacarpals II to V and the carpal bones are much less mobile than the carpometacarpal joint of the thumb, allowing only limited gliding movements. Movement of the joints increases medially, so metacarpal V slides to the greatest degree. This can be best observed on the dorsal surface of the hand as it makes a fist.

Metacarpophalangeal joints

The joints between the distal heads of the metacarpals and the proximal phalanges of the digits are condylar joints, which allow flexion, extension, abduction, adduction, circumduction, and limited rotation. The capsule of each joint is reinforced by the **palmar ligament** and by **medial** and **lateral collateral ligaments** (Fig. 7.82).

Deep transverse metacarpal ligaments

The three deep **transverse metacarpal ligaments** (Fig. 7.82) are thick bands of connective tissue connecting the palmar ligaments of the metacarpophalangeal joints of the fingers to each other. They are important because, by linking the heads of the metacarpal bones together, they restrict the movement of these bones relative to each other. As a result, they help form a unified skeletal framework for the palm of the hand.

Significantly, a deep transverse metacarpal ligament does not occur between the palmar ligament of the metacarpophalangeal joint of the thumb and the palmar ligament of the index finger. The absence of this ligament and the presence of a saddle joint between metacarpal I and the trapezium are responsible for the increased mobility of the thumb relative to the rest of the digits of the hand.

Interphalangeal joints of hand

The interphalangeal joints of the hand are hinge joints that allow mainly flexion and extension. They are reinforced by medial and lateral **collateral ligaments** and **palmar ligaments.**

Clinical app

Fracture of the scaphoid and avascular necrosis of the proximal scaphoid

The most common carpal injury is a fracture across the waist of the scaphoid bone (Fig. 7.83B). In approximately 10% of individuals, the scaphoid bone has a sole blood supply from the radial artery, which enters through the distal portion of the bone to supply the proximal portion. When a fracture occurs across the waist of the scaphoid, the proximal portion therefore undergoes avascular necrosis.

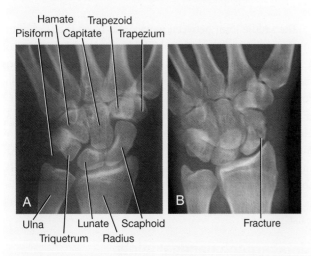

Fig. 7.83 Wrist radiographs (posterior–anterior view).

Double jointed

Double jointed refers to hypermobility of a joint due to increased range of motion. Increased range of motion can be caused by permissive shapes of joint surfaces and more flexible capsule and ligaments. It can also be related to pathology.

Clinical app

Knuckle cracking

Knuckle cracking refers to the sound made when the metacarpophalangeal joints are forcefully flexed. The sound is made by the explosive formation of a gas bubble in the joint during the flexion.

Carpal tunnel and structures at the wrist

The carpal tunnel is formed anteriorly at the wrist by a deep arch formed by the carpal bones and the flexor retinaculum (Fig. 7.84).

The base of the carpal arch is formed medially by the pisiform and the hook of the hamate and laterally by the tubercles of the scaphoid and trapezium.

The flexor retinaculum is a thick connective tissue ligament that bridges the space between the medial and lateral sides of the base of the arch and converts the carpal arch into the carpal tunnel.

The four tendons of the flexor digitorum profundus, the four tendons of the flexor digitorum superficialis, and the tendon of the flexor pollicis longus pass through the carpal tunnel, as does the median nerve (Fig. 7.84).

The flexor retinaculum holds the tendons to the bony plane at the wrist and prevents them from "bowing."

Free movement of the tendons in the carpal tunnel is facilitated by synovial sheaths, which surround the tendons. All the tendons of the flexor digitorum profundus and flexor digitorum superficialis are surrounded by a single synovial sheath; a separate sheath surrounds the tendon of the flexor pollicis longus. The median nerve is anterior to the tendons in the carpal tunnel.

The tendon of the flexor carpi radialis is surrounded by a synovial sheath and passes through a tubular compartment formed by the attachment of the lateral aspect of the flexor retinaculum to the margins of a groove on the medial side of the tubercle of trapezium.

The ulnar artery, ulnar nerve, and the tendon of the palmaris longus pass into the hand anterior to the flexor retinaculum and therefore do not pass through the carpal tunnel (Fig. 7.84). The tendon of the palmaris longus is not surrounded by a synovial sheath.

The radial artery passes dorsally around the lateral side of the wrist and lies adjacent to the external surface of the scaphoid.

The extensor tendons pass into the hand on the medial, lateral, and posterior surfaces of the wrist in six compartments defined by an extensor retinaculum and lined by synovial sheaths (Fig. 7.84):

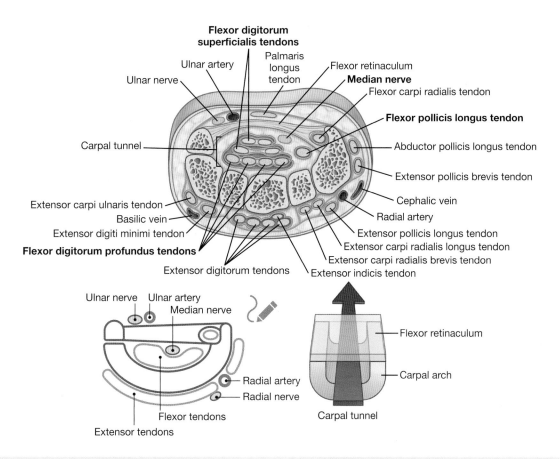

Fig. 7.84 Carpal tunnel. Structure and relations.

- The tendons of the extensor digitorum and extensor indicis share a compartment and synovial sheath on the posterior surface of the wrist.
- The tendons of the extensor carpi ulnaris and extensor digiti minimi have separate compartments and sheaths on the medial side of the wrist.
- The tendons of the abductor pollicis longus and extensor pollicis brevis muscles, the extensor carpi radialis longus and extensor carpi radialis brevis muscles, and the extensor pollicis longus muscle pass through three compartments on the lateral surface of the wrist.

Clinical app

De Quervain syndrome

De Quervain syndrome is an inflammatory disorder that occurs within the first dorsal extensor compartment and involves the extensor pollicis brevis and abductor pollicis longus tendon and their common tendon sheath. Patients typically present with significant wrist pain preventing appropriate flexion/extension and abduction of the thumb. The cause of this disorder is often overuse. For example, the syndrome is common in young mothers who are constantly lifting young children. Other causes include inflammatory disorders such as rheumatoid arthritis.

Palmar aponeurosis

The **palmar aponeurosis** is a triangular condensation of deep fascia that covers the palm and is anchored to the skin in distal regions (Fig. 7.86).

Surface anatomy

Position of the flexor retinaculum and the recurrent branch of the median nerve

The proximal margin of the flexor retinaculum can be determined using two bony landmarks (Fig. 7.85).

The pisiform bone is readily palpable at the distal end of the flexor carpi ulnaris tendon.

The tubercle of the scaphoid can be palpated at the distal end of the flexor carpi radialis tendon as it enters the wrist.

An imaginary line between these two points marks the proximal margin of the flexor retinaculum. The distal margin of the flexor retinaculum is approximately deep to the point where the anterior margin of the thenar eminence meets the hypothenar eminence near the base of the palm.

The recurrent branch of the median nerve lies deep to the skin and deep fascia overlying the anterior margin of the thenar eminence near the midline of the palm (Fig. 7.85).

Continued

Surface anatomy—cont'd

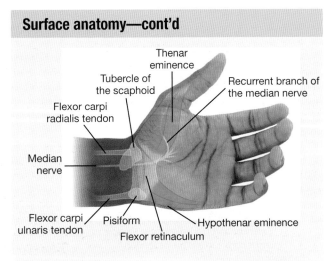

Fig. 7.85 Anterior hand to show the position of the flexor retinaculum and recurrent branch of the median nerve in the left hand.

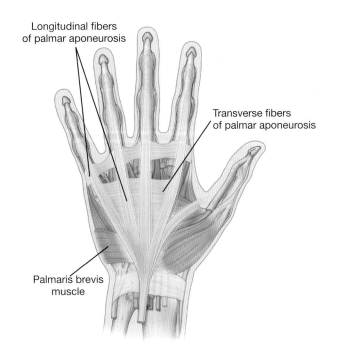

Fig. 7.86 Palmar aponeurosis, right hand.

Clinical app

Carpal tunnel syndrome

Carpal tunnel syndrome is an entrapment syndrome caused by pressure on the median nerve within the carpal tunnel.

Patients typically report pain and pins and needles in the distribution of the median nerve in the hand. Weakness and loss of muscle bulk of the thenar muscles may also occur. Gently tapping over the median nerve (in the region of the flexor retinaculum) readily produces these symptoms (Tinel's sign).

The apex of the triangle is continuous with the palmaris longus tendon when present; otherwise it is anchored to the flexor retinaculum. From this point, fibers radiate to extensions at the base of the digits that project into each of the index, middle, ring, and little fingers and, to a lesser extent, the thumb.

Transverse fibers interconnect the more longitudinally arranged bundles that continue into the digits.

Vessels, nerves, and long flexor tendons lie deep to the palmar aponeurosis in the palm.

Anatomical snuffbox

The *anatomical snuffbox* is a term given to the triangular depression formed on the posterolateral side of the wrist and metacarpal I by the extensor tendons passing into the thumb (Fig. 7.87). Historically, ground tobacco (snuff) was placed in this depression before being inhaled into the nose. The base of the triangle is at

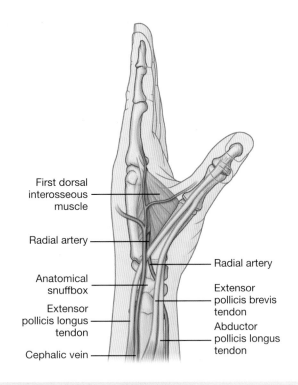

Fig. 7.87 Anatomical snuffbox, left hand.

the wrist, and the apex is directed into the thumb. The impression is most apparent when the thumb is extended:

- The lateral border is formed by the tendons of the abductor pollicis longus and extensor pollicis brevis.
- The medial border is formed by the tendon of the extensor pollicis longus.

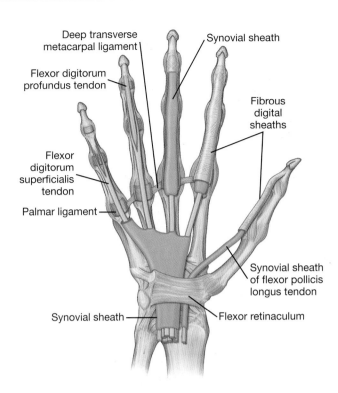

Deep transverse metacarpal ligament

Synovial sheath

Flexor digitorum profundus tendon

Fibrous digital sheaths

Flexor digitorum superficialis tendon

Palmar ligament

Synovial sheath of flexor pollicis longus tendon

Synovial sheath

Flexor retinaculum

Fig. 7.88 Fibrous digital sheaths and synovial sheaths of the right hand.

- The floor of the impression is formed by the scaphoid, trapezium, and the distal ends of the tendons of the extensor carpi radialis longus and extensor carpi radialis brevis.

The radial artery passes obliquely through the anatomical snuffbox deep to the extensor tendons of the thumb and lies adjacent to the scaphoid and trapezium.

Terminal parts of the superficial branch of the radial nerve pass subcutaneously over the snuffbox as does the origin of the cephalic vein from the dorsal venous arch of the hand.

Fibrous digital sheaths

After exiting the carpal tunnel, the tendons of the flexor digitorum superficialis and profundus muscles cross the palm and enter fibrous sheaths on the palmar aspect of the digits (Fig. 7.88). These fibrous sheaths:

- begin proximally, anterior to the metacarpophalangeal joints, and extend to the distal phalanges;
- are formed by fibrous arches and cruciate (cross-shaped) ligaments, which are attached posteriorly to the margins of the phalanges and to the palmar ligaments associated with the metacarpophalangeal and interphalangeal joints; and
- hold the tendons to the bony plane and prevent the tendons from bowing when the digits are flexed.

Within each tunnel, the tendons are surrounded by a synovial sheath. The synovial sheaths of the thumb and little finger are continuous with the sheaths associated with the tendons in the carpal tunnel (Fig. 7.88).

Clinical app

Tenosynovitis

Tenosynovitis is inflammation of a tendon and its sheath. The condition may be due to overuse; however, it can also be associated with other disorders such as rheumatoid arthritis and connective tissue pathologies. If the inflammation becomes severe and ensuing fibrosis occurs, the tendon will not run smoothly within the tendon sheath and typically within the fingers, the tendon may stick or may require excess force to fully extend and flex, producing a "triggering" phenomenon.

Clinical app

Trigger finger

Trigger finger is a common disorder of late childhood and adulthood and is typically characterized by catching or snapping and occasionally locking of the flexor tendon(s) in the hand. Trigger finger can be associated with significant dysfunction and pain. The triggering is usually related to fibrosis and tightening of the flexor tendon sheath at the level of the metacarpophalangeal joint.

Extensor hoods

The tendons of the extensor digitorum and extensor pollicis longus muscles pass onto the dorsal aspect of the digits and expand over the proximal phalanges to form complex **"extensor hoods"** or **"dorsal digital expansions"** (Fig. 7.89). The tendons of the extensor digiti minimi, extensor indicis, and extensor pollicis brevis muscles join these hoods.

Each extensor hood is triangular with:

- the apex attached to the distal phalanx;
- the central region attached to the middle phalanx (index, middle, ring, and little fingers) or proximal phalanx (thumb); and
- each corner of the base wrapped around the sides of the metacarpophalangeal joint—in the index, middle, ring, and little fingers, the corners of the hoods attach mainly to the deep transverse metacarpal ligaments; in the thumb, the hood is attached on each side to muscles.

Fig. 7.89 Extensor hood, left hand.

In addition to other attachments, many of the intrinsic muscles of the hand insert into the free margin of the hood on each side. By inserting into the extensor hood, these intrinsic muscles are responsible for complex delicate movements of the digits that could not be accomplished with the long flexor and extensor tendons alone.

In the index, middle, ring, and little fingers, the lumbrical, interossei, and abductor digiti minimi muscles attach to the extensor hoods. In the thumb, the adductor pollicis and abductor pollicis brevis muscles insert into and anchor the extensor hood.

Because force from the small intrinsic muscles of the hand is applied to the extensor hood distal to the fulcrum of the metacarpophalangeal joints, the muscles flex these joints (Fig. 7.89). Simultaneously, the force is transferred dorsally through the hood to extend the interphalangeal joints. This ability to flex the metacarpophalangeal joints while extending the interphalangeal joints is entirely due to the intrinsic

muscles of the hand working through the extensor hoods. This type of precision movement is used in the upstroke when writing a *t* (Fig. 7.89).

Muscles

The intrinsic muscles of the hand are the palmaris brevis, interossei, adductor pollicis, thenar, hypothenar, and lumbrical muscles (Table 7.15, Figs. 7.90 to 7.94). Unlike the extrinsic muscles that originate in the forearm, insert in the hand, and function in forcefully gripping ("power grip") with the hand, the intrinsic muscles occur entirely in the hand and mainly execute precision movements ("precision grip") with the fingers and thumb.

All of the intrinsic muscles of the hand are innervated by the deep branch of the ulnar nerve except for the three thenar and two lateral lumbrical muscles, which are innervated by the median nerve. The intrinsic muscles are predominantly

Table 7.15 Intrinsic muscles of the hand (spinal segments indicated in **bold** are the major segments innervating the muscle)

Muscles	Origin	Insertion	Innervation	Function
Palmaris brevis	Palmar aponeurosis and flexor retinaculum	Dermis of skin on the medial margin of the hand	Superficial branch of the ulnar nerve [C8, **T1**]	Improves grip
Dorsal interossei (four muscles)	Adjacent sides of metacarpals	Extensor hood and base of proximal phalanges of index, middle, and ring fingers	Deep branch of ulnar nerve [C8, **T1**]	Abduction of index, middle, and ring fingers at the metacarpophalangeal joints
Palmar interossei (four muscles)	Sides of metacarpals	Extensor hoods of the thumb, index, ring, and little fingers and the proximal phalanx of thumb	Deep branch of ulnar nerve [C8, **T1**]	Adduction of the thumb, index, ring, and little fingers at the metacarpophalangeal joints
Adductor pollicis	Transverse head—metacarpal III; oblique head—capitate and bases of metacarpals II and III	Base of proximal phalanx and extensor hood of thumb	Deep branch of ulnar nerve [C8, **T1**]	Adducts thumb
Lumbricals (four muscles)	Tendons of flexor digitorum profundus	Extensor hoods of index, ring, middle, and little fingers	Medial two by the deep branch of the ulnar nerve; lateral two by digital branches of the median nerve	Flex metacarpophalangeal joints while extending interphalangeal joints
Thenar muscles				
Opponens pollicis	Tubercle of trapezium and flexor retinaculum	Lateral margin and adjacent palmar surface of metacarpal I	Recurrent branch of median nerve [C8, **T1**]	Medially rotates thumb
Abductor pollicis brevis	Tubercles of scaphoid and trapezium and adjacent flexor retinaculum	Proximal phalanx and extensor hood of thumb	Recurrent branch of median nerve [C8, **T1**]	Abducts thumb at metacarpophalangeal joint
Flexor pollicis brevis	Tubercle of the trapezium and flexor retinaculum	Proximal phalanx of the thumb	Recurrent branch of median nerve [C8, **T1**]	Flexes thumb at metacarpophalangeal joint
Hypothenar muscles				
Opponens digiti minimi	Hook of hamate and flexor retinaculum	Medial aspect of metacarpal V	Deep branch of ulnar nerve [C8, **T1**]	Laterally rotates metacarpal V
Abductor digiti minimi	Pisiform, the pisohamate ligament, and tendon of flexor carpi ulnaris	Proximal phalanx of little finger	Deep branch of ulnar nerve [C8, **T1**]	Abducts little finger at metacarpophalangeal joint
Flexor digiti minimi brevis	Hook of the hamate and flexor retinaculum	Proximal phalanx of little finger	Deep branch of ulnar nerve [C8, **T1**]	Flexes little finger at metacarpophalangeal joint

innervated by spinal cord segment T1 with a contribution from C8.

Interossei

The four bipennate **dorsal interossei** are the most posterior of all of the intrinsic muscles and can be palpated through the skin on the posterior aspect of the hand (Fig. 7.90). The muscles lie between and are attached to the shafts of adjacent metacarpal bones (Fig. 7.90). Each muscle inserts both into the base of the proximal phalanx and into the extensor hood of its related digit.

The four **palmar interossei** are anterior to the dorsal interossei and are unipennate muscles originating from the metacarpals of the digits with which each is associated (Fig. 7.91).

The first palmar interosseous muscle is rudimentary and often considered part of either the adductor pollicis or the flexor pollicis brevis. When present, it originates from the medial side of the palmar surface of metacarpal I and inserts into both the base of the proximal phalanx of the thumb and into the extensor hood. A sesamoid bone often occurs in the tendon attached to the base of the phalanx.

Thenar muscles

The three thenar muscles (the **opponens pollicis, flexor pollicis brevis,** and **abductor pollicis brevis** muscles) are associated with opposition of the thumb to the fingers and with delicate movements of the thumb (Table 7.15, Fig. 7.93) and are responsible for the prominent swelling (**thenar eminence**) on the lateral side of the palm at the base of the thumb.

Hypothenar muscles

The hypothenar muscles (the **opponens digiti minimi, abductor digiti minimi,** and **flexor digiti minimi brevis**) contribute to the swelling (**hypothenar eminence**) on the

Upper Limb

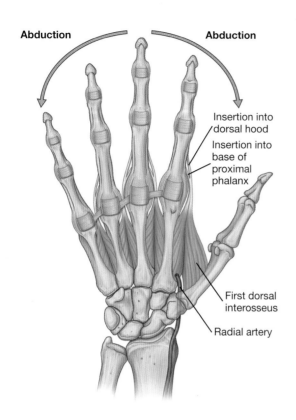

Fig. 7.90 Dorsal interossei (palmar view), right hand.

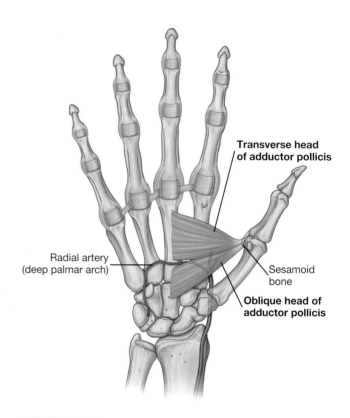

Fig. 7.92 Adductor pollicis, right hand.

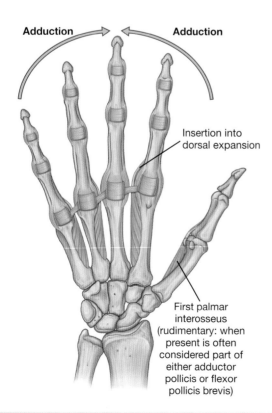

Fig. 7.91 Palmar interossei (palmar view), right hand.

medial side of the palm at the base of the little finger (Table 7.15, Fig. 7.93). The hypothenar muscles are similar to the thenar muscles in name and in organization.

Lumbrical muscles

There are four lumbrical (worm-like) muscles, each of which is associated with one of the fingers (Fig. 7.94). The muscles originate from the tendons of the flexor digitorum profundus in the palm and insert into the extensor hoods. The lumbricals are unique because they link flexor tendons with extensor tendons. Through their insertion into the extensor hoods, they participate in flexing the metacarpophalangeal joints and extending the interphalangeal joints.

Arteries and veins

The blood supply to the hand is by the radial and ulnar arteries, which form two interconnected vascular arches (superficial and deep) in the palm (Fig. 7.95). Vessels to the digits, muscles, and joints originate from the two arches and the parent arteries:

- The radial artery contributes substantially to the supply of the thumb and the lateral side of the index finger.
- The remaining digits and the medial side of the index finger are supplied mainly by the ulnar artery.

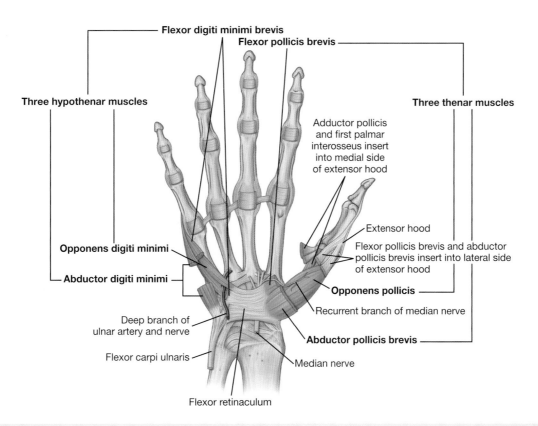

Flexor digiti minimi brevis

Flexor pollicis brevis

Three hypothenar muscles

Adductor pollicis and first palmar interosseus insert into medial side of extensor hood

Three thenar muscles

Extensor hood

Flexor pollicis brevis and abductor pollicis brevis insert into lateral side of extensor hood

Opponens digiti minimi

Opponens pollicis

Abductor digiti minimi

Recurrent branch of median nerve

Deep branch of ulnar artery and nerve

Abductor pollicis brevis

Flexor carpi ulnaris

Median nerve

Flexor retinaculum

Fig. 7.93 Thenar and hypothenar muscles, right hand.

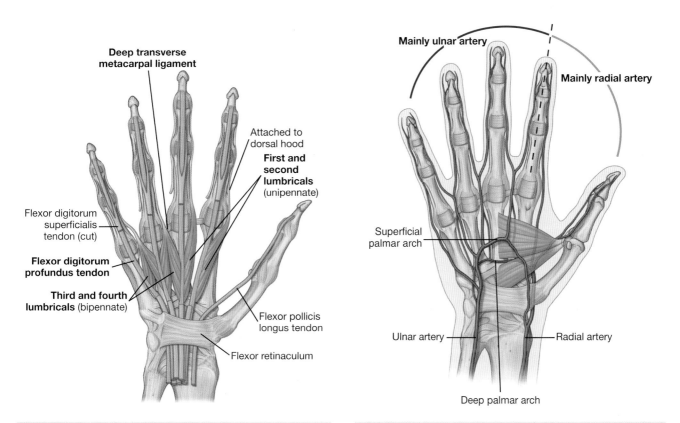

Deep transverse metacarpal ligament

Attached to dorsal hood

First and second lumbricals (unipennate)

Flexor digitorum superficialis tendon (cut)

Flexor digitorum profundus tendon

Third and fourth lumbricals (bipennate)

Flexor pollicis longus tendon

Flexor retinaculum

Fig. 7.94 Lumbrical muscles, right hand.

Mainly ulnar artery

Mainly radial artery

Superficial palmar arch

Ulnar artery

Radial artery

Deep palmar arch

Fig. 7.95 Arterial supply of the right hand.

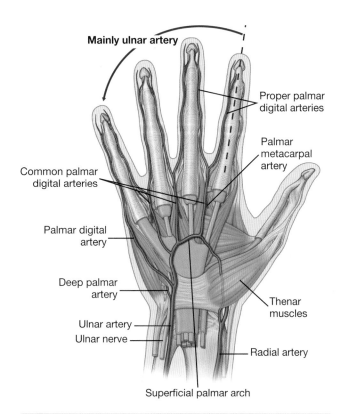

Fig. 7.96 Superficial palmar arch, right hand.

Ulnar artery and superficial palmar arch

The **ulnar artery** and ulnar nerve enter the hand on the medial side of the wrist (Figs. 7.95, 7.96). The vessel lies between the palmaris brevis and the flexor retinaculum and is lateral to the ulnar nerve and the pisiform bone. Distally, the ulnar artery is medial to the hook of the hamate bone and then swings laterally across the palm, forming the **superficial palmar arch** (Fig. 7.96), which is superficial to the long flexor tendons of the digits and just deep to the palmar aponeurosis. On the lateral side of the palm, the arch communicates with a palmar branch of the radial artery.

One branch of the ulnar artery in the hand is the **deep palmar branch** (Figs. 7.96, 7.97), which arises from the medial aspect of the ulnar artery just distal to the pisiform, and penetrates the origin of the hypothenar muscles. It curves medially around the hook of the hamate to access the deep plane of the palm and to anastomose with the deep palmar arch derived from the radial artery.

Branches from the superficial palmar arch include (Fig. 7.96):

- a **palmar digital artery** to the medial side of the little finger; and
- three large, **common palmar digital arteries,** which ultimately provide the principal blood supply to the lateral side of the little finger, both sides of the ring and middle fingers, and the medial side of the index finger; they are

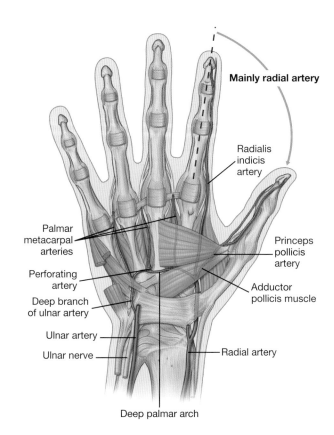

Fig. 7.97 Deep palmar arch, right hand.

joined by palmar metacarpal arteries from the deep palmar arch before bifurcating into the **proper palmar digital arteries,** which enter the fingers.

Radial artery and deep palmar arch

The **radial artery** curves around the lateral side of the wrist, passes over the floor of the anatomical snuffbox and into the deep plane of the palm by penetrating anteriorly through the back of the hand (Fig. 7.95). It passes between the two heads of the first dorsal interosseous muscle and then between the two heads of the adductor pollicis to access the deep plane of the palm and form the deep palmar arch.

The **deep palmar arch** passes medially through the palm between the metacarpal bones and the long flexor tendons of the digits. On the medial side of the palm, it communicates with the deep palmar branch of the ulnar artery (Fig. 7.97).

Before penetrating the back of the hand, the radial artery gives rise to two vessels (Fig. 7.98):

- a **dorsal carpal branch,** which passes medially as the **dorsal carpal arch** across the wrist and gives rise to **dorsal metacarpal arteries,** which subsequently divide to become small dorsal digital arteries that enter the fingers; and
- the **first dorsal metacarpal artery,** which supplies adjacent sides of the index finger and thumb.

Two vessels, the **princeps pollicis artery** and the **radialis indicis artery,** arise from the radial artery in the plane between the first dorsal interosseus and adductor pollicis (Fig. 7.97). The princeps pollicis artery is the major blood supply to the thumb, and the radialis indicis artery supplies the lateral side of the index finger.

The deep palmar arch gives rise to (Fig. 7.97):

- three **palmar metacarpal arteries,** which join the common palmar digital arteries from the superficial palmar arch, and
- three **perforating branches,** which pass posteriorly between the heads of origin of the dorsal interossei to anastomose with the dorsal metacarpal arteries from the dorsal carpal arch.

Clinical app

Allen's test

To test for adequate anastomoses between the radial and ulnar arteries, compress both the radial and ulnar arteries at the wrist, then release pressure from one or the other and determine the filling pattern of the hand. If there is little connection between the deep and superficial palmar arches, only the thumb and lateral side of the index finger will fill with blood (become red) when pressure on the radial artery alone is released.

Veins

As generally found in the upper limb, the hand contains interconnected networks of deep and superficial veins. The deep veins follow the arteries; the superficial veins drain into a dorsal venous network on the back of the hand over the metacarpal bones (Fig. 7.99).

The cephalic vein originates from the lateral side of the dorsal venous network and passes over the anatomical snuffbox into the forearm.

The basilic vein originates from the medial side of the dorsal venous network and passes into the dorsomedial aspect of the forearm.

Nerves

The hand is supplied by the ulnar, median, and radial nerves (Figs. 7.100, 7.102, 7.104). All three nerves contribute to cutaneous or general sensory innervation. The ulnar nerve innervates all intrinsic muscles of the hand except for the three thenar muscles and the two lateral lumbricals, which are innervated by the median nerve. The radial nerve only innervates skin on the dorsolateral side of the hand.

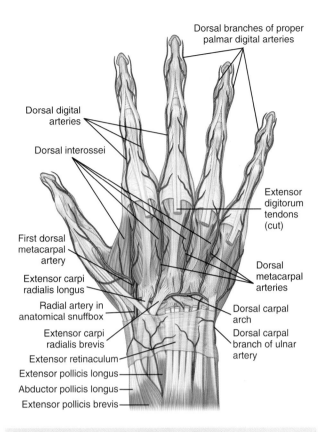

Fig. 7.98 Arteries on the dorsum of the right hand.

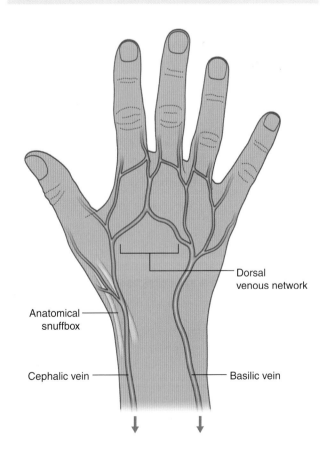

Fig. 7.99 Dorsal venous arch of the right hand.

Ulnar nerve

The ulnar nerve enters the hand lateral to the pisiform and posteromedially to the ulnar artery (Fig. 7.100). Immediately distal to the pisiform, it divides into a deep branch, which is mainly motor, and a superficial branch, which is mainly sensory.

The **deep branch** of the ulnar nerve passes with the deep branch of the ulnar artery (Fig. 7.100). It penetrates and supplies the hypothenar muscles to reach the deep aspect of the palm, arches laterally across the palm deep to the long flexors of the digits, and supplies the interossei, adductor pollicis, and the two medial lumbricals. In addition, the deep branch of the ulnar nerve contributes small articular branches to the wrist joint.

As the deep branch of the ulnar nerve passes across the palm, it lies in a fibro-osseous tunnel (Guyon's canal) between the hook of the hamate and the flexor tendons. Occasionally, small outpouchings of synovial membrane (ganglia) from the joints of the carpus compress the nerve within this canal, producing sensory and motor symptoms.

The superficial branch of the ulnar nerve innervates the palmaris brevis muscle and continues across the palm to supply skin on the palmar surface of the little finger and the medial half of the ring finger (Fig. 7.100).

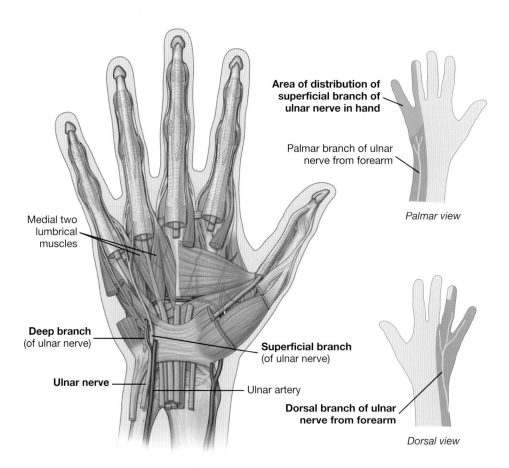

Fig. 7.100 Ulnar nerve in the right hand.

Clinical app

Ulnar nerve injury

The ulnar nerve is most commonly injured at two sites: the elbow and the wrist.

At the elbow, the nerve lies posterior to the medial epicondyle.

At the wrist, the ulnar nerve passes superficial to the flexor retinaculum and lies lateral to the pisiform bone.

Ulnar nerve lesions are characterized by "clawing" of the hand in which the metacarpophalangeal joints of the fingers are hyperextended and the interphalangeal joints are flexed because the function of most of the intrinsic muscles of the hand is lost (Fig. 7.101).

Clawing is most pronounced in the medial fingers because the function of all intrinsic muscles of these digits is lost, whereas in the lateral two digits, the lumbricals are innervated by the median nerve. Function of the adductor pollicis muscle is also lost.

In lesions of the ulnar nerve at the elbow, function of the flexor carpi ulnaris muscle and flexor digitorum profundus to the medial two digits is lost as well. Clawing of the hand, particularly of the little and ring fingers, is worse with lesions of the ulnar nerve at the wrist than at the elbow because interruption of the nerve at the elbow paralyzes the ulnar half of the flexor digitorum profundus, which leads to lack of flexion at the distal interphalangeal joints in these fingers.

Ulnar nerve lesions at the elbow and wrist result in impaired sensory innervation on the palmar aspect of the medial one and one-half digits.

Damage to the ulnar nerve at the wrist or at a site proximal to the wrist can be distinguished by evaluating the status of

function of the **dorsal branch** (cutaneous) of the ulnar nerve, which originates in distal regions of the forearm. This branch innervates skin over the dorsal surface of the hand on the medial side.

Fig. 7.101 Typical appearance of a "clawed hand" due to a lesion of the ulnar nerve.

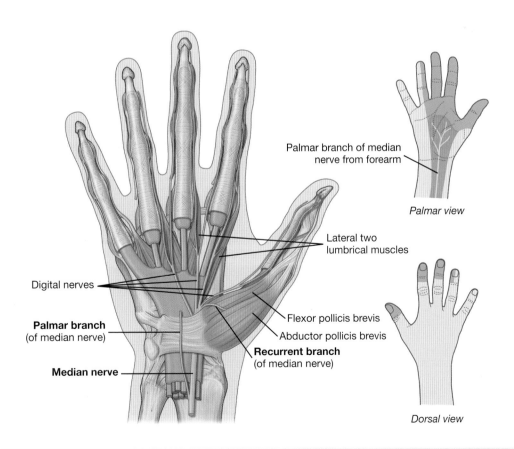

Palmar branch of median nerve from forearm

Palmar view

Lateral two lumbrical muscles

Digital nerves

Palmar branch
(of median nerve)

Flexor pollicis brevis

Abductor pollicis brevis

Recurrent branch
(of median nerve)

Median nerve

Dorsal view

Fig. 7.102 Median nerve in the right hand.

Median nerve

The median nerve is the most important sensory nerve in the hand because it innervates skin on the thumb, index, and middle fingers, and on the lateral side of the ring finger (Fig. 7.102). The nervous system, using touch, gathers information about the environment from this area, particularly from the skin on the thumb and index finger. In addition, sensory information from the lateral three and one-half digits enables the fingers to be positioned with the appropriate amount of force when using precision grip.

The median nerve also innervates the thenar muscles that are responsible for opposition of the thumb to the other digits.

The median nerve enters the hand by passing through the carpal tunnel and divides into a recurrent branch and palmar digital branches (Fig. 7.102).

The **recurrent branch** of the median nerve innervates the three thenar muscles. Originating from the lateral side of the median nerve near the distal margin of the flexor retinaculum, it curves around the margin of the retinaculum and passes proximally over the flexor pollicis brevis muscle. The recurrent branch then passes between the flexor pollicis brevis and abductor pollicis brevis to end in the opponens pollicis.

The **palmar digital nerves** cross the palm deep to the palmar aponeurosis and the superficial palmar arch and enter the digits. They innervate skin on the palmar surfaces of the lateral three and one-half digits and cutaneous regions over the dorsal aspects of the distal phalanges (nail beds) of the same digits. In addition to skin, the digital nerves supply the lateral two lumbrical muscles.

Superficial branch of the radial nerve

The only part of the radial nerve that enters the hand is the superficial branch (Fig. 7.104). It enters the hand by passing over the anatomical snuffbox on the dorsolateral side of the wrist.

The superficial branch of the radial nerve innervates skin over the dorsolateral aspect of the palm and the dorsal aspects of the lateral three and one-half digits distally to approximately the terminal interphalangeal joints.

Surface anatomy

Motor function of the median and ulnar nerves in the hand

The ability to flex the metacarpophalangeal joints while extending the interphalangeal joints of the fingers is entirely dependent on the intrinsic muscles of the hand (Fig. 7.103). These muscles are mainly innervated by the deep branch of the ulnar nerve, which carries fibers from spinal cord level (C8)T1.

Adducting the fingers to grasp an object placed between them is caused by the palmar interossei muscles, which are innervated by the deep branch of the ulnar nerve carrying fibers from spinal cord level (C8)T1.

The ability to grasp an object between the pad of the thumb and the pad of one of the fingers depends on normal functioning of the thenar muscles, which are innervated by the recurrent branch of the median nerve carrying fibers from spinal cord level C8(T1).

Fig. 7.103 Flexing the metacarpophalangeal joints and extending the interphalangeal joints: the "ta-ta" position.

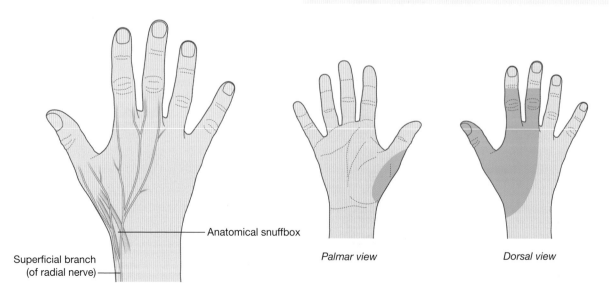

Anatomical snuffbox

Superficial branch (of radial nerve)

Palmar view   *Dorsal view*

Fig. 7.104 Radial nerve in the right hand.

Clinical app

Radial nerve injury

Around the elbow joint the radial nerve divides into its two terminal branches—the superficial branch and the deep branch.

The most common radial nerve injury is damage to the nerve in the radial groove of the humerus, which produces a global paralysis of the muscles of the posterior compartment resulting in "**wrist drop.**" Radial nerve damage can result from fracture of the shaft of the humerus as the radial nerve spirals around in the radial groove. The typical injury produces reduction of sensation in the cutaneous distribution, predominantly over the posterior aspect of the hand. Severing the posterior interosseous nerve (continuation of deep branch of radial nerve) may paralyze the muscles of the posterior compartment of the forearm, but the nerve supply is variable. Typically, the patient may not be able to extend the fingers.

The distal branches of the superficial branch of the radial nerve can be readily palpated as "cords" passing over the tendon of the extensor pollicis longus in the anatomical snuffbox. Damage to these branches is of little consequence because they supply only a small area of skin.

Clinical app

Dermatomes and myotomes in the upper limb

Innervation of the upper limb is by the brachial plexus, which is formed by the anterior rami of cervical spinal nerves C5 to C8 and T1. This plexus is initially formed in the neck and then continues into the upper limb. Major nerves that ultimately innervate the arm, forearm, and hand originate from the brachial plexus.

As a consequence of this innervation pattern, clinical testing of lower cervical and T1 nerves is carried out by examining dermatomes, myotomes, and tendon reflexes in the upper limb. Another consequence is that the clinical signs of problems related to lower cervical nerves—pain, pins-and-needles sensations or paresthesia, and muscle twitching—appear in the upper limb.

Importantly, the major spinal cord level associated with innervation of the diaphragm, C4, is immediately above the spinal cord levels associated with the upper limb. Evaluation of dermatomes and myotomes in the upper limb can provide important information about potential breathing problems that might develop as complications of damage to the spinal cord in regions just below the C4 spinal level.

Dermatomes of the upper limb are shown in Fig. 7.105A. Areas where overlap of dermatomes is minimal and can be clinically tested include the:

- upper lateral region of the arm for spinal cord level C5,
- palmar pad of the thumb for spinal cord level C6,

Clinical app—cont'd

- pad of the index finger for spinal cord level C7,
- pad of the little finger for spinal cord level C8, and
- skin on the medial aspect of the elbow for spinal cord level T1.

Select joint movements are used to test myotomes (Fig. 7.105B):

- Abduction of the arm at the glenohumeral joint is controlled predominantly by C5.
- Flexion of the forearm at the elbow joint is controlled primarily by C6.
- Extension of the forearm at the elbow joint is controlled mainly by C7.
- Flexion of the fingers is controlled mainly by C8.
- Abduction and adduction of the index, middle, and ring fingers is controlled predominantly by T1.

Fig. 7.105 Dermatomes and myotomes in the upper limb. **A.** Dermatomes. **B.** Movements produced by myotomes.

Clinical app

Tendon taps in the upper limb

In an unconscious patient, both somatic sensory and motor functions of spinal cord levels can be tested using tendon reflexes:

- A tap on the tendon of the biceps in the cubital fossa tests mainly for spinal cord level C6.
- A tap on the tendon of the triceps posterior to the elbow tests mainly for C7.

Upper Limb

Clinical app

Testing sensory innervation carried by major peripheral nerves in the upper limb

In addition to innervating major muscle groups, each of the major peripheral nerves originating from the brachial plexus carries somatic sensory information from patches of skin quite different from dermatomes. Sensation in these areas can be used to test for peripheral nerve lesions:

- The axillary nerve innervates skin on the superior lateral surface on the arm.

- The musculocutaneous nerve innervates skin on the anterolateral side of the forearm.
- The median nerve innervates the palmar surface of the lateral three and one-half digits.
- The ulnar nerve innervates the medial one and one-half digits.
- The radial nerve supplies skin on the posterior surface of the forearm and the dorsolateral surface of the hand.

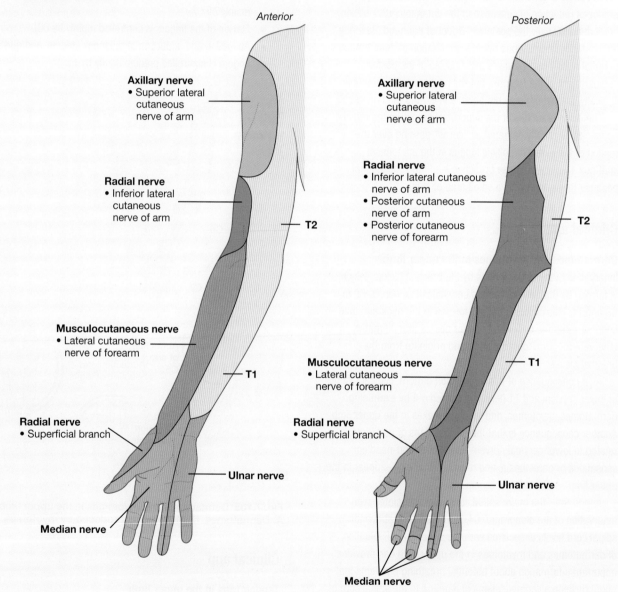

Fig. 7.106 Anterior and posterior areas of skin innervated by major peripheral nerves in the arm and forearm.

Surface anatomy

Pulse points

Peripheral pulses can be felt at six locations in the upper limb (Fig. 7.107A):

Axillary pulse: axillary artery in the axilla lateral to the apex of the dome of skin covering the floor of the axilla.

Brachial pulse in midarm: brachial artery on the medial side of the arm in the cleft between the biceps brachii and triceps brachii muscles. This is the position where a blood pressure cuff is placed (Fig. 7.107B).

Brachial pulse in the cubital fossa: brachial artery medial to the tendon of the biceps brachii muscle. This is the position where a stethoscope is placed to hear the pulse of the vessel when taking a blood pressure reading (Fig. 7.107B).

Radial pulse in the distal forearm: radial artery immediately lateral to the tendon of the flexor carpi radialis muscle. This is the most common site for "taking a pulse."

Ulnar pulse in the distal forearm: ulnar artery immediately under the lateral margin of the flexor carpi ulnaris tendon and proximal to the pisiform.

Radial pulse in the anatomical snuffbox: radial artery as it crosses the lateral side of the wrist between the tendon of the extensor pollicis longus muscle and the tendons of the extensor pollicis brevis and abductor pollicis longus muscles.

Axillary pulse

Brachial pulse in mid-arm

Radial pulse in distal forearm

Brachial pulse in the cubital fossa

A Radial pulse in the anatomical snuffbox

Ulnar pulse in distal forearm

B

Fig. 7.107 Where to take peripheral artery pulses in the upper limb. **A.** Pulse points. **B.** Placement of blood pressure cuff and stethoscope.

8

Head and Neck

ADDITIONAL LEARNING RESOURCES FOR CHAPTER 8, *HEAD AND NECK,* CAN BE FOUND ON THE ACCOMPANYING EBOOK:

- Self-Assessment — National Board style multiple-choice questions, Chapter 8
- Short Questions — These are questions requiring short responses, Chapter 8
- Clinical Cases
  Pancoast tumor
  Subclavian steal syndrome
  Branchial cyst
  Epiglottitis
  Otosclerosis
  Scalp laceration
  Scaphocephaly
  Temporal arteritis
  Tonsillitis
  Multinodular goiter
  Parotid duct calculus
  Extradural hematoma
  Stenosis of the internal carotid artery
  Posterior communicating artery aneurysm
  Recurrent epistaxis
  Complication of orbital fracture
  Brainstem tumor
  Pituitary macroadenoma

Regional anatomy **445**

Head **446**
Neck **446**
Skull **446**
   Anterior view   446
   Lateral view   448
   Posterior view   451
   Superior view   451
   Inferior view   452
Cranial cavity **454**
   Roof   455
   Floor   455
Meninges **462**
   Cranial dura mater   462
   Arachnoid mater   465
   Pia mater   465
   Meningeal spaces   465
Brain and its blood supply **466**
   Brain   466
   Blood supply   467
   Venous drainage   469
Cranial nerves **475**
   Olfactory nerve [I]   475
   Optic nerve [II]   475
   Oculomotor nerve [III]   477
   Trochlear nerve [IV]   478
   Trigeminal nerve [V]   478
   Ophthalmic nerve [V_1]   478
   Maxillary nerve [V_2]   479
   Mandibular nerve [V_3]   479
   Abducent nerve [VI]   479
   Facial nerve [VII]   479
   Vestibulocochlear nerve [VIII]   479
   Glossopharyngeal nerve [IX]   480
   Vagus nerve [X]   480
   Accessory nerve [XI]   480
   Hypoglossal nerve [XII]   484

Face 484
    Muscles 484
    Parotid gland 487
    Innervation 489
    Vessels 492
Scalp 496
    Layers 496
    Innervation 498
    Vessels 499
    Lymphatic drainage 500
Orbit 501
    Bony orbit 501
    Eyelids 502
    Lacrimal apparatus 505
    Sensory innervation 506
    Fissures and foramina 507
    Fascial specializations 509
    Muscles 510
    Vessels 513
    Innervation 515
    Eyeball 519
Ear 522
    External ear 522
    Middle ear 526
    Internal ear 530
Temporal and infratemporal fossae 535
    Bony framework 536
    Temporomandibular joints 538
    Masseter muscle 540
    Temporal fossa 540
    Infratemporal fossa 541
Pterygopalatine fossa 550
    Skeletal framework 551
    Gateways 551
    Contents 552
Neck 557
    Fascia 558
    Superficial venous drainage 560
    Anterior triangle of the neck 561
    Posterior triangle of the neck 572
    Root of the neck 577
Pharynx 584
    Skeletal framework 585
    Pharyngeal wall 586

    Fascia 587
    Gaps in the pharyngeal wall and structures passing through them 587
    Nasopharynx 588
    Oropharynx 590
    Laryngopharynx 590
    Tonsils 590
    Vessels 590
    Nerves 591
Larynx 592
    Laryngeal cartilages 593
    Extrinsic ligaments 595
    Intrinsic ligaments 596
    Laryngeal joints 597
    Cavity of the larynx 598
    Intrinsic muscles 600
    Function of the larynx 601
    Vessels 602
    Nerves 603
Nasal cavities 604
    Lateral wall 605
    Regions 605
    Skeletal framework 606
    External nose 606
    Paranasal sinuses 607
    Walls, floor, and roof 609
    Nares 611
    Choanae 611
    Gateways 611
    Vessels 613
    Innervation 614
Oral cavity 616
    Skeletal framework 617
    Walls: the cheeks 620
    Floor 621
    Salivary glands 627
    Roof—palate 629
    Oral fissure and lips 633
    Oropharyngeal isthmus 634
    Teeth and gingivae 634

Regional anatomy

The head and neck are anatomically complex areas of the body. The **head** is composed of a series of compartments, which are formed by bone and soft tissues (Fig. 8.1). They are:

- the cranial cavity,
- two ears,
- two orbits,
- two nasal cavities, and
- an oral cavity.

The **neck** extends from the head above to the shoulders and thorax below (Fig. 8.1). The neck has four major compartments (Fig. 8.2), which are enclosed by an outer musculofascial collar:

- The vertebral compartment contains the cervical vertebrae and associated postural muscles.

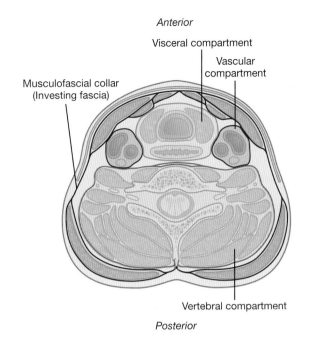

Fig. 8.2 Major compartments of the neck.

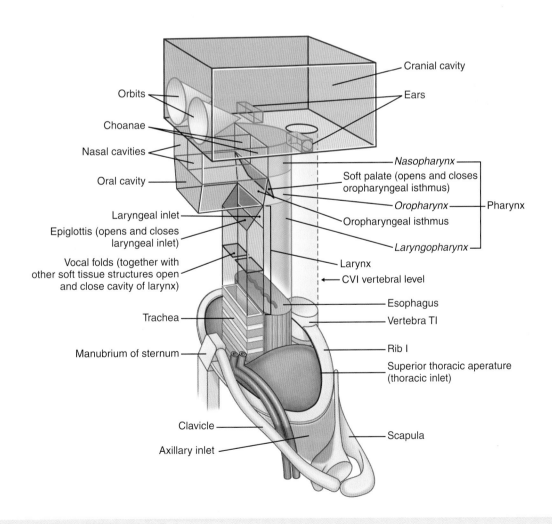

Fig. 8.1 Overall design of head and neck.

- The visceral compartment contains important glands (thyroid, parathyroid, and thymus) and parts of the respiratory and digestive tracts (larynx and pharynx) that pass between the head and thorax.
- The two vascular compartments, one on each side, contain the major blood vessels and the vagus nerve.

HEAD

- Houses and protects the brain and all the receptor systems associated with the special senses—the nasal cavities associated with smell, the orbits with vision, the ears with hearing and balance, and the oral cavity with taste.
- Contains the upper parts of the respiratory and digestive systems—the nasal and oral cavities—which have structural features for modifying the air or food passing into each system.

NECK

- Supports and positions the head. Importantly, it enables an individual to position sensory systems in the head relative to environmental cues without moving the entire body.
- Contains specialized structures (pharynx and larynx) that connect the upper parts of the digestive and respiratory tracts (nasal and oral cavities) in the head with the esophagus and trachea, which begin relatively low in the neck and pass into the thorax.

The head and neck together function in communication. Sounds produced by the larynx are modified in the pharynx and oral cavity to produce speech. In addition, the muscles of facial expression adjust the contours of the face to relay nonverbal signals.

SKULL

The skull has 22 bones, excluding the ossicles of the ear. Except for the mandible, which forms the lower jaw, the bones of the skull are attached to each other by sutures, are immobile, and form the **cranium.**

The cranium can be subdivided into:

- an upper domed part (the **calvaria**), which covers the cranial cavity containing the brain;
- a base that consists of the floor of the cranial cavity; and
- a lower anterior part—the **facial skeleton (viscerocranium).**

The bones forming the calvaria are mainly the paired temporal and parietal bones and parts of the unpaired frontal, sphenoid, and occipital bones.

The bones forming the base of the cranium are mainly parts of the sphenoid, temporal, and occipital bones.

The bones forming the facial skeleton are the paired nasal bones, palatine bones, lacrimal bones, zygomatic bones, maxillae, inferior nasal conchae, and the unpaired vomer.

The mandible is not part of the cranium nor part of the facial skeleton.

Anterior view

The anterior view of the skull includes the **forehead** superiorly, and, inferiorly, the orbits, the **nasal region,** the part of the face between the orbit and the upper jaw, the upper jaw, and the lower jaw (Fig. 8.3; also see Fig. 8.4).

Frontal bone

The forehead consists of the **frontal bone,** which also forms the superior part of the rim of each orbit (Fig. 8.3).

Just superior to the rim of the orbit on each side are the raised **superciliary arches.** These are more pronounced in men than in women. Between these arches is a small depression (the **glabella**).

Clearly visible in the medial part of the superior rim of each orbit is the **supra-orbital foramen (supra-orbital notch;** Table 8.1).

Medially, the frontal bone projects inferiorly, forming a part of the medial rim of the orbit.

Laterally, the **zygomatic process** of the frontal bone projects inferiorly, forming the upper lateral rim of the orbit. This process articulates with the **frontal process** of the zygomatic bone.

Zygomatic and nasal bones

The lower lateral rim of the orbit, as well as the lateral part of the inferior rim of the orbit, is formed by the **zygomatic bone** (the cheekbone) (Fig. 8.3).

Superiorly, in the nasal region, the paired nasal bones articulate with each other in the midline and with the frontal bone superiorly. The center of the **frontonasal suture** formed by the articulation of the nasal bones and the frontal bone is the **nasion.**

Laterally, each nasal bone articulates with the **frontal process** of each maxilla.

Inferiorly, the **piriform aperture** is the large opening in the nasal region and the anterior opening of the nasal cavities. It is bounded superiorly by the nasal bones and laterally and inferiorly by each maxilla.

Visible through the piriform aperture are the fused **nasal crests,** forming the lower part of the bony **nasal septum** and ending anteriorly as the **anterior nasal spine,** and the paired **inferior nasal conchae.**

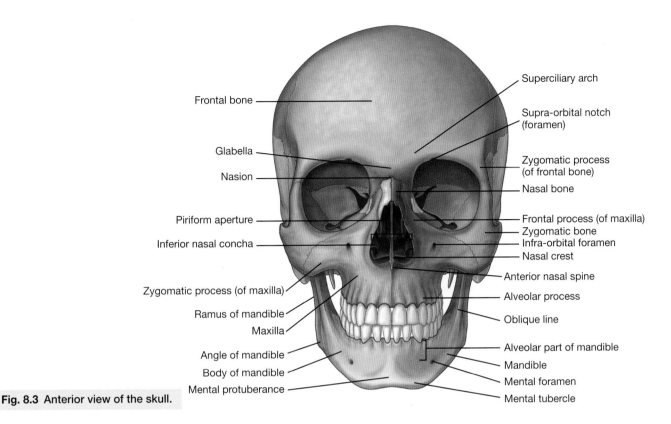

Fig. 8.3 Anterior view of the skull.

Labels (clockwise from top):
Superciliary arch
Supra-orbital notch (foramen)
Zygomatic process (of frontal bone)
Nasal bone
Frontal process (of maxilla)
Zygomatic bone
Infra-orbital foramen
Nasal crest
Anterior nasal spine
Alveolar process
Oblique line
Alveolar part of mandible
Mandible
Mental foramen
Mental tubercle
Mental protuberance
Body of mandible
Angle of mandible
Maxilla
Ramus of mandible
Zygomatic process (of maxilla)
Inferior nasal concha
Piriform aperture
Nasion
Glabella
Frontal bone

Visualizing the skull—anterior view

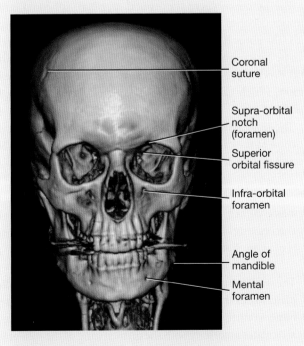

Coronal suture
Supra-orbital notch (foramen)
Superior orbital fissure
Infra-orbital foramen
Angle of mandible
Mental foramen

Fig. 8.4 Volume-rendered anterior view using multidetector computed tomography.

Maxillae

The part of the face between the orbit and the upper teeth and each upper jaw is formed by the paired maxillae (Fig. 8.3).

Superiorly, each maxilla contributes to the inferior and medial rims of the orbit.

Laterally, the **zygomatic process** of each maxilla articulates with the zygomatic bone, and medially, the frontal process of each maxilla articulates with the frontal bone.

Inferiorly, the part of each maxilla, lateral to the opening of the nasal cavity, is the **body of maxilla.**

On the anterior surface of the body of maxilla, just below the inferior rim of the orbit, is the **infra-orbital foramen** (Table 8.1).

Inferiorly, each maxilla ends as the **alveolar process,** which contains the teeth and forms the upper jaw.

Mandible

The lower jaw (mandible) is the most inferior structure in the anterior view of the skull (see Fig. 8.3). It consists of the **body of mandible** anteriorly and the **ramus of mandible** posteriorly. These meet posteriorly at the **angle of mandible.** All these parts of the mandible are visible, to some extent, in the anterior view.

The body of mandible is arbitrarily divided into two parts:

- The lower part is the **base of mandible.**
- The upper part is the **alveolar part of mandible.**

Table 8.1 External foramina of the skull

Foramen	Structures passing through foramen
Anterior view	
Supra-orbital foramen	Supra-orbital nerve and vessels
Infra-orbital foramen	Infra-orbital nerve and vessels
Mental foramen	Mental nerve and vessels
Lateral view	
Zygomaticofacial foramen	Zygomaticofacial nerve
Superior view	
Parietal foramen	Emissary veins
Inferior view	
Incisive foramina	Nasopalatine nerve; sphenopalatine vessels
Greater palatine foramen	Greater palatine nerve and vessels
Lesser palatine foramina	Lesser palatine nerve and vessels
Pterygoid canal	Nerve of pterygoid canal and vessels
Foramen ovale	Mandibular nerve [V$_3$]; lesser petrosal nerve
Foramen spinosum	Middle meningeal artery
Foramen lacerum	Filled with cartilage
Carotid canal	Internal carotid artery and nerve plexus
Foramen magnum	Continuation of brain and spinal cord; vertebral arteries and nerve plexuses; anterior spinal artery; posterior spinal arteries; roots of accessory nerve [XI]; meninges
Condylar canal	Emissary veins
Hypoglossal canal	Hypoglossal nerve [XII] and vessels
Jugular foramen	Internal jugular vein; inferior petrosal sinus; glossopharyngeal nerve [IX]; vagus nerve [X]; accessory nerve [XI]
Stylomastoid foramen	Facial nerve [VII]

The alveolar part of mandible contains the teeth and is resorbed when the teeth are removed. The base of mandible has a midline swelling (the **mental protuberance**) on its anterior surface where the two sides of the mandible come together. Just lateral to the mental protuberance, on either side, are slightly more pronounced bumps (**mental tubercles**).

Laterally, a **mental foramen** (see Table 8.1) is visible halfway between the upper border of the alveolar part of mandible and the lower border of the base of mandible. Continuing past this foramen is a ridge (the **oblique line**) passing from the front of the ramus onto the body of mandible. The oblique line is a point of attachment for muscles that depress the lower lip.

Lateral view

The lateral view of the skull consists of the lateral wall of the cranium, which includes lateral portions of the calvaria and the facial skeleton, and half of the lower jaw (Fig. 8.5; see also Fig. 8.6):

- Bones forming the lateral portion of the calvaria include the frontal, parietal, occipital, sphenoid, and temporal bones.
- Bones forming the visible part of the facial skeleton include the nasal, maxilla, and zygomatic bones.
- The mandible forms the visible part of the lower jaw.

Lateral portion of the calvaria

The lateral portion of the calvaria begins anteriorly with the frontal bone. In upper regions, the frontal bone articulates with the parietal bone at the **coronal suture** (Fig. 8.5). The parietal bone then articulates with the occipital bone at the **lambdoid suture**.

In lower parts of the lateral portion of the calvaria, the frontal bone articulates with the **greater wing of sphenoid bone** (Fig. 8.5), which then articulates with the parietal bone at the **sphenoparietal suture,** and with the anterior edge of the temporal bone at the **sphenosquamous suture.**

The junction where the frontal, parietal, sphenoid, and temporal bones are in close proximity is the **pterion** (Fig. 8.5). The clinical consequences of a skull fracture in this area can be very serious. The bone in this area is particularly thin and overlies the anterior division of the middle meningeal artery, which can be torn by a skull fracture in this area, resulting in an extradural hematoma.

The final articulation across the lower part of the lateral portion of the calvaria is between the temporal bone and the occipital bone at the **occipitomastoid suture** (Fig. 8.5).

Temporal bone

A major contributor to the lower portion of the lateral wall of the cranium is the temporal bone (Fig. 8.5), which consists of several parts:

- The **squamous part** has the appearance of a large, flat plate, forms the anterior and superior parts of the temporal bone, contributes to the lateral wall of the cranium, and articulates anteriorly with the greater wing of the sphenoid bone at the sphenosquamous suture and with the parietal bone superiorly at the squamous suture.
- The **zygomatic process** is an anterior bony projection from the lower surface of the squamous part of the temporal bone

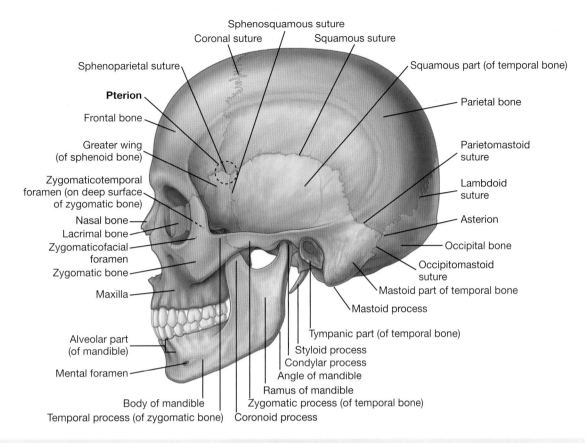

Fig. 8.5 Lateral view of the skull.

Imaging app

Visualizing the skull—lateral view

Fig. 8.6 Volume-rendered lateral view using multidetector computed tomography.

that initially projects laterally and then curves anteriorly to articulate with the temporal process of the zygomatic bone to form the **zygomatic arch.**

■ Immediately below the origin of the zygomatic process from the squamous part of the temporal bone is the **tympanic part** of the temporal bone, and clearly visible on the surface of this part is the **external acoustic opening** leading to the **external acoustic meatus** (ear canal).

■ The petromastoid part is usually separated into a **petrous part** and a **mastoid part** for descriptive purposes.

The mastoid part is the most posterior part of the temporal bone and is the only part of the petromastoid part of the temporal bone seen on a lateral view of the skull. It is continuous with the squamous part of the temporal bone anteriorly and articulates with the parietal bone superiorly at the **parietomastoid suture** and with the occipital bone posteriorly at the occipitomastoid suture. These two sutures are continuous with each other, and the parietomastoid suture is continuous with the squamous suture.

Inferiorly, a large bony prominence (the **mastoid process**) projects from the inferior border of the mastoid part of the temporal bone (Fig. 8.5). This is a point of attachment for several muscles.

Medial to the mastoid process, the **styloid process** projects from the lower border of the temporal bone.

449

Surface anatomy
Anatomical position of the head and major landmarks

The head is in the anatomical position when the inferior margins of the bony orbits and the superior margins of the external acoustic meatuses are in the same horizontal plane (Frankfort plane).

In addition to the external acoustic meatus and the bony margin of the orbit, other features that are palpable include the head of mandible, zygomatic arch, zygomatic bone, mastoid process, and external occipital protuberance (Fig. 8.7).

The head of mandible is anterior to the external ear and behind and inferior to the posterior end of the zygomatic arch. It is best found by opening and closing the jaw and palpating the head of mandible as it moves forward onto the articular tubercle and then back into the mandibular fossa, respectively.

The zygomatic arch extends forward from the region of the temporomandibular joint to the zygomatic bone, which forms a bony prominence lateral to the inferior margin of the anterior opening of the orbit.

The mastoid process is a large bony protuberance that is easily palpable posterior to the inferior aspect of the external acoustic meatus. The superior end of the sternocleidomastoid muscle attaches to the mastoid process.

The external occipital protuberance is palpable in the midline posteriorly where the contour of the skull curves sharply forward. This landmark marks the point superficially where the back of the neck joins the head.

Another clinically useful feature of the head is the vertex. This is the highest point of the head in the anatomical position and marks the approximate point on the scalp where there is a transition from cervical to cranial innervation of the scalp. Anterior to the vertex, the scalp and face are innervated by the trigeminal nerve [V]. Posterior to the vertex, the scalp is innervated by branches from cervical spinal nerves.

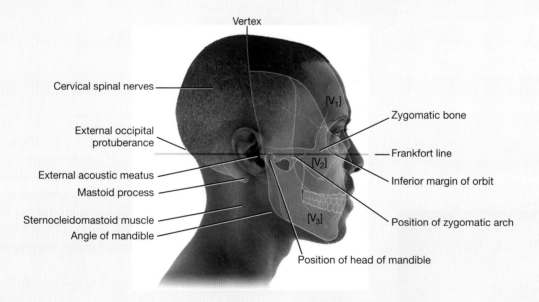

Fig. 8.7 Anatomical position of the head and major landmarks. Lateral head and neck of a man.

Visible part of the facial skeleton

The bones of the viscerocranium visible in a lateral view of the skull include the nasal, maxilla, and zygomatic bones (Fig. 8.5) as follows:

- a nasal bone anteriorly;
- the maxilla with its alveolar process containing teeth forming the upper jaw; anteriorly, it articulates with the nasal bone; superiorly, it contributes to the formation of the inferior and medial borders of the orbit; medially, its frontal process articulates with the frontal bone; laterally,

its zygomatic process articulates with the zygomatic bone; and

- the zygomatic bone, an irregularly shaped bone with a rounded lateral surface that forms the prominence of the cheek, is a visual centerpiece in this view; medially, it assists in the formation of the inferior rim of the orbit through its articulation with the zygomatic process of the maxilla; superiorly, its frontal process articulates with the zygomatic process of the frontal bone, assisting in the formation of the lateral rim of the orbit; laterally, seen prominently in this view of the skull, the horizontal temporal process of the zygomatic bone projects backward to articulate with the zygomatic process of the temporal bone and so form the zygomatic arch.

Usually a small foramen (the **zygomaticofacial foramen;** see Table 8.1) is visible on the lateral surface of the zygomatic bone. A **zygomaticotemporal foramen** is present on the medial deep surface of the bone.

Mandible

The final bony structure visible in a lateral view of the skull is the mandible. Inferiorly in the anterior part of this view, it consists of the anterior body of mandible, a posterior ramus of mandible, and the angle of mandible where the inferior margin of the mandible meets the posterior margin of the ramus (Fig. 8.5).

The teeth are in the alveolar part of the body of mandible, and the mental protuberance is visible in this view.

The mental foramen is on the lateral surface of the body and on the superior part of the ramus, and a **condylar** and **coronoid process** extend upward.

The condylar process is involved in articulation of the mandible with the temporal bone, and the coronoid process is the point of attachment for the temporalis muscle.

Posterior view

The occipital, parietal, and temporal bones are seen in the posterior view of the skull (Fig. 8.8).

Occipital bone

Centrally the flat or **squamous part of occipital bone** is the main structure in this view of the skull (Fig. 8.8). It articulates superiorly with the paired parietal bones at the lambdoid suture and laterally with each temporal bone at the occipitomastoid sutures. Along the lambdoid suture, small islands of bone (**sutural bones** or wormian bones) may be observed.

Several bony landmarks are visible on the occipital bone. There is a midline projection (the **external occipital protuberance**) with curved lines extending laterally from it (**superior nuchal lines**). The most prominent point of the external occipital protuberance is the **inion**. About 1 inch (2.5 cm) below the superior nuchal lines, two additional lines (the **inferior nuchal lines**) curve laterally. Extending downward from the external occipital protuberance is the **external occipital crest.**

Temporal bones

Laterally, the temporal bones are visible in the posterior view of the skull, with the mastoid processes being the prominent feature (Fig. 8.8). On the inferomedial border of each mastoid process is a notch (the **mastoid notch**), which is a point of attachment for the posterior belly of the digastric muscle.

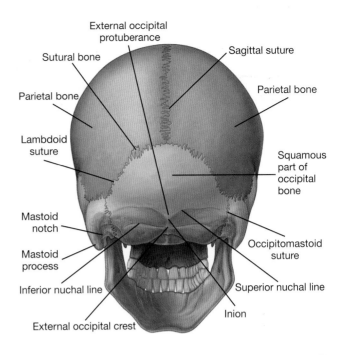

Fig. 8.8 Posterior view of the skull.

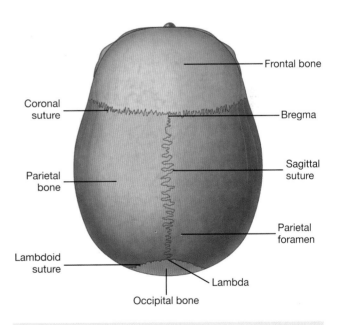

Fig. 8.9 Superior view of the skull.

Superior view

The frontal bone, parietal bones, and occipital bone are seen in a superior view of the skull (Fig. 8.9). These bones make up the superior part of the calvaria, or the **calva** (skullcap).

In an anterior to posterior direction:

■ The unpaired frontal bone articulates with the paired parietal bones at the coronal suture.

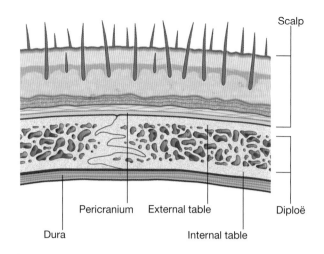

Scalp

Pericranium   External table

Dura   Internal table   Diploë

Fig. 8.10 Calvaria.

- The two parietal bones articulate with each other in the midline at the sagittal suture.
- The parietal bones articulate with the unpaired occipital bone at the lambdoid suture.

The junction of the sagittal and coronal sutures is the **bregma,** and the junction of the sagittal and lambdoid sutures is the **lambda.**

The only foramena visible in this view of the skull may be the parietal foramina located posteriorly, one on each parietal bone just lateral to the sagittal suture (Fig. 8.9).

The bones making up the calvaria (Fig. 8.10) are unique in their structure, consisting of dense internal and external tables of compact bone separated by a layer of spongy bone (the **diploë**).

Inferior view

The base of the skull is seen in the inferior view and extends anteriorly from the middle incisor teeth posteriorly to the superior nuchal lines and laterally to the mastoid processes and zygomatic arches (Fig. 8.11).

For descriptive purposes, the base of the skull is often divided into:

- an anterior part, which includes the teeth and the hard palate;
- a middle part, which extends from behind the hard palate to the anterior margin of the foramen magnum; and
- a posterior part, which extends from the anterior edge of the foramen magnum to the superior nuchal lines.

Anterior part

The main features of the anterior part of the base of the skull are the teeth and the hard palate.

The teeth project from the **alveolar processes** of the two maxillae. These processes are arranged together in a U-shaped alveolar arch that borders the hard palate on three sides (Fig. 8.11).

The **hard palate** is composed of the **palatine processes** of each maxilla anteriorly and the **horizontal plates** of each **palatine bone** posteriorly.

The paired palatine processes of each maxilla meet in the midline at the **intermaxillary suture,** the paired maxilla and the paired palatine bones meet at the **palatomaxillary suture,** and the paired horizontal plates of each palatine bone meet in the midline at the **interpalatine suture.**

Several additional features are also visible when the hard palate is examined:

- The **incisive fossa** in the anterior midline immediately posterior to the teeth, the walls of which contain **incisive foramina** (the openings of the **incisive canals,** which are passageways between the hard palate and nasal cavity).
- The **greater palatine foramina** near the posterolateral border of the hard palate on each side, which lead to **greater palatine canals**.
- Just posterior to the greater palatine foramina, the **lesser palatine foramina** in the **pyramidal process** of each palatine bone, which lead to **lesser palatine canals.**
- A midline pointed projection (the **posterior nasal spine**) in the free posterior border of the hard palate.

Middle part

The middle part of the base of the skull is complex:

- Forming the anterior half are the vomer and sphenoid bones.
- Forming the posterior half are the occipital and paired temporal bones.

Anterior half

Vomer

Anteriorly, the small vomer is in the midline, resting on the sphenoid bone (Fig. 8.11). It contributes to the formation of the bony nasal septum separating the two choanae.

Sphenoid

Most of the anterior part of the middle part of the base of the skull consists of the sphenoid bone.

The sphenoid bone is made up of a centrally placed **body,** paired **greater and lesser wings** projecting laterally from the body, and two downward-projecting **pterygoid processes** immediately lateral to each choana.

Three parts of the sphenoid bone, the body, greater wings, and pterygoid processes, are seen in the inferior view of the skull (Fig. 8.11). The lesser wing of the sphenoid is not seen in the inferior view.

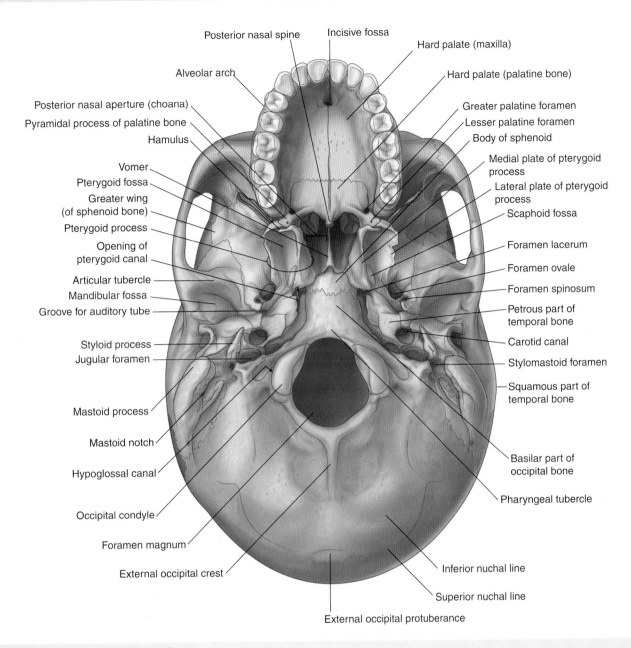

Posterior nasal spine
Incisive fossa
Hard palate (maxilla)
Alveolar arch
Hard palate (palatine bone)
Posterior nasal aperture (choana)
Greater palatine foramen
Pyramidal process of palatine bone
Lesser palatine foramen
Hamulus
Body of sphenoid
Vomer
Medial plate of pterygoid process
Pterygoid fossa
Lateral plate of pterygoid process
Greater wing (of sphenoid bone)
Scaphoid fossa
Pterygoid process
Foramen lacerum
Opening of pterygoid canal
Foramen ovale
Articular tubercle
Foramen spinosum
Mandibular fossa
Petrous part of temporal bone
Groove for auditory tube
Styloid process
Carotid canal
Jugular foramen
Stylomastoid foramen
Squamous part of temporal bone
Mastoid process
Mastoid notch
Hypoglossal canal
Basilar part of occipital bone
Occipital condyle
Pharyngeal tubercle
Foramen magnum
External occipital crest
Inferior nuchal line
Superior nuchal line
External occipital protuberance

Fig. 8.11 Inferior view of the skull.

Body

The body of the sphenoid is a centrally placed cube of bone containing two large air sinuses separated by a septum.

It articulates anteriorly with the vomer, ethmoid, and palatine bones, posterolaterally with the temporal bones, and posteriorly with the occipital bone.

Pterygoid processes

Extending downward from the junction of the body and the greater wings are the pterygoid processes (Fig. 8.11). Each of these processes consists of a narrow **medial plate** and broader **lateral plate** separated by the **pterygoid fossa.**

Each medial plate of the pterygoid process ends inferiorly with a hook-like projection, the **pterygoid hamulus,** and divides superiorly to form the small, shallow **scaphoid fossa.**

Just superior to the scaphoid fossa, at the root of the medial plate of the pterygoid process is the opening of the **pterygoid canal,** which passes forward from near the anterior margin of the foramen lacerum.

Greater wing

Lateral to the lateral plate of the pterygoid process is the greater wing of the sphenoid (Fig. 8.11), which not only forms a part of the base of the skull, but also continues laterally to form part of the lateral wall of the skull. It articulates laterally and posteriorly with parts of the temporal bone.

Important features visible on the surface of the greater wing in an inferior view of the skull are the foramen ovale and the foramen spinosum on the posterolateral border extending outward from the upper end of the lateral plate of the pterygoid process.

Head and Neck

Posterior half of middle part

In the posterior half of the middle part of the base of the skull are the occipital bone and the paired temporal bones (Fig. 8.11).

Occipital bone

The occipital bone, or more specifically its **basilar part,** is in the midline immediately posterior to the body of the sphenoid. It extends posteriorly to the **foramen magnum** and is bounded laterally by the temporal bones.

Prominent on the basilar part of the occipital bone is the **pharyngeal tubercle,** a bony protuberance for the attachment of parts of the pharynx to the base of the skull (Fig. 8.11).

Temporal bone

Immediately lateral to the basilar part of the occipital bone is the petrous part of the petromastoid part of each temporal bone.

Wedge-shaped in its appearance, with its **apex** anteromedial, the petrous part of the temporal bone is between the greater wing of the sphenoid anteriorly and the basilar part of the occipital bone posteriorly. The apex forms one of the boundaries of the **foramen lacerum,** an irregular opening filled in life with cartilage (Fig. 8.11).

The other boundaries of the foramen lacerum are the basilar part of the occipital bone medially and the body of the sphenoid anteriorly.

Posterolateral from the foramen lacerum along the petrous part of the temporal bone is the large circular opening for the **carotid canal.**

Between the petrous part of the temporal bone and the greater wing of the sphenoid is a groove for the cartilaginous part of the **pharyngotympanic tube (auditory tube).** This groove continues posterolaterally into a bony canal in the petrous part of the temporal bone for the pharyngotympanic tube.

Just lateral to the greater wing of the sphenoid is the squamous part of the temporal bone, which participates in the temporomandibular joint. It contains the **mandibular fossa,** which is a concavity where the head of the mandible articulates with the base of the skull. An important feature of this articulation is the prominent **articular tubercle,** which is the downward projection of the anterior border of the mandibular fossa (Fig. 8.11).

Posterior part

The posterior part of the base of the skull extends from the anterior edge of the foramen magnum posteriorly to the superior nuchal lines (Fig. 8.11). It consists of parts of the occipital bone centrally and the temporal bones laterally.

Occipital bone

The occipital bone is the major bony element of this part of the base of the skull (Fig. 8.11). It has four parts organized around the foramen magnum, which is a prominent feature of this part of the base of the skull and through which the brain and spinal cord are continuous.

The parts of the occipital bone are the squamous part, which is posterior to the foramen magnum, the **lateral parts,** which are lateral to the foramen magnum, and the **basilar part,** which is anterior to the foramen magnum (Fig. 8.11).

The squamous and lateral parts are components of the posterior part of the base of the skull.

The most visible feature of the squamous part of the occipital bone, when examining the inferior view of the skull, is a ridge of bone (the external occipital crest) that extends downward from the external occipital protuberance toward the foramen magnum. The inferior nuchal lines arc laterally from the midpoint of the crest.

Immediately lateral to the foramen magnum are the lateral parts of the occipital bones, which contain numerous important structural features.

On each anterolateral border of the foramen magnum are the rounded **occipital condyles** (Fig. 8.11). These paired structures articulate with the atlas (vertebra CI). Posterior to each condyle is a depression (the **condylar fossa**) containing a **condylar canal,** and anterior and superior to each condyle is the large **hypoglossal canal.** Lateral to each hypoglossal canal is a large, irregular, **jugular foramen** formed by opposition of the **jugular notch** of the occipital bone and **jugular notch** of the temporal bone.

Temporal bone

Laterally, on each side, in the posterior part of the base of the skull is the temporal bone. The parts of the temporal bone seen in this location are the mastoid part of the petromastoid part and the styloid process (see Fig. 8.11).

The lateral edge of the mastoid part is identified by the large cone-shaped mastoid process projecting from its inferior surface. This prominent bony structure is the point of attachment for several muscles. On the medial aspect of the mastoid process is the deep mastoid notch, which is also an attachment point for a muscle.

Anteromedial to the mastoid process is the needle-shaped styloid process projecting from the lower border of the temporal bone. The styloid process is also a point of attachment for numerous muscles and ligaments.

Finally, between the styloid process and the mastoid process is the stylomastoid foramen.

CRANIAL CAVITY

The cranial cavity is the space within the cranium that contains the brain, meninges, proximal parts of the cranial nerves, blood vessels, and cranial venous sinuses.

454

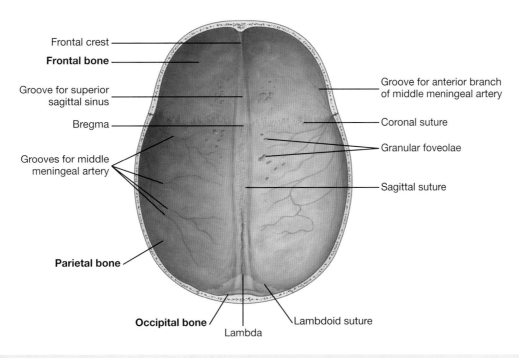

Fig. 8.12 Roof of the cranial cavity.

Labels on figure:
- Frontal crest
- **Frontal bone**
- Groove for superior sagittal sinus
- Bregma
- Grooves for middle meningeal artery
- **Parietal bone**
- **Occipital bone**
- Lambda
- Groove for anterior branch of middle meningeal artery
- Coronal suture
- Granular foveolae
- Sagittal suture
- Lambdoid suture

Roof

The calvaria is the dome-shaped roof that protects the superior aspect of the brain. It consists mainly of the frontal bone anteriorly, the paired parietal bones in the middle, and the occipital bone posteriorly (Fig. 8.12).

Sutures visible internally include:

- the coronal suture between the frontal and parietal bones,
- the sagittal suture between the paired parietal bones, and
- the lambdoid suture between the parietal and occipital bones.

Visible junctions of these sutures are the bregma, where the coronal and sagittal sutures meet, and the lambda, where the lambdoid and sagittal sutures meet.

Other markings on the internal surface of the calva include bony ridges and numerous grooves and pits (Fig. 8.12).

From anterior to posterior, features seen on the bony roof of the cranial cavity are (Fig. 8.12):

- a midline ridge of bone extending from the surface of the frontal bone (the **frontal crest**), which is a point of attachment for **the falx cerebri** (a specialization of the dura mater that partially separates the two cerebral hemispheres);
- a **groove for the superior sagittal sinus,** which widens and deepens posteriorly and marks the position of the superior sagittal sinus (an intradural venous structure);

- on either side of the groove for the superior sagittal sinus throughout its course, a small number of depressions and pits (the **granular foveolae**), which mark the location of arachnoid granulations (prominent structures readily identifiable when a brain with its meningeal coverings is examined; the arachnoid granulations are involved in the reabsorption of cerebrospinal fluid [CSF]); and
- on the lateral aspects of the roof of the cranial cavity, smaller grooves created by various meningeal vessels.

Floor

The floor of the cranial cavity is divided into anterior, middle, and posterior cranial fossae.

Anterior cranial fossa

Parts of the frontal, ethmoid, and sphenoid bones form the anterior cranial fossa (Fig. 8.13). Its floor is composed of:

- frontal bone in the anterior and lateral direction;
- ethmoid bone in the midline; and
- two parts of the sphenoid bone (posteriorly), the body (midline), and the lesser wings (laterally).

The anterior cranial fossa is above the nasal cavity and the orbits and is filled by the frontal lobes of the cerebral hemispheres.

Anteriorly, a small wedge-shaped midline crest of bone (the frontal crest) projects from the frontal bone. This is a point of attachment for the falx cerebri. Immediately

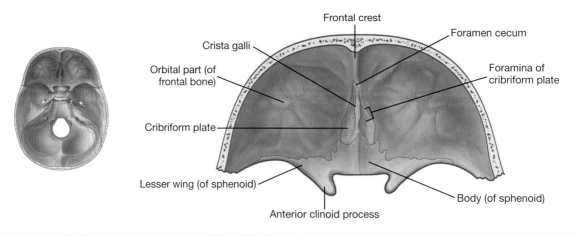

Fig. 8.13 Anterior cranial fossa.

Table 8.2 Internal foramina of the skull

Foramen	Structures passing through foramen
Anterior cranial fossa	
Foramen cecum	Emissary veins to nasal cavity
Olfactory foramina in cribriform plate	Olfactory nerves [I]
Middle cranial fossa	
Optic canal	Optic nerve [II]; ophthalmic artery
Superior orbital fissure	Oculomotor nerve [III]; trochlear nerve [IV]; ophthalmic division of the trigeminal nerve [V$_1$]; abducent nerve [VI]; ophthalmic veins
Foramen rotundum	Maxillary division of the trigeminal nerve [V$_2$]
Foramen ovale	Mandibular division of the trigeminal nerve [V$_3$]; lesser petrosal nerve
Foramen spinosum	Middle meningeal artery
Hiatus for the greater petrosal nerve	Greater petrosal nerve
Hiatus for the lesser petrosal nerve	Lesser petrosal nerve
Posterior cranial fossa	
Foramen magnum	End of brainstem/beginning of spinal cord; vertebral arteries; spinal roots of the accessory nerve; meninges
Internal acoustic meatus	Facial nerve [VII]; vestibulocochlear nerve [VIII]; labyrinthine artery
Jugular foramen	Glossopharyngeal nerve [IX]; vagus nerve [X]; accessory nerve [XI]; inferior petrosal sinus, sigmoid sinus (forming internal jugular vein)
Hypoglossal canal	Hypoglossal nerve [XII]; meningeal branch of the ascending pharyngeal artery
Condylar canal	Emissary vein

posterior to the frontal crest is the **foramen cecum** (Table 8.2). This foramen between the frontal and ethmoid bones may transmit emissary veins connecting the nasal cavity with the superior sagittal sinus.

Posterior to the frontal crest is a prominent wedge of bone projecting superiorly from the **ethmoid** (the **crista galli**). This is another point of attachment for the falx cerebri, which is the vertical extension of dura mater partially separating the two cerebral hemispheres.

Lateral to the crista galli is the **cribriform plate** of the ethmoid bone (see Fig. 8.13). This is a sieve-like structure,

which allows small olfactory nerve fibers to pass through its foramina from the nasal mucosa to the olfactory bulb. The olfactory nerves are commonly referred to collectively as the olfactory nerve [I].

On each side of the ethmoid, the floor of the anterior cranial fossa is formed by relatively thin plates of frontal bone (the **orbital part** of the frontal bone), which also forms the roof of the orbit below. Posterior to both the frontal and ethmoid bones, the rest of the floor of the anterior cranial fossa is formed by the body and lesser wings of the sphenoid. In the midline the body extends anteriorly between the

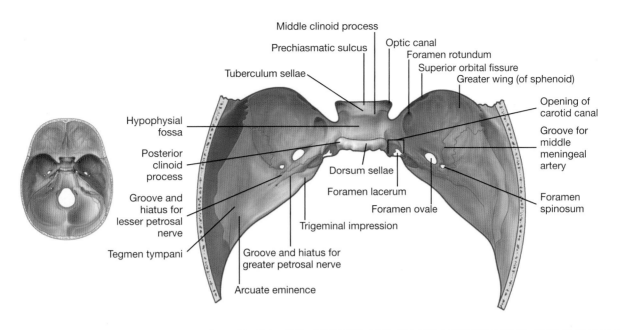

Middle clinoid process
Prechiasmatic sulcus
Optic canal
Foramen rotundum
Superior orbital fissure
Greater wing (of sphenoid)
Tuberculum sellae
Opening of carotid canal
Hypophysial fossa
Groove for middle meningeal artery
Posterior clinoid process
Dorsum sellae
Foramen lacerum
Foramen ovale
Foramen spinosum
Groove and hiatus for lesser petrosal nerve
Trigeminal impression
Tegmen tympani
Groove and hiatus for greater petrosal nerve
Arcuate eminence

Fig. 8.14 Middle cranial fossa.

orbital parts of the frontal bone to reach the ethmoid bone and posteriorly into the middle cranial fossa.

The boundary between the anterior and middle cranial fossae in the midline is the anterior edge of the prechiasmatic sulcus, a smooth groove stretching between the optic canals across the body of the sphenoid.

Lesser wings of the sphenoid

The two lesser wings of the sphenoid project laterally from the body of the sphenoid and form a distinct boundary between the lateral parts of the anterior and middle cranial fossae (see Fig. 8.13).

Overhanging the anterior part of the middle cranial fossae, each lesser wing ends laterally as a sharp point at the junction of the frontal bone and the greater wing of the sphenoid near the upper lateral edge of the superior orbital fissure that is formed between the greater and lesser wings.

Medially each lesser wing widens, curves posteriorly, and ends as a rounded **anterior clinoid process** (see Fig. 8.13). These processes serve as the anterior point of attachment for the **tentorium cerebelli,** which is a sheet of dura that separates the posterior part of the cerebral hemispheres from the cerebellum. Just anterior to each anterior clinoid process is a circular opening in the lesser wing of the sphenoid (the **optic canal**), through which the ophthalmic artery and optic nerve [II] pass as they exit the cranial cavity to enter the orbit. The optic canals are usually included in the middle cranial fossa.

Middle cranial fossa

The middle cranial fossa consists of parts of the sphenoid and temporal bones (Fig. 8.14).

The boundary between the anterior and middle cranial fossae in the midline is the anterior edge of the prechiasmatic sulcus, which is a smooth groove stretching between the optic canals across the body of the sphenoid.

The posterior boundaries of the middle cranial fossa are formed on each side by the anterior surface, as high as the superior border of the petrous part of the petromastoid part of the temporal bone.

Sphenoid

The floor in the midline of the middle cranial fossa is elevated and formed by the body of the sphenoid. Lateral to this are large depressions formed on either side by the greater wing of the sphenoid and the squamous part of the temporal bone. These depressions contain the temporal lobes of the brain.

Sella turcica

Just posterior to the chiasmatic sulcus is the uniquely modified remainder of the body of the sphenoid (the **sella turcica**), which consists of a deep central area (the **hypophysial fossa**) containing the pituitary gland with anterior and posterior vertical walls of bone (Fig. 8.14).

The anterior wall of the sella is vertical in position with its superior extent visible as a slight elevation (the **tuberculum sellae**) at the posterior edge of the chiasmatic sulcus.

Lateral projections from the corners of the tuberculum sellae (the **middle clinoid processes**) are sometimes evident.

The posterior wall of the sella turcica is the **dorsum sellae,** a large ridge of bone projecting upward and forward. At the top of this bony ridge, the lateral edges contain rounded projections (the **posterior clinoid processes**), which are points of attachment, like the anterior clinoid processes, for the tentorium cerebelli.

Fissures and foramina

A diagonal gap, the **superior orbital fissure,** separates the greater wing of the sphenoid from the lesser wing and is a major passageway between the middle cranial fossa and the orbit (Fig. 8.14; also see Table 8.2). Passing through the fissure are the oculomotor nerve [III], the trochlear nerve [IV], the ophthalmic nerve [V_1], the abducent nerve [VI], and ophthalmic veins.

Posterior to the medial end of the superior orbital fissure on the floor of the middle cranial fossa is a rounded foramen projecting in an anterior direction (the **foramen rotundum**) through which the maxillary nerve [V_2] passes from the middle cranial fossa to the pterygopalatine fossa (Fig. 8.14; also see Table 8.2).

Posterolateral to the **foramen rotundum** is a large oval opening (the **foramen ovale**), which allows structures to pass between the extracranial infratemporal fossa and the middle cranial fossa (Fig. 8.14; also see Table 8.2). The mandibular nerve [V_3], lesser petrosal nerve (carrying fibers from the tympanic plexus that originally came from the glossopharyngeal nerve [IX]), and occasionally a small vessel (the accessory middle meningeal artery) pass through this foramen.

Posterolateral from the foramen ovale is the small **foramen spinosum** (Fig. 8.14). This opening also connects the infratemporal fossa with the middle cranial fossa. The middle meningeal artery and its associated veins pass through this foramen, and, once inside, the groove for the middle meningeal artery across the floor and lateral wall of the middle cranial fossa clearly marks their path.

Posteromedial to the foramen ovale is the **rounded intracranial opening** of the **carotid canal**. Directly inferior to this opening is an irregular foramen (the **foramen lacerum**) (Fig. 8.14; also see Table 8.2). Clearly observed in the inferior view of the skull, the foramen lacerum is closed in life by a cartilaginous plug and no structures pass through it completely.

Temporal bone

The posterior boundary of the middle cranial fossa is formed by the anterior surface of the petrous part of the petromastoid part of the temporal bone.

Medially, there is a slight depression (**trigeminal impression**) in the anterior surface of the petrous part of the temporal bone (Fig. 8.14), which marks the location of the sensory ganglion for the trigeminal nerve [V].

Lateral to the trigeminal impression and on the anterior surface of the petrous part of the temporal bone is a small linear groove that passes in a superolateral direction and ends in a foramen (the **groove** and **hiatus for the greater petrosal nerve**) (Fig. 8.14). The greater petrosal nerve is a branch of the facial nerve [VII].

Anterolateral to the groove for the greater petrosal nerve is a second, smaller **groove** and **hiatus for the lesser petrosal nerve**, a branch from the tympanic plexus carrying fibers that originally came from the glossopharyngeal nerve [IX] (Fig. 8.14).

Above and lateral to the small openings for the greater and lesser petrosal nerves, near the superior ridge of the petrous part of the temporal bone, is a rounded protrusion of bone (the **arcuate eminence**) produced by the underlying anterior semicircular canal of the inner ear (Fig. 8.14).

Just anterior and lateral to the arcuate eminence, the anterior surface of the petrous part of the temporal bone is slightly depressed. This region is the **tegmen tympani,** which marks the thin bony roof of the middle ear cavity.

Posterior cranial fossa

The posterior cranial fossa consists mostly of parts of the temporal and occipital bones, with small contributions from the sphenoid and parietal bones (Fig. 8.15). It is the largest and deepest of the three cranial fossae and contains the brainstem (midbrain, pons, and medulla) and the cerebellum.

Boundaries

The anterior boundaries of the posterior cranial fossa in the midline are the dorsum sellae and the **clivus** (Fig. 8.15). The clivus is a slope of bone that extends upward from the foramen magnum. It is formed by contributions from the body of the sphenoid and from the basilar part of the occipital bone.

Laterally the anterior boundaries of the posterior cranial fossa are the superior border of the petrous part of the petromastoid part of the temporal bone.

Posteriorly the squamous part of the occipital bone to the level of the transverse groove is the major boundary, and laterally the petromastoid part of the temporal bone and small parts of the occipital and parietal bones border the fossa.

Foramen magnum

Centrally, in the deepest part of the posterior cranial fossa, is the largest foramen in the skull, the foramen magnum (Fig. 8.15; also see Table 8.2). It is surrounded by the basilar part of the occipital bone anteriorly, the lateral parts of the occipital bone on either side, and the squamous part of the occipital bone posteriorly.

The spinal cord passes superiorly through the foramen magnum to continue as the brainstem.

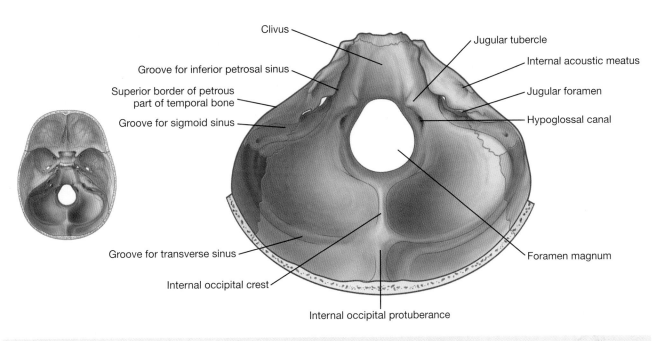

Clivus

Jugular tubercle

Groove for inferior petrosal sinus

Internal acoustic meatus

Superior border of petrous part of temporal bone

Jugular foramen

Groove for sigmoid sinus

Hypoglossal canal

Groove for transverse sinus

Foramen magnum

Internal occipital crest

Internal occipital protuberance

Fig. 8.15 Posterior cranial fossa.

Also passing through the foramen magnum are the vertebral arteries, the meninges, and the spinal roots of the accessory nerve [XI].

Grooves and foramina

The clivus slopes upward from the foramen magnum. Lateral to the clivus is a **groove for the inferior petrosal sinus** between the basilar part of the occipital bone and the petrous part of the petromastoid part of the temporal bone (Fig. 8.15).

Laterally, across the upper half of the posterior surface of the petrous part of the temporal bone, is an oval foramen (the **internal acoustic meatus**) (Fig. 8.15; also see Table 8.2). The facial [VII] and vestibulocochlear [VIII] nerves and the labyrinthine artery pass through it.

Inferior to the internal acoustic meatus, the temporal bone is separated from the occipital bone by the large jugular foramen (Fig. 8.15). Leading to this foramen from the medial side is the groove for the inferior petrosal sinus and from the lateral side is the **groove for the sigmoid sinus.** The sigmoid sinus passes into the jugular foramen and is continuous with the internal jugular vein, while the inferior petrosal sinus empties into the internal jugular vein in the area of the jugular foramen. Also passing through the jugular foramen are the glossopharyngeal nerve [IX], the vagus nerve [X], and the accessory nerve [XI].

Medial to the jugular foramen is a large rounded mound of the occipital bone (the **jugular tubercle**). Just inferior to this, and superior to the foramen magnum, is the

hypoglossal canal through which the hypoglossal nerve [XII] leaves the posterior cranial fossa and a meningeal branch of the ascending pharyngeal artery enters the posterior cranial fossa (Fig. 8.15).

Just posterolateral to the hypoglossal canal is the small **condylar canal** that, when present, transmits an emissary vein.

Squamous part of the occipital bone

The squamous part of the occipital bone has several prominent features (Fig. 8.15):

- Running upward in the midline from the foramen magnum is the **internal occipital crest.**
- On either side of the internal occipital crest, the floor of the posterior cranial fossa is concave to accommodate the cerebellar hemispheres.
- The internal occipital crest ends superiorly in a bony prominence (the internal occipital protuberance).
- Extending laterally from the internal occipital protuberance are grooves produced by the transverse sinuses, which continue laterally, eventually joining a groove for each sigmoid sinus. Each of these grooves then turns inferiorly toward the jugular foramina.

The transverse and sigmoid sinuses are intradural venous sinuses.

Foramina and fissures through which major structures pass between the cranial cavity and other regions are summarized in Fig. 8.16.

Foramen rotundum:
(*middle cranial fossa/
pterygopalatine fossa*)
- [V_2] Maxillary division
  of [V] (trigeminal nerve)

Foramen ovale:
(*middle cranial fossa/
infratemporal fossa*)
- [V_3] Mandibular division
  of [V] (trigeminal nerve)
- Lesser petrosal nerve

Carotid canal:
(*middle cranial fossa/neck*)
- Internal carotid artery

Foramen spinosum:
(*middle cranial fossa/
infratemporal fossa*)
- Middle meningeal artery

Jugular foramen:
(*posterior cranial fossa/neck*)
- [IX] Glossopharyngeal nerve
- [X] Vagus nerve
- [XI] Accessory nerve
- Internal jugular vein

Foramen magnum:
(*posterior cranial fossa/neck*)
- Spinal cord
- Vertebral arteries
- Roots of accessory nerve [XI] pass from
  upper region of spinal cord through the foramen
  magnum into the cranial cavity and then leave
  the cranial cavity through the jugular foramen

A

Cribiform plate:
(*anterior cranial fossa/nasal cavity*)
- [I] Olfactory nerves

Optic canal:
(*middle cranial fossa/orbit*)
- [II] Optic nerve
- Ophthalmic artery

Superior orbital fissure:
(*middle cranial fossa/orbit*)
- [V_1] Ophthalmic division
  of [V] (trigeminal nerve)
- [III] Oculomotor nerve
- [IV] Trochlear nerve
- [VI] Abducent nerve
- Superior ophthalmic vein

Foramen lacerum
(filled with cartilage in life)

Internal acoustic meatus:
(*posterior cranial fossa/ear, and neck
via stylomastoid foramen*)
- [VII] Facial nerve
- [VIII] Vestibulocochlear nerve
- Labrynthine artery and vein

Hypoglossal canal:
(*posterior cranial fossa/neck*)
- [XII] Hypoglossal nerve

Carotid canal:
- Internal carotid artery

Stylomastoid foramen:
- [VII] Facial nerve

Foramen magnum:
- Spinal cord
- Vertebral arteries
- Roots of accessory nerve [XI] pass from
  upper region of spinal cord through the
  foramen magnum into the cranial cavity
  and then leave the cranial cavity through
  the jugular foramen

B

Foramen ovale:
- [V_3] Mandibular division
  of [V] (trigeminal nerve)
- Lesser petrosal nerve

Foramen spinosum:
- Middle meningeal artery

Hypoglossal canal:
- [XII] Hypoglossal nerve

Jugular foramen:
- [IX] Glossopharyngeal nerve
- [X] Vagus nerve
- [XI] Accessory nerve
- Internal jugular vein

Fig. 8.16 Summary of foramina and fissures through which major structures enter and leave the cranial cavity. **A.** Floor of cranial cavity. **B.** Inferior aspect of cranium.

Clinical app

Medical imaging of the head

Radiography

Until recently the standard method of imaging the head was plain radiography. The radiographs are taken in three standard projections—namely the posteroanterior view, the lateral view, and the Towne's view.

Computed tomography

Since the development of computed tomography (CT), cerebral computed tomography has become the "workhorse" of neuroradiological examination. It is ideally used for head injury because the brain and its coverings can be easily and quickly examined and blood is easily detected.

With intravenous contrast, CT angiography can be used to demonstrate the position and the size of an intracerebral aneurysm before endovascular treatment.

Magnetic resonance imaging

Magnetic resonance imaging (MRI) is unsurpassed by other imaging techniques in its ability for contrast resolution. The brain and its coverings, cerebrospinal fluid (CSF), and the vertebral column can be easily and quickly examined.

Magnetic resonance angiography has been extremely useful in determining the completeness of the intracranial vasculature (circle of Willis), which is necessary in some surgical conditions.

Ultrasonography

Initial work using ultrasound to assess the brain appeared fruitless, but with increasing probe technology it is now possible to carry out intracranial Doppler studies, which enable a surgeon to detect whether a patient is experiencing cerebral embolization from a carotid plaque.

Clinical app

Fractures of the skull vault

The skull vault is a remarkably strong structure because it protects our most vital organ, the brain. From a clinical standpoint, skull fractures alert clinicians to the nature and force of an injury and potential complications. Of key importance is the need to minimize the extent of primary brain injury and to treat potential secondary complications rather than focusing on the skull fracture. Skull fractures that have particular significance include depressed skull fractures, compound fractures, and pterion fractures.

Depressed skull fractures

In a depressed skull fracture, a bony fragment is depressed below the normal skull convexity. This may lead to secondary arterial and venous damage with hematoma formation. Furthermore, a primary brain injury can also result from this type of fracture.

Clinical app—cont'd

Compound fractures

In a compound fracture there is a fracture of the bone together with a breach of the skin, which may allow an infection to enter. Typically these fractures are associated with scalp lacerations and can usually be treated with antibiotics.

Pterion fractures

The **pterion** is an important circular area on the lateral aspect of the skull where the frontal, parietal, sphenoid, and temporal bones come together. Importantly, deep to the pterion is the middle meningeal artery. An injury to this point of the skull is extremely serious because damage to this vessel may produce a significant extradural hematoma, which can be fatal.

Surface anatomy
Estimating the position of the middle meningeal artery

The middle meningeal artery (Fig. 8.17) is a branch of the maxillary artery in the infratemporal fossa. It enters the skull through the foramen spinosum and is within the dura mater lining the cranial cavity.

In lateral blows to the head, the middle meningeal artery can be ruptured, leading to extradural hemorrhage and eventual death if not treated.

The anterior branch of the middle meningeal artery is the part of the vessel most often torn. This branch is in the temple region of the head, approximately midway between the superior margin of the orbit and the upper part of the external ear in what is termed the *pterion*.

Lateral blows to the head can fracture the internal table of bone of the skull and tear the middle meningeal artery in the outer layer of dura mater that is fused to the cranium. Blood under pulsatile arterial pressure leaks out of the vessel and gradually separates the dura from the bone, forming a progressively larger extradural hematoma.

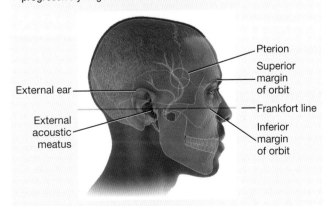

Fig. 8.17 Estimating the position of the middle meningeal artery. Lateral head and neck of a man.

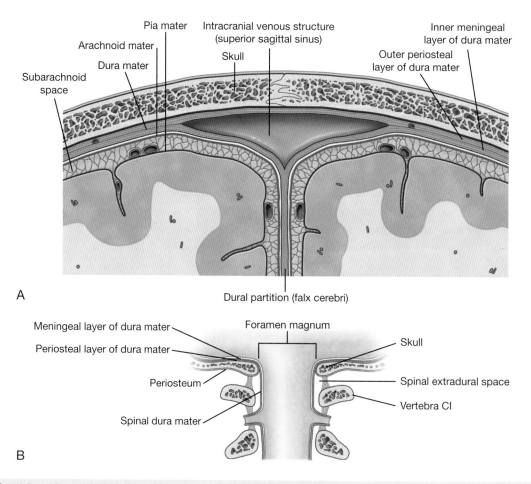

Fig. 8.18 Cranial meninges. **A.** Superior coronal view. **B.** Continuity with the spinal meninges.

MENINGES

The brain, as well as the spinal cord, is surrounded by three layers of memebranes (the **meninges;** Fig. 8.18A): a tough outer layer—the **dura mater,** a delicate middle layer—the **arachnoid mater,** and an inner layer firmly attached to the surface of the brain—the **pia mater.**

The cranial meninges are continuous with, and similar to, the spinal meninges through the foramen magnum, with one important distinction—the cranial dura mater consists of two layers, and only one of these is continuous through the foramen magnum (Fig. 8.18B).

Cranial dura mater

The cranial dura mater is a thick, tough, outer covering of the brain. It consists of an outer periosteal layer and an inner meningeal layer (Fig. 8.18A):

- The outer **periosteal layer** is firmly attached to the skull, is the periosteum of the cranial cavity, contains the meningeal arteries, and is continuous with the periosteum

on the outer surface of the skull at the foramen magnum and other intracranial foramina (Fig. 8.18B).
- The inner **meningeal layer** is in close contact with the arachnoid mater and is continuous with the spinal dura mater through the foramen magnum.

The two layers of dura separate from each other at numerous locations to form two unique types of structures (Fig. 8.18A):

- dural partitions, which project inward and incompletely separate parts of the brain; and
- intracranial venous structures (cranial venous sinuses, see pp. 469 to 472).

Dural partitions

The dural partitions project into the cranial cavity and partially subdivide the cranial cavity. They include the falx cerebri, tentorium cerebelli, falx cerebelli, and diaphragma sellae.

Falx cerebri

The falx cerebri (Fig. 8.19) is a crescent-shaped downward projection of meningeal dura mater from the dura lining the

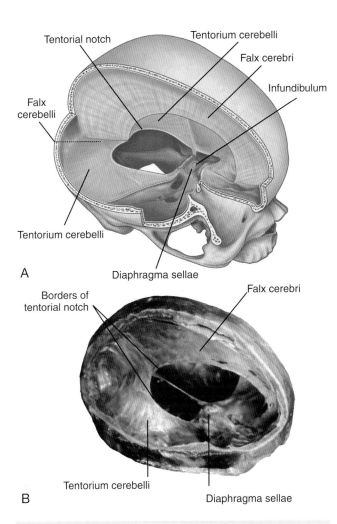

A

B

Fig. 8.19 Dural partitions. A. Diagram. B. Dissection.

Labels for image A:
- Tentorial notch
- Tentorium cerebelli
- Falx cerebri
- Infundibulum
- Falx cerebelli
- Tentorium cerebelli
- Diaphragma sellae

Labels for image B:
- Borders of tentorial notch
- Falx cerebri
- Tentorium cerebelli
- Diaphragma sellae

calva that passes between the two cerebral hemispheres. It is attached anteriorly to the crista galli of the ethmoid bone and frontal crest of the frontal bone. Posteriorly it is attached to and blends with the tentorium cerebelli.

Tentorium cerebelli

The tentorium cerebelli (Fig. 8.19) is a horizontal projection of the meningeal dura mater that covers and separates the cerebellum in the posterior cranial fossa from the posterior parts of the cerebral hemispheres. It is attached posteriorly to the occipital bone along the grooves for the transverse sinuses. Laterally, it is attached to the superior border of the petrous part of the temporal bone, ending anteriorly at the anterior and posterior clinoid processes.

The anterior and medial borders of the tentorium cerebelli are free, forming an oval opening in the midline (the **tentorial notch**) through which the midbrain passes.

Falx cerebelli

The falx cerebelli (Fig. 8.19) is a small midline projection of meningeal dura mater in the posterior cranial fossa. It

is attached posteriorly to the internal occipital crest of the occipital bone and superiorly to the tentorium cerebelli. Its anterior edge is free and is between the two cerebellar hemispheres.

Diaphragma sellae

The final dural projection is the diaphragma sellae (Fig. 8.19). This small horizontal shelf of meningeal dura mater covers the hypophysial fossa in the sella turcica of the sphenoid bone. There is an opening in the center of the diaphragma sellae through which passes the **infundibulum,** which connects the pituitary gland with the base of the brain and any accompanying blood vessels.

Arterial supply

The arterial supply to the dura mater (Fig. 8.20) travels in the outer periosteal layer of the dura and consists of:

- **anterior meningeal arteries** in the anterior cranial fossa,
- the **middle** and **accessory meningeal arteries** in the middle cranial fossa, and
- the **posterior meningeal artery** and other meningeal branches in the posterior cranial fossa.

All are small arteries except for the middle meningeal artery, which is much larger and supplies the greatest part of the dura.

The anterior meningeal arteries are branches of the **ethmoidal arteries** (Fig. 8.20).

The middle meningeal artery is a branch of the maxillary artery (Fig. 8.20). It enters the middle cranial fossa through the foramen spinosum and divides into anterior and posterior branches:

- The anterior branch passes in an almost vertical direction to reach the vertex of the skull, crossing the pterion during its course.
- The posterior branch passes in a posterosuperior direction, supplying this region of the middle cranial fossa.

The accessory meningeal artery is usually a small branch of the maxillary artery that enters the middle cranial fossa through the foramen ovale and supplies areas medial to this foramen.

The posterior meningeal artery and other meningeal branches supplying the dura mater in the posterior cranial fossa come from several sources (Fig. 8.20):

- The posterior meningeal artery, the terminal branch of the **ascending pharyngeal artery,** enters the posterior cranial fossa through the jugular foramen.

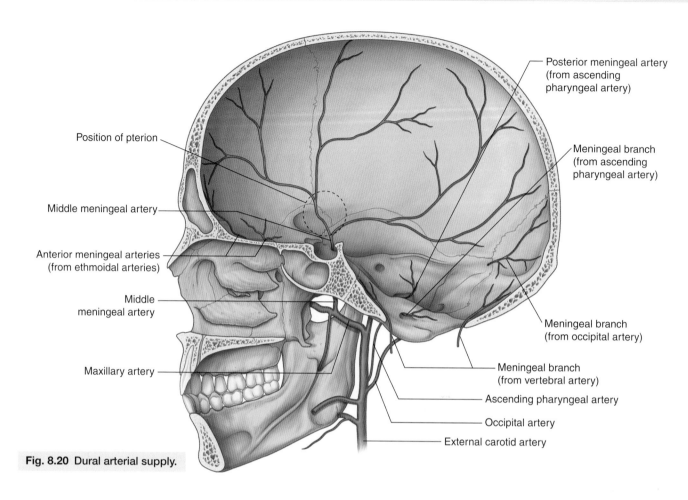

Position of pterion

Middle meningeal artery

Anterior meningeal arteries
(from ethmoidal arteries)

Middle
meningeal artery

Maxillary artery

Posterior meningeal artery
(from ascending
pharyngeal artery)

Meningeal branch
(from ascending
pharyngeal artery)

Meningeal branch
(from occipital artery)

Meningeal branch
(from vertebral artery)

Ascending pharyngeal artery

Occipital artery

External carotid artery

Fig. 8.20 Dural arterial supply.

- A meningeal branch from the ascending pharyngeal artery enters the posterior cranial fossa through the hypoglossal canal.
- Meningeal branches from the **occipital artery** enter the posterior cranial fossa through the jugular foramen and the mastoid foramen.
- A meningeal branch from the **vertebral artery** arises as the vertebral artery enters the posterior cranial fossa through the foramen magnum.

Innervation

Innervation of the dura mater (Fig. 8.21) is by small meningeal branches of all three divisions of the trigeminal nerve [V₁, V₂, and V₃], the vagus nerve [X], and the first, second, and, sometimes third cervical nerves. (Possible involvement of the glossopharyngeal [IX] and hypoglossal nerves [XII] in the posterior cranial fossa has also been reported.)

In the anterior cranial fossa, meningeal branches from the ethmoidal nerves, which are branches of the ophthalmic nerve [V₁], supply the floor and the anterior part of the falx cerebri (Fig. 8.21).

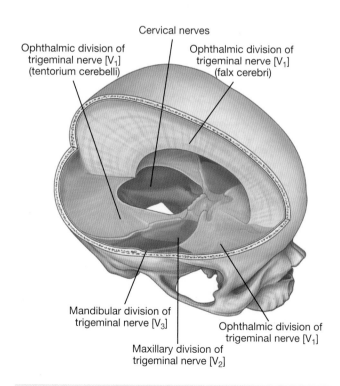

Cervical nerves

Ophthalmic division of
trigeminal nerve [V₁]
(tentorium cerebelli)

Ophthalmic division of
trigeminal nerve [V₁]
(falx cerebri)

Mandibular division of
trigeminal nerve [V₃]

Maxillary division of
trigeminal nerve [V₂]

Ophthalmic division of
trigeminal nerve [V₁]

Fig. 8.21 Dural innervation.

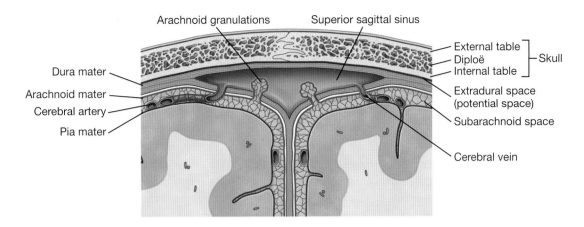

Arachnoid granulations   Superior sagittal sinus

External table ⎤
Diploë ⎬ Skull
Internal table ⎦

Dura mater

Arachnoid mater

Cerebral artery

Pia mater

Extradural space
(potential space)

Subarachnoid space

Cerebral vein

Fig. 8.22 Arrangement of the meninges and spaces.

Additionally, a meningeal branch of the ophthalmic nerve [V₁] turns and runs posteriorly, supplying the tentorium cerebelli and the posterior part of the falx cerebri (Fig. 8.21).

The middle cranial fossa is supplied medially by meningeal branches from the maxillary nerve [V₂] and laterally, along the distribution of the middle meningeal artery, by meningeal branches from the mandibular nerve [V₃] (Fig. 8.21).

The posterior cranial fossa is supplied by meningeal branches from the first, second, and, sometimes, the third cervical nerves, which enter the fossa through the foramen magnum, the hypoglossal canal, and the jugular foramen (Fig. 8.21). Meningeal branches of the vagus nerve [X] have also been described. (Possible contributions from the glossopharyngeal [IX] and hypoglossal [XII] nerves have also been reported.)

Arachnoid mater

The arachnoid mater is a thin, avascular membrane that lines, but is not adherent to, the inner surface of the dura mater (Fig. 8.22). From its inner surface, thin processes or trabeculae extend downward, cross the subarachnoid space, and become continuous with the pia mater.

Unlike the pia, the arachnoid does not enter the grooves or fissures of the brain, except for the longitudinal fissure between the two cerebral hemispheres.

Pia mater

The pia mater is a thin, delicate membrane that closely invests the surface of the brain (Fig. 8.22). It follows the contours of the brain, entering the grooves and fissures on its surface, and is closely applied to the roots of the cranial nerves at their origins.

Meningeal spaces

Extradural space

The potential space between dura mater and bone is the **extradural space.** Normally, the outer or periosteal layer of dura mater is firmly attached to the bones surrounding the cranial cavity (Fig. 8.22).

Subdural space

Anatomically, a true subdural space does not exist. Blood collecting in this region (subdural hematoma) due to injury represents a dissection of the dural border cell layer, which is the innermost lining of the meningeal dura. Dural border cells are flattened cells surrounded by extracellular spaces filled with amorphous material. While very infrequent, an occasional cell junction may be seen between these cells and the underlying arachnoid layer.

Subarachnoid space

Deep to the arachnoid mater is the only normally occurring fluid-filled space associated with the meninges. It occurs because the arachnoid mater clings to the inner surface of the dura mater and does not follow the contour of the brain, while the pia mater, being against the surface of the brain, closely follows the grooves and fissures on the surface of the brain. A narrow space (the **subarachnoid space**) is therefore created between these two membranes (Fig. 8.22).

The subarachnoid space surrounds the brain and spinal cord, and in certain locations it enlarges into expanded areas (subarachnoid **cisterns**). It contains CSF and blood vessels.

CSF is produced by the choroid plexus, primarily in the ventricles of the brain. It is a clear, colorless, cell-free fluid that circulates through the subarachnoid space surrounding the brain and spinal cord.

The CSF returns to the venous system through **arachnoid villi**. These project as clumps (**arachnoid granulations**) into the superior sagittal sinus, which is a dural venous sinus, and its lateral extensions, the **lateral lacunae**.

Clinical app

Cerebrospinal fluid leak

Leakage of CSF from the subarachnoid space may occur after any procedure in and around the brain, spinal cord, and meningeal membranes. These procedures include lumbar spine surgery, epidural injection, and CSF aspiration.

In "cerebrospinal fluid leak syndrome," CSF leaks out of the subarachnoid space and through dura mater for no apparent reason. The clinical consequences of this include dizziness, nausea, fatigue, and metallic taste in the mouth. Other effects also include facial nerve weakness and double vision.

Clinical app

Hydrocephalus

Hydrocephalus is a dilatation of the cerebral ventricular system, which is due to either an obstruction to the flow of CSF, overproduction of CSF, or a failure of reabsorption of CSF.

CSF is secreted by the epithelial cells of the choroid plexus within ventricles of the brain. The CSF passes from the ventricles through foramina into the subarachnoid space.

The CSF circulates around the spinal cord inferiorly, envelops the brain superiorly, and is absorbed through the arachnoid granulations in the walls of the dural venous sinuses. In adults almost half a liter of CSF is produced a day.

In adults the commonest cause of hydrocephalus is an interruption of the normal CSF absorption through the arachnoid granulations. This occurs when blood enters the subarachnoid space after subarachnoid hemorrhage, passes over the brain, and interferes with normal CSF absorption. To prevent severe hydrocephalus, it may be necessary to place a small catheter through the brain into the ventricular system to drain the CSF to relieve the pressure.

In children, hydrocephalus is always dramatic in its later stages. The hydrocephalus increases the size and dimensions of the ventricle, and as a result the brain enlarges. Because the skull sutures are not fused, the head expands. Cranial enlargement in utero may make a vaginal delivery impossible, and delivery then has to be by caesarean section.

Both computed tomography and MRI enable a radiologist to determine the site of obstruction and, in most cases, the cause of the obstruction.

Clinical app

Meningitis

Meningitis is a rare infection of the leptomeninges (the **leptomeninges** are a combination of the arachnoid mater and the pia mater). Infection of the meninges typically occurs via a blood-borne route, though in some cases it may be by direct spread (e.g., trauma) or from the nasal cavities through the cribriform plate in the ethmoid bone.

The typical history of meningitis is nonspecific at first. The patient may have a mild headache, fever, drowsiness, and nausea. As the infection progresses, photophobia (light intolerance) and ecchymosis may ensue. Straight leg raising causes marked neck pain and discomfort (Kernig's sign) and an emergency hospital admission is warranted.

BRAIN AND ITS BLOOD SUPPLY

Brain

The brain is a component of the central nervous system (CNS).

During development the brain can be divided into five continuous parts (Figs. 8.23, 8.24). From rostral (or cranial) to caudal they are:

- the **telencephalon (cerebrum),** which becomes the large cerebral hemispheres, the surface of which consists of elevations (gyri) and depressions (sulci) and is partially separated by a deep longitudinal fissure, and which fills the area of the cranial cavity above the tentorium cerebelli and is subdivided into lobes based on their position;
- the **diencephalon,** which is hidden from view in the adult brain by the cerebral hemispheres, consists of the thalamus, hypothalamus, and other related structures and classically

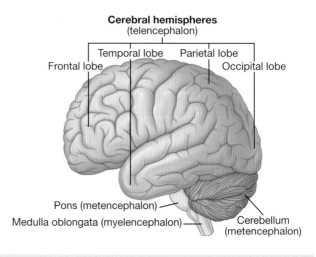

Fig. 8.23 Lateral view of the brain.

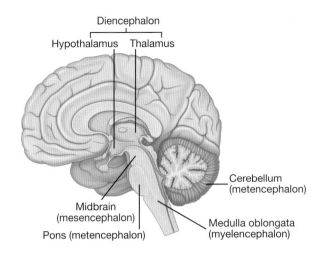

Fig. 8.24 Sagittal section of the brain.

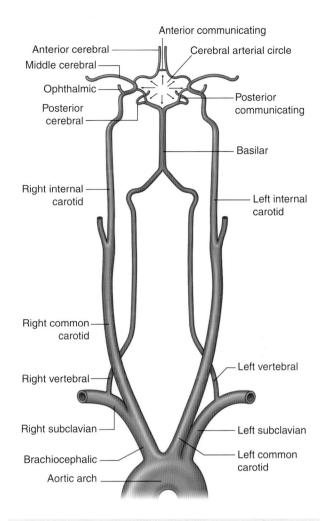

Fig. 8.25 Arterial supply to the brain.

is considered to be the most rostral part of the brainstem. (However, in common use today, the term *brainstem* usually refers to the midbrain, pons, and medulla);

- the **mesencephalon (midbrain),** which is the first part of the brainstem seen when an intact adult brain is examined and spans the junction between the middle and posterior cranial fossae;
- the **metencephalon,** which gives rise to the cerebellum (consisting of two lateral hemispheres and a midline part in the posterior cranial fossa below the tentorium cerebelli) and the pons (anterior to the cerebellum, a bulging part of the brainstem in the most anterior part of the posterior cranial fossa against the clivus and dorsum sellae); and
- the **myelencephalon (medulla oblongata),** the caudal most part of the brainstem, which ends at the foramen magnum or the uppermost rootlets of the first cervical nerve and to which cranial nerves VI to XII are attached.

Blood supply

The brain receives its arterial supply from two pairs of vessels, the **vertebral** and **internal carotid arteries** (Figs. 8.25, 8.26), which are interconnected in the cranial cavity to produce a **cerebral arterial circle** (of Willis).

Vertebral arteries

Each vertebral artery arises from the first part of each **subclavian artery** in the lower part of the neck and passes superiorly through the foramen transversarium of the upper six cervical vertebrae. On entering the cranial cavity through the foramen magnum, each vertebral artery gives off a small meningeal branch.

Continuing forward, the vertebral artery gives rise to three additional branches before joining with its companion vessel to form the **basilar artery** (Fig. 8.27):

- The largest branch is a **posterior inferior cerebellar artery.**
- Another branch joins with its companion from the other side to form the single **anterior spinal artery,** which then descends in the anterior median fissure of the spinal cord.
- A third branch is the **posterior spinal artery,** which passes posteriorly around the medulla then descends on the posterior surface of the spinal cord in the area of the attachment of the posterior roots—there are two posterior spinal arteries, one on each side (although the posterior spinal arteries can originate directly from the vertebral arteries, they more commonly branch from the posterior inferior cerebellar arteries).

The basilar artery travels in a rostral direction along the anterior aspect of the pons (Fig. 8.27). Its branches, in a caudal to rostral direction, include the **anterior inferior cerebellar arteries,** several small **pontine arteries,** and the **superior cerebellar arteries.** The basilar artery ends as a bifurcation, giving rise to two **posterior cerebral arteries.**

467

Imaging app

Visualizing the internal carotid and vertebral arteries

Basilar

Right internal carotid

Right vertebral

Right common carotid

Left internal carotid

Left vertebral

Left common carotid

Fig. 8.26 Magnetic resonance angiogram showing normal carotid and vertebral arteries.

Internal carotid arteries

The two internal carotid arteries arise as one of the two terminal branches of the common carotid arteries (see Figs. 8.25, 8.26). They proceed superiorly to the base of the skull where they enter the carotid canal.

Entering the cranial cavity, each internal carotid artery gives off the **ophthalmic artery,** the **posterior communicating artery,** the **middle cerebral artery,** and the **anterior cerebral artery** (Fig. 8.27).

Cerebral arterial circle

The cerebral arterial circle (of Willis) is formed at the base of the brain by the interconnecting vertebrobasilar and internal carotid systems of vessels (see Fig. 8.25). This anastomotic interconnection is accomplished by:

- an anterior communicating artery connecting the left and right anterior cerebral arteries to each other (Fig. 8.27; also see Fig. 8.25); and

- two posterior communicating arteries, one on each side, connecting the internal carotid artery with the posterior cerebral artery (Fig. 8.27; also see Fig. 8.25).

Clinical app

Endarterectomy
Endarterectomy is a surgical procedure to remove atheromatous plaques from arteries.

Atheromatous plaques occur in the subendothelial layer of vessels and consist of lipid-laden macrophages and cholesterol debris. The developing plaques eventually accumulate fibrous connective tissue and calcify. Plaques commonly occur around vessel bifurcations, limiting blood flow, and may embolize to distal organs.

During endarterectomy, the plaque is removed and the vessel reopened. In many instances a patch of material is sewn over the hole in the vessel, enabling improved flow and preventing narrowing from the suturing of the vessel.

Clinical app

Stroke
A stroke is the acute development of a focal neurological deficit as a result of localized or diffuse cerebral hypoperfusion.

The causes of stroke include cerebral thrombosis, cerebral hemorrhage, subarachnoid hemorrhage, and cerebral embolus. In the case of most strokes, small vessel cerebrovascular obstruction is caused by emboli from an atherosclerotic plaque within more proximal vessels in the neck and thorax.

Less severe strokes—transient ischemic attacks (TIAs)—are caused in the same way as strokes, but recovery is usually complete within 24 hours. They serve as a warning that treatment may be necessary.

Clinical app

Intracerebral aneurysms
Cerebral aneurysms most commonly arise from the vessels in and around the cerebral arterial circle (of Willis). They typically occur in and around the anterior communicating artery, the posterior communicating artery, the branches of the middle cerebral artery, the distal end of the basilar artery, and the posterior inferior cerebellar artery.

If the aneurysm ruptures, the patient complains of a sudden-onset "thunderclap" headache that produces neck stiffness and may induce vomiting. An initial CT scan demonstrates blood within the subarachnoid space, and this may be associated with an intracerebral bleed. Further management usually includes cerebral angiography, which enables the radiologist to determine the site, size, and origin of the aneurysm.

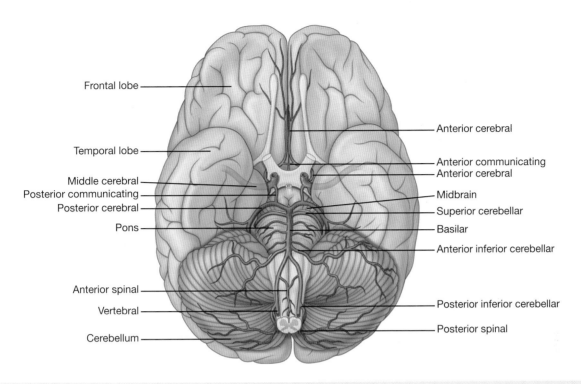

Frontal lobe

Temporal lobe

Middle cerebral
Posterior communicating
Posterior cerebral
Pons

Anterior spinal
Vertebral
Cerebellum

Anterior cerebral

Anterior communicating
Anterior cerebral

Midbrain
Superior cerebellar
Basilar
Anterior inferior cerebellar

Posterior inferior cerebellar

Posterior spinal

Fig. 8.27 Arteries on the base of the brain.

Venous drainage

Venous drainage of the brain begins internally as networks of small venous channels lead to larger cerebral veins, cerebellar veins, and veins draining the brainstem, which eventually empty into **dural venous sinuses.** The dural venous sinuses are endothelial-lined spaces between the outer periosteal and the inner meningeal layers of the dura mater and eventually lead to the **internal jugular veins.**

Also emptying into the dural venous sinuses are **diploic veins,** which run between the internal and external tables of compact bone in the roof of the cranial cavity, and **emissary veins,** which pass from outside the cranial cavity to the dural venous sinuses (Fig. 8.28).

Dural venous sinuses

The dural venous sinuses include the superior sagittal, inferior sagittal, straight, transverse, sigmoid, and occipital sinuses; the confluence of sinuses; and the cavernous, sphenoparietal, superior petrosal, inferior petrosal, and basilar sinuses (Table 8.3, Fig. 8.29).

Superior sagittal sinus

The superior sagittal sinus is in the superior border of the falx cerebri (Fig. 8.29). It begins anteriorly at the foramen cecum where it may receive a small emissary vein from the nasal cavity and ends posteriorly in the confluence of sinuses, usually bending to the right to empty into the right transverse sinus. The superior sagittal sinus communicates

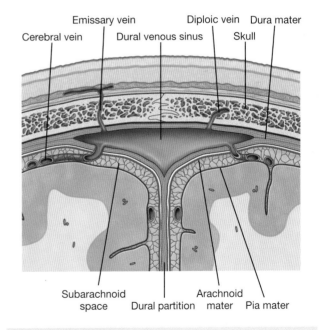

Emissary vein   Diploic vein   Dura mater
Cerebral vein   Dural venous sinus   Skull

Subarachnoid   Arachnoid
space   Dural partition   mater   Pia mater

Fig. 8.28 Dural venous sinuses.

with lateral extensions (lateral lacunae) of the sinus containing numerous arachnoid granulations.

Inferior sagittal and straight sinuses

The inferior sagittal sinus is in the inferior margin of the falx cerebri (Fig. 8.29). It receives a few cerebral veins and veins from the falx cerebri and ends posteriorly at the anterior edge of the tentorium cerebelli where it is joined by the

Table 8.3 Dural venous sinuses

Dural sinus	Location	Receives
Superior sagittal	Superior border of falx cerebri	Superior cerebral, diploic, and emissary veins and cerebrospinal fluid
Inferior sagittal	Inferior margin of falx cerebri	A few cerebral veins and veins from the falx cerebri
Straight	Junction of falx cerebri and tentorium cerebelli	Inferior sagittal sinus, great cerebral vein, posterior cerebral veins, superior cerebellar veins, and veins from the falx cerebri
Occipital	In falx cerebelli against occipital bone	[Communicates inferiorly with vertebral plexus of veins]
Confluence of sinuses	Dilated space at the internal occipital protuberance	Superior sagittal, straight, and occipital sinuses
Transverse (right and left)	Horizontal extensions from the confluence of sinuses along the posterior and lateral attachments of the tentorium cerebelli	Drainage from confluence of sinuses (the right transverse sinus usually receives the superior sagittal sinus; the left transverse sinus usually receives the straight sinus.
Sigmoid (right and left)	Continuation of transverse sinuses to internal jugular vein; groove of parietal, temporal, and occipital bones	Transverse sinuses, and cerebral, cerebellar, diploic, and emissary veins
Cavernous (paired)	Lateral aspect of body of sphenoid	Cerebral and ophthalmic veins, sphenoparietal sinuses, and emissary veins from pterygoid plexus of veins
Intercavernous	Crossing sella turcica	[Interconnects cavernous sinuses]
Sphenoparietal (paired)	Inferior surface of lesser wings of sphenoid	Diploic and meningeal veins
Superior petrosal (paired)	Superior margin of petrous part of temporal bone	Cavernous sinus and cerebral and cerebellar veins
Inferior petrosal (paired)	Groove between petrous part of temporal bone and occipital bone ending in internal jugular vein	Cavernous sinus, cerebellar veins, and veins from the internal ear and brainstem
Basilar	Clivus, just posterior to sella turcica of sphenoid	[Connect bilateral inferior petrosal sinuses and communicate with vertebral plexus of veins]

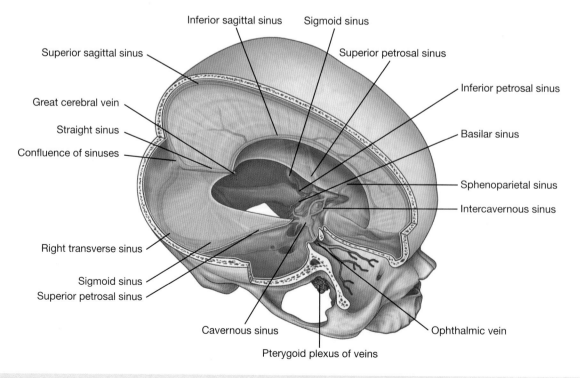

Fig. 8.29 Veins and dural venous sinuses.

great cerebral vein and, together with the great cerebral vein, forms the straight sinus (Fig. 8.29).

The straight sinus continues posteriorly along the junction of the falx cerebri and the tentorium cerebelli and ends in the confluence of sinuses, usually bending to the left to empty into the left transverse sinus (Fig. 8.29).

Confluence of sinuses, transverse and sigmoid sinuses

The superior sagittal and straight sinuses and the occipital sinus (in the falx cerebelli) empty into the confluence of sinuses, which is a dilated space at the internal occipital protuberance (Fig. 8.29) and is drained by the right and left transverse sinuses.

The paired transverse sinuses extend in horizontal directions from the confluence of sinuses where the tentorium cerebelli joins the lateral and posterior walls of the cranial cavity (Fig. 8.29).

The right transverse sinus usually receives blood from the superior sagittal sinus, and the left transverse sinus usually receives blood from the straight sinus.

The transverse sinuses also receive blood from the superior petrosal sinus, veins from the inferior parts of the cerebral hemispheres and the cerebellum, and diploic and emissary veins.

As the transverse sinuses leave the surface of the occipital bone, they become the sigmoid sinuses (Fig. 8.29), which turn inferiorly, grooving the parietal, temporal, and occipital bones before ending at the beginning of the internal jugular veins. The sigmoid sinuses also receive blood from cerebral, cerebellar, diploic, and emissary veins.

Cavernous sinuses

The paired cavernous sinuses are against the lateral aspect of the body of the sphenoid bone on either side of the sella turcica (Figs. 8.29, 8.30, 8.31). They are of great clinical importance because of their connections and the structures that pass through them.

The cavernous sinuses receive blood not only from cerebral veins, but also from the ophthalmic veins (from the orbit) and emissary veins (from the pterygoid plexus of veins in the infratemporal fossa). These connections provide pathways for infections to pass from extracranial sites into intracranial locations.

Structures passing through each cavernous sinus are (Fig. 8.30):

- the internal carotid artery, and
- the abducent nerve [VI].

Structures in the lateral wall of each cavernous sinus are, from superior to inferior (Fig. 8.30):

- the oculomotor nerve [III],
- the trochlear nerve [IV],

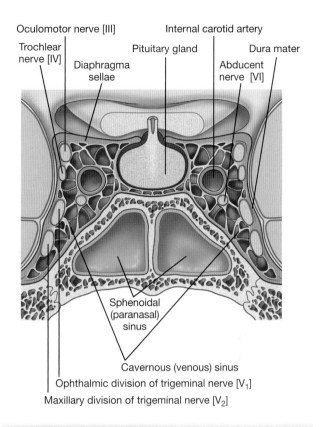

Fig. 8.30 Cavernous sinus.

- the ophthalmic nerve [V₁], and
- the maxillary nerve [V₂].

These structures passing through the cavernous sinus and lateral walls are vulnerable to injury due to inflammation.

Connecting the right and left cavernous sinuses are the intercavernous sinuses on the anterior and posterior sides of the pituitary stalk (Fig. 8.29).

Sphenoparietal sinuses drain into the anterior ends of each cavernous sinus. These small sinuses are along the inferior surface of the lesser wings of the sphenoid and receive blood from the diploic and meningeal veins.

Superior and inferior petrosal sinuses

The superior petrosal sinuses drain the cavernous sinuses into the transverse sinuses. Each superior petrosal sinus begins at the posterior end of the cavernous sinus, passes posterolaterally along the superior margin of the petrous part of each temporal bone, and connects to the transverse sinus (Fig. 8.29). The superior petrosal sinuses also receive cerebral and cerebellar veins.

The inferior petrosal sinuses also begin at the posterior ends of the cavernous sinuses. These bilateral sinuses pass posteroinferiorly in a groove between the petrous part of the temporal bone and the basal part of the occipital bone, ending in the internal jugular veins. They assist in draining the cavernous sinuses and receive blood from cerebellar veins and veins from the internal ear and brainstem.

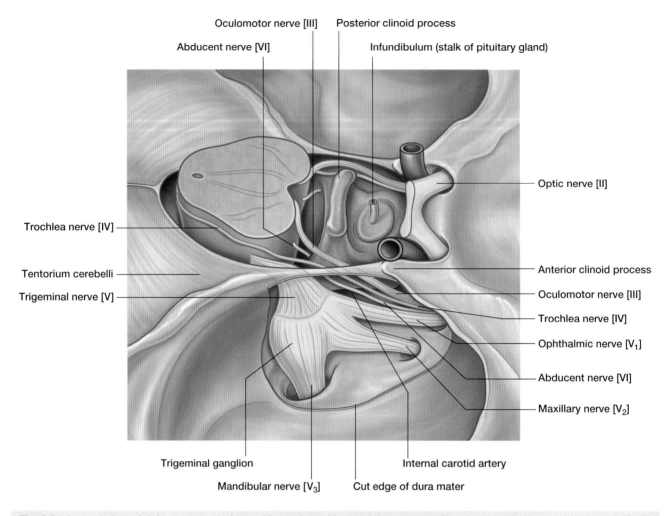

Fig. 8.31 Lateral view of right cavernous sinus with meningeal layer of dura removed to show contents.

Basilar sinuses connect the inferior petrosal sinuses to each other and to the vertebral plexus of veins. They are on the clivus, just posterior to the sella turcica of the sphenoid bone (Fig. 8.29).

Clinical app

Emissary veins

Emissary veins connect extracranial veins with intracranial veins and are important clinically because they can be a conduit through which infections can enter the cranial cavity. Emissary veins lack valves, as do the majority of veins in the head and neck.

Clinical app

Head injury

Head trauma is a common injury and is a significant cause of morbidity and death. At the time of the initial head injury two processes take place.

- First the primary brain injury may involve primary axonal and cellular damage, which results from the shearing deceleration forces within the brain. These injuries are generally not repairable. Further primary brain injuries

include intracerebral hemorrhage and penetrating injuries, which may directly destroy gray and white matter.

- The secondary injuries are sequelae of the initial trauma. They include scalp laceration, fracture of the cranial vault, disruption of intracerebral arteries and veins, intracerebral edema, and infection. In most cases these can be treated if diagnosed early, and rapid and effective treatment will significantly improve the patient's recovery and prognosis.

Clinical app

Concussion

Concussion (mild traumatic brain injury [MTBI]) is the most common type of traumatic brain injury. The injury typically results from a rapid deceleration of the head or by a rotation of the brain within the cranial cavity. General symptoms of MTBI can include posttraumatic amnesia, confusion, loss of consciousness, headache, dizziness, vomiting, lack of motor coordination, and light sensitivity. The diagnosis of concussion, MTBI, is based on the event, the current neurological status, and the state of consciousness of the patient.

Clinical app

Types of intracranial hemorrhage

Extradural hemorrhage

An extradural hemorrhage (Fig. 8.32) is caused by arterial damage and results from tearing of the branches of the middle meningeal artery, which typically occurs in the region of the pterion. Blood collects between the periosteal layer of the dura and the calvaria and, under arterial pressure, slowly expands.

The typical history is of a blow to the head (often during a sporting activity) that produces a minor loss of consciousness. Following the injury, the patient usually regains consciousness and has a lucid interval for a period of hours. After this, rapid drowsiness and unconsciousness ensue, which may lead to death.

Subdural hematoma

Subdural hematoma

A subdural hematoma (Fig. 8.33) is created by a hemorrhage within the dural border cell layer. The hematoma results from venous bleeding, usually from torn cerebral veins where they enter the superior sagittal sinus.

Patients at most risk of developing a subdural hematoma are the young and elderly. The clinical history usually includes a trivial injury followed by an insidious loss of consciousness or alteration of personality.

Subarachnoid hemorrhage

Subarachnoid hemorrhage

Subarachnoid hemorrhage (Fig. 8.34) typically results from a ruptured intracerebral aneurysm arising from the vessels supplying and around the arterial circle (of Willis) but may occur in patients who have undergone significant cerebral trauma.

Subdural hematoma   Lateral ventricles shifted

Fig. 8.33 Chronic (low-density) subdural hematoma. Axial CT scan of brain.

Subarachnoid basal cisterns containing blood

Fig. 8.34 Subarachnoid hemorrhage. Axial CT scan of brain.

Shift of the falx cerebri
Extradural hematoma

Fig. 8.32 Extradural hematoma. Axial CT scan of brain.

Clinical app

Scalp and meninges

Summary of relationships and clinical significance of the scalp and meninges

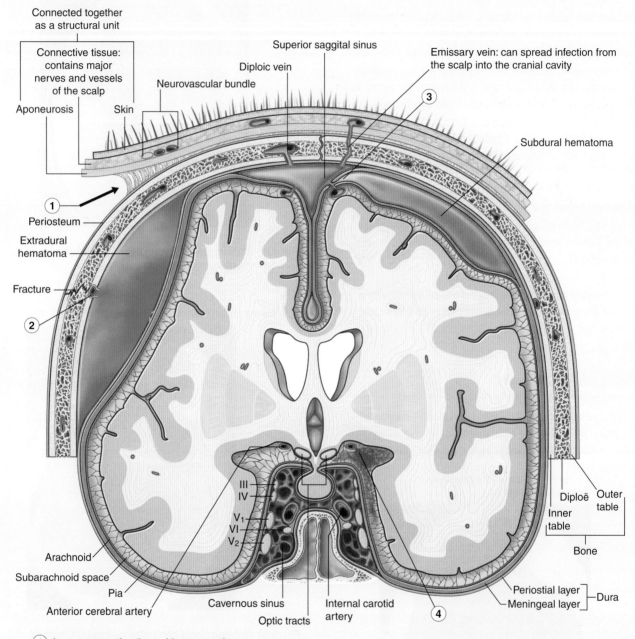

Connected together as a structural unit

Connective tissue: contains major nerves and vessels of the scalp

Aponeurosis

Skin

Neurovascular bundle

Diploic vein

Superior saggital sinus

Emissary vein: can spread infection from the scalp into the cranial cavity

3

Subdural hematoma

1

Periosteum

Extradural hematoma

Fracture

2

III
IV
V₁
VI
V₂

Diploë

Inner table

Outer table

Bone

Arachnoid

Subarachnoid space

Pia

Anterior cerebral artery

Cavernous sinus

Optic tracts

Internal carotid artery

4

Periostial layer
Meningeal layer

Dura

1 Loose connective tissue (danger area)
  • In scalping injuries, this is the layer in which separation occurs.
  • Infection can easily spread in this layer.
  • Blunt trauma can result in hemorrhage in this layer (blood can spread forward into the face, resulting in "black eyes").

2 Rupture of the middle meningeal artery (branches) by fracture of the inner table of bone results in extradural hematoma. Under pressure, the blood progressively separates dura from the bone.

3 Tear to cerebral vein where it crosses dura to enter cranial venous sinus can result in subdural hematoma. The tear separates a thin layer of meningeal dura from that which remains attached to the periosteal layer. As a result, the hematoma is covered by an inner limiting membrane derived from part of the meningeal dura.

4 Aneurysm
  • Ruptured aneurysms of vessels of the cerebral arterial circle hemorrhage directly into the subarachnoid space and CSF.

CRANIAL NERVES

The 12 pairs of cranial nerves are part of the peripheral nervous system (PNS) and pass through foramina or fissures in the cranial cavity. All nerves except one, the accessory nerve [XI], originate from the brain.

In addition to having similar somatic and visceral components as spinal nerves, some cranial nerves also contain special sensory and motor components (Tables 8.4, 8.5).

The special sensory components are associated with hearing, seeing, smelling, balancing, and tasting.

Special motor components include those that innervate skeletal muscles derived embryologically from the pharyngeal arches and not from somites.

In human embryology, six pharyngeal arches are designated, but the fifth pharyngeal arch never develops. Each of the pharyngeal arches that does develop is associated with a developing cranial nerve or one of its branches. These cranial nerves carry efferent fibers that innervate the skeletal musculature derived from the pharyngeal arch.

Innervation of the musculature derived from the five pharyngeal arches that do develop is as follows:

- first arch—trigeminal nerve [V₃],
- second arch—facial nerve [VII],
- third arch—glossopharyngeal nerve [IX],
- fourth arch—superior laryngeal branch of the vagus nerve [X],

- sixth arch—recurrent laryngeal branch of the vagus nerve [X], and
- posterior arches—accessory nerve [XI].

Olfactory nerve [I]

The **olfactory nerve [I]** carries special afferent (SA) fibers for the sense of smell. Its sensory neurons have:

- peripheral processes that act as olfactory receptors in the nasal mucosa, and
- central processes that return information to the brain.

The receptors are in the roof and upper parts of the nasal cavity and the central processes. After joining into small bundles, axons of the receptors enter the cranial cavity by passing through the cribriform plate of the ethmoid bone (Fig. 8.35). They terminate by synapsing with secondary neurons in the olfactory bulbs (Fig. 8.36).

Optic nerve [II]

The **optic nerve [II]** carries SA fibers for vision. These fibers return information to the brain from photoreceptors in the retina. Neuronal processes leave the retinal receptors, join into small bundles, and are carried by the optic nerves to other components of the visual system in the brain. The optic nerves enter the cranial cavity through the optic canals (Fig. 8.35).

Table 8.4 Cranial nerve functional components

Functional component	Abbreviation	General function	Cranial nerves containing component
General somatic afferent	GSA	Perception of touch, pain, temperature	Trigeminal nerve [V]; facial nerve [VII]; glossopharyngeal nerve [IX]; vagus nerve [X]
General visceral afferent	GVA	Sensory input from viscera	Glossopharyngeal nerve [IX]; vagus nerve [X]
Special afferent*	SA	Smell, taste, vision, hearing, and balance	Olfactory nerve [I]; optic nerve [II]; facial nerve [VII]; vestibulocochlear nerve [VIII]; glossopharyngeal nerve [IX]; vagus nerve [X]
General somatic efferent	GSE	Motor innervation to skeletal (voluntary) muscles	Oculomotor nerve [III]; trochlear nerve [IV]; abducent nerve [VI]; hypoglossal nerve [XII]
General visceral efferent	GVE	Motor innervation to smooth muscle, heart muscle, and glands	Oculomotor nerve [III]; facial nerve [VII]; glossopharyngeal nerve [IX]; vagus nerve [X]
Branchial efferent†	BE	Motor innervation to skeletal muscles derived from pharyngeal arch mesoderm	Trigeminal nerve [V]; facial nerve [VII]; glossopharyngeal nerve [IX]; vagus nerve [X]; accessory nerve [XI] (see Diogo et al. 2015 *Nature* 520:466–473)

Other terminology used when describing functional components:
*Special sensory, or special visceral afferent (SVA): smell, taste. Special somatic afferent (SSA): vision, hearing, balance.
†Special visceral efferent (SVE) or branchial motor.

Table 8.5 Cranial nerves (see Table 8.4 for abbreviations)

| Nerve | COMPONENT | | Exit from skull | Function |
	Afferent	Efferent		
Olfactory nerve [I]	SA		Cribriform plate of ethmoid bone	Smell
Optic nerve [II]	SA		Optic canal	Vision
Oculomotor nerve [III]		GSE, GVE	Superior orbital fissure	GSE—innervates levator palpebrae superioris, superior rectus, inferior rectus, medial rectus, and inferior oblique muscles GVE—innervates sphincter pupillae for pupillary constriction; ciliary muscles for accommodation of the lens for near vision
Trochlear nerve [IV]		GSE	Superior orbital fissure	Innervates superior oblique muscle
Trigeminal nerve [V]	GSA	BE	Superior orbital fissure—ophthalmic division [V$_1$] Foramen rotundum—maxillary nerve [V$_2$] Foramen ovale—mandibular division [V$_3$]	GSA—sensory from: ophthalmic division [V$_1$]—eyes, conjunctiva, orbital contents, nasal cavity, frontal sinus, ethmoidal cells, upper eyelid, dorsum of nose, anterior part of scalp, dura in anterior cranial fossa, superior part of tentorium cerebelli; maxillary nerve [V$_2$]—dura in middle cranial fossa, nasopharynx, palate, nasal cavity, upper teeth, maxillary sinus, skin covering the side of the nose, lower eyelid, cheek, upper lip; mandibular division [V$_3$]—skin of lower face, cheek, lower lip, anterior part of external ear, part of external acoustic meatus, temporal fossa, anterior two-thirds of tongue, lower teeth, mastoid air cells, mucous membranes of cheek, mandible, dura in middle cranial fossa BE—innervates temporalis, masseter, medial and lateral pterygoids, tensor tympani, tensor veli palatini, anterior belly of digastric, and mylohyoid muscles
Abducent nerve [VI]		GSE	Superior orbital fissure	Innervates lateral rectus muscle
Facial nerve [VII]	GSA, SA	GVE, BE	Stylomastoid foramen [nerve leaves cranial cavity through internal acoustic meatus and gives rise to branches in the facial canal of the temporal bone before exiting through the stylomastoid foramen. These branches leave the skull through other fissures and canals.]	GSA—sensory from part of external acoustic meatus and deeper parts of auricle SA—taste from anterior two-thirds of tongue GVE—innervates lacrimal gland, submandibular and sublingual salivary glands, and mucous membranes of nasal cavity, hard and soft palates BE—innervates muscles of face (muscles of facial expression) and scalp derived from the second pharyngeal arch, and stapedius, posterior belly of digastric, stylohyoid muscles
Vestibulocochlear nerve [VIII]	SA		[Nerve leaves cranial cavity through internal acoustic meatus]	Vestibular division—balance Cochlear division—hearing
Glossopharyngeal nerve [IX]	GVA, SA, GSA	GVE, BE	Jugular foramen	GVA—sensory from carotid body and sinus GSA—posterior one-third of tongue, palatine tonsils, oropharynx, mucosa of middle ear, pharyngotympanic tube, and mastoid air cells SA—taste from posterior one-third of tongue GVE—innervates parotid salivary gland BE—innervates stylopharyngeus muscle
Vagus nerve [X]	GSA, GVA, SA	GVE, BE	Jugular foramen	GSA—sensory from larynx, laryngopharynx, deeper parts of auricle, part of external acoustic meatus, and dura in posterior cranial fossa GVA—sensory from aortic body chemoreceptors and aortic arch baroreceptors, esophagus, bronchi, lungs, heart, and abdominal viscera of the foregut and midgut SA—taste from the epiglottis and pharynx GVE—innervates smooth muscle and glands in the pharynx, larynx, thoracic viscera, and abdominal viscera of the foregut and midgut BE—innervates one tongue muscle (palatoglossus), muscles of soft palate (except tensor veli palatini), pharynx (except stylopharyngeus), and larynx
Accessory nerve [XI]		BE	Jugular foramen	Innervates sternocleidomastoid and trapezius muscles
Hypoglossal nerve [XII]		GSE	Hypoglossal canal	Innervates hyoglossus, genioglossus, and styloglossus muscles and all intrinsic muscles of the tongue

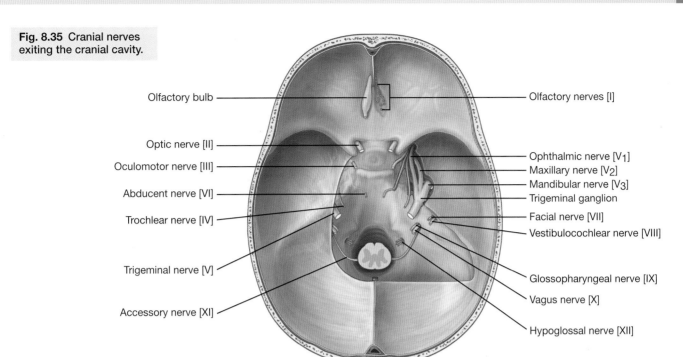

Fig. 8.35 Cranial nerves exiting the cranial cavity.

Olfactory bulb

Optic nerve [II]

Oculomotor nerve [III]

Abducent nerve [VI]

Trochlear nerve [IV]

Trigeminal nerve [V]

Accessory nerve [XI]

Olfactory nerves [I]

Ophthalmic nerve [V₁]

Maxillary nerve [V₂]

Mandibular nerve [V₃]

Trigeminal ganglion

Facial nerve [VII]

Vestibulocochlear nerve [VIII]

Glossopharyngeal nerve [IX]

Vagus nerve [X]

Hypoglossal nerve [XII]

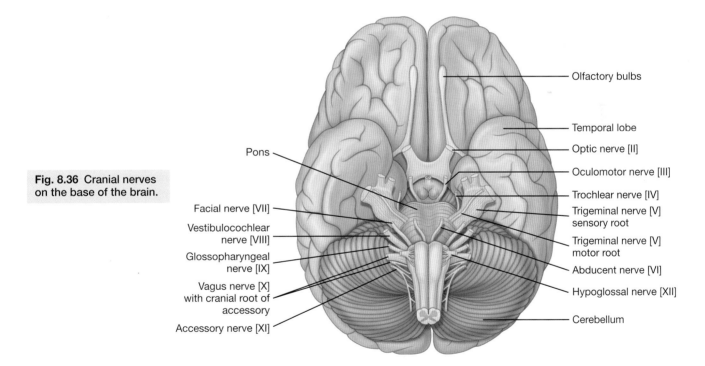

Fig. 8.36 Cranial nerves on the base of the brain.

Pons

Facial nerve [VII]

Vestibulocochlear nerve [VIII]

Glossopharyngeal nerve [IX]

Vagus nerve [X] with cranial root of accessory

Accessory nerve [XI]

Olfactory bulbs

Temporal lobe

Optic nerve [II]

Oculomotor nerve [III]

Trochlear nerve [IV]

Trigeminal nerve [V] sensory root

Trigeminal nerve [V] motor root

Abducent nerve [VI]

Hypoglossal nerve [XII]

Cerebellum

Oculomotor nerve [III]

The **oculomotor nerve [III]** carries two types of fibers:

■ General somatic efferent (GSE) fibers innervate most of the extra-ocular muscles.

■ General visceral efferent (GVE) fibers are part of the parasympathetic part of the autonomic division of the PNS.

The oculomotor nerve [III] leaves the anterior surface of the brainstem between the midbrain and the pons

477

Table 8.6 Parasympathetic ganglia of the head

Ganglion	Input	Cranial nerve origin of preganglionic fibers	Function
Ciliary	Oculomotor nerve [III]	Oculomotor nerve [III]	Innervation of sphincter pupillae muscle for pupillary constriction and ciliary muscles for accommodation of the lens for near vision
Pterygopalatine	Greater petrosal nerve	Facial nerve [VII]	Innervation of lacrimal gland and mucous glands of nasal cavity, maxillary sinus, and palate
Otic	Lesser petrosal nerve	Glossopharyngeal nerve [IX]	Innervation of parotid gland
Submandibular	Chorda tympani to lingual	Facial nerve [VII]	Innervation of submandibular and sublingual glands

(Fig. 8.36). It enters the anterior edge of the tentorium cerebelli, continues in an anterior direction in the lateral wall of the cavernous sinus (Figs. 8.35, 8.36; also see Fig. 8.34), and leaves the cranial cavity through the superior orbital fissure.

In the orbit, the GSE fibers in the oculomotor nerve innervate levator palpebrae superioris, superior rectus, inferior rectus, medial rectus, and inferior oblique muscles.

The GVE fibers are preganglionic parasympathetic fibers that synapse in the ciliary ganglion and ultimately innervate the sphincter pupillae muscle responsible for pupillary constriction and the ciliary muscles responsible for accommodation of the lens for near vision (Table 8.6).

Trochlear nerve [IV]

The **trochlear nerve [IV]** is a cranial nerve that carries GSE fibers to innervate the superior oblique muscle, an extraocular muscle in the orbit. It arises in the midbrain and is the only cranial nerve to exit from the posterior surface of the brainstem (Fig. 8.36). After curving around the midbrain, it enters the inferior surface of the free edge of the tentorium cerebelli, continues in an anterior direction in the lateral wall of the cavernous sinus (Figs. 8.35, 8.36; also see Fig. 8.34), and enters the orbit through the superior orbital fissure.

Trigeminal nerve [V]

The **trigeminal nerve [V]** is the major sensory nerve of the head and innervates muscles that move the lower jaw. It carries general somatic afferent (GSA) and branchial efferent (BE) fibers:

- The GSA fibers provide sensory input from the face, anterior one-half of the scalp, mucous membranes of the oral and nasal cavities and the paranasal sinuses, the nasopharynx, part of the ear and external acoustic meatus, part of the tympanic membrane, orbital contents and conjunctiva, the dura mater in the anterior and middle cranial fossae, and possibly the mastoid air cells.

- The BE fibers innervate the muscles of mastication, the tensor tympani, the tensor veli palatini, the mylohyoid, and the anterior belly of the digastric.

The trigeminal nerve exits from the anterolateral surface of the pons as a large sensory root and a small motor root (Fig. 8.36). These roots continue forward out of the posterior cranial fossa and into the middle cranial fossa by passing over the medial tip of the petrous part of the temporal bone (Fig. 8.35).

In the middle cranial fossa the sensory root expands into the **trigeminal ganglion** (Fig. 8.35), which contains cell bodies for the sensory neurons in the trigeminal nerve and is comparable to a spinal ganglion. The ganglion is in a depression (the trigeminal depression) on the anterior surface of the petrous part of the temporal bone in a dural cave (the **trigeminal cave**). The motor root is below and completely separate from the sensory root at this point.

Arising from the anterior border of the trigeminal ganglion are the three terminal divisions of the trigeminal nerve, which, in descending order, are:

- the **ophthalmic nerve (ophthalmic division [V$_1$])**,
- the **maxillary nerve (maxillary division [V$_2$])**, and
- the **mandibular nerve (mandibular division [V$_3$])**.

Ophthalmic nerve [V$_1$]

The ophthalmic nerve [V$_1$] passes forward in the dura of the lateral wall of the cavernous sinus (see Fig. 8.34), leaves the cranial cavity, and enters the orbit through the superior orbital fissure.

The ophthalmic nerve [V$_1$] carries sensory branches from the eyes, conjunctiva, and orbital contents, including the lacrimal gland. It also receives sensory branches from the nasal cavity, frontal sinus, ethmoidal cells, falx cerebri, dura in the anterior cranial fossa and superior parts of the tentorium cerebelli, upper eyelid, dorsum of the nose, and the anterior part of the scalp.

Maxillary nerve [V₂]

The maxillary nerve [V$_2$] passes forward in the dura mater of the lateral wall of the cavernous sinus just inferior to the ophthalmic nerve [V$_1$] (see Fig. 8.34), leaves the cranial cavity through the foramen rotundum, and enters the pterygopalatine fossa.

The maxillary nerve [V$_2$] receives sensory branches from the dura in the middle cranial fossa, the nasopharynx, the palate, the nasal cavity, teeth of the upper jaw, maxillary sinus, skin covering the side of the nose, the lower eyelid, the cheek, and the upper lip.

Mandibular nerve [V₃]

The mandibular nerve [V$_3$] leaves the inferior margin of the trigeminal ganglion and leaves the skull through the foramen ovale and enters the infratemporal fossa.

The motor root of the trigeminal nerve also passes through the foramen ovale and unites with the sensory component of the mandibular nerve [V$_3$] outside the skull. Thus the mandibular nerve [V$_3$] is the only division of the trigeminal nerve that contains a motor component.

Outside the skull the motor fibers innervate the four muscles of mastication (temporalis, masseter, and medial and lateral pterygoids), as well as the tensor tympani, the tensor veli palatini, the anterior belly of the digastric, and the mylohyoid muscles.

The mandibular nerve [V$_3$] also receives sensory branches from the skin of the lower face, cheek, lower lip, anterior part of the external ear, part of the external acoustic meatus and the temporal region, the anterior two-thirds of the tongue, the teeth of the lower jaw, the mastoid air cells, the mucous membranes of the cheek, the mandible, and dura in the middle cranial fossa.

Abducent nerve [VI]

The **abducent nerve [VI]** carries GSE fibers to innervate the lateral rectus muscle in the orbit. It arises from the brainstem between the pons and medulla and passes forward, piercing the dura covering the clivus (see Figs. 8.35, 8.36). Continuing upward in a dural canal, it crosses the superior edge of the petrous temporal bone, enters and crosses the cavernous sinus (see Fig. 8.34) just inferolateral to the internal carotid artery, and enters the orbit through the superior orbital fissure.

Facial nerve [VII]

The **facial nerve [VII]** carries GSA, SA, GVE, and BE fibers:

- The GSA fibers provide sensory input from part of the external acoustic meatus and deeper parts of the auricle.
- The SA fibers are for taste from the anterior two-thirds of the tongue.
- The GVE fibers are part of the parasympathetic part of the autonomic division of the PNS and stimulate secretomotor activity in the lacrimal gland, submandibular and sublingual salivary glands, glands in the mucous membranes of the nasal cavity, and hard and soft palates.
- The BE fibers innervate the muscles of the face (muscles of facial expression) and scalp derived from the second pharyngeal arch and the stapedius, the posterior belly of the digastric, and the stylohyoid muscles.

The facial nerve [VII] attaches to the lateral surface of the brainstem between the pons and medulla oblongata (see Fig. 8.36). It consists of a large motor root and a smaller sensory root (the **intermediate nerve**):

- The intermediate nerve contains the SA fibers for taste, the parasympathetic GVE fibers, and the GSA fibers.
- The larger motor root contains the BE fibers.

The motor and sensory roots cross the posterior cranial fossa and leave the cranial cavity through the internal acoustic meatus (see Fig. 8.35). After entering the facial canal in the petrous part of the temporal bone, the two roots fuse and form the facial nerve [VII]. Near this point the nerve enlarges as the **geniculate ganglion,** which is similar to a spinal ganglion containing cell bodies for sensory neurons.

At the geniculate ganglion, the facial nerve [VII] turns and gives off the **greater petrosal nerve,** which carries mainly preganglionic parasympathetic (GVE) fibers (Table 8.6).

The facial nerve [VII] continues along the bony canal, giving off the **nerve to stapedius** and the **chorda tympani** before exiting the skull through the stylomastoid foramen.

The chorda tympani carries taste (SA) fibers from the anterior two-thirds of the tongue and preganglionic parasympathetic (GVE) fibers destined for the submandibular ganglion (Table 8.6).

Vestibulocochlear nerve [VIII]

The vestibulocochlear nerve [VIII] carries SA fibers for hearing and balance and consists of two divisions:

- a vestibular component for balance, and
- a cochlear component for hearing.

The vestibulocochlear nerve [VIII] attaches to the lateral surface of the brainstem between the pons and medulla after emerging from the internal acoustic meatus and crossing the posterior cranial fossa (see Figs. 8.35, 8.36). The two divisions combine into the single nerve seen in the posterior cranial fossa within the substance of the petrous part of the temporal bone.

Glossopharyngeal nerve [IX]

The glossopharyngeal nerve [IX] carries GVA, GSA, SA, GVE, and BE fibers:

- The GVA fibers provide sensory input from the carotid body and sinus.
- The GSA fibers provide sensory input from the posterior one-third of the tongue, palatine tonsils, oropharynx, mucosa of the middle ear, mastoid air cells, and pharyngotympanic tube.
- The SA fibers are for taste from the posterior one-third of the tongue.
- The GVE fibers are part of the parasympathetic part of the autonomic division of the PNS and stimulate secretomotor activity in the parotid salivary gland.
- The BE fibers innervate the muscle derived from the third pharyngeal arch (the stylopharyngeus muscle).

The glossopharyngeal nerve [IX] arises as several rootlets on the anterolateral surface of the upper medulla oblongata (see Fig. 8.36). The rootlets cross the posterior cranial fossa and enter the jugular foramen (see Fig. 8.35). Within the jugular foramen, and before exiting from it, the rootlets merge to form the glossopharyngeal nerve.

Within or immediately outside the jugular foramen are two ganglia (the **superior** and **inferior ganglia**), which contain the cell bodies of the sensory neurons in the glossopharyngeal nerve [IX].

Tympanic nerve

Branching from the glossopharyngeal nerve [IX] either within or immediately outside the jugular foramen is the **tympanic nerve.** This branch re-enters the temporal bone, enters the middle ear cavity, and participates in the formation of the **tympanic plexus.** Within the middle ear cavity it provides sensory innervation to the mucosa of the cavity, pharyngotympanic tube, and mastoid air cells.

The tympanic nerve also contributes GVE fibers, which leave the tympanic plexus in the **lesser petrosal nerve**—a small nerve that exits the temporal bone, enters the middle cranial fossa, and descends through the foramen ovale to exit the cranial cavity carrying preganglionic parasympathetic fibers to the otic ganglion (see Table 8.6).

Vagus nerve [X]

The vagus nerve [X] carries GSA, GVA, SA, GVE, and BE fibers:

- The GSA fibers provide sensory input from the larynx, laryngopharynx, deeper parts of the auricle, part of the external acoustic meatus, and the dura mater in the posterior cranial fossa.
- The GVA fibers provide sensory input from the aortic body chemoreceptors, aortic arch baroreceptors, and the esophagus, bronchi, lungs, heart, and abdominal viscera in the foregut and midgut.
- The SA fibers are for taste around the epiglottis and pharynx.
- The GVE fibers are part of the parasympathetic part of the autonomic division of the PNS and stimulate smooth muscle and glands in the pharynx, larynx, thoracic viscera, and abdominal viscera of the foregut and midgut.
- The BE fibers innervate one muscle of the tongue (palatoglossus) and the muscles of the soft palate (except tensor veli palatini), pharynx (except stylopharyngeus), and larynx.

The vagus nerve arises as a group of rootlets on the anterolateral surface of the medulla oblongata just inferior to the rootlets arising to form the glossopharyngeal nerve [IX] (see Fig. 8.36). The rootlets cross the posterior cranial fossa and enter the jugular foramen (see Fig. 8.35). Within this foramen, and before exiting from it, the rootlets merge to form the vagus nerve [X]. Within or immediately outside the jugular foramen are two ganglia, the **superior** (jugular) and **inferior** (nodose) **ganglia,** which contain the cell bodies of the sensory neurons in the vagus nerve [X].

Accessory nerve [XI]

The accessory nerve [XI] is a cranial nerve that carries BE fibers to innervate the sternocleidomastoid and trapezius muscles. It is a unique cranial nerve because its roots arise from motor neurons in the upper five segments of the cervical spinal cord. These fibers leave the lateral surface of the spinal cord and, joining together as they ascend, enter the cranial cavity through the foramen magnum (see Fig. 8.36). The accessory nerve [XI] continues through the posterior cranial fossa and exits through the jugular foramen (see Fig. 8.35). It then descends in the neck to innervate the sternocleidomastoid and trapezius muscles from their deep surfaces.

Cranial root of the accessory nerve

Some descriptions of the accessory nerve [XI] refer to a few rootlets arising from the caudal part of the medulla

Clinical app

Cranial nerve lesions

Cranial nerve	Clinical findings	Example of lesion
Olfactory nerve [I]	Loss of smell (anosmia)	Injury to the cribriform plate; congenital absence
Optic nerve [II]	Blindness/visual field abnormalities, loss of pupillary constriction	Direct trauma to the orbit; disruption of the optic pathway
Oculomotor nerve [III]	Dilated pupil, ptosis, loss of normal pupillary reflex, eye moves inferiorly and laterally (down and out)	Pressure from an aneurysm arising from the posterior communicating, posterior cerebral, or superior cerebellar artery; pressure from a herniating cerebral uncus (false localizing sign); cavernous sinus mass or thrombosis
Trochlear nerve [IV]	Inability to look inferiorly when the eye is adducted (down and in)	Along the course of the nerve around the brainstem; orbital fracture
Trigeminal nerve [V]	Loss of sensation and pain in the region supplied by the three divisions of the nerve over the face; loss of motor function of the muscles of mastication on the side of the lesion	Typically in the region of the trigeminal ganglion, though local masses around the foramina through which the divisions pass can produce symptoms
Abducent nerve [VI]	Inability of lateral eye movement	Brain lesion or cavernous sinus lesion extending onto the orbit
Facial nerve [VII]	Paralysis of facial muscles Abnormal taste sensation from the anterior two-thirds of the tongue and dry conjunctivae Paralysis of contralateral facial muscles below the eye	Damage to the branches within the parotid gland; injury to temporal bone; viral inflammation of nerve; brainstem injury
Vestibulocochlear nerve [VIII]	Progressive unilateral hearing loss and tinnitus (ringing in the ear)	Tumor at the cerebellopontine angle
Glossopharyngeal nerve [IX]	Loss of taste to the posterior one-third of the tongue and sensation of the soft palate	Brainstem lesion; penetrating neck injury
Vagus nerve [X]	Soft palate deviation with deviation of the uvula to the normal side; vocal cord paralysis	Brainstem lesion; penetrating neck injury
Accessory nerve [XI]	Paralysis of sternocleidomastoid and trapezius muscles	Penetrating injury to the posterior triangle of the neck
Hypoglossal nerve [XII]	Atrophy of ipsilateral muscles of the tongue and deviation toward the affected side; speech disturbance	Penetrating injury to the neck and skull base pathology

Clinical app

Overview of cranial nerves

Cranial nerve reflexes	
Corneal (blink) reflex ■ Afferent—Trigeminal nerve (CN V) ■ Efferent—Facial nerve (CN VII) Gag reflex ■ Afferent—Glossopharyngeal nerve (CN IX) ■ Efferent—Vagus nerve (CN X)	Pupillary (light) reflex ■ Afferent—optic nerve (CN II) ■ Efferent—oculomotor nerve (CN III)

Continued

Olfactory nerve [I]

Special sensory – smell

Optic nerve [II]

Special sensory – vision

Oculomotor nerve [III]

Somatic motor – five extra-ocular muscles (superior rectus, medial rectus, inferior oblique, inferior rectus, and levator palpebrae superioris)
Visceral motor – ciliary muscles and sphincter pupillae muscles

Trochlear nerve [IV]

Somatic motor – one extra-ocular muscle (superior oblique)

Abducent nerve [VI]

Somatic motor – one extra-ocular muscle (lateral rectus)

Trigeminal nerve [V] sensory root

Somatic sensory – eyes, orbital contents, face, sinuses, teeth, nasal cavities, oral cavity, nasopharynx, dura, anterior part of external ear, and part of external acoustic meatus

Trigeminal nerve [V] motor root

Branchial motor – the four muscles of mastication (medial pterygoid, lateral pterygoid, masseter, temporalis) and mylohyoid, anterior belly of digastric, tensor tympani, and tensor veli palatini

V_1

V_2

V_3

V_3

—— Efferent (motor) fibers

—— Afferent (sensory) fibers

Facial nerve [VII]

Branchial motor – all muscles of facial expression and stapedius, stylohyoid, and posterior belly of digastric

Facial nerve [VII] (intermediate nerve)

Special sensory – taste (anterior 2/3 of tongue)
Somatic sensory – part of external acoustic meatus and deeper parts of auricle
Visceral motor (parasympathetic) – secretomotor to all salivary glands except for parotid gland; all mucous glands associated with the oral and nasal cavities; lacrimal gland

Vestibulocochlear nerve [VIII]

Special sensory – hearing and balance

Glossopharyngeal nerve [IX]

Special sensory – taste (posterior 1/3 of tongue)
Somatic sensory – posterior 1/3 of tongue, oropharynx, palatine tonsil, middle ear, pharyngotympanic tube, and mastoid air cells
Branchial motor – stylopharyngeus
Visceral motor – (parasympathetic) – secretomotor to the parotid gland
Visceral sensory – from carotid body and sinus

Vagus nerve [X]

Somatic sensory – larynx, laryngopharynx, deeper parts of auricle, and part of external acoustic meatus
Special sensory – taste from epiglottis and pharynx
Branchial motor – all muscles of pharynx except for stylopharyngeus; all muscles of the soft palate except for tensor veli palatini, all intrinsic muscles of larynx
Visceral motor – (parasympathetic) – thoracic viscera and abdominal viscera to end of midgut
Visceral sensory – thoracic viscera and abdominal viscera to end of midgut, chemo- and baroreceptors (and in some cases carotid body)

Hypoglossal nerve [XII]

Somatic motor – all muscles of the tongue except palatoglossus

Accessory nerve [XI]

Branchial motor – sternocleidomastoid and trapezius

483

oblongata on the anterolateral surface just inferior to the rootlets arising to form the vagus nerve [X] as the "cranial" root of the accessory nerve (see Fig. 8.36). Leaving the medulla, the cranial roots course with the "spinal" roots of the accessory nerve [XI] into the jugular foramen at which point the cranial roots join the vagus nerve [X]. As part of the vagus nerve [X], they are distributed to the pharyngeal musculature innervated by the vagus nerve [X] and are therefore described as being part of the vagus nerve [X].

Hypoglossal nerve [XII]

The hypoglossal nerve [XII] carries GSE fibers to innervate all intrinsic and most of the extrinsic muscles of the tongue. It arises as several rootlets from the anterior surface of the medulla, passes laterally across the posterior cranial fossa and exits through the hypoglossal canal (see Figs. 8.35, 8.36). This nerve innervates the hyoglossus, styloglossus, and genioglossus muscles and all intrinsic muscles of the tongue.

FACE

A face-to-face meeting is an important initial contact between individuals. Part of this exchange is the use of facial expressions to convey emotions. In fact, a physician can gain important information about an individual's general health by observing a patient's face.

Thus an understanding of the unique organization of the various structures between the superciliary arches superiorly, the lower edge of the mandible inferiorly, and as far back as the ears on either side—the area defined as the face—is particularly useful in the practice of medicine.

Muscles

The muscles of the face (Table 8.7, Fig. 8.37) develop from the second pharyngeal arch and are innervated by branches of the facial nerve [VII]. They are in the superficial fascia, with origins from either bone or fascia and insertions into the skin.

Because these muscles control expressions of the face, they are sometimes referred to as muscles of "facial expression." They also act as sphincters and dilators of the orifices of the face (i.e., the orbits, nose, and mouth). This organizational arrangement into functional groups provides a logical approach to understanding these muscles.

Orbital group

Two muscles are associated with the orbital group—the orbicularis oculi and the corrugator supercilii.

The **orbicularis oculi** is a large muscle that completely surrounds each orbital orifice and extends into each eyelid

(Table 8.7; also see Fig. 8.38). It closes the eyelids. It has two major parts:

- the outer **orbital part;** and
- the inner **palpebral part.**

The second muscle in the orbital group is the much smaller **corrugator supercilii** (Table 8.7; also see Fig. 8.38), which is deep to the eyebrows and the orbicularis oculi muscle and is active when frowning.

Nasal group

Three muscles are associated with the nasal group—the nasalis, the procerus, and the depressor septi nasi (Table 8.7, Fig. 8.39). The largest and best developed of the muscles of the nasal group is the **nasalis,** which is active when the nares are flared (Table 8.7, Fig. 8.39).

The **procerus** is a small muscle superficial to the nasal bone and is active when an individual frowns (Table 8.7, Fig. 8.39).

The final muscle in the nasal group is the **depressor septi nasi,** another muscle that assists in widening the nares (see Table 8.7, Fig. 8.39).

Oral group

The muscles in the oral group move the lips and cheek. They include the orbicularis oris and buccinator muscles and a lower and upper group of muscles (Fig. 8.40; also see Table 8.7). Many of these muscles intersect just lateral to the corner of the mouth on each side at a structure termed the *modiolus.* The **orbicularis oris** is a complex muscle consisting of fibers that completely encircle the mouth (Fig. 8.40; also see Table 8.7). Its function is apparent when pursing the lips, as occurs during whistling.

The **buccinator** forms the muscular component of the cheek and is used every time air expanding the cheeks is forcefully expelled (Table 8.7, Figs. 8.40, 8.41).

Lower group of oral muscles

The muscles in the lower group consist of the depressor anguli oris, depressor labii inferioris, and mentalis (Table 8.7, Fig. 8.40). The **depressor anguli oris** is active during frowning. The **depressor labii inferioris** depresses the lower lip and moves it laterally, and the **mentalis** helps position the lip when drinking from a cup or when pouting.

Upper group of oral muscles

The muscles of the upper group of oral muscles consist of risorius, zygomaticus major, zygomaticus minor, levator labii superioris, levator labii superioris alaeque nasi, and levator anguli oris (Table 8.7, Fig. 8.40). The **risorius** helps produce a grin; the **zygomaticus major** and **zygomaticus minor** help produce a smile; the **levator labii superioris**

Table 8.7 Muscles of the face

Muscle	Origin	Insertion	Innervation	Function
Orbital group				
Orbicularis oculi —Palpebral part	Medial palpebral ligament	Lateral palpebral raphe	Facial nerve [VII]	Closes the eyelids gently
—Orbital part	Nasal part of frontal bone; frontal process of maxilla; medial palpebral ligament	Fibers form an uninterrupted ellipse around orbit	Facial nerve [VII]	Closes the eyelids forcefully
Corrugator supercilii	Medial end of the superciliary arch	Skin of the medial half of eyebrow	Facial nerve [VII]	Draws the eyebrows medially and downward
Nasal group				
Nasalis —Transverse part	Maxilla just lateral to nose	Aponeurosis across dorsum of nose with muscle fibers from the other side	Facial nerve [VII]	Compresses nasal aperture
—Alar part	Maxilla over lateral incisor	Alar cartilage of nose	Facial nerve [VII]	Draws cartilage downward and laterally, opening nostril
Procerus	Nasal bone and upper part of lateral nasal cartilage	Skin of lower forehead between eyebrows	Facial nerve [VII]	Draws down medial angle of eyebrows, producing transverse wrinkles over bridge of nose
Depressor septi	Maxilla above medial incisor	Mobile part of the nasal septum	Facial nerve [VII]	Pulls nose inferiorly
Oral group				
Depressor anguli oris	Oblique line of mandible below canine, premolar, and first molar teeth	Skin at the corner of mouth and blending with orbicularis oris	Facial nerve [VII]	Draws corner of mouth down and laterally
Depressor labii inferioris	Anterior part of oblique line of mandible	Lower lip at midline; blends with muscle from opposite side	Facial nerve [VII]	Draws lower lip downward and laterally
Mentalis	Mandible inferior to incisor teeth	Skin of chin	Facial nerve [VII]	Raises and protrudes lower lip as it wrinkles skin on chin
Risorius	Fascia over masseter muscle	Skin at the corner of the mouth	Facial nerve [VII]	Retracts corner of mouth
Zygomaticus major	Posterior part of lateral surface of zygomatic bone	Skin at the corner of the mouth	Facial nerve [VII]	Draws the corner of the mouth upward and laterally
Zygomaticus minor	Anterior part of lateral surface of zygomatic bone	Upper lip just medial to corner of mouth	Facial nerve [VII]	Draws the upper lip upward
Levator labii superioris	Infra-orbital margin of maxilla	Skin of upper lateral half of upper lip	Facial nerve [VII]	Raises upper lip; helps form nasolabial furrow
Levator labii superioris alaeque nasi	Frontal process of maxilla	Alar cartilage of nose and upper lip	Facial nerve [VII]	Raises upper lip and opens nostril
Levator anguli oris	Maxilla below infra-orbital foramen	Skin at the corner of mouth	Facial nerve [VII]	Raises corner of mouth; helps form nasolabial furrow
Orbicularis oris	From muscles in area; maxilla and mandible in midline	Forms ellipse around mouth	Facial nerve [VII]	Closes lips; protrudes lips
Buccinator	Posterior parts of maxilla and mandible; pterygomandibular raphe	Blends with orbicularis oris and into lips	Facial nerve [VII]	Presses the cheek against teeth; compresses distended cheeks
Other muscles or groups				
Anterior auricular	Anterior part of temporal fascia	Into helix of ear	Facial nerve [VII]	Draws ear upward and forward
Superior auricular	Epicranial aponeurosis on side of head	Upper part of auricle	Facial nerve [VII]	Elevates ear
Posterior auricular	Mastoid process of temporal bone	Convexity of concha of ear	Facial nerve [VII]	Draws ear upward and backward
Occipitofrontalis —Frontal belly	Skin of eyebrows	Into galea aponeurotica	Facial nerve [VII]	Wrinkles forehead; raises eyebrows

Continued

Table 8.7 Muscles of the face—cont'd

Muscle	Origin	Insertion	Innervation	Function
—Occipital belly	Lateral part of superior nuchal line of occipital bone and mastoid process of temporal bone	Into galea aponeurotica	Facial nerve [VII]	Draws scalp backward
Platysma	Below the clavicle in the upper part of the thorax	Ascends through the neck to the mandible. The more medial fibers insert on the mandible, more lateral fibers join muscles around mouth	Facial nerve [VII]	Tenses skin of neck and moves lower lip and corners of mouth down

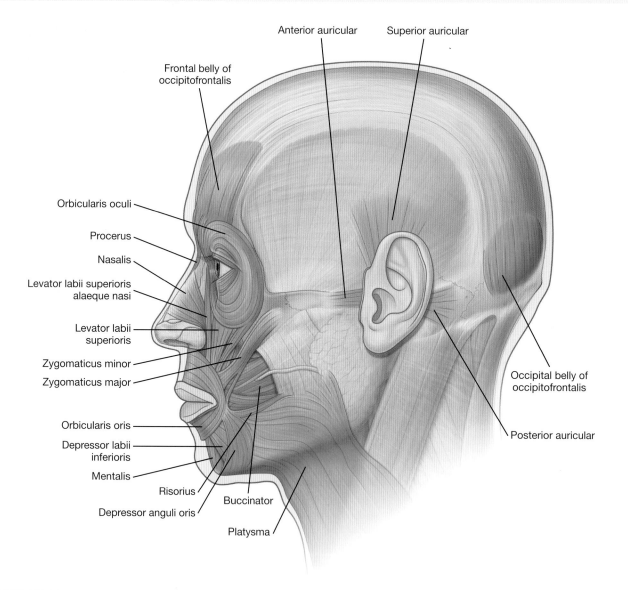

Fig. 8.37 Facial muscles.

deepens the furrow between the nose and the corner of the mouth during sadness; the **levator labii superioris alaeque nasi** may assist in flaring the nares; and the **levator anguli oris** elevates the corner of the mouth and may help deepen the furrow between the nose and the corner of the mouth during sadness.

Other muscles or muscle groups

Several additional muscles or groups of muscles not in the area defined as the face, but derived from the second pharyngeal arch and innervated by the facial nerve [VII], are considered muscles of facial expression. They include the platysma, auricular, and occipitofrontalis muscles (Table 8.7,

Fig. 8.38 Orbital group of facial muscles.

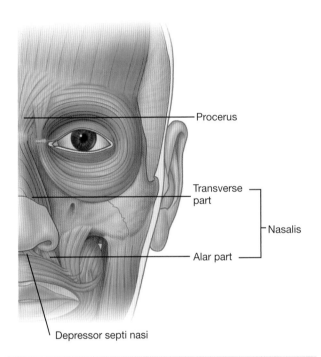

Fig. 8.39 Nasal group of facial muscles.

Fig. 8.37). The **platysma** is a large, thin sheet of muscle in the superficial fascia of the neck. It tenses the skin of the neck and can move the lower lip and corners of the mouth down.

Three muscles associated with the ear are also in the group of "other muscles of facial expression." These are the anterior, superior, and posterior **auricular muscles** (Table 8.7, Fig. 8.42; see Fig. 8.37).

The **occipitofrontalis** is the final muscle in this category and is associated with the scalp (Table 8.7; see Fig. 8.37). It consists of a frontal belly anteriorly and an occipital belly posteriorly. An aponeurotic tendon connects the two.

Parotid gland

The **parotid glands** are the largest of the three pairs of main salivary glands in the head and numerous structures pass through them. They are anterior to and below the lower half of the ear, superficial, posterior, and deep to the ramus of mandible (Fig. 8.43). They extend down to the lower border of the mandible and up to the zygomatic arch. Posteriorly they cover the anterior part of the sternocleidomastoid muscle and continue anteriorly to halfway across the masseter muscle.

The **parotid duct** leaves the anterior edge of the parotid gland midway between the zygomatic arch and the corner of the mouth (see Fig. 8.43). It crosses the face in a transverse direction and, after crossing the medial border of the masseter muscle, turns deeply into the buccal fat pad and pierces the buccinator muscle. It opens into the oral cavity near the second upper molar tooth.

Important relationships

Several major structures enter and pass through or pass just deep to the parotid gland. These include the facial nerve [VII], the external carotid artery and its branches, and the retromandibular vein and its tributaries (see Fig. 8.43).

Facial nerve

The facial nerve [VII] exits the skull through the stylomastoid foramen and then passes into the parotid gland where it usually divides into upper and lower trunks. These pass through the substance of the parotid gland where there may be further branching and anastomosing of the nerves.

Five terminal groups of branches of the facial nerve [VII]—the **temporal, zygomatic, buccal, marginal mandibular,** and **cervical branches**—emerge from the upper, anterior, and lower borders of the parotid gland (see Fig. 8.43).

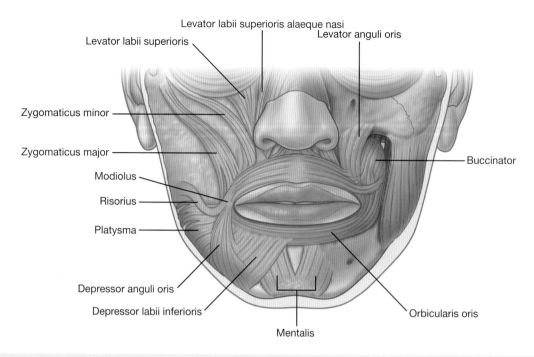

Levator labii superioris alaeque nasi

Levator labii superioris

Levator anguli oris

Zygomaticus minor

Zygomaticus major

Modiolus

Risorius

Platysma

Buccinator

Depressor anguli oris

Depressor labii inferioris

Orbicularis oris

Mentalis

Fig. 8.40 Oral group of facial muscles.

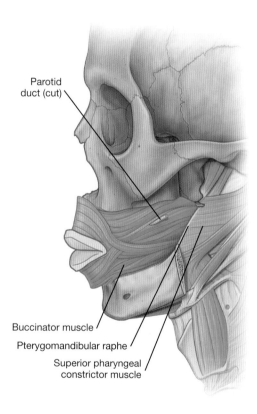

Parotid
duct (cut)

Buccinator muscle

Pterygomandibular raphe

Superior pharyngeal
constrictor muscle

Fig. 8.41 Buccinator muscle.

External carotid artery and its branches

The external carotid artery enters into or passes deep to the inferior border of the parotid gland (see Fig. 8.43). As it continues in a superior direction, it gives off the

Superior auricular

Anterior auricular   Posterior auricular

Fig. 8.42 Auricular muscles.

posterior auricular artery before dividing into its two terminal branches (the **maxillary** and **superficial temporal arteries**) near the lower border of the ear:

- The maxillary artery passes horizontally, deep to the mandible.
- The superficial temporal artery continues in a superior direction and emerges from the upper border of the gland after giving off the **transverse facial artery**.

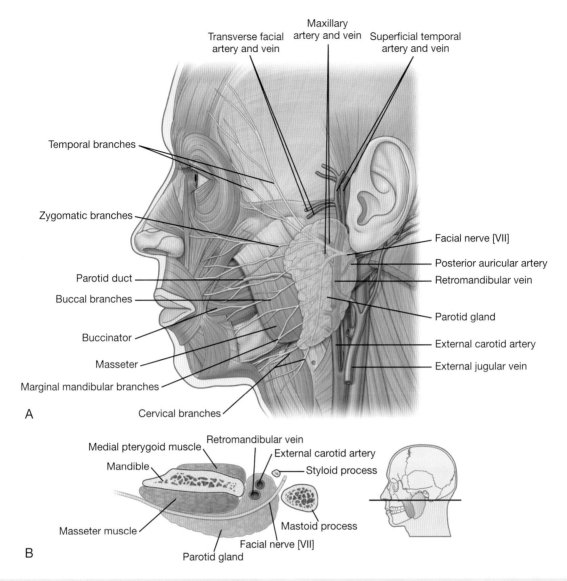

Fig. 8.43 Parotid gland. A. Lateral view. B. Cross-section.

Retromandibular vein and its tributaries

The retromandibular vein is formed in the substance of the parotid gland when the **superficial temporal** and **maxillary veins** join together (see Fig. 8.43) and pass inferiorly in the substance of the parotid gland. It usually divides into anterior and posterior branches just below the inferior border of the gland.

Arterial supply

The parotid gland receives its arterial supply from the numerous arteries that pass through its substance (see above).

Innervation

Sensory innervation of the parotid gland is provided by the **auriculotemporal nerve,** which is a branch of the mandibular nerve [V₃]. This division of the trigeminal nerve exits the skull through the foramen ovale.

The auriculotemporal nerve also carries secretomotor fibers to the parotid gland. These postganglionic parasympathetic fibers have their origin in the otic ganglion associated with the mandibular nerve [V₃] and are just inferior to the foramen ovale.

Preganglionic parasympathetic fibers to the otic ganglion come from the glossopharyngeal nerve [IX].

Innervation

During development a cranial nerve becomes associated with each of the pharyngeal arches. Because the face is primarily derived from the first and second pharyngeal arches, innervation of neighboring facial structures varies as follows:

- The trigeminal nerve [V] innervates facial structures derived from the first arch.

Clinical app

Parotid gland—tumors and stones

The parotid gland is the largest of the paired salivary glands and is enclosed within the investing layer of deep cervical fascia.

The parotid gland produces a watery saliva and salivary amylase, which are necessary for food bolus formation, oral digestion, and smooth passage of the bolus into the upper gastrointestinal tract.

Tumors of the parotid gland

The commonest tumors of the parotid gland (Fig. 8.44) are benign and typically involve the superficial gland. These include pleomorphic adenoma and part of the adenolymphoma. Their importance is in relation to their anatomical position. Critically, the relationship of the tumor to the branches of the facial nerve [VII] must be defined because resection may damage the facial nerve [VII].

Parotid gland stones

It is not uncommon for stones to develop within the parotid gland. They typically occur within the main confluence of the ducts and within the main parotid duct. The patient usually complains of intense pain when salivating and tends to avoid foods that produce this symptom. The pain can be easily reproduced in the clinic by squirting lemon juice into the patient's mouth.

Parotid gland | Right internal carotid artery | Maxilla | Body of mandible

Styloid process | Right jugular vein | Tumor in left parotid gland

Fig. 8.44 Tumor in parotid gland. Axial CT scan.

- The facial nerve [VII] innervates facial structures derived from the second arch.

Sensory innervation

Because the face is derived developmentally from a number of structures originating from the first pharyngeal arch, cutaneous innervation of the face is by branches of the trigeminal nerve [V].

The trigeminal nerve [V] divides into three major divisions—the ophthalmic [V_1], maxillary [V_2], and mandibular [V_3] nerves—before leaving the middle cranial fossa (Fig. 8.45). Each of these divisions passes out of the cranial cavity to innervate a part of the face, so most of the skin covering the face is innervated by branches of the trigeminal nerve [V]. The exception is a small area covering the angle and lower border of the ramus of mandible and parts of the ear, which are innervated by the trigeminal [V], facial [VII], vagus [X], and cervical nerves.

Ophthalmic nerve [V_1]

The ophthalmic nerve [V_1] exits the skull through the superior orbital fissure and enters the orbit (Fig. 8.45). Its branches that innervate the face include (Fig. 8.46):

- the **supra-orbital** and **supratrochlear nerves,** which leave the orbit superiorly and innervate the upper eyelid, forehead, and scalp;
- the **infratrochlear nerve,** which exits the orbit in the medial angle to innervate the medial half of the upper eyelid, the skin in the area of the medial angle, and the side of the nose;
- the **lacrimal nerve,** which exits the orbit in the lateral angle to innervate the lateral half of the upper eyelid and the skin in the area of the lateral angle; and
- the **external nasal nerve,** which supplies the anterior part of the nose.

Maxillary nerve [V_2]

The maxillary nerve [V_2] exits the skull through the foramen rotundum. Branches (see Fig. 8.45) that innervate the face include (Fig. 8.46):

- a small **zygomaticotemporal branch,** which exits the zygomatic bone and supplies a small area of the anterior temple above the zygomatic arch;
- a small **zygomaticofacial branch,** which exits the zygomatic bone and supplies a small area of skin over the zygomatic bone; and
- the large **infra-orbital nerve,** which exits the maxilla through the infra-orbital foramen and immediately divides into multiple branches to supply the lower eyelid, cheek, side of the nose, and upper lip (Fig. 8.46).

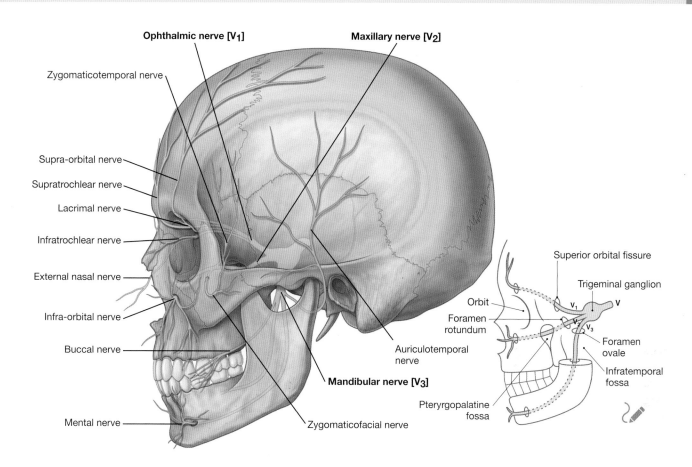

Ophthalmic nerve [V₁]

Maxillary nerve [V₂]

Zygomaticotemporal nerve

Supra-orbital nerve

Supratrochlear nerve

Lacrimal nerve

Infratrochlear nerve

External nasal nerve

Infra-orbital nerve

Buccal nerve

Mental nerve

Zygomaticofacial nerve

Auriculotemporal nerve

Mandibular nerve [V₃]

Pteryrgopalatine fossa

Superior orbital fissure

Trigeminal ganglion

Orbit

Foramen rotundum

Foramen ovale

Infratemporal fossa

Fig. 8.45 Trigeminal nerve [V] leaving the skull.

Mandibular nerve [V₃]

The mandibular nerve [V₃] exits the skull through the foramen ovale. Branches (see Fig. 8.45) innervating the face include (Fig. 8.46):

- the auriculotemporal nerve, which enters the face just posterior to the temporomandibular joint, passes through the parotid gland, and ascends just anterior to the ear to supply the external acoustic meatus, the surface of the tympanic membrane (eardrum), and a large area of the temple;
- the **buccal nerve,** which is on the surface of the buccinator muscle supplying the cheek; and
- the **mental nerve,** which exits the mandible through the mental foramen and immediately divides into multiple branches to supply the skin and mucous membrane of the lower lip and skin of the chin.

Motor innervation

The muscles of the face, as well as those associated with the ear and the scalp, are derived from the second pharyngeal arch. The cranial nerve associated with this arch is the facial nerve [VII] and therefore branches of the facial nerve [VII] innervate all these muscles (Fig. 8.47A).

Clinical app

Trigeminal neuralgia

Trigeminal neuralgia (tic douloureux) is a complex sensory disorder of the sensory root of the trigeminal nerve. Typically the pain is in the region of the mandibular [V₃] and maxillary [V₂] nerves. Usually the pain is of sudden onset, excruciating in nature, and triggered by touching a sensitive region of skin.

The facial nerve [VII] exits the posterior cranial fossa through the internal acoustic meatus. It passes through the temporal bone, giving off several branches, and emerges from the base of the skull through the stylomastoid foramen (Fig. 8.47B). At this point it gives off the **posterior auricular nerve.** This branch passes upward, behind the ear, to supply the occipital belly of the occipitofrontalis muscle of the scalp and the posterior auricular muscle of the ear.

The main stem of the facial nerve [VII] then gives off another branch, which innervates the posterior belly of the digastric muscle and the stylohyoid muscle. At this point, the facial nerve [VII] enters the deep surface of the parotid gland (Fig. 8.47B).

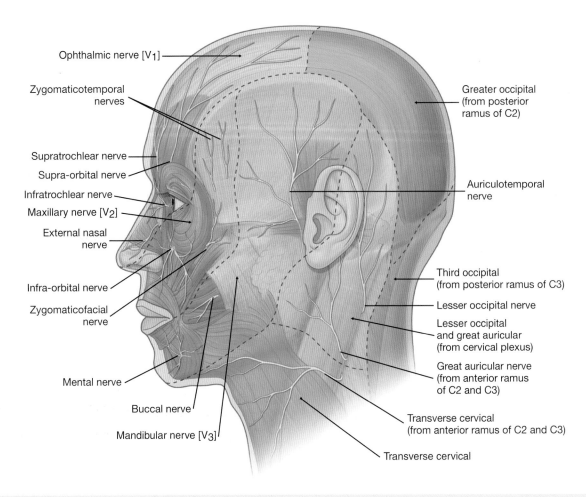

Fig. 8.46 Cutaneous distribution of the trigeminal nerve [V].

Once in the parotid gland, the main stem of the facial nerve [VII] usually divides into upper (temporofacial) and lower (cervicofacial) trunks or branches. As these branches pass through the substance of the parotid gland, they may branch further or take part in an anastomotic network (the parotid plexus).

Whatever types of interconnections occur, five terminal groups of branches of the facial nerve [VII]—the temporal, zygomatic, buccal, marginal mandibular, and cervical branches—emerge from the parotid gland (Fig. 8.47A).

Although there are variations in the pattern of distribution of the five terminal groups of branches, the basic pattern is as follows:

- Temporal branches exit from the superior border of the parotid gland to supply muscles in the area of the temple, forehead, and supra-orbital area.
- Zygomatic branches emerge from the anterosuperior border of the parotid gland to supply muscles in the infra-orbital area, the lateral nasal area, and the upper lip.
- Buccal branches emerge from the anterior border of the parotid gland to supply muscles in the cheek, the upper lip, and the corner of the mouth.

- Marginal mandibular branches emerge from the anteroinferior border of the parotid gland to supply muscles of the lower lip and chin.
- Cervical branches emerge from the inferior border of the parotid gland to supply the platysma.

Vessels

The arterial supply to the face is primarily from branches of the external carotid artery, though there is some limited supply from a branch of the internal carotid artery.

Similarly, most of the venous return is back to the internal jugular vein, though some important connections from the face result in venous return through a clinically relevant intracranial pathway involving the cavernous sinus.

Arteries

Facial artery

The facial artery is the major vessel supplying the face (Fig. 8.48A). It branches from the anterior surface of the external carotid artery (Fig. 8.48B), passes up through the deep structures of the neck, and appears at the lower border of

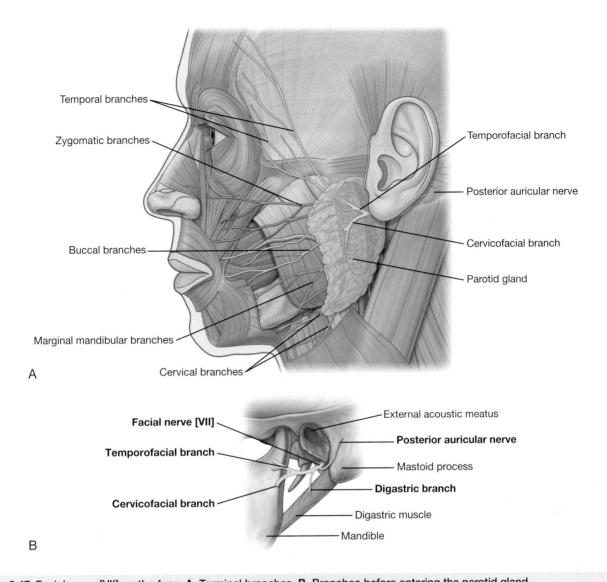

Fig. 8.47 Facial nerve [VII] on the face. **A.** Terminal branches. **B.** Branches before entering the parotid gland.

the mandible after passing posterior to the submandibular gland. Curving around the inferior border of the mandible just anterior to the masseter where its pulse can be felt, the facial artery then enters the face (Fig. 8.48B). From this point, the facial artery runs upward and medially in a tortuous course. It passes along the side of the nose and terminates as the **angular artery** at the medial corner of the eye.

Along its path the facial artery is deep to the platysma, risorius, and zygomaticus major and minor, superficial to the buccinator and levator anguli oris, and may pass superficially to or through the levator labii superioris.

Branches of the facial artery include the superior and inferior labial branches and the lateral nasal branch (Fig. 8.48B).

The labial branches arise near the corner of the mouth:

- The **inferior labial branch** supplies the lower lip.
- The **superior labial branch** supplies the upper lip and provides a branch to the nasal septum.

Near the midline, the superior and inferior labial branches anastomose with their companion arteries from the opposite side of the face. This provides an important connection between the facial arteries and the external carotid arteries of opposite sides.

The **lateral nasal branch** is a small branch arising from the facial artery as it passes along the side of the nose. It supplies the lateral surface and dorsum of the nose.

Transverse facial artery

Another contributor to the vascular supply of the face is the transverse facial artery (Fig. 8.48A,B), which is a branch of the superficial temporal artery (the smaller of the two terminal branches of the external carotid artery).

The transverse facial artery arises from the superficial temporal artery within the substance of the parotid gland, passes through the gland, and crosses the face in a transverse direction. Lying on the superficial surface of the

493

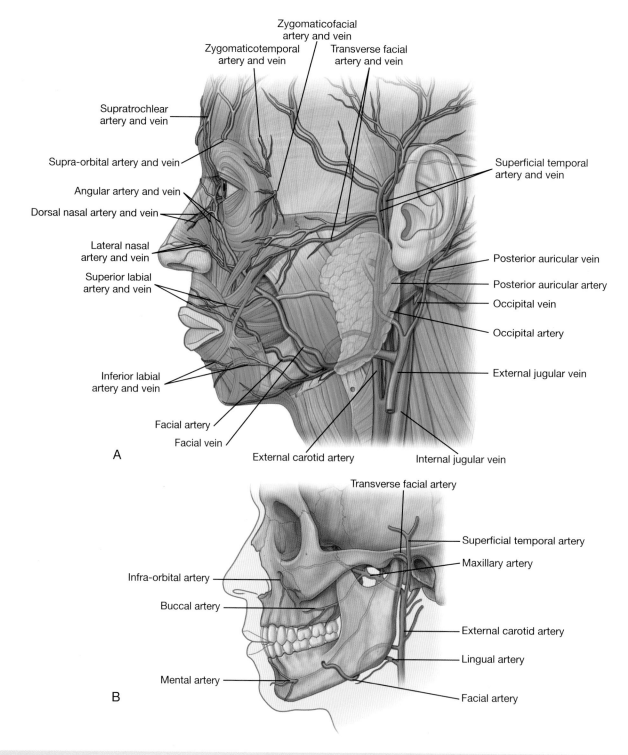

Fig. 8.48 Vasculature of the face. **A.** Lateral view. **B.** Branches of the maxillary artery.

masseter muscle, it is between the zygomatic arch and the parotid duct.

Branches of the maxillary artery

The maxillary artery, the larger of the two terminal branches of the external carotid artery, gives off several small branches that contribute to the arterial supply to the face (Fig. 8.48):

- The **infra-orbital artery** enters the face through the infra-orbital foramen and supplies the lower eyelid, upper lip, and the area between these structures.
- The **buccal artery** enters the face on the superficial surface of the buccinator muscle and supplies structures in this area.
- The **mental artery** enters the face through the mental foramen and supplies the chin.

Branches of the ophthalmic artery

Three small arteries from the internal carotid artery also contribute to the arterial supply of the face. These vessels arise from the **ophthalmic artery,** a branch of the internal carotid artery, after the ophthalmic artery enters the orbit:

- The **zygomaticofacial** and **zygomaticotemporal arteries** come from the lacrimal branch of the ophthalmic artery (Fig. 8.48A), enter the face through the zygomaticofacial and zygomaticotemporal foramina, and supply the area of the face over the zygomatic bone.
- The **dorsal nasal artery,** a terminal branch of the ophthalmic artery, exits the orbit in the medial corner and supplies the dorsum of the nose (Fig. 8.48A).
- The supra-orbital and supratrochlear arteries supply the anterior scalp.

Veins

Facial vein

The facial vein is the major vein draining the face (Fig. 8.49). Its point of origin is near the medial corner of the orbit as the **supratrochlear** and **supra-orbital veins** come together to form the **angular vein.** This vein becomes the facial vein as it proceeds inferiorly and assumes a position just posterior to the facial artery. The facial vein descends across the face with the facial artery until it reaches the inferior border of the mandible. Here the artery and vein part company, and the facial vein passes superficial to the submandibular gland to enter the internal jugular vein.

Throughout its course, the facial vein receives tributaries from veins draining the eyelids, external nose, lips, cheek, and chin that accompany the various branches of the facial artery.

Transverse facial vein

The transverse facial vein is a small vein that accompanies the transverse facial artery in its journey across the face (see Fig. 8.48A). It empties into the superficial temporal vein within the substance of the parotid gland.

Intracranial venous connections

As it crosses the face, the facial vein has numerous connections with venous channels passing into deeper regions of the head (see Fig. 8.49):

- Near the medial corner of the orbit, it communicates with ophthalmic veins.
- In the area of the cheek, it communicates with veins passing into the infra-orbital foramen.
- It communicates with veins passing into deeper regions of the face (i.e., the deep facial vein connecting with the pterygoid plexus of veins).

All these venous channels have interconnections with the intracranial cavernous sinus through emissary veins that connect intracranial with extracranial veins. There are no valves in the facial vein or any other venous channels in the head, so blood can move in any direction. Because of the interconnections between the veins, infections of the face, primarily above the mouth (i.e., the "danger area") should be handled with great care to prevent the dissemination of infectious material in an intracranial direction.

Lymphatic drainage

Lymphatic drainage from the face primarily moves toward three groups of lymph nodes (Fig. 8.50):

- **submental nodes** inferior and posterior to the chin, which drain lymphatics from the medial part of the lower lip and chin bilaterally;
- **submandibular nodes** superficial to the submandibular gland and inferior to the body of the mandible, which drain the lymphatics from the medial corner of the orbit, most of the external nose, medial part of the cheek, the upper lip and the lateral part of the lower lip that follow the course of the facial artery; and

Ophthalmic veins   Cavernous sinus

Infra-orbital vein

Facial vein

Deep facial vein

Pterygoid plexus of veins

Fig. 8.49 Intracranial venous connections.

■ **pre-auricular** and **parotid** nodes anterior to the ear, which drain lymphatics from most of the eyelids, a part of the external nose, and the lateral part of the cheek.

Facial nerve [VII] palsy (Bell's palsy)

The complexity of the facial nerve [VII] is demonstrated by the different pathological processes and sites at which these processes occur.

Central lesions

A primary brainstem lesion affecting the motor nucleus of the facial nerve (VII) would lead to ipsilateral (same side) weakness of the whole face. However, because the upper part of the nucleus receives motor input from the left and right cerebral hemispheres, a lesion occurring above the nucleus leads to contralateral lower facial weakness. In this example, motor innervation to the upper face is spared because the upper part of the nucleus receives input from both hemispheres. Preservation and loss of the special functions are determined by the extent of the lesion.

Lesions at and around the geniculate ganglion

Typically lesions at and around the geniculate ganglion are accompanied by loss of motor function on the whole of the ipsilateral (same) side of the face. Taste to the anterior two-thirds of the tongue, lacrimation, and some salivation also are likely to be affected because the lesion is proximal to the greater petrosal and chorda tympani branches of the nerve.

Lesions at and around the stylomastoid foramen

Lesions at and around the stylomastoid foramen are the commonest abnormality of the facial nerve [VII] and usually result from a viral inflammation of the nerve within the bony canal before exiting through the stylomastoid foramen. Typically the patient has an ipsilateral loss of motor function that produces an unusual appearance: one side of the face looks normal and the affected side sags and lacks tone. Lacrimation and taste may not be affected if the lesion remains distal to the greater petrosal and chorda tympani branches that originate deep in the temporal bone.

SCALP

The scalp is the part of the head that extends from the superciliary arches anteriorly to the external occipital protuberance and superior nuchal lines posteriorly. Laterally it continues inferiorly to the zygomatic arch.

The scalp is a multilayered structure with layers that can be defined by the word itself (Fig. 8.52):

■ S—skin,
■ C—connective tissue (dense),

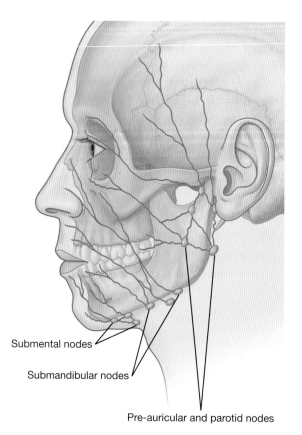

Submental nodes

Submandibular nodes

Pre-auricular and parotid nodes

Fig. 8.50 Lymphatic drainage of the face.

■ A—aponeurotic layer,
■ L—loose connective tissue, and
■ P—pericranium.

Layers

Examining the layers of the scalp reveals that the first three layers are tightly held together, forming a single unit. This unit is sometimes referred to as the *scalp proper* and is the tissue torn away during serious "scalping" injuries.

Skin

The skin is the outer layer of the scalp (Figs. 8.52 and 8.53). It is similar structurally to skin throughout the body with the exception that hair is present on a large amount of it.

Connective tissue (dense)

Deep to the skin is dense connective tissue (Figs. 8.52, 8.53). This layer anchors the skin to the third layer and contains the arteries, veins, and nerves supplying the scalp.

Aponeurotic layer

The deepest layer of the first three layers is the aponeurotic layer (Fig. 8.53; also see Fig. 8.52). Firmly attached to the skin by the dense connective tissue of the second layer,

Surface anatomy
Major features of the face

The major features of the face are those related to the anterior openings of the orbit, the nasal cavities, and the oral cavity (Fig. 8.51).

The palpebral fissures are between the upper and lower eyelids and can be opened and closed. The oral fissure is the gap between the upper and lower lips and can also be opened and closed.

The sphincter muscles of the oral and palpebral fissures are the orbicularis oris and orbicularis oculi muscles, respectively. These muscles are innervated by the facial nerve [VII].

The nares are the anterior apertures of the nasal cavities and are continuously open.

The vertical groove in the midline between the external nose and the upper lip is the philtrum.

Sensory innervation of the face is carried by the trigeminal nerve [V]. The three divisions of this nerve are represented on the face and can be tested by touching the forehead (the ophthalmic nerve [V$_1$]), the anterior cheek (the maxillary nerve [V$_2$]), and skin over the anterior body of the mandible (the mandibular nerve [V$_3$]).

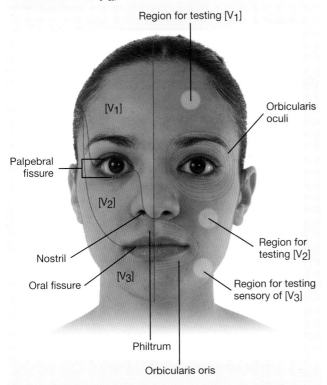

Fig. 8.51 Major features of the face. Anterior head and neck of a woman.

this layer consists of the occipitofrontalis muscle, which has a frontal belly anteriorly, an occipital belly posteriorly, and an aponeurotic tendon—the **epicranial aponeurosis (galea aponeurotica)**—connecting the two (Fig. 8.54).

Fig. 8.52 SCALP.

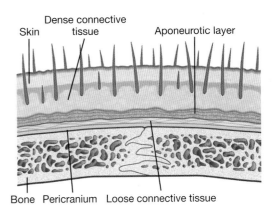

Fig. 8.53 Layers of the scalp.

The frontal belly of occipitofrontalis begins anteriorly where it is attached to the skin of the eyebrows. It passes upward, across the forehead, to become continuous with the aponeurotic tendon (Fig. 8.54A).

Posteriorly, each occipital belly of occipitofrontalis arises from the lateral part of the superior nuchal line of the occipital bone and the mastoid process of the temporal bone (Fig. 8.54B). It also passes superiorly to attach to the aponeurotic tendon.

The occipitofrontalis muscles move the scalp, wrinkle the forehead, and raise the eyebrows. The frontal belly is

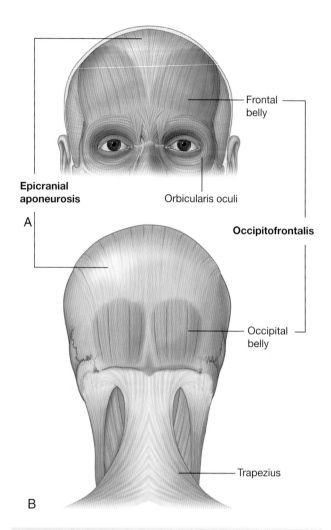

Epicranial
aponeurosis

Frontal
belly

Orbicularis oculi

Occipitofrontalis

A

Occipital
belly

Trapezius

B

Fig. 8.54 Occipitofrontalis muscle. A. Frontal belly.
B. Occipital belly.

innervated by temporal branches of the facial nerve [VII] and the posterior belly by the posterior auricular branch.

Loose connective tissue

A layer of loose connective tissue separates the aponeurotic layer from the pericranium and facilitates movement of the scalp proper over the calvaria (Fig. 8.53; also see Fig. 8.52). Because of its consistency, infections tend to localize and spread through the loose connective tissue.

Pericranium

The pericranium is the deepest layer of the scalp and is the periosteum on the outer surface of the calvaria (Fig. 8.53; also see Fig. 8.52). It is attached to the bones of the calvaria but is removable, except in the area of the sutures.

Innervation

Sensory innervation of the scalp is from two major sources, cranial nerves or cervical nerves, depending on whether it is

anterior or posterior to the ears and the vertex of the head (Fig. 8.55). The occipitofrontalis muscle is innervated by branches of the facial nerve [VII].

Anterior to the ears and the vertex

Branches of the trigeminal nerve [V] supply the scalp anterior to the ears and the vertex of the head (Fig. 8.55). These branches are the supratrochlear, supra-orbital, zygomatic-temporal, and auriculotemporal nerves:

- The **supratrochlear nerve** exits the orbit, passes through the frontalis muscle, continues superiorly across the front of the forehead, and supplies the front of the forehead near the midline.
- The **supra-orbital nerve** exits the orbit through the supra-orbital notch or foramen, passes through the frontalis muscle, and continues superiorly across the scalp as far back as the vertex of the head.
- The **zygomaticotemporal nerve** exits the skull through a foramen in the zygomatic bone and supplies the scalp over a small anterior area of the temple.
- The **auriculotemporal nerve** exits from the skull deep to the parotid gland, passes just anterior to the ear, continues superiorly anterior to the ear until nearly reaching the vertex of the head, and supplies the scalp over the temporal region and anterior to the ear to near the vertex.

Posterior to the ears and the vertex

Posterior to the ears and vertex, sensory innervation of the scalp is by cervical nerves, specifically branches from spinal cord levels C2 and C3 (Fig. 8.55). These branches are the great auricular, the lesser occipital, the greater occipital, and the third occipital nerves:

- The **great auricular nerve** is a branch of the cervical plexus, arises from the anterior rami of the C2 and C3 spinal nerves, ascends on the surface of the sternocleidomastoid muscle, and innervates a small area of the scalp just posterior to the ear.
- The **lesser occipital nerve** is also a branch of the cervical plexus, arises from the anterior ramus of the C2 spinal nerve, ascends on the posterior border of the sternocleidomastoid muscle, and supplies an area of the scalp posterior and superior to the ear.
- The **greater occipital nerve** is a branch of the posterior ramus of the C2 spinal nerve, emerges just inferior to the obliquus capitis inferior muscle, ascends superficial to the suboccipital triangle, pierces the semispinalis capitis and trapezius muscles, and then spreads out to supply a large part of the posterior scalp as far superiorly as the vertex.
- The **third occipital nerve** is a branch of the posterior ramus of the C3 spinal nerve, pierces the semispinalis capitis and trapezius muscles, and supplies a small area of the lower part of the scalp.

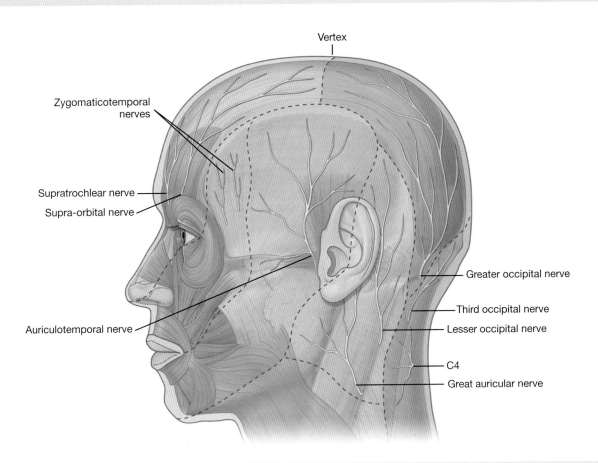

Vertex

Zygomaticotemporal nerves

Supratrochlear nerve

Supra-orbital nerve

Auriculotemporal nerve

Greater occipital nerve

Third occipital nerve

Lesser occipital nerve

C4

Great auricular nerve

Fig. 8.55 Innervation of the scalp.

Vessels

Arteries

Arteries supplying the scalp (Fig. 8.56) are branches of either the external carotid artery or the ophthalmic artery, which is a branch of the internal carotid artery.

Branches from the ophthalmic artery

The supratrochlear and supra-orbital arteries supply the anterior and superior aspects of the scalp (Fig. 8.56). They branch from the ophthalmic artery while it is in the orbit, continue through the orbit, and exit onto the forehead in association with the supratrochlear and supra-orbital nerves. Like the nerves, the arteries ascend across the forehead to supply the scalp as far posteriorly as the vertex of the head.

Branches from the external carotid artery

Three branches of the external carotid artery supply the largest part of the scalp—the posterior auricular, occipital, and superficial temporal arteries supply the lateral and posterior aspects of the scalp (Fig. 8.56):

- The smallest branch (the **posterior auricular artery**) leaves the posterior aspect of the external carotid artery, passes through deeper structures, and emerges to supply an area of the scalp posterior to the ear.

- Also arising from the posterior aspect of the external carotid artery is the **occipital artery,** which ascends in a posterior direction, passes through several layers of back musculature, and emerges to supply a large part of the posterior aspect of the scalp.

- The third arterial branch supplying the scalp is the **superficial temporal artery,** a terminal branch of the external carotid artery that passes superiorly just anterior to the ear, divides into anterior and posterior branches, and supplies almost the entire lateral aspect of the scalp.

Veins

Veins draining the scalp follow a pattern similar to the arteries (Fig. 8.56):

- The **supratrochlear** and **supra-orbital veins** drain the anterior part of the scalp from the superciliary arches to the vertex of the head, pass inferior to the superciliary arches, communicate with the ophthalmic veins in the orbit, and continue inferiorly to participate in the formation of the angular vein, which is the upper tributary to the facial vein.

- The **superficial temporal vein** drains the entire lateral area of the scalp before passing inferiorly to join in the formation of the retromandibular vein.

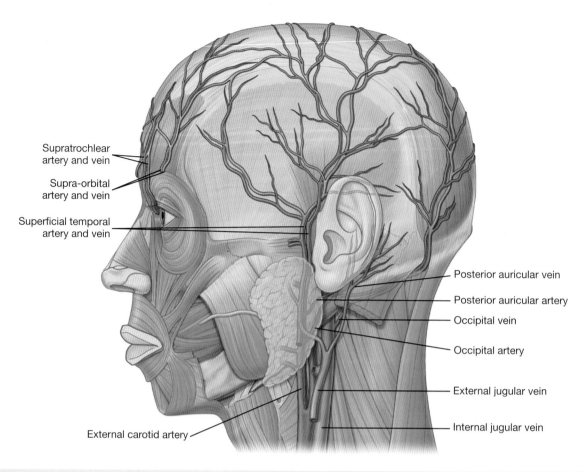

Supratrochlear
artery and vein

Supra-orbital
artery and vein

Superficial temporal
artery and vein

Posterior auricular vein

Posterior auricular artery

Occipital vein

Occipital artery

External jugular vein

Internal jugular vein

External carotid artery

Fig. 8.56 Vasculature of the scalp.

- The **posterior auricular vein** drains the area of the scalp posterior to the ear and eventually empties into a tributary of the retromandibular vein.
- The **occipital vein** drains the posterior aspect of the scalp from the external occipital protuberance and superior nuchal lines to the vertex of the head; deeper, it passes through the musculature in the posterior neck to join in the formation of the plexus of veins in the suboccipital triangle.

Clinical app

Scalp laceration
The scalp has an extremely rich blood supply from the external carotid arteries, so lacerations of the scalp tend to bleed profusely. Importantly, scalp bleeding is predominantly arterial because of two reasons. First, in the erect position the venous pressure is extremely low. Second, the vessels do not retract when lacerated because the dense connective tissue layer in which they are found prevents retraction.

Lymphatic drainage

Lymphatic drainage of the scalp generally follows the pattern of arterial distribution.

The lymphatics in the occipital region initially drain to occipital nodes near the attachment of the trapezius muscle at the base of the skull (Fig. 8.57). Further along the pathway occipital nodes drain into upper deep cervical nodes. There is also some direct drainage to upper deep cervical nodes from this part of the scalp.

Lymphatics from the upper part of the scalp drain in two directions:

- Posterior to the vertex of the head, they drain to **mastoid nodes** (retro-auricular/posterior auricular nodes) posterior to the ear near the mastoid process of the temporal bone, and efferent vessels from these nodes drain into upper deep cervical nodes.
- Anterior to the vertex of the head they drain to **pre-auricular** and **parotid nodes** anterior to the ear on the surface of the parotid gland.

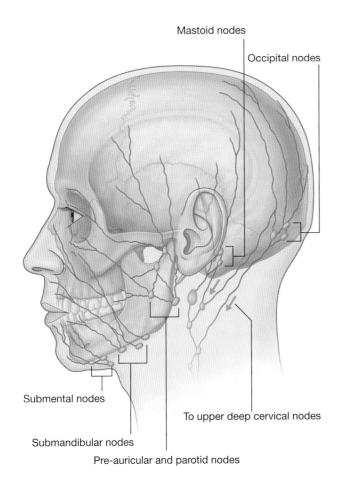

Fig. 8.57 Lymphatic drainage of the scalp.

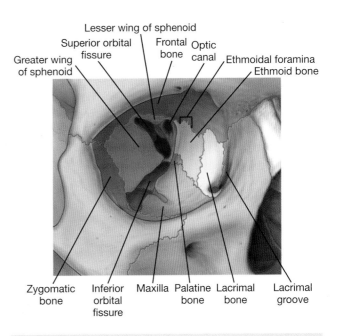

Fig. 8.58 Bones of the orbit.

Finally, there may be some lymphatic drainage from the forehead to the submandibular nodes through efferent vessels that follow the facial artery.

ORBIT

The orbits are bilateral structures in the upper half of the face below the anterior cranial fossa and anterior to the middle cranial fossa that contain the eyeball, the optic nerve, the extra-ocular muscles, the lacrimal apparatus, adipose tissue, fascia, and the nerves and vessels that supply these structures.

Bony orbit

Seven bones contribute to the framework of each orbit (Fig. 8.58). They are the maxilla, zygomatic, frontal, ethmoid, lacrimal, sphenoid, and palatine bones. Together they give the bony orbit the shape of a pyramid, with its wide base opening anteriorly onto the face, and its apex extending in a posteromedial direction. Completing the pyramid configuration are medial, lateral, superior, and inferior walls.

The apex of the pyramid-shaped bony orbit is the optic canal, whereas the base (the orbital rim) is formed (Fig. 8.58):

- superiorly by the frontal bone,
- medially by the frontal process of the maxilla,
- inferiorly by the zygomatic process of the maxilla and the zygomatic bone, and
- laterally by the zygomatic bone, the frontal process of the zygomatic bone, and the zygomatic process of the frontal bone.

Roof

The **roof (superior wall)** of the bony orbit is made up of the orbital part of the frontal bone with a small contribution from the sphenoid bone (Fig. 8.58). This thin plate of bone separates the contents of the orbit from the brain in the anterior cranial fossa.

Unique features of the roof include:

- anteromedially, the **trochlear fovea** for the attachment of a pulley through which the superior oblique muscle passes and the possible intrusion of part of the frontal sinus; and
- anterolaterally, a depression (the **lacrimal fossa**) for the orbital part of the lacrimal gland.

Posteriorly, the lesser wing of the sphenoid bone completes the roof.

Medial wall

The **medial walls** of the paired bony orbits are parallel to each other, and each consists of four bones—the maxilla, lacrimal, ethmoid, and sphenoid bones (Fig. 8.58).

501

The largest contributor to the medial wall is the orbital plate of the ethmoid bone. This part of the ethmoid bone contains collections of ethmoidal cells, which are clearly visible in a dried skull.

Also visible at the junction between the roof and the medial wall, usually associated with the fronto-ethmoidal suture, are the **anterior** and **posterior ethmoidal foramina.** The anterior and posterior ethmoidal nerves and vessels leave the orbit through these openings.

Anterior to the ethmoid bone is the small lacrimal bone, and completing the anterior part of the medial wall is the frontal process of the maxilla. These two bones participate in the formation of the **lacrimal groove,** which contains the lacrimal sac and is bound by the **posterior lacrimal crest** (part of the lacrimal bone) and the **anterior lacrimal crest** (part of the maxilla).

Posterior to the ethmoid bone the medial wall is completed by a small part of the sphenoid bone, which forms a part of the medial wall of the optic canal.

Floor

The **floor (inferior wall)** of the bony orbit, which is also the roof of the maxillary sinus, consists primarily of the orbital surface of the maxilla (see Fig. 8.58), with small contributions from the zygomatic and palatine bones.

Beginning posteriorly and continuing along the lateral boundary of the floor of the bony orbit is the inferior orbital fissure. Beyond the anterior end of the fissure, the zygomatic bone completes the floor of the bony orbit.

Posteriorly, the orbital process of the palatine bone makes a small contribution to the floor of the bony orbit near the junction of the maxilla, ethmoid, and sphenoid bones.

Lateral wall

The **lateral wall** of the bony orbit consists of contributions from two bones—anteriorly the zygomatic bone and posteriorly the greater wing of the sphenoid bone (see Fig. 8.58).

Clinical app

Orbital fracture

Fractures of the orbit are not uncommon and may involve the orbital margins with extension into the maxilla, frontal, and zygomatic bones. These fractures are often part of complex facial fractures. Fractures within the orbit frequently occur within the floor and the medial wall; however, superior and lateral wall fractures also occur. Inferior orbital floor fractures are one of the commonest types of injuries. These fractures may drag the inferior oblique muscle and associated tissues into the fracture line. In these instances, patients may have upward gaze failure (upward gaze diplopia) in the affected eye.

Clinical app—cont'd

Medial wall fractures characteristically show air within the orbit in radiographs. This is due to fracture of the ethmoidal labyrinth permitting direct continuity between the orbit and the ethmoidal paranasal sinuses. Occasionally, patients feel a "full" sensation within the orbit when blowing their nose.

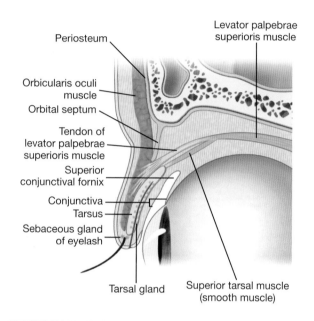

Fig. 8.59 Eyelids.

Eyelids

The upper and lower eyelids are anterior structures that, when closed, protect the surface of the eyeball.

The space between the eyelids, when they are open, is the **palpebral fissure**.

The layers of the eyelids, from anterior to posterior, consist of skin, subcutaneous tissue, voluntary muscle, the orbital septum, the tarsus, and conjunctiva (Fig. 8.59).

The upper and lower eyelids are basically similar in structure except for the addition of two muscles (levator palpebrae superioris and superior tarsal) in the upper eyelid.

Skin and subcutaneous tissue

The skin of the eyelids is not particularly substantial and only a thin layer of connective tissue separates the skin from the underlying voluntary muscle layer (Fig. 8.59).

Orbicularis oculi

The muscle fibers encountered next in an anteroposterior direction through the eyelid belong to the **palpebral part** of **orbicularis oculi** (Fig. 8.59). This muscle is part of the larger orbicularis oculi muscle, which consists primarily of two

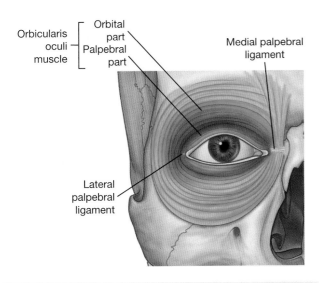

Fig. 8.60 Orbicularis oculi muscle.

parts—an **orbital part,** which surrounds the orbit, and the palpebral part, which is in the eyelids (Fig. 8.60). Orbicularis oculi is innervated by the facial nerve [VII] and closes the eyelids.

The palpebral part is thin and anchored medially by the **medial palpebral ligament,** which attaches to the anterior lacrimal crest, and laterally blends with fibers from the muscle in the lower eyelid at the **lateral palpebral ligament.**

Orbital septum

Deep to the palpebral part of the orbicularis oculi is an extension of periosteum into both the upper and lower eyelids from the margin of the orbit (Fig. 8.61). This is the **orbital septum,** which extends downward into the upper eyelid and upward into the lower eyelid and is continuous with the periosteum outside and inside the orbit (Fig. 8.61). The orbital septum attaches to the tendon of levator palpebrae superioris muscle in the upper eyelid and attaches to the tarsus in the lower eyelid.

Tarsus and levator palpebrae superioris

Providing major support for each eyelid is the tarsus (Fig. 8.62). There is a large **superior tarsus** in the upper eyelid and a smaller **inferior tarsus** in the lower eyelid. These plates of dense connective tissue are attached medially to the anterior lacrimal crest of the maxilla by the medial palpebral ligament and laterally to the orbital tubercle on the zygomatic bone by the lateral palpebral ligament.

Although the tarsal plates in the upper and lower eyelids are generally similar in structure and function, there is one unique difference. Associated with the tarsus in the upper eyelid is the **levator palpebrae superioris** muscle (Fig. 8.62; also see Table 8.8, pg. 511), which raises the eyelid. In companion with the levator palpebrae superioris muscle is a collection of smooth muscle fibers passing from the inferior

Fig. 8.61 Orbital septum.

Fig. 8.62 Tarsal plates.

surface of the levator to the upper edge of the superior tarsus (Fig. 8.59). Innervated by postganglionic sympathetic fibers from the superior cervical ganglion, this muscle is the **superior tarsal muscle.**

Conjunctiva

The structure of the eyelid is completed by a thin membrane (the **conjunctiva**), which covers the posterior surface of each eyelid (Fig. 8.59) and then reflects onto the outer surface (**sclera**) of the eyeball. It extends on the eyeball to the junction between the sclera and the cornea. With this membrane in place, a **conjunctival sac** is formed when the eyelids are closed, and the upper and lower extensions of this sac are the **superior** and **inferior conjunctival fornices** (Fig. 8.59).

Glands

Embedded in the tarsal plates are tarsal glands, which empty onto the free margin of each eyelid (Fig. 8.59). These glands are modified sebaceous glands and secrete an oily substance that increases the viscosity of the tears and decreases the rate of evaporation of tears from the surface of the eyeball. Blockage and inflammation of a tarsal gland is a **chalazion** and is on the inner surface of the eyelid.

The tarsal glands are not the only glands associated with the eyelids (see Fig. 8.59). Associated with the eyelash follicles are sebaceous and sweat glands. Blockage and inflammation of either of these is a **stye** and is on the edge of the eyelid.

Vessels

The arterial supply to the eyelids is from the numerous vessels in the area. They include (Fig. 8.63):

- the supratrochlear, supra-orbital, lacrimal, and dorsal nasal arteries from the ophthalmic artery,
- the angular artery from the facial artery,
- the transverse facial artery from the superficial temporal artery, and
- branches from the superficial temporal artery itself.

Venous drainage follows an external pattern through veins associated with the various arteries and an internal pattern moving into the orbit through connections with the ophthalmic veins.

Lymphatic drainage is primarily to the parotid nodes, with some drainage from the medial corner of the eye along lymphatic vessels associated with the angular and facial arteries to the submandibular nodes.

Innervation

Innervation of the eyelids includes both sensory and motor components.

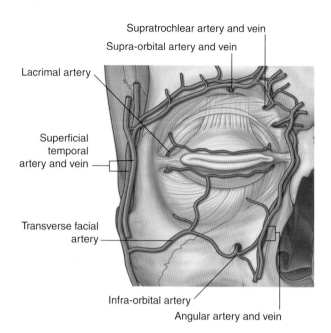

Fig. 8.63 Vasculature of the eyelids.

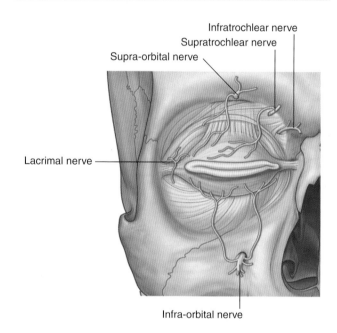

Fig. 8.64 Innervation of the eyelids.

The sensory nerves are all branches of the trigeminal nerve [V]. Palpebral branches arise from (Fig. 8.64):

- the supra-orbital, supratrochlear, infratrochlear, and lacrimal branches of the ophthalmic nerve [V$_1$], and
- the infra-orbital branch of the maxillary nerve [V$_2$].

Motor innervation is from:

- the facial nerve [VII], which innervates the palpebral part of the orbicularis oculi;

- the oculomotor nerve [III], which innervates the levator palpebrae superioris; and
- sympathetic fibers, which innervate the superior tarsal muscle.

Clinical app

Full and partial ptosis

Loss of innervation of the orbicularis oculi by the facial nerve [VII] causes an inability to close the eyelids tightly and the lower eyelid droops away, resulting in a spillage of tears.

Loss of innervation of the levator palpebrae superioris by the oculomotor nerve causes an inability to open the superior eyelid voluntarily, producing a complete ptosis.

Loss of innervation of the superior tarsal muscle by sympathetic fibers causes a constant partial ptosis.

Clinical app

Horner's syndrome

Horner's syndrome is caused by a lesion in the sympathetic trunk in the neck that results in sympathetic dysfunction. It is characterized by three typical features:

- pupillary constriction due to paralysis of the dilator pupillae muscle;
- partial ptosis (drooping of the upper eyelid) due to paralysis of the superior tarsal muscle; and
- absence of sweating on the ipsilateral side of the face and the neck due to absence of innervation of the sweat glands. Secondary changes may also include:
- ipsilateral vasodilation due to loss of the normal sympathetic control of the subcutaneous blood vessels; and
- enophthalmos (sinking of the eye)—believed to result from paralysis of the orbitalis muscle (a smooth muscle that spans the inferior orbital fissure and may contribute to maintaining the normal position of the eyeball), though this is an uncommon feature of Horner's syndrome.

The commonest cause for Horner's syndrome is an apical lung tumor eroding the cervicothoracic ganglion.

Lacrimal apparatus

The lacrimal apparatus is involved in the production, movement, and drainage of fluid from the surface of the eyeball. It is made up of the **lacrimal gland** and its ducts, the **lacrimal canaliculi**, the **lacrimal sac**, and the **nasolacrimal duct.**

The lacrimal gland is anterior in the superolateral region of the orbit (Fig. 8.65) and is divided into two parts by the levator palpebrae superioris (Fig. 8.66):

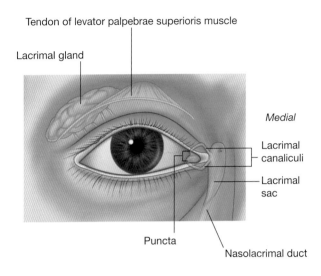

Fig. 8.65 Lacrimal gland, anterior view.

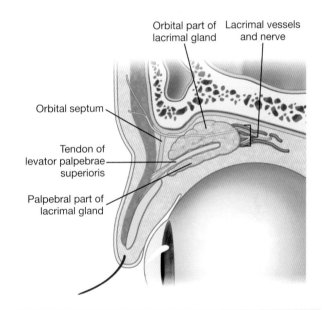

Fig. 8.66 Lacrimal gland and levator palpebrae superioris.

- The larger **orbital part** is in a depression, and the lacrimal fossa is in the frontal bone.
- The smaller **palpebral part** is inferior to levator palpebrae superioris in the superolateral part of the eyelid.

Numerous ducts empty the glandular secretions into the lateral part of the superior fornix of the conjunctiva.

Fluid is continually being secreted by the lacrimal gland and moved across the surface of the eyeball from lateral to medial as the eyelids blink.

The fluid accumulates medially in the **lacrimal lake** and is drained from the lake by the lacrimal canaliculi, one canaliculus is associated with each eyelid (Fig. 8.65). The

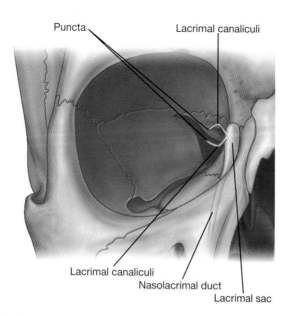

Fig. 8.67 Formation of the lacrimal sac.

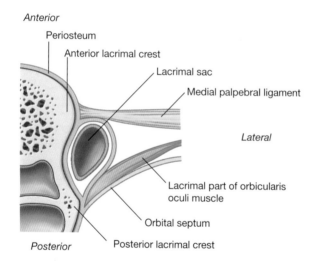

Fig. 8.68 Position of lacrimal sac.

lacrimal punctum is the opening through which fluid enters each canaliculus.

Passing medially, the lacrimal canaliculi eventually join the lacrimal sac between the anterior and posterior lacrimal crests posterior to the medial palpebral ligament and anterior to the lacrimal part of the orbicularis oculi muscle (Figs. 8.67 and 8.68). When the orbicularis oculi muscle contracts during blinking, the small lacrimal part of the muscle may dilate the lacrimal sac and draw tears into it through the canaliculi from the conjunctival sac.

Innervation

The innervation of the lacrimal gland involves three different components (Fig. 8.70).

Sensory innervation

Sensory neurons from the lacrimal gland return to the CNS through the lacrimal branch of the ophthalmic nerve [V$_1$].

Secretomotor (parasympathetic) innervation

Secretomotor fibers from the parasympathetic part of the autonomic division of the PNS stimulate fluid secretion from the lacrimal gland. These preganglionic parasympathetic neurons leave the CNS in the facial nerve [VII], enter the greater petrosal nerve (a branch of the facial nerve [VII]), and continue with this nerve until it becomes the **nerve of the pterygoid canal** (Fig. 8.70).

Surface anatomy
The eye and lacrimal apparatus

Major features of the eye include the sclera, cornea, iris, and pupil (Fig. 8.69A). The cornea is continuous with the sclera and is the clear circular region of the external covering of the eye through which the pupil and iris are visible. The sclera is not transparent and is normally white.

The upper and lower eyelids of each eye (Fig. 8.69B) enclose between them the palpebral fissure. The eyelids come together at the medial and lateral palpebral commissures on either side of each eye (Fig. 8.69A).

At the medial side of the palpebral fissure and lateral to the medial palpebral commissure is a small triangular area, the lacrimal lake (Fig. 8.69A).

The elevated mound of tissue on the medial side of the lacrimal lake is the lacrimal caruncle, and the lateral margin overlying the sclera is the lacrimal fold (Fig. 8.69B).

The lacrimal apparatus consists of the lacrimal gland and the system of ducts and channels that collect the tears and drain them into the nasal cavity (Fig. 8.69C). Tears hydrate and maintain the transparency of the cornea.

The lacrimal gland is associated with the upper eyelid and is in a small depression in the lateral roof of the orbit just posterior to the orbital margin. The multiple small ducts of the gland open into the upper margin of the conjunctival sac, which is the thin gap between the deep surface of the eyelid and the cornea.

Tears are swept medially over the eye by blinking and are collected in small openings (lacrimal puncta), one on each of the upper and lower eyelids near the lacrimal lake (Fig. 8.69C).

Each punctum is on a small raised mound of tissue (a lacrimal papilla) and is the opening of a small canal (lacrimal canaliculus) that connects with the lacrimal sac (Fig. 8.69C).

The lacrimal sac is in the lacrimal fossa on the medial side of the orbit. From the lacrimal sac, tears drain via the nasolacrimal duct into the nasal cavity (Fig. 8.69C).

Surface anatomy
The eye and lacrimal apparatus—cont'd

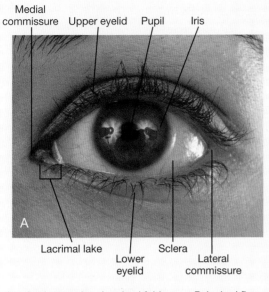

Medial commissure · Upper eyelid · Pupil · Iris

Lacrimal lake · Lower eyelid · Sclera · Lateral commissure

A

Lacrimal caruncle · Lacrimal fold · Palpebral fissure

Lacrimal papilla · Lacrimal punctum

B

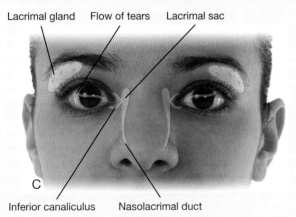

Lacrimal gland · Flow of tears · Lacrimal sac

Inferior canaliculus · Nasolacrimal duct

C

Fig. 8.69 Eye and lacrimal apparatus. **A.** Left eye and surrounding structures. **B.** Left eye with surrounding structures with lower eyelid pulled down to reveal the lacrimal papilla and lacrimal punctum. **C.** Face of a woman. Lacrimal apparatus and the flow of tears are indicated.

The nerve of the pterygoid canal eventually joins the pterygopalatine ganglion where the preganglionic parasympathetic neurons synapse on postganglionic parasympathetic neurons (Fig. 8.70). The postganglionic neurons join the maxillary nerve [V_2] and continue with it until the zygomatic nerve branches from it and travel with the zygomatic nerve until it gives off the zygomaticotemporal nerve, which eventually distributes postganglionic parasympathetic fibers in a small branch that joins the lacrimal nerve. The lacrimal nerve passes to the lacrimal gland.

Sympathetic innervation

Sympathetic innervation of the lacrimal gland follows a similar path as parasympathetic innervation. Postganglionic sympathetic fibers originating in the superior cervical ganglion travel along the plexus surrounding the internal carotid artery (Fig. 8.70). They leave this plexus as the deep petrosal nerve and join the parasympathetic fibers in the nerve of the pterygoid canal. Passing through the pterygopalatine ganglion, the sympathetic fibers from this point onward follow the same path as the parasympathetic fibers to the lacrimal gland.

Vessels

The arterial supply to the lacrimal gland is by branches from the ophthalmic artery, and venous drainage is through the ophthalmic veins.

Fissures and foramina

Numerous structures enter and leave the orbit through a variety of openings (Fig. 8.71).

Optic canal

When the bony orbit is viewed from an anterolateral position, the round opening at the apex of the pyramidal-shaped orbit is the optic canal, which opens into the middle cranial fossa and is bounded medially by the body of the sphenoid and laterally by the lesser wing of the sphenoid. Passing through the optic canal are the optic nerve and the ophthalmic artery (Fig. 8.72).

Superior orbital fissure

Just lateral to the optic canal is a triangular-shaped gap between the roof and lateral wall of the bony orbit. This is the superior orbital fissure and allows structures to pass between the orbit and the middle cranial fossa (see Fig. 8.71).

Passing through the superior orbital fissure are the superior and inferior branches of the oculomotor nerve [III]; the trochlear nerve [IV]; the abducent nerve [VI]; the lacrimal, frontal, and nasociliary branches of the ophthalmic nerve [V_1]; and the superior ophthalmic vein (Fig. 8.72).

Fig. 8.70 Innervation of the lacrimal gland.

Inferior orbital fissure

Separating the lateral wall of the orbit from the floor of the orbit is a longitudinal opening, the inferior orbital fissure (see Fig. 8.71). Its borders are the greater wing of the sphenoid and the maxilla, palatine, and zygomatic bones. This long fissure allows communication between:

- the orbit and the pterygopalatine fossa posteriorly,
- the orbit and the infratemporal fossa in the middle, and
- the orbit and the temporal fossa posterolaterally.

Passing through the inferior orbital fissure are the maxillary nerve [V$_2$] and its zygomatic branch, the infra-orbital vessels, and a vein communicating with the pterygoid plexus of veins.

Infra-orbital foramen

Beginning posteriorly and crossing about two-thirds of the inferior orbital fissure, a groove (the **infra-orbital groove**) is encountered that continues anteriorly across the floor of the orbit (see Fig. 8.71). This groove connects with the **infra-orbital canal** that opens onto the face at the **infra-orbital foramen.**

The infra-orbital nerve, a branch of the maxillary nerve [V$_2$], and vessels pass through this structure as they exit onto the face.

Other openings

Associated with the medial wall of the bony orbit are several smaller openings (see Fig. 8.71).

The **anterior** and **posterior ethmoidal foramina** are at the junction between the superior and medial walls (see

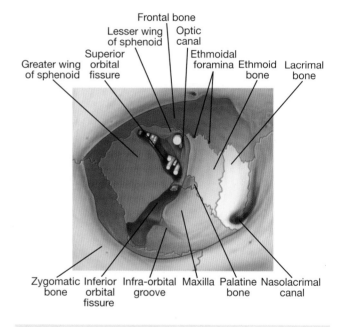

Fig. 8.71 Openings into the bony orbit.

Fig. 8.71). These openings provide exits from the orbit into the ethmoid bone for the anterior and posterior ethmoidal nerves and vessels.

Completing the openings on the medial wall is a canal in the lower part of the wall anteriorly. Clearly visible is the depression for the lacrimal sac formed by the lacrimal bone and the frontal process of the maxilla. This depression is continuous with the nasolacrimal canal (see Fig. 8.71), which leads to the inferior nasal meatus. Contained within the nasolacrimal canal is the nasolacrimal duct, a part of the lacrimal apparatus.

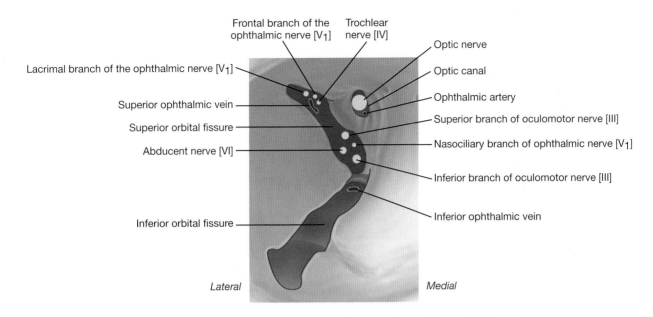

Fig. 8.72 Optic canal and superior orbital fissure.

Fascial specializations

Periorbita

The periosteum lining the bones that form the orbit is the **periorbita** (Fig. 8.73A). It is continuous at the margins of the orbit with the periosteum on the outer surface of the skull and sends extensions into the upper and lower eyelids (the **orbital septa**).

At the various openings where the orbit communicates with the cranial cavity, the periorbita is continuous with the periosteal layer of dura mater. In the posterior part of the orbit, the periorbita thickens around the optic canal and the central part of the superior orbital fissure. This is the point of origin of the four rectus muscles and is the **common tendinous ring** (Fig. 8.73B).

Fascial sheath of the eyeball

The **fascial sheath of the eyeball** (bulbar sheath) is a layer of fascia that encloses a major part of the eyeball (Figs. 8.74, 8.75):

- Posteriorly, it is firmly attached to the sclera (the white part of the eyeball) around the point of entrance of the optic nerve into the eyeball.
- Anteriorly, it is firmly attached to the sclera near the edge of the cornea (the clear part of the eyeball).
- Additionally, as the muscles approach the eyeball, the investing fascia surrounding each muscle blends with the fascial sheath of the eyeball as the muscles pass through and continue to their point of attachment.

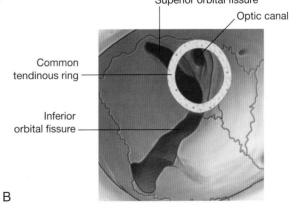

Fig. 8.73 Periorbita. **A.** Lateral view. **B.** Common tendinous ring.

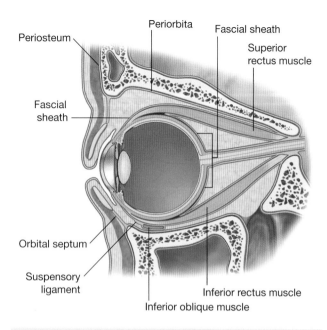

Fig. 8.74 Fascial sheath of the eyeball.

A

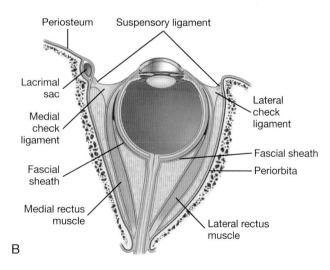

B

Fig. 8.75 Check ligaments. **A. Anterior view. B. Superior view.**

A specialized lower part of the fascial sheath of the eyeball is the **suspensory ligament** (Figs. 8.74, 8.75A), which supports the eyeball. This "sling-like" structure is made up of the fascial sheath of the eyeball and contributions from the two inferior ocular muscles and the medial and lateral ocular muscles.

Check ligaments of the medial and lateral rectus muscles

Other fascial specialization in the orbit are the check ligaments (see Fig. 8.75B). These are expansions of the investing fascia covering the medial and lateral rectus muscles, which attach to the medial and lateral walls of the bony orbit and may assist in maintaining the normal position of the eyeball:

- The medial check ligament attaches immediately posterior to the posterior lacrimal crest of the lacrimal bone.
- The lateral check ligament attaches to the orbital tubercle of the zygomatic bone.

Muscles

There are two groups of muscles within the orbit:

- **extrinsic muscles of the eyeball (extra-ocular muscles)** involved in movements of the eyeball or raising upper eyelids, and
- **intrinsic muscles** within the eyeball, which control the shape of the lens and size of the pupil.

The extrinsic muscles include the levator palpebrae superioris, superior rectus, inferior rectus, medial rectus, lateral rectus, superior oblique, and inferior oblique.

The intrinsic muscles include the **ciliary muscle,** the **sphincter pupillae,** and the **dilator pupillae.**

Extrinsic muscles

Of the seven muscles in the extrinsic group of muscles, one raises the eyelids, whereas the other six move the eyeball itself (Table 8.8).

The movements of the eyeball, in three dimensions, (Fig. 8.76) are:

- elevation—moving the pupil superiorly,
- depression—moving the pupil inferiorly,
- abduction—moving the pupil laterally,
- adduction—moving the pupil medially,
- internal rotation (intorsion)—rotating the upper part of the pupil medially (or toward the nose), and
- external rotation (extorsion)—rotating the upper part of the pupil laterally (or toward the temple).

Table 8.8 Extrinsic (extra-ocular) muscles

Muscle	Origin	Insertion	Innervation	Function
Levator palpebrae superioris	Lesser wing of sphenoid anterior to optic canal	Anterior surface of tarsal plate; a few fibers to skin and superior conjunctival fornix	Oculomotor nerve [III]—superior branch	Elevation of upper eyelid
Superior rectus	Superior part of common tendinous ring	Anterior half of eyeball superiorly	Oculomotor nerve [III]—superior branch	Elevation, adduction, internal rotation of eyeball
Inferior rectus	Inferior part of common tendinous ring	Anterior half of eyeball inferiorly	Oculomotor nerve [III]—inferior branch	Depression, adduction, external rotation of eyeball
Medial rectus	Medial part of common tendinous ring	Anterior half of eyeball medially	Oculomotor nerve [III]—inferior branch	Adduction of eyeball
Lateral rectus	Lateral part of common tendinous ring	Anterior half of eyeball laterally	Abducent nerve [VI]	Abduction of eyeball
Superior oblique	Body of sphenoid, superior and medial to optic canal	Outer posterior quadrant of eyeball (superior surface)	Trochlear nerve [IV]	Depression, abduction, internal rotation of eyeball
Inferior oblique	Medial floor of orbit posterior to rim; maxilla lateral to nasolacrimal groove	Outer posterior quadrant of eyeball (inferior surface)	Oculomotor nerve [III]—inferior branch	Elevation, abduction, external rotation of eyeball

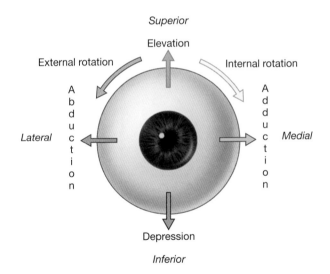

Fig. 8.76 Movements of the eyeball.

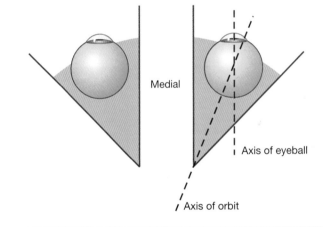

Fig. 8.77 Axes of the eyeball and orbit.

The axis of each orbit is directed slightly laterally from back to front, but each eyeball is directed anteriorly (Fig. 8.77). Therefore the pull of some muscles has multiple effects on the movement of the eyeball, whereas that of others has a single effect.

The levator palpebrae superioris raises the upper eyelid and is the most superior muscle in the orbit (Table 8.8, Fig. 8.78B).

A unique feature of levator palpebrae superioris is that a collection of smooth muscle fibers passes from its inferior surface to the upper edge of the superior tarsus (see Fig. 8.59). This group of smooth muscle fibers (the superior tarsal muscle) help maintain eyelid elevation and are innervated by

postganglionic sympathetic fibers from the superior cervical ganglion.

The four rectus muscles occupy medial, lateral, inferior, and superior positions as they pass from their origins posteriorly to their points of attachment on the anterior half of the eyeball (Table 8.8, Figs. 8.78, 8.80, 8.81; also see Fig. 8.79).

The superior and inferior rectus muscles have complicated actions because the apex of the orbit, where the muscles originate, is medial to the central axis of the eyeball when looking directly forward (Table 8.8, Fig. 8.81A).

To isolate the function of and to test the superior and inferior rectus muscles, a patient is asked to track a physician's finger laterally and then either upward or downward (Fig. 8.81B). The first movement brings the axis of the eyeball into alignment with the long axis of the superior and inferior rectus muscles. Moving the finger upward tests the

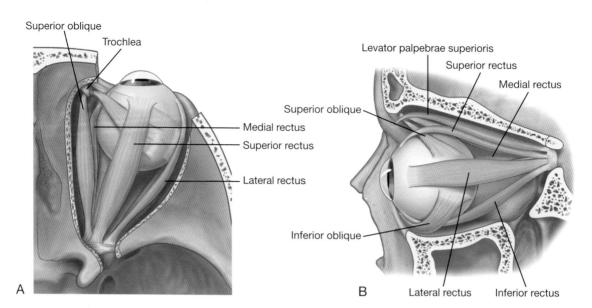

Fig. 8.78 Muscles of the eyeball. **A.** Superior view. **B.** Lateral view.

Imaging app

Visualizing the muscles of the eyeball

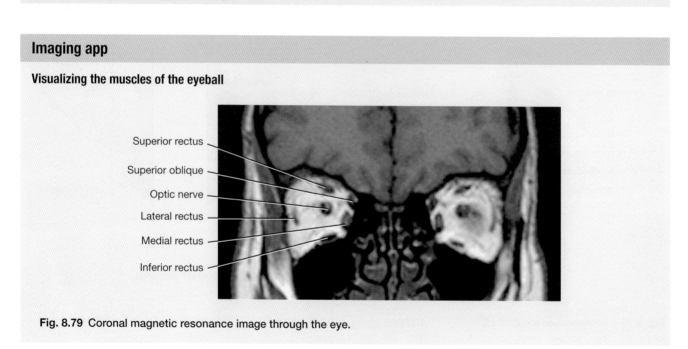

Fig. 8.79 Coronal magnetic resonance image through the eye.

superior rectus muscle and moving it downward tests the inferior rectus muscle (Fig. 8.81B).

The orientation and actions of the medial and lateral rectus muscles are more straightforward than those of the superior and inferior rectus muscles (Table 8.8, Fig. 8.81A).

To isolate the function of and test the medial and lateral rectus muscles, a patient is asked to track a physician's finger medially and laterally, respectively, in the horizontal plane (Fig. 8.81B).

The oblique muscles are in the superior and inferior parts of the orbit, do not originate from the common tendinous ring, are angular in their approaches to the eyeball, and,

unlike the rectus muscles, attach to the posterior half of the eyeball (Table 8.8; also see Figs. 8.78, 8.79, 8.80).

A unique feature of the superior oblique is that the tendon of this muscle passes through the trochlea and turns laterally to cross the eyeball in a posterolateral direction (see Fig. 8.78A). It continues deep to the superior rectus muscle and inserts into the outer posterior quadrant of the eyeball.

To isolate the function of and to test the superior oblique muscle, a patient is asked to track a physician's finger medially to bring the axis of the tendon of the muscle into alignment with the axis of the eyeball and then to look down, which tests the muscle (Fig. 8.81B).

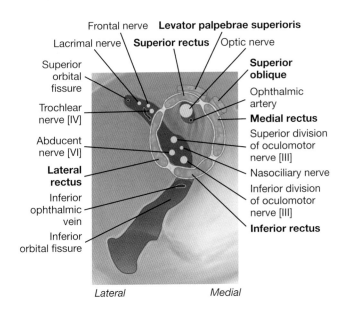

Fig. 8.80 Origins of muscles of the eyeball, coronal view.

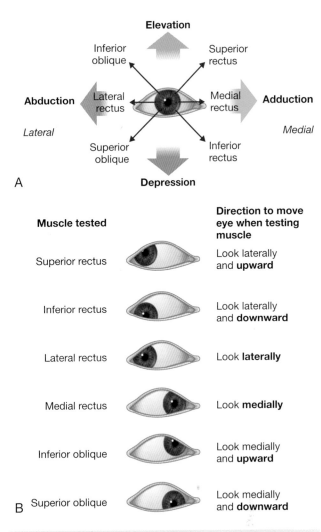

Fig. 8.81 Actions of muscles of the eyeball. **A.** Action of individual muscles (anatomical action). **B.** Movement of eye when testing specific muscle (clinical testing).

A unique feature of the inferior oblique muscle is that it is the only extrinsic muscle that does not take origin from the posterior part of the orbit (Table 8.8; see Fig. 8.78B). It crosses the floor of the orbit in a posterolateral direction between the inferior rectus and the floor of the orbit before inserting into the outer posterior quadrant just under the lateral rectus.

To isolate the function of and to test the inferior oblique muscle, a patient is asked to track a physician's finger medially to bring the axis of the eyeball into alignment with the axis of the muscle and then to look up, which tests the muscle (Fig. 8.81B).

Extrinsic muscles and eyeball movements

Six of the seven extrinsic muscles of the orbit are directly involved in movements of the eyeball.

For each of the rectus muscles, the medial, lateral, inferior, and superior, and the superior and inferior obliques, a specific action or group of actions can be described (see Table 8.8). However, these muscles do not act in isolation. They work as teams of muscles in the coordinated movement of the eyeball to position the pupil as needed.

For example, although the lateral rectus is the muscle primarily responsible for moving the eyeball laterally, it is assisted in this action by the superior and inferior oblique muscles.

Vessels

Arteries

The arterial supply to the structures in the orbit, including the eyeball, is by the **ophthalmic artery** (Fig. 8.83). This vessel is a branch of the internal carotid artery given off immediately after the internal carotid artery leaves the cavernous sinus. The ophthalmic artery passes into the orbit through the optic canal with the optic nerve (Fig. 8.83).

In the orbit the ophthalmic artery initially lies inferior and lateral to the optic nerve (Fig. 8.83). As it passes forward in the orbit, it crosses superior to the optic nerve and proceeds anteriorly on the medial side of the orbit.

In the orbit the ophthalmic artery gives off numerous branches as follows (Fig. 8.83):

- the **lacrimal artery,** which arises from the ophthalmic artery on the lateral side of the optic nerve and passes anteriorly on the lateral side of the orbit, supplying the lacrimal gland, muscles, the anterior ciliary branch to the eyeball, and the lateral sides of the eyelid;
- the **central retinal artery,** which enters the optic nerve, proceeds down the center of the nerve to the retina, and is clearly seen when viewing the retina with an

The H–test

A simple "formula' for remembering the nerves that innervate the extraocular muscles is "LR6SO4 and all the rest are 3" (lateral rectus [VI], superior oblique [IV], all the rest including levator palpebrae superioris are [III]).

The function of all extrinsic muscles and their nerves [III, IV, VI] that move the eyeball in both orbits can all easily be tested at the same time by having the patient track, without moving his or her head, an object such as the tip of a pen or a finger moved in an "H" pattern—starting from the midline between the two eyes (Fig. 8.82).

	Right eye	Left eye
1.	Lateral rectus [VI]	Medial rectus [III]
2.	Superior rectus [III]	Inferior oblique [III]
3.	Inferior rectus [III]	Superior oblique [IV]
4.	Medial rectus [III]	Lateral rectus [VI]
5.	Superior oblique [IV]	Inferior rectus [III]
6.	Inferior oblique [III]	Superior rectus [III]

Fig. 8.82 The "H-test."

ophthalmoscope—occlusion of this vessel or of the parent artery leads to blindness;

■ the **long** and **short posterior ciliary arteries,** which are branches that enter the eyeball posteriorly, piercing the sclera and supplying structures inside the eyeball;

■ the **muscular arteries,** which are branches supplying the intrinsic muscles of the eyeball;

■ the **supra-orbital artery,** which usually arises from the ophthalmic artery immediately after it has crossed the optic nerve, proceeds anteriorly, and exits the orbit through the supra-orbital foramen with the supra-orbital nerve—it supplies the forehead and scalp as it passes across these areas to the vertex of the skull;

■ the **posterior ethmoidal artery,** which exits the orbit through the posterior ethmoidal foramen to supply the ethmoidal cells and nasal cavity;

■ the **anterior ethmoidal artery,** which exits the orbit through the anterior ethmoidal foramen, enters the cranial

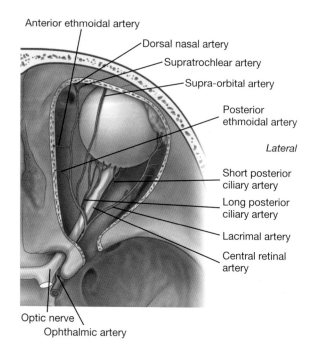

Fig. 8.83 Arterial supply to the orbit and eyeball.

cavity, giving off the anterior meningeal branch, and continues into the nasal cavity, supplying the septum and lateral wall, and ending as the dorsal nasal artery;

■ the **medial palpebral arteries,** which are small branches supplying the medial area of the upper and lower eyelids;

■ the **dorsal nasal artery,** which is one of the two terminal branches of the ophthalmic artery, leaves the orbit to supply the upper surface of the nose; and

■ the **supratrochlear artery,** which is the other terminal branch of the ophthalmic artery and leaves the orbit with the supratrochlear nerve, supplying the forehead as it passes across it in a superior direction.

Veins

There are two venous channels in the orbit—the superior and inferior ophthalmic veins (Fig. 8.84).

The **superior ophthalmic vein** begins in the anterior area of the orbit as connecting veins from the supra-orbital vein and the angular vein join together. It passes across the superior part of the orbit, receiving tributaries from the companion veins to the branches of the ophthalmic artery and veins draining the posterior part of the eyeball. Posteriorly, it leaves the orbit through the superior orbital fissure and enters the cavernous sinus.

The **inferior ophthalmic vein** is smaller than the superior ophthalmic vein, begins anteriorly, and passes across the inferior part of the orbit. It receives various tributaries from muscles and the posterior part of the eyeball as it crosses the orbit.

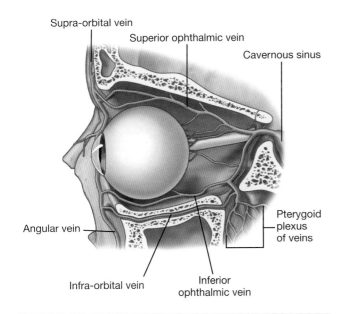

Supra-orbital vein
Superior ophthalmic vein
Cavernous sinus
Angular vein
Pterygoid plexus of veins
Infra-orbital vein
Inferior ophthalmic vein

Fig. 8.84 Venous drainage of the orbit and eyeball.

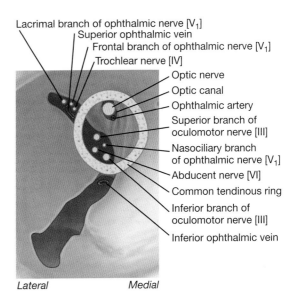

Lacrimal branch of ophthalmic nerve [V₁]
Superior ophthalmic vein
Frontal branch of ophthalmic nerve [V₁]
Trochlear nerve [IV]
Optic nerve
Optic canal
Ophthalmic artery
Superior branch of oculomotor nerve [III]
Nasociliary branch of ophthalmic nerve [V₁]
Abducent nerve [VI]
Common tendinous ring
Inferior branch of oculomotor nerve [III]
Inferior ophthalmic vein

Lateral   *Medial*

Fig. 8.85 Innervation of the orbit and eyeball.

The inferior ophthalmic vein leaves the orbit posteriorly by:

- joining with the superior ophthalmic vein,
- passing through the superior orbital fissure on its own to join the cavernous sinus, or
- passing through the inferior orbital fissure to join with the pterygoid plexus of veins in the infratemporal fossa.

Because the ophthalmic veins communicate with the cavernous sinus, they act as a route by which infections can spread from outside to inside the cranial cavity.

Innervation

Numerous nerves pass into the orbit and innervate structures within its bony walls. They include the optic nerve [II], the oculomotor nerve [III], the trochlear nerve [IV], the abducent nerve [VI], and autonomic nerves. Other nerves such as the ophthalmic nerve [V₁] innervate orbital structures and then travel out of the orbit to innervate other regions.

Optic nerve

The optic nerve [II] is not a true cranial nerve, but rather an extension of the brain carrying afferent fibers from the retina of the eyeball to the visual centers of the brain. The optic nerve is surrounded by the cranial meninges, including the subarachnoid space, which extend as far forward as the eyeball.

Any increase in intracranial pressure therefore results in increased pressure in the subarachnoid space surrounding the optic nerve. This may impede venous return along the retinal veins, causing edema of the optic disc (papilledema), which can be seen when the retina is examined using an ophthalmoscope.

The optic nerve leaves the orbit through the optic canal (Fig. 8.85). It is accompanied in the optic canal by the ophthalmic artery.

Oculomotor nerve

The oculomotor nerve [III] leaves the anterior surface of the brainstem between the midbrain and the pons. It passes forward in the lateral wall of the cavernous sinus.

Just before entering the orbit the oculomotor nerve [III] divides into superior and inferior branches (Fig. 8.86). These branches enter the orbit through the superior orbital fissure, lying within the common tendinous ring (Fig. 8.85).

Inside the orbit the small superior branch passes upward over the lateral side of the optic nerve to innervate the superior rectus and levator palpebrae superioris muscles (Fig. 8.86).

The large inferior branch divides into three branches (Fig. 8.86):

- one passing below the optic nerve as it passes to the medial side of the orbit to innervate the medial rectus muscle,
- a second descending to innervate the inferior rectus muscle, and
- the third descends as it runs forward along the floor of the orbit to innervate the inferior oblique muscle.

As the third branch descends, it gives off the **branch to the ciliary ganglion** (Fig. 8.86). This is the parasympathetic root to the ciliary ganglion and carries preganglionic parasympathetic fibers that will synapse in the ciliary ganglion

515

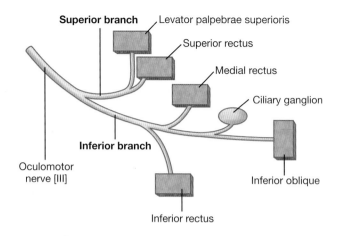

Fig. 8.86 Oculomotor nerve [III] and its divisions.

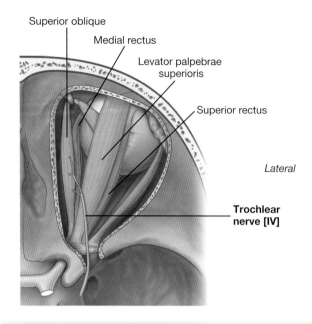

Fig. 8.87 Trochlear nerve [IV] in the orbit.

with postganglionic parasympathetic fibers. The postganglionic fibers are distributed to the eyeball through short ciliary nerves and innervate the sphincter pupillae and ciliary muscles.

Trochlear nerve

The trochlear nerve [IV] arises from the posterior surface of the midbrain and passes around the midbrain to enter the edge of the tentorium cerebelli. It continues on an intradural path, arriving in and passing through the lateral wall of the cavernous sinus just below the oculomotor nerve [III].

Just before entering the orbit, the trochlear nerve ascends, passing across the oculomotor nerve [III] and enters the orbit through the superior orbital fissure above the common tendinous ring (Fig. 8.85). In the orbit the trochlear nerve [IV] ascends and turns medially, crossing above the levator palpebrae superioris muscle to enter the upper border of the superior oblique muscle (Fig. 8.87).

Abducent nerve

The abducent nerve [VI] arises from the brainstem between the pons and medulla. It enters the dura covering the clivus and continues in a dural canal until it reaches the cavernous sinus.

The abducent nerve enters the cavernous sinus and runs through the sinus lateral to the internal carotid artery. It passes out of the sinus and enters the orbit through the superior orbital fissure within the common tendinous ring (Fig. 8.85). Once in the orbit it courses laterally to supply the lateral rectus muscle.

Postganglionic sympathetic fibers

Preganglionic sympathetic fibers arise from the upper segments of the thoracic spinal cord, mainly T1. They enter the sympathetic chain through white rami communicantes, and ascend to the **superior cervical ganglion** where they synapse with postganglionic sympathetic fibers.

The postganglionic fibers are distributed along the internal carotid artery and its branches.

The postganglionic sympathetic fibers destined for the orbit travel with the ophthalmic artery. Once in the orbit the fibers are distributed to the eyeball either by:

- passing through the ciliary ganglion, without synapsing, and joining the short ciliary nerves, which pass from the ganglion to the eyeball; or
- passing through long ciliary nerves to reach the eyeball.

In the eyeball postganglionic sympathetic fibers innervate the dilator pupillae muscle.

Ophthalmic nerve [V₁]

The ophthalmic nerve [V_1] is the smallest and most superior of the three divisions of the trigeminal nerve [V]. This purely sensory nerve receives input from structures in the orbit and from additional branches on the face and scalp.

Leaving the trigeminal ganglion, the ophthalmic nerve [V_1] passes forward in the lateral wall of the cavernous sinus inferior to the trochlear [IV] and oculomotor [III] nerves. Just before it enters the orbit it divides into three branches—the lacrimal, frontal, and nasociliary nerves (Fig. 8.88). These branches enter the orbit through the superior orbital fissure with the frontal and lacrimal nerves outside the common tendinous ring and the nasociliary nerve within the common tendinous ring (Fig. 8.85).

Lacrimal nerve

The lacrimal nerve is the smallest of the three branches of the ophthalmic nerve [V_1]. Once in the orbit it passes

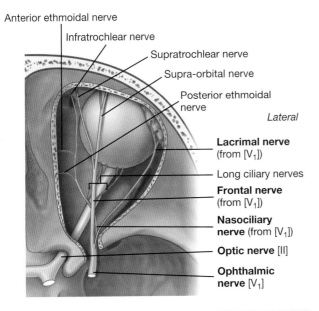

Fig. 8.88 Ophthalmic nerve [V₁] and its divisions.

forward along the upper border of the lateral rectus muscle (Figs. 8.89, 8.90). It receives a branch from the zygomaticotemporal nerve, which carries parasympathetic and sympathetic postganglionic fibers for distribution to the lacrimal gland.

Reaching the anterolateral aspect of the orbit, the lacrimal nerve supplies the lacrimal gland, conjunctiva, and lateral part of the upper eyelid.

Frontal nerve

The frontal nerve is the largest branch of the ophthalmic nerve [V₁] and receives sensory input from areas outside the orbit. Exiting the superior orbital fissure, this branch passes forward between the levator palpebrae superioris and the periorbita on the roof of the orbit (Fig. 8.89). About midway across the orbit, it divides into its two terminal branches—the supra-orbital and supratrochlear nerves (Fig. 8.89; also see Fig. 8.88):

■ The supratrochlear nerve continues forward in an anteromedial direction, passing above the trochlea, and exits the orbit medial to the supra-orbital foramen and supplies the conjunctiva and skin of the upper eyelid and the skin on the lower medial part of the forehead.

■ The supra-orbital nerve is the larger of the two branches; it continues forward, passing between the levator palpebrae superioris muscle and the periorbita covering the roof of the orbit (Fig. 8.89), exits the orbit through the supra-orbital notch, and ascends across the forehead and scalp, supplying the upper eyelid and conjunctiva, the forehead, and as far posteriorly as the middle of the scalp.

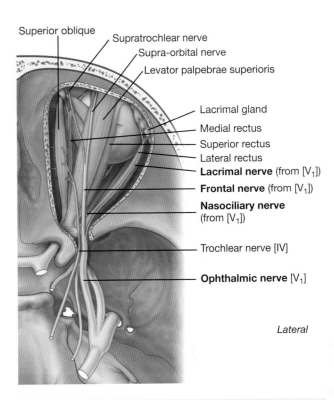

Fig. 8.89 Relationship of the ophthalmic nerve [V₁] and its divisions to the muscles of the eyeball.

Nasociliary nerve

The nasociliary nerve is intermediate in size between the frontal and lacrimal nerves and is usually the first branch from the ophthalmic nerve [V₁] (Fig. 8.88). It is most deeply placed in the orbit, entering the area within the common tendinous ring between the superior and inferior branches of the oculomotor nerve [III] (Fig. 8.90; also see Fig. 8.85).

Once in the orbit, the nasociliary nerve crosses the superior surface of the optic nerve as it passes in a medial direction below the superior rectus muscle (Figs. 8.88, 8.90). Its first branch, the **communicating branch with the ciliary ganglion (sensory root to the ciliary ganglion)**, is given off early in its path through the orbit (Fig. 8.91).

The nasociliary nerve continues forward along the medial wall of the orbit between the superior oblique and the medial rectus muscles, giving off several branches (Figs. 8.89, 8.91). These include:

■ the **long ciliary nerves,** which are sensory to the eyeball but may also carry sympathetic fibers for pupillary dilation;

■ the **posterior ethmoidal nerve,** which exits the orbit through the posterior ethmoidal foramen to supply posterior ethmoidal cells and the sphenoidal sinus;

■ the **infratrochlear nerve,** which distributes to the medial part of the upper and lower eyelids, the lacrimal sac, and skin of the upper half of the nose; and

517

Fig. 8.90 Course of the nasociliary nerve [V₁] in the orbit.

- the **anterior ethmoidal nerve,** which exits the orbit through the anterior ethmoidal foramen to supply the anterior cranial fossa, nasal cavity, and skin of the lower half of the nose.

Ciliary ganglion

The ciliary ganglion is a parasympathetic ganglion of the oculomotor nerve [III]. It is associated with the nasociliary branch of the ophthalmic nerve [V₁] and is the site where preganglionic and postganglionic parasympathetic neurons synapse as fibers from this part of the autonomic division of the PNS make their way to the eyeball. The ciliary ganglion is also traversed by postganglionic sympathetic fibers and sensory fibers as they travel to the eyeball.

The ciliary ganglion is a very small ganglion, in the posterior part of the orbit immediately lateral to the optic nerve and between the optic nerve and the lateral rectus muscle (Fig. 8.90). It is usually described as receiving at least two, and possibly three, branches or roots from other nerves in the orbit.

Parasympathetic root

As the inferior branch of the oculomotor nerve [III] passes the area of the ciliary ganglion, it sends a branch to the ganglion (the parasympathetic root). The parasympathetic branch carries preganglionic parasympathetic fibers, which enter the ganglion and synapse with postganglionic parasympathetic fibers within the ganglion (Fig. 8.91).

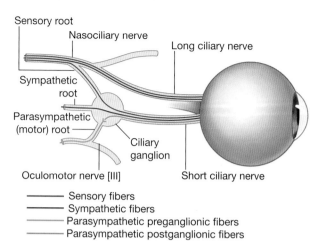

Fig. 8.91 Ciliary ganglion.

The postganglionic parasympathetic fibers leave the ganglion through short ciliary nerves, which enter the posterior aspect of the eyeball around the optic nerve.

In the eyeball the parasympathetic fibers innervate:

- the sphincter pupillae muscle, responsible for pupillary constriction, and
- the ciliary muscle, responsible for accommodation of the lens of the eye for near vision.

Sensory root

A second branch (the sensory root) passes from the nasociliary nerve to the ganglion (Fig. 8.91). This branch enters the posterosuperior aspect of the ganglion and carries sensory fibers, which pass through the ganglion and continue along the short ciliary nerves to the eyeball. These fibers are responsible for sensory innervation to all parts of the eyeball.

Sympathetic root

The third branch to the ciliary ganglion is the most variable. This branch, when present, is the sympathetic root and contains postganglionic sympathetic fibers from the superior cervical ganglion (Fig. 8.91). These fibers travel up the internal carotid artery, leave the plexus surrounding the artery in the cavernous sinus, and enter the orbit through the common tendinous ring. In the orbit they enter the posterior aspect of the ciliary ganglion, cross the ganglion, and continue along the short ciliary nerves to the eyeball.

Sympathetic fibers to the eyeball may not enter the ganglion as a separate sympathetic root. Rather, the postganglionic sympathetic fibers may leave the plexus associated with the internal carotid artery in the cavernous sinus, join the ophthalmic nerve (V₁), and course into the ciliary ganglion in the sensory root from the nasociliary nerve. In addition, the sympathetic fibers carried in the nasociliary nerve may not enter the ganglion at all and course directly into the eyeball in the long ciliary nerves (Fig. 8.91).

Whatever their path, postganglionic sympathetic fibers reach the eyeball and innervate the dilator pupillae muscle.

Eyeball

The globe-shaped eyeball occupies the anterior part of the orbit. Its rounded shape is disrupted anteriorly where it bulges outward. This outward projection represents about one-sixth of the total area of the eyeball and is the transparent cornea (Fig. 8.92).

Posterior to the cornea and in order from front to back are the anterior chamber, the iris and pupil, the posterior chamber, the lens, the postremal (vitreous) chamber, and the retina.

Anterior and posterior chambers

The **anterior chamber** is the area directly posterior to the cornea and anterior to the colored part of the eye (**iris**) (Fig. 8.92).

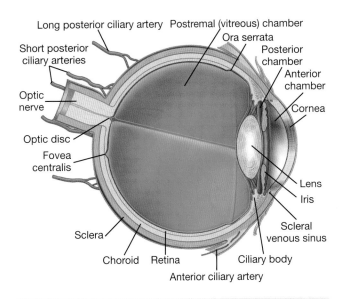

Fig. 8.92 Eyeball.

Clinical app

Ophthalmoscopy

Direct visualization of the postremal (vitreous) chamber of the eye and the posterior wall of the eye through the pupil and the lens is possible using an ophthalmoscope (Fig. 8.93).

The optic nerve, observed as the optic disc, is easily seen. The typical four branches of the retinal artery and the fovea are also seen.

Using ophthalmoscopy, the physician can look for diseases of the optic nerve, vascular abnormalities, and changes within the retina (Fig. 8.93).

Fig. 8.93 Ophthalmoscopic view of posterior chamber of the right eye.

The central opening in the iris is the **pupil.** Posterior to the iris and anterior to the lens is the smaller **posterior chamber.**

The anterior and posterior chambers are continuous with each other through the pupillary opening. They are filled with a fluid **(aqueous humor),** which is secreted into the posterior chamber, flows into the anterior chamber through the pupil, and is absorbed into the **scleral venous sinus** (the canal of Schlemm), which is a circular venous channel at the junction between the cornea and the iris (see Fig. 8.92).

The aqueous humor supplies nutrients to the avascular cornea and lens and maintains the intra-ocular pressure. If the normal cycle of its production and absorption is disturbed so that the amount of fluid increases, intra-ocular pressure will increase.

Lens and vitreous humor

The **lens** separates the anterior one-fifth of the eyeball from the posterior four-fifths (see Fig. 8.92). It is a transparent, biconvex elastic disc attached circumferentially to muscles associated with the outer wall of the eyeball. This lateral attachment provides the lens with the ability to change its refractive ability to maintain visual acuity. The clinical term for opacity of the lens is a cataract.

The posterior four-fifths of the eyeball, from the lens to the retina, is occupied by the postremal (vitreous) chamber (see Fig. 8.92). This segment is filled with a transparent, gelatinous substance—the **vitreous body (vitreous humor).** This substance, unlike aqueous humor, cannot be replaced.

Walls of the eyeball

Surrounding the internal components of the eyeball are the walls of the eyeball. They consist of three layers: an outer fibrous layer, a middle vascular layer, and an inner retinal layer (see Fig. 8.92).

- The outer fibrous layer consists of the **sclera** posteriorly and the **cornea** anteriorly.
- The middle vascular layer consists of the **choroid** posteriorly and is continuous with the ciliary body and iris anteriorly.
- The inner layer consists of the optic part of the **retina** posteriorly and the nonvisual retina that covers the internal surface of the ciliary body and iris anteriorly.

Vessels

Arterial supply

The arterial supply to the eyeball is from several sources (see Fig. 8.92):

- The **short posterior ciliary arteries** are branches from the ophthalmic artery that pierce the sclera around the optic nerve and enter the choroid layer (see Fig. 8.92).

- The **long posterior ciliary arteries,** usually two, enter the sclera on the medial and lateral sides of the optic nerve and proceed anteriorly in the choroid layer to anastomose with the anterior ciliary arteries (see Fig. 8.92).
- The **anterior ciliary arteries** are branches of the arteries supplying the muscles (see Fig. 8.92); as the muscles attach to the sclera, these arteries pierce the sclera to anastomose with the long posterior ciliary arteries in the choroid layer.
- The **central retinal artery** that has traversed the optic nerve and enters the area of the retina at the optic disc (Fig. 8.93).

Venous drainage

Venous drainage of the eyeball is primarily related to drainage of the choroid layer. Four large veins (the **vorticose veins**) are involved in this process. They exit through the sclera from each of the posterior quadrants of the eyeball and enter the superior and inferior ophthalmic veins. There is also a central retinal vein accompanying the central retinal artery.

> ### Clinical app
>
> #### Glaucoma
>
> Intraocular pressure will rise if the normal cycle of aqueous humor fluid production and absorption is disturbed so that the amount of fluid increases. This condition is glaucoma and can lead to a variety of visual problems including blindness, which results from compression of the retina and its blood supply.

> ### Clinical app
>
> #### Cataracts
>
> With increasing age and in certain disease states the lens of the eye becomes opaque. Increasing opacity results in increasing visual impairment. A common operation is excision of the cloudy lens and replacement with a new man-made lens.

Fibrous layer of the eyeball

The fibrous layer of the eyeball consists of two components—the sclera covers the posterior and lateral parts of the eyeball, about five-sixths of the surface, and the cornea covers the anterior part (see Fig. 8.92).

Sclera

The sclera is an opaque layer of dense connective tissue that can be seen anteriorly through its conjunctival covering as the "white of the eye" (see Fig. 8.92). It is pierced by numerous vessels and nerves, including the optic nerve posteriorly, and provides attachment for the various muscles involved in eyeball movements.

The fascial sheath of the eyeball covers the surface of the sclera externally from the entrance of the optic nerve to the corneoscleral junction while internally the surface of the sclera is loosely attached to the choroid of the vascular layer.

Cornea

Continuous with the sclera anteriorly is the transparent cornea. It covers the anterior one-sixth of the surface of the eyeball and, being transparent, allows light to enter the eyeball (see Fig. 8.92).

Vascular layer of the eyeball

The vascular layer of the eyeball consists of three continuous parts—the choroid, the ciliary body, and the iris from posterior to anterior (see Fig. 8.92).

Choroid

The choroid is posterior and represents approximately two-thirds of the vascular layer (see Fig. 8.92). It is a thin, highly vascular, pigmented layer consisting of smaller vessels adjacent to the retina and larger vessels more peripherally. It is firmly attached to the retina internally and loosely attached to the sclera externally.

Ciliary body

Extending from the anterior border of the choroid is the ciliary body (Figs. 8.92, 8.94). This triangular-shaped structure between the choroid and the iris forms a complete ring around the eyeball. Its components include the ciliary muscle and the ciliary processes (see Fig. 8.94).

The **ciliary muscle** consists of smooth muscle fibers arranged longitudinally, circularly, and radially. Controlled by parasympathetics traveling to the orbit in the oculomotor nerve [III], these muscle fibers, on contraction, decrease the size of the ring formed by the ciliary body (Table 8.9, see Fig. 8.94).

The **ciliary processes** are longitudinal ridges projecting from the inner surface of the ciliary body (see Fig. 8.94). Extending from them are **zonular fibers** attached to the lens of the eyeball, which suspend the lens in its proper position and collectively form the **suspensory ligament of the lens.**

Contraction of the ciliary muscle decreases the size of the ring formed by the ciliary body. This reduces tension on the suspensory ligament of the lens. The lens therefore becomes more rounded (relaxed), resulting in accommodation of the lens for near vision.

Ciliary processes also contribute to the formation of aqueous humor.

Iris

Completing the vascular layer of the eyeball anteriorly is the iris (see Fig. 8.94). This circular structure, projecting outward from the ciliary body, is the colored part of the eye with a

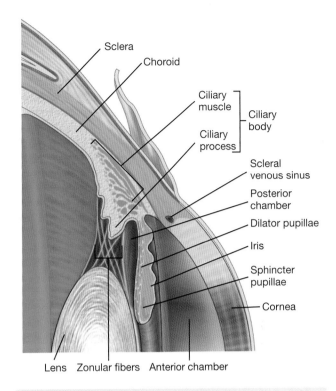

Fig. 8.94 Ciliary body.

central opening (the pupil). Controlling the size of the pupil are smooth muscle fibers (sphincter pupillae) and myoepithelial cells (dilator pupillae) within the iris (see Fig. 8.94):

- Fibers arranged in a circular pattern make up the **sphincter pupillae** muscle (Table 8.9), which is innervated by parasympathetics—contraction of its fibers decreases or constricts the pupillary opening.
- Contractile fibers arranged in a radial pattern make up the **dilator pupillae** muscle (Table 8.9), which is innervated by sympathetics—contraction of its fibers increases or dilates the pupillary opening.

Inner layer of the eyeball

The inner layer of the eyeball is the retina (see Fig. 8.92). It consists of two parts. Posteriorly and laterally is the **optic part of the retina,** which is sensitive to light, and anteriorly is the **nonvisual part,** which covers the internal surface of the ciliary body and the iris. The junction between these parts is an irregular line (the **ora serrata**).

Optic part of the retina

The optic part of the retina consists of two layers, an outer pigmented layer and an inner neural layer:

- The **pigmented layer** is firmly attached to the choroid and continues anteriorly over the internal surface of the ciliary body and iris.

Table 8.9 Intrinsic muscles of the eye

Muscle	Location	Innervation	Function
Ciliary	Muscle fibers in the ciliary body	Parasympathetics from the oculomotor nerve [III]	Constricts ciliary body, relaxes tension on lens, lens become more rounded
Sphincter pupillae	Circularly arranged fibers in the iris	Parasympathetics from the oculomotor nerve [III]	Constricts pupil
Dilator pupillae	Radially arranged fibers in the iris	Sympathetics from the superior cervical ganglion (T1)	Dilates pupil

- The **neural layer,** which can be further subdivided into its various neural components, is only attached to the pigmented layer around the optic nerve and at the ora serrata.

It is the neural layer that separates in the case of a detached retina.

Several obvious features are visible on the posterior surface of the optic part of the retina.

The **optic disc** is where the optic nerve leaves the retina (see Fig. 8.93). It is lighter than the surrounding retina, and branches of the central retinal artery spread from this point outward to supply the retina. As there are no light-sensitive receptor cells in the optic disc, it is referred to as a blind spot in the retina.

Lateral to the optic disc, a small area with a hint of yellowish coloration is the **macula lutea** with its central depression, the **fovea centralis** (see Fig. 8.93). This is the thinnest area of the retina and visual sensitivity here is higher than elsewhere in the retina because it has fewer **rods** (light-sensitive receptor cells that function in dim light and are insensitive to color) and more **cones** (light-sensitive receptor cells that respond to bright light and are sensitive to color).

EAR

The ear is the organ of hearing and balance. It has three parts (Fig. 8.95):

- The first part is the **external ear** consisting of the part attached to the lateral aspect of the head and the canal leading inward.
- The second part is the **middle ear**—a cavity in the petrous part of the temporal bone bounded laterally and separated from the external canal by a membrane and connected internally to the pharynx by a narrow tube.
- The third part is the **internal ear** consisting of a series of cavities within the petrous part of the temporal bone between the middle ear laterally and the internal acoustic meatus medially.

The internal ear converts the mechanical signals received from the middle ear, which start as sound captured by the external ear into electrical signals to transfer information to the brain. The internal ear also contains receptors that detect motion and position.

External ear

The external ear consists of two parts (Fig. 8.95). The part projecting from the side of the head is the **auricle (pinna)**, and the canal leading inward is the **external acoustic meatus.**

Auricle

The auricle is on the side of the head and assists in capturing sound. It consists of cartilage covered with skin and arranged in a pattern of various elevations and depressions (Fig. 8.96).

The large outside rim of the auricle is the **helix.** It ends inferiorly at the fleshy **lobule,** the only part of the auricle not supported by cartilage.

The hollow center of the auricle is the **concha of auricle.** The external acoustic meatus leaves from the depths of this area.

Just anterior to the opening of the external acoustic meatus, in front of the concha, is an elevation (the **tragus**). Opposite the tragus, and above the fleshy lobule, is another elevation (the **antitragus**). A smaller curved rim, parallel and anterior to the helix, is the **antihelix.**

Muscles

Numerous intrinsic and extrinsic muscles are associated with the auricle:

- The intrinsic muscles pass between the cartilaginous parts of the auricle and may change the shape of the auricle.
- The extrinsic muscles, the anterior, superior, and posterior auricular muscles, pass from the scalp or skull to the auricle and may also play a role in positioning of the auricle (see Fig. 8.35).

Both groups of muscles are innervated by the facial nerve [VII].

Innervation

Sensory innervation of the auricle is from many sources (Fig. 8.97):

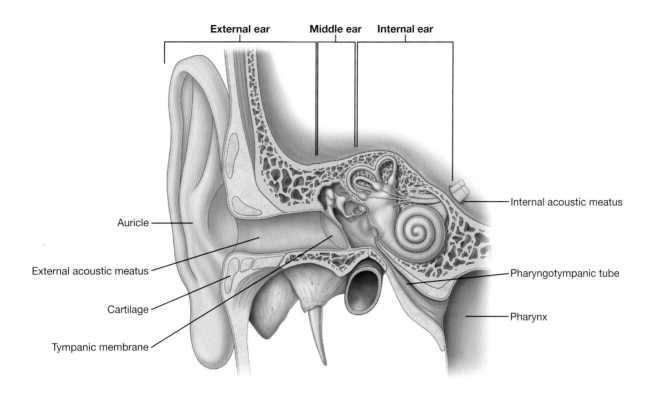

External ear   Middle ear   Internal ear

Auricle

External acoustic meatus

Cartilage

Tympanic membrane

Internal acoustic meatus

Pharyngotympanic tube

Pharynx

Fig. 8.95 Right ear.

Depression

Helix

Concha

Antihelix

External acoustic meatus

Triangular fossa

Cymba conchae

Tragus

Intertragic incisure

Antitragus

Lobule

Fig. 8.96 Auricle.

- The outer more superficial surfaces of the auricle are supplied by the great auricular nerve (anterior and posterior inferior portions) and the lesser occipital nerve (posterior superior portion) from the cervical plexus and the auriculotemporal branch of the mandibular nerve [V$_3$] (anterior superior portion).

- The deeper parts of the auricle are supplied by the vagus nerve [X] (the auricular branch) and the facial nerve [VII]

(which sends a branch to the auricular branch of the vagus nerve [X]).

Vessels

The arterial supply to the auricle is from numerous sources. The external carotid artery supplies the posterior auricular artery, the superficial temporal artery supplies anterior auricular branches, and the occipital artery supplies a branch.

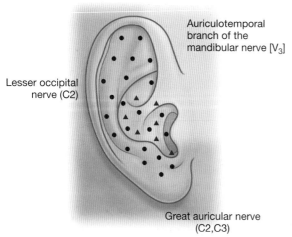

Fig. 8.97 Sensory innervation of the auricle.

Throughout its length the external acoustic meatus is covered with skin, some of which contains hair and modified sweat glands producing **cerumen** (earwax). Its diameter varies, being wider laterally and narrow medially.

The external acoustic meatus does not follow a straight course. From the external opening it passes upward in an anterior direction, then turns slightly posteriorly—still passing upward—and finally turns again in an anterior direction with a slight descent.

Clinical app

Swimmer's ear

Swimmer's ear, often called otitis externa, is a painful condition resulting from an infection in the external acoustic meatus. It frequently occurs in swimmers.

Clinical app

Surfer's ear

Surfer's ear, which is prevalent among individuals who surf or swim in cold water, results from the development of a "bony lump" in the external acoustic meatus. Growth of the lump eventually constricts the meatus and reduces hearing by the affected ear.

Innervation

Sensory innervation of the external acoustic meatus is from several of the cranial nerves. The major sensory input travels through branches of the auriculotemporal nerve, a branch of the mandibular nerve [V_3] (anterior and superior walls), and in the auricular branch of the vagus nerve [X] (posterior and inferior walls). A minor sensory input may also come from a branch of the facial nerve [VII] to the auricular branch of the vagus nerve [X].

Tympanic membrane

The tympanic membrane separates the external acoustic meatus from the middle ear (Figs. 8.99, 8.100). It is at an angle, sloping medially from top to bottom and posteriorly to anteriorly. Its lateral surface therefore faces inferiorly and anteriorly. It consists of a connective tissue core lined with skin on the outside and mucous membrane on the inside.

Around the periphery of the tympanic membrane a **fibrocartilaginous ring** attaches it to the tympanic part of the temporal bone. At its center, a concavity is produced by the attachment on its internal surface of the lower end of the **handle of malleus,** part of the malleus bone in the middle ear. This point of attachment is the **umbo of tympanic membrane.**

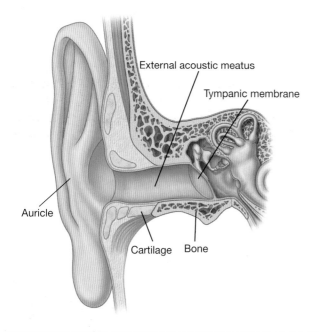

Fig. 8.98 External acoustic meatus.

Venous drainage is through vessels following the arteries.

Lymphatic drainage of the auricle passes anteriorly into parotid nodes, posteriorly into mastoid nodes, and possibly into the upper deep cervical nodes.

External acoustic meatus

The external acoustic meatus extends from the deepest part of the concha to the **tympanic membrane** (eardrum) a distance of approximately 1 inch (2.5 cm) (Fig. 8.98). Its walls consist of cartilage and bone. The lateral one-third is formed from cartilaginous extensions from some of the auricular cartilages, and the medial two-thirds is a bony tunnel in the temporal bone.

Middle ear

Malleus

External acoustic meatus

Tympanic membrane

Pharyngotympanic tube

Fig. 8.99 Middle ear.

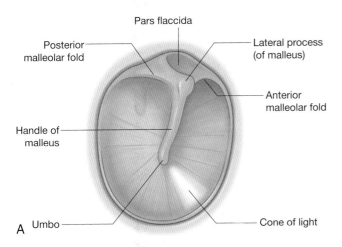

Pars flaccida

Posterior malleolar fold

Lateral process (of malleus)

Anterior malleolar fold

Handle of malleus

A Umbo

Cone of light

B

Fig. 8.100 Tympanic membrane (right ear). **A.** Diagram. **B.** Otoscopic view.

Anteroinferior to the umbo of tympanic membrane a bright reflection of light, referred to as the cone of light, is usually visible when examining the tympanic membrane with an otoscope (Fig. 8.100).

Superior to the umbo in an anterior direction is the attachment of the rest of the handle of malleus (Fig. 8.100). At the most superior extent of this line of attachment, a small bulge in the membrane marks the position of the **lateral process** of the malleus as it projects against the internal surface of the tympanic membrane. Extending away from this elevation, on the internal surface of the membrane, are the **anterior** and **posterior malleolar folds.** Superior to these folds the tympanic membrane is thin and slack (the **pars flaccida**), whereas the rest of the membrane is thick and taut (the **pars tensa**).

Innervation

Innervation of the external and internal surfaces of the tympanic membrane is by several cranial nerves:

- Sensory innervation of the skin on the outer surface of the tympanic membrane is primarily by the auriculotemporal nerve, a branch of the mandibular nerve [V$_3$] with additional participation of the auricular branch of the vagus nerve [X], a small contribution by a branch of the facial nerve [VII] to the auricular branch of the vagus nerve [X], and possibly a contribution from the glossopharyngeal nerve [IX].
- Sensory innervation of the mucous membrane on the inner surface of the tympanic membrane is carried entirely by the glossopharyngeal [IX] nerve.

Clinical app

Examination of the ear
External ear
The external ear is easily examined. The external acoustic meatus and the tympanic membrane require otoscopic examination (see Fig. 8.100B). An otoscope is a device through which light can be shone and the image magnified to inspect the external acoustic meatus and the tympanic membrane.

The examination begins by grasping the posterosuperior aspect of the ear and gently pulling it superiorly, posteriorly and slightly laterally to straighten the external acoustic meatus. The normal tympanic membrane is relatively translucent and has a gray-reddish tinge. The handle of the malleus is visible near the center of the membrane. In the 5 o'clock position, a cone of light is always demonstrated.

Middle and inner ears
In addition to a functional assessment, the middle and inner ear can also be evaluated by computed tomography and MRI.

Tympanic membrane perforation
Although perforation of the tympanic membrane (eardrum) has many causes, trauma and infection are the commonest.

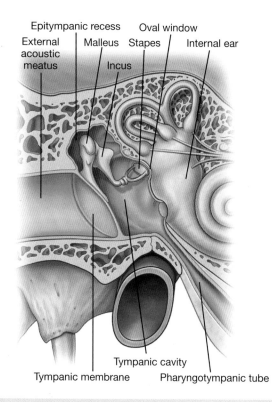

Fig. 8.101 Parts of the middle ear.

Middle ear

The middle ear is an air-filled, mucous membrane–lined space in the temporal bone between the tympanic membrane laterally and the lateral wall of the internal ear medially. It is described as consisting of two parts (Fig. 8.101):

- the **tympanic cavity** immediately adjacent to the tympanic membrane; and
- the **epitympanic recess** superiorly.

The middle ear communicates with the mastoid area posteriorly (via the aditus to the mastoid antrum) and the nasopharynx anteriorly (via the pharyngotympanic tube)(Fig. 8.101). Its basic function is to transmit vibrations of the tympanic membrane across the cavity of the middle ear to the internal ear. It accomplishes this through three interconnected but movable bones that bridge the space between the tympanic membrane and the internal ear. These bones are the malleus (connected to the tympanic membrane), the incus (connected to the malleus by a synovial joint), and the stapes (connected to the incus by a synovial joint and attached to the lateral wall of the internal ear at the oval window).

Boundaries

The middle ear has a roof and a floor and anterior, posterior, medial, and lateral walls (Fig. 8.102).

Roof (tegmental wall)

The tegmental wall of the middle ear consists of a thin layer of bone, which separates the middle ear from the middle cranial fossa. This layer of bone is the **tegmen tympani** on the anterior surface of the petrous part of the temporal bone (Fig. 8.102).

Floor (jugular wall)

The jugular wall of the middle ear consists of a thin layer of bone that separates it from the internal jugular vein (Fig. 8.102). Occasionally the floor is thickened by the presence of mastoid air cells.

Near the medial border of the floor is a small aperture through which the tympanic branch from the glossopharyngeal nerve [IX] enters the middle ear.

Lateral wall (membranous wall)

The membranous wall of the middle ear consists almost entirely of the tympanic membrane (Fig. 8.102), but because the tympanic membrane does not extend superiorly into the epitympanic recess, the upper part of the membranous wall of the middle ear is the bony lateral wall of the epitympanic recess.

Posterior wall (mastoid wall)

The mastoid wall of the middle ear is only partially complete. The lower part of this wall consists of a bony partition between the tympanic cavity and mastoid air cells. Superiorly, the epitympanic recess is continuous with the **aditus to the mastoid antrum** (Figs. 8.102, 8.103).

Associated with the mastoid wall are (Fig. 8.102):

- the pyramidal eminence, a small elevation through which the tendon of the stapedius muscle enters the middle ear; and
- the opening through which the chorda tympani nerve, a branch of the facial nerve [VII], enters the middle ear.

Anterior wall

The anterior wall of the middle ear is only partially complete. The lower part consists of a thin layer of bone that

Prominence of lateral semicircular canal

Prominence of facial canal

Promontory

Tegmen tympani

Tensor tympani muscle

Aditus to mastoid antrum

Pharyngotympanic tube

Oval window

Lesser petrosal nerve

Branch from internal carotid plexus

Pyramidal eminence

Chorda tympani nerve

Sympathetic plexus

Round window

Internal carotid artery

Facial nerve [VII]

Chorda tympani nerve

Tympanic branch of the glossopharyngeal nerve [IX]

Internal jugular vein

Fig. 8.102 Boundaries of the middle ear.

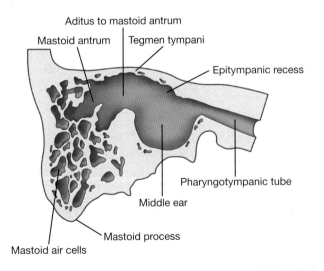

Aditus to mastoid antrum

Mastoid antrum   Tegmen tympani

Epitympanic recess

Pharyngotympanic tube

Middle ear

Mastoid process

Mastoid air cells

Fig. 8.103 Mastoid antrum and surrounding bone.

separates the tympanic cavity from the internal carotid artery. Superiorly, the wall is deficient because of the presence of (Fig. 8.102):

■ a large opening for the entrance of the pharyngotympanic tube into the middle ear; and

■ a smaller opening for the canal containing the tensor tympani muscle.

The foramen for the exit of the chorda tympani nerve from the middle ear is also associated with this wall (Fig. 8.102).

Medial wall (labyrinthine wall)

The labyrinthine wall of the middle ear is also the lateral wall of the internal ear. A prominent structure on this wall is a rounded bulge (the **promontory**) produced by the basal coil of the **cochlea,** which is an internal ear structure involved with hearing (see Fig. 8.102).

Associated with the mucous membrane covering the promontory is a plexus of nerves (the **tympanic plexus**), which consists primarily of contributions from the tympanic branch of the glossopharyngeal nerve [IX] and branches from the internal carotid plexus. It supplies the mucous membrane of the middle ear, the mastoid area, and the pharyngotympanic tube and gives rise to the lesser petrosal nerve that enters the middle cranial fossa (see pp. 491, 507). Other structures associated with the labyrinthine wall are two openings, the oval and round windows, and two prominent elevations (see Fig. 8.102):

Head and Neck

- The **oval window** is posterosuperior to the promontory, is the point of attachment for the **base of stapes (footplate),** and ends the chain of bones that transfer vibrations initiated by the tympanic membrane to the cochlea of the internal ear.
- The **round window** is posteroinferior to the promontory.
- Posterior and superior to the oval window on the medial wall is the **prominence of facial canal,** which is a ridge of bone produced by the facial nerve [VII] in its canal as it passes through the temporal bone.
- Just above and posterior to the prominence of facial canal is a broader ridge of bone (**prominence of lateral semicircular canal**) produced by the lateral semicircular canal, which is a structure involved in detecting motion.

Mastoid area

Posterior to the epitympanic recess of the middle ear is the aditus to mastoid antrum, which is the opening to the mastoid antrum (see Fig. 8.103).

The **mastoid antrum** is a cavity continuous with collections of air-filled spaces (the **mastoid cells**) throughout the mastoid part of the temporal bone, including the mastoid process. The mastoid antrum is separated from the middle cranial fossa above by only the thin tegmen tympani.

The mucous membrane lining the mastoid air cells is continuous with the mucous membrane throughout the middle ear. Therefore infections in the middle ear can easily spread into the mastoid area.

Clinical app

Mastoiditis
Infection within the mastoid antrum and mastoid cells is usually secondary to infection in the middle ear. The mastoid cells provide an excellent culture chamber for infection. Infection of the bone (osteomyelitis) may also develop, spreading into the middle cranial fossa.

Pharyngotympanic tube

The pharyngotympanic tube connects the middle ear with the nasopharynx (Fig. 8.104) and equalizes pressure on both sides of the tympanic membrane. Its opening in the middle ear is on the anterior wall, and from here it extends forward, medially, and downward to enter the nasopharynx just posterior to the inferior meatus of the nasal cavity. It consists of:

- a **bony part** (the one-third nearest the middle ear), and
- a **cartilaginous part** (the remaining two-thirds).

The opening of the bony part is clearly visible on the inferior surface of the skull at the junction of the squamous and

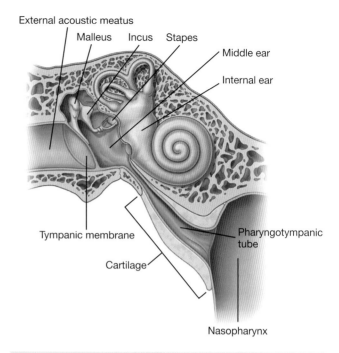

Fig. 8.104 Pharyngotympanic tube.

petrous parts of the temporal bone immediately posterior to the foramen ovale and foramen spinosum.

Vessels

The arterial supply to the pharyngotympanic tube is from several sources. Branches arise from the **ascending pharyngeal artery** (a branch of the external carotid artery) and from two branches of the maxillary artery (the middle meningeal artery and the artery of the pterygoid canal).

Venous drainage of the pharyngotympanic tube is to the pterygoid plexus of veins in the infratemporal fossa.

Innervation

Innervation of the mucous membrane lining the pharyngotympanic tube is primarily from the tympanic plexus because it is continuous with the mucous membrane lining the tympanic cavity, the internal surface of the tympanic membrane, and the mastoid antrum and mastoid cells. This plexus receives its major contribution from the tympanic nerve, a branch of the glossopharyngeal nerve [IX].

Auditory ossicles

The bones of the middle ear consist of the malleus, incus, and stapes. They form an osseous chain across the middle ear from the tympanic membrane to the oval window of the internal ear (Fig. 8.105).

Muscles associated with the auditory ossicles modulate movement during the transmission of vibrations.

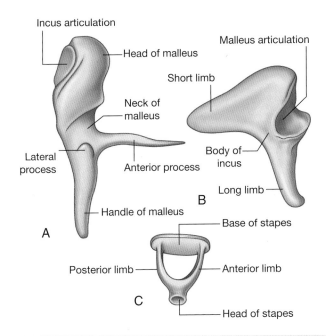

Fig. 8.105 Auditory ossicles. **A.** Malleus. **B.** Incus. **C.** Stapes.

Malleus

The malleus is the largest of the auditory ossicles and is attached to the tympanic membrane. Identifiable parts include the **head of malleus, neck of malleus, anterior and lateral processes,** and **handle of malleus** (Fig. 8.105). The head of malleus is the rounded upper part of the malleus in the epitympanic recess. Its posterior surface articulates with the incus.

Inferior to the head of malleus is the constricted neck of malleus, and below this are the anterior and lateral processes:

■ The anterior process is attached to the anterior wall of the middle ear by a ligament.
■ The lateral process is attached to the anterior and posterior malleolar folds of the tympanic membrane.

The downward extension of the malleus, below the anterior and lateral processes, is the handle of malleus, which is attached to the tympanic membrane.

Incus

The second bone in the series of auditory ossicles is the incus. It consists of the **body of incus** and **long** and **short limbs** (Fig. 8.105):

■ The enlarged body of incus articulates with the head of malleus and is in the epitympanic recess.
■ The long limb extends downward from the body, paralleling the handle of the malleus, and ends by bending medially to articulate with the stapes.
■ The short limb extends posteriorly and is attached by a ligament to the upper posterior wall of the middle ear.

Stapes

The stapes is the most medial bone in the osseous chain and is attached to the oval window. It consists of the **head of stapes, anterior** and **posterior limbs,** and the **base of stapes** (Fig. 8.105):

■ The head of stapes is directed laterally and articulates with the long process of the incus.
■ The two limbs separate from each other and attach to the oval base.
■ The base of stapes fits into the oval window on the labyrinthine wall of the middle ear.

Muscles associated with the ossicles

Two muscles are associated with the bony ossicles of the middle ear—the tensor tympani and stapedius (Table 8.10, Fig. 8.106).

Vessels

Numerous arteries supply the structures in the middle ear:

■ The two largest branches are the **tympanic branch** of the maxillary artery and the **mastoid branch** of the occipital or posterior auricular arteries.
■ Smaller branches come from the middle meningeal artery, the ascending pharyngeal artery, the artery of the pterygoid canal, and tympanic branches from the internal carotid artery.

Table 8.10	Muscles of the middle ear			
Muscle	**Origin**	**Insertion**	**Innervation**	**Function**
Tensor tympani	Cartilaginous part of pharyngotympanic tube, greater wing of sphenoid, its own bony canal	Upper part of handle of malleus	Branch from mandibular nerve [V₃]	Contraction pulls handle of malleus medially, tensing tympanic membrane
Stapedius	Attached to inside of pyramidal eminence	Neck of stapes	Branch of facial nerve [VII]	Contraction pulls stapes posteriorly, preventing excessive oscillation

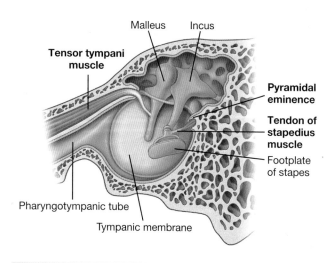

Fig. 8.106 Muscles associated with the auditory ossicles.

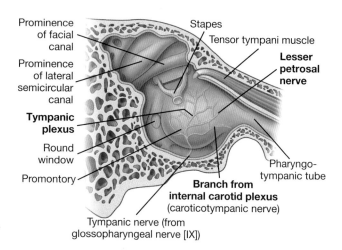

Fig. 8.107 Innervation of the middle ear.

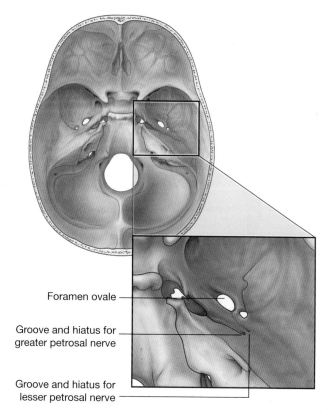

Fig. 8.108 Grooves and hiatuses for the greater and lesser petrosal nerves.

Venous drainage of the middle ear returns to the pterygoid plexus of veins and the superior petrosal sinus.

Innervation

The tympanic plexus innervates the mucous membrane lining the walls and contents of the middle ear, which includes the mastoid area and the pharyngotympanic tube. It is formed by the **tympanic nerve,** a branch of the glossopharyngeal nerve [IX], and from branches of the internal carotid plexus. The tympanic plexus occurs in the mucous membrane covering the promontory, which is the rounded bulge on the labyrinthine wall of the middle ear (Fig. 8.107).

As the glossopharyngeal nerve [IX] exits the skull through the jugular foramen, it gives off the tympanic nerve. This branch re-enters the skull through a small foramen and passes through the bone to the middle ear.

Once in the middle ear, the tympanic nerve forms the **tympanic plexus,** along with branches from the plexus of nerves surrounding the internal carotid artery

(caroticotympanic nerves). Branches from the tympanic plexus supply the mucous membranes of the middle ear, including the pharyngotympanic tube and the mastoid area.

The tympanic plexus also gives off a major branch (the lesser petrosal nerve), which supplies preganglionic parasympathetic fibers to the otic ganglion (Fig. 8.107).

The **lesser petrosal nerve** leaves the area of the promontory, exits the middle ear, travels through the petrous part of the temporal bone, and exits onto the anterior surface of the petrous part of the temporal bone through a hiatus just below the hiatus for the greater petrosal nerve (Fig. 8.108). It continues diagonally across the anterior surface of the temporal bone before exiting the middle cranial fossa through the foramen ovale. Once outside the skull, it enters the otic ganglion.

Internal ear

The internal ear consists of a series of bony cavities (the **bony labyrinth**) and membranous ducts and sacs (the **membranous labyrinth**) within these cavities. All these structures are in the petrous part of the temporal bone between the middle ear laterally and the internal acoustic meatus medially (Figs. 8.109, 8.110).

The bony labyrinth consists of the **vestibule,** three **semicircular canals,** and the **cochlea** (Fig. 8.110). These bony cavities are lined with periosteum and contain a clear fluid (the **perilymph**).

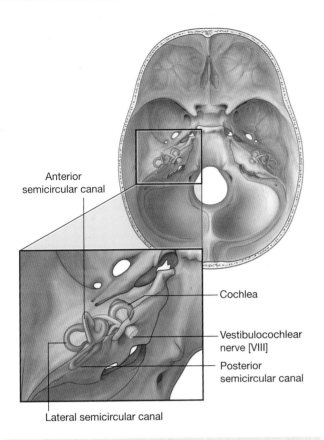

Fig. 8.109 Location of the internal ear in temporal bone.

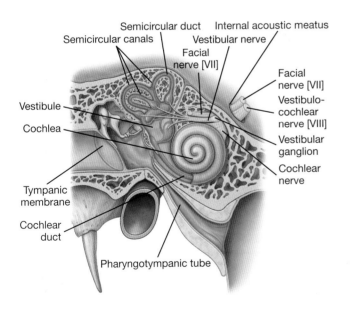

Fig. 8.110 Internal ear.

Suspended within the perilymph but not filling all spaces of the bony labyrinth is the membranous labyrinth, which consists of the **semicircular ducts,** the **cochlear duct,** and two sacs (the **utricle** and the **saccule**). These membranous spaces are filled with **endolymph.**

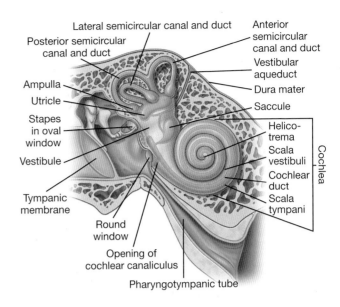

Fig. 8.111 Bony labyrinth.

The structures in the internal ear convey information to the brain about balance and hearing:

■ The cochlear duct is the organ of hearing.
■ The semicircular ducts, utricle, and saccule are the organs of balance.

The nerve responsible for these functions is the vestibulocochlear nerve [VIII], which divides into vestibular (balance) and cochlear (hearing) parts after entering the internal acoustic meatus (Fig. 8.110).

Bony labyrinth

The vestibule, which contains the oval window in its lateral wall, is the central part of the bony labyrinth (Fig. 8.111). It communicates anteriorly with the cochlea and posterosuperiorly with the semicircular canals.

A narrow canal (the **vestibular aqueduct**) leaves the vestibule and passes through the temporal bone to open on the posterior surface of the petrous part of the temporal bone.

Semicircular canals

Projecting in a posterosuperior direction from the vestibule are the **anterior, posterior,** and **lateral semicircular canals** (Fig. 8.111). Each of these canals forms two-thirds of a circle connected at both ends to the vestibule and with one end dilated to form the **ampulla.** The canals are oriented so that each canal is at right angles to the other two.

Cochlea

Projecting in an anterior direction from the vestibule is the cochlea, which is a bony structure that twists on itself two

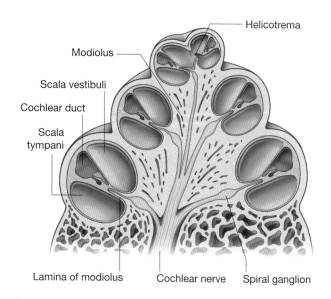

Helicotrema

Modiolus

Scala vestibuli

Cochlear duct

Scala tympani

Lamina of modiolus Cochlear nerve Spiral ganglion

Fig. 8.112 Cochlea.

and one-half to two and three-quarters times around a central column of bone (the **modiolus**). This arrangement produces a cone-shaped structure with a **base of cochlea** that faces posteromedially and an apex that faces anterolaterally (Fig. 8.112). This positions the wide base of the modiolus near the internal acoustic meatus where it is entered by branches of the cochlear part of the vestibulocochlear nerve [VIII].

Extending laterally throughout the length of the modiolus is a thin lamina of bone (the **lamina of modiolus**, or **spiral lamina**) (Fig. 8.112). Circling around the modiolus and held in a central position by its attachment to the lamina of

modiolus is the cochlear duct, which is a component of the membranous labyrinth.

Attached peripherally to the outer wall of the cochlea, the cochlear duct creates two canals (the **scala vestibuli** and the **scala tympani**) (Figs. 8.112, 8.113), which extend throughout the cochlea and are continuous with each other at the apex through a narrow slit (the **helicotrema**):

- The scala vestibuli is continuous with the vestibule.
- The scala tympani is separated from the middle ear by the secondary tympanic membrane covering the round window (Fig. 8.113).

Finally, near the round window is a small channel (the **cochlear canaliculus**), which passes through the temporal bone and opens on its inferior surface into the posterior cranial fossa. This provides a connection between the perilymph-containing cochlea and the subarachnoid space (Fig. 8.113).

Membranous labyrinth

The membranous labyrinth is a continuous system of ducts and sacs within the bony labyrinth. It is filled with endolymph and separated from the periosteum that covers the walls of the bony labyrinth by perilymph (Fig. 8.113).

Consisting of two sacs (the utricle and the saccule) and four ducts (the three semicircular ducts and the cochlear duct), the membranous labyrinth has unique functions related to balance and hearing (Fig. 8.113):

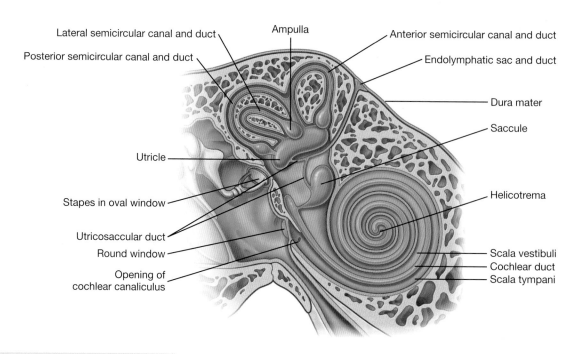

Lateral semicircular canal and duct

Posterior semicircular canal and duct

Ampulla

Anterior semicircular canal and duct

Endolymphatic sac and duct

Dura mater

Saccule

Utricle

Stapes in oval window

Helicotrema

Utricosaccular duct

Round window

Opening of cochlear canaliculus

Scala vestibuli
Cochlear duct
Scala tympani

Fig. 8.113 Membranous labyrinth.

- The utricle, saccule, and three semicircular ducts are part of the vestibular apparatus (i.e., organs of balance).
- The cochlear duct is the organ of hearing.

The general organization of the parts of the membranous labyrinth (Fig. 8.113) places:

- the cochlear duct within the cochlea of the bony labyrinth anteriorly;
- the three semicircular ducts within the three semicircular canals of the bony labyrinth posteriorly; and
- the saccule and utricle within the vestibule of the bony labyrinth in the middle.

Organs of balance

Five of the six components of the membranous labyrinth are concerned with balance. These are the two sacs (the utricle and the saccule) and three ducts (the anterior, posterior, and lateral semicircular ducts).

Utricle, saccule, and endolymphatic duct

The utricle is the larger of the two sacs (Fig. 8.113). It is oval, elongated, and irregular in shape and is in the posterosuperior part of the vestibule of the bony labyrinth.

The three semicircular ducts empty into the utricle (Fig. 8.113). Each semicircular duct is similar in shape, including a dilated end forming the ampulla, to its complementary bony semicircular canal, only much smaller.

The saccule is a smaller, rounded sac lying in the antero-inferior part of the vestibule of the bony labyrinth (Fig. 8.113). The cochlear duct empties into it.

The utriculosaccular duct establishes continuity between all components of the membranous labyrinth and connects the utricle and saccule (Fig. 8.113). Branching from this small duct is the **endolymphatic duct,** which enters the vestibular aqueduct (a channel through the temporal bone) to emerge onto the posterior surface of the petrous part of the temporal bone in the posterior cranial fossa. Here the endolymphatic duct expands into the **endolymphatic sac,** which is an extradural pouch that functions in resorption of endolymph.

Sensory receptors

Functionally, sensory receptors for balance are organized into unique structures that are located in each of the components of the vestibular apparatus. In the utricle and saccule, the sense organ is the **macula of utricle** and the **macula of saccule,** respectively, and in the ampulla of each of the three semicircular ducts it is the **crista.**

The utricle responds to linear acceleration in the horizontal plane and sideways head tilts, while the saccule responds to linear acceleration in the vertical plane, such as forward–backward and upward–downward movements. In contrast,

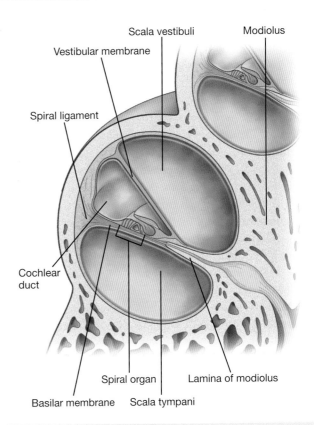

Fig. 8.114 Membranous labyrinth, cross-section.

the receptors in the three semicircular ducts respond to rotational movement in any direction.

Organ of hearing
Cochlear duct

The cochlear duct has a central position in the cochlea of the bony labyrinth dividing it into two canals (the scala vestibuli and the scala tympani). It is maintained in this position by being attached centrally to the lamina of modiolus, which is a thin lamina of bone extending from the modiolus (the central bony core of the cochlea), and peripherally to the outer wall of the cochlea (Figs. 8.113, 8.114).

Thus the triangular-shaped cochlear duct has (Fig. 8.114):

- an outer wall against the bony cochlea consisting of thickened, epithelial-lined periosteum (the **spiral ligament**);
- a roof (the **vestibular membrane**), which separates the endolymph in the cochlear duct from the perilymph in the scala vestibuli and consists of a membrane with a connective tissue core lined on either side with epithelium; and
- a floor, which separates the endolymph in the cochlear duct from the perilymph in the scala tympani and consists of the free edge of the lamina of modiolus and a membrane (the **basilar membrane**) extending from this free edge of the lamina of modiolus to an extension of the spiral ligament covering the outer wall of the cochlea.

The **spiral organ** is the organ of hearing, rests on the basilar membrane, and projects into the enclosed, endolymph-filled cochlear duct (Fig. 8.114).

Vessels

The arterial supply to the internal ear is divided between vessels supplying the bony labyrinth and the membranous labyrinth.

The bony labyrinth is supplied by the same arteries that supply the surrounding temporal bone. These include an anterior tympanic branch from the maxillary artery, a stylomastoid branch from the posterior auricular artery, and a petrosal branch from the middle meningeal artery.

The membranous labyrinth is supplied by the **labyrinthine artery,** which either arises from the anterior inferior cerebellar artery or is a direct branch of the basilar artery. Whatever its origin, it enters the internal acoustic meatus with the facial [VII] and vestibulocochlear [VIII] nerves and eventually divides into:

- a **cochlear branch**, which passes through the modiolus and supplies the cochlear duct; and
- one or two **vestibular branches,** which supply the vestibular apparatus.

Venous drainage of the membranous labyrinth is through vestibular veins and cochlear veins, which follow the arteries. These come together to form a **labyrinthine vein,** which eventually empties into either the inferior petrosal sinus or the sigmoid sinus.

Innervation

The vestibulocochlear nerve [VIII] carries SA fibers for hearing (the cochlear component) and balance (the vestibular component). It enters the lateral surface of the brainstem, between the pons and medulla, after exiting the temporal bone through the internal acoustic meatus and crossing the posterior cranial fossa.

Inside the temporal bone, at the distal end of the internal acoustic meatus, the vestibulocochlear nerve divides to form:

- the **cochlear nerve,** and
- the **vestibular nerve**.

The vestibular nerve enlarges to form the **vestibular ganglion** before dividing into **superior and inferior parts,** which distribute to the three semicircular ducts and the utricle and saccule (see Fig. 8.110).

The cochlear nerve enters the base of the cochlea and passes upward through the modiolus. The ganglion cells of the cochlear nerve are in the **spiral ganglion** at the base of the lamina of modiolus as it winds around the modiolus (see Fig. 8.112). Branches of the cochlear nerve pass through the

lamina of modiolus to innervate the receptors in the spiral organ.

Facial nerve [VII] in the temporal bone

The facial nerve [VII] is closely associated with the vestibulocochlear nerve [VIII] as it enters the internal acoustic meatus of the temporal bone. Traveling through the temporal bone, its path and several of its branches are directly related to the internal and middle ears.

The facial nerve [VII] enters the internal acoustic meatus in the petrous part of the temporal bone (Fig. 8.115A). The vestibulocochlear nerve and the labyrinthine artery accompany it.

At the distal end of the internal acoustic meatus, the facial nerve [VII] enters the facial canal and continues laterally between the internal and middle ears. At this point the facial nerve [VII] enlarges and bends posteriorly and laterally. The enlargement is the sensory **geniculate ganglion.** As the facial canal continues, the facial nerve [VII] turns sharply downward and running in an almost vertical direction, it exits the skull through the stylomastoid foramen (Fig. 8.115A).

Branches

Greater petrosal nerve. At the geniculate ganglion, the facial nerve [VII] gives off the greater petrosal nerve (Fig. 8.115A). This is the first branch of the facial nerve [VII]. The greater petrosal nerve leaves the geniculate ganglion, travels anteromedially through the temporal bone, and emerges through the hiatus for the greater petrosal nerve on the anterior surface of the petrous part of the temporal bone (see Fig. 8.108). The greater petrosal nerve carries preganglionic parasympathetic fibers to the pterygopalatine ganglion.

Continuing beyond the bend, the position of the facial nerve [VII] is indicated on the medial wall of the middle ear by a bulge (see Fig. 8.107).

Nerve to stapedius and chorda tympani. Near the beginning of its vertical descent, the facial nerve [VII] gives off a small branch, the nerve to stapedius (Fig. 8.115A), which innervates the stapedius muscle, and just before it exits the skull, the facial nerve [VII] gives off the chorda tympani nerve (Fig. 8.115).

The chorda tympani does not immediately exit the temporal bone, but ascends to enter the middle ear through its posterior wall, passing near the upper aspect of the tympanic membrane between the malleus and incus (Fig. 8.115B). It then exits the middle ear through a canal leading to the **petrotympanic fissure** and exits the skull through this fissure to join the lingual nerve in the infratemporal fossa.

Transmission of sound

A sound wave enters the external acoustic meatus and strikes the tympanic membrane moving it medially (Fig. 8.116). As

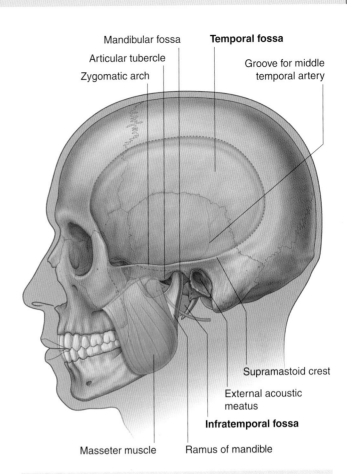

Fig. 8.117 Temporal and infratemporal fossae.

Fig. 8.115 A. Facial nerve in the temporal bone. **B.** Chorda tympani in the temporal bone.

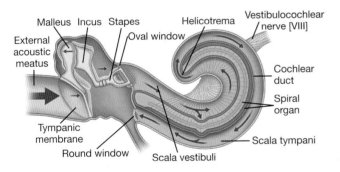

Fig. 8.116 Transmission of sound.

the handle of malleus is attached to this membrane, the handle of malleus also moves medially. This moves the head of the malleus laterally. Because the heads of the malleus and incus articulate with each other, the head of the incus is also moved laterally. This pushes the long process of the incus medially. The long process articulates with the stapes, so its movement causes the stapes to move medially. In turn, because the base of stapes is attached to the oval window, the oval window is also moved medially.

This action completes the transfer of a large-amplitude, low-force, airborne wave that vibrates the tympanic membrane into a small-amplitude, high-force vibration of the

oval window, which generates a wave in the fluid-filled scala vestibuli of the cochlea.

The wave established in the perilymph of the scala vestibuli moves through the cochlea and causes an outward bulging of the secondary tympanic membrane covering the round window at the lower end of the scala tympani (Fig. 8.116). This wave causes the basilar membrane to vibrate, which in turn leads to stimulation of receptor cells in the spiral organ.

The receptor cells send impulses back to the brain through the cochlear part of the vestibulocochlear nerve [VIII] where they are interpreted as sound.

If the sounds are too loud, causing excessive movement of the tympanic membrane, contraction of the tensor tympani muscle (attached to the malleus) and/or the stapedius muscle (attached to the stapes) dampens the vibrations of the ossicles and decreases the force of the vibrations reaching the oval window.

TEMPORAL AND INFRATEMPORAL FOSSAE

The temporal and infratemporal fossae are interconnected spaces on the lateral side of the head (Fig. 8.117). Their boundaries are formed by bone and soft tissues.

The temporal fossa is superior to the infratemporal fossa, above the zygomatic arch, and communicates with the infratemporal fossa below through the gap between the zygomatic arch and the more medial surface of the skull.

The infratemporal fossa is a wedge-shaped space deep to the masseter muscle and the underlying ramus of mandible. Structures that travel between the cranial cavity, neck, pterygopalatine fossa, floor of the oral cavity, floor of the orbit, temporal fossa, and superficial regions of the head pass through it.

Of the four muscles of mastication (masseter, temporalis, medial pterygoid, and lateral pterygoid) that move the lower jaw at the temporomandibular joint, one (masseter) is lateral to the infratemporal fossa, two (medial and lateral pterygoid) are in the infratemporal fossa, and one (temporalis) fills the temporal fossa.

Bony framework

Bones that contribute significantly to the boundaries of the temporal and infratemporal fossae include the temporal, zygomatic, and sphenoid bones and the maxilla and mandible (Figs. 8.118, 8.119).

Parts of the frontal and parietal bones are also involved.

Temporal bone

The squamous part of the temporal bone forms part of the bony framework of the temporal and infratemporal fossae (Fig. 8.118).

The tympanic part of the temporal bone forms the posteromedial corner of the roof of the infratemporal fossa and articulates with the head of mandible to form the temporomandibular joint.

The lateral surface of the squamous part of the temporal bone is marked by two surface features on the medial wall of the temporal fossa (Fig. 8.118):

- a transversely oriented **supramastoid crest,** which extends posteriorly from the base of the zygomatic process and marks the posteroinferior border of the temporal fossa; and
- a vertically oriented **groove for middle temporal artery,** a branch of the superficial temporal artery.

Two features that participate in forming the temporomandibular joint on the inferior aspect of the root of the zygomatic process of the temporal bone are the articular tubercle and the mandibular fossa (Fig. 8.118). Both are elongate from medial to lateral. Posterior to the mandibular fossa is the external acoustic meatus. The tympanic part of the temporal bone is a flat concave plate of bone that curves inferiorly from the back of the mandibular fossa and forms part of the wall of the external acoustic meatus.

When viewed from inferiorly, there is a distinct **tympanosquamous fissure** between the tympanic and squamous parts of the temporal bone. Medially, a small slip of bone from the petrous part of the temporal bone insinuates itself into the fissure and forms a **petrotympanic fissure** between it and the tympanic part (Fig. 8.118).

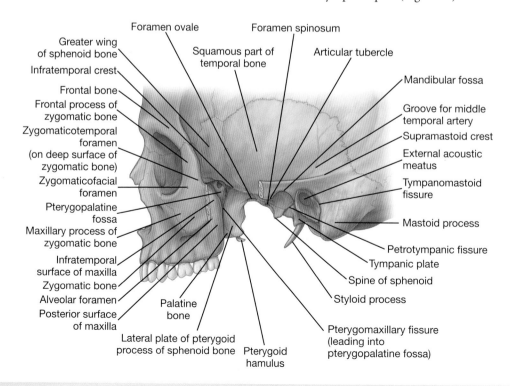

Fig. 8.118 Bony features related to the temporal and infratemporal fossae.

The chorda tympani nerve exits the skull and enters the infratemporal fossa through the medial end of the petrotympanic fissure.

Sphenoid bone

The parts of the sphenoid bone that form part of the bony framework of the infratemporal fossa are the lateral plate of the pterygoid process and the greater wing (Fig. 8.118). The greater wing also forms part of the medial wall of the temporal fossa.

The greater wings extend one on each side from the body of sphenoid. They project laterally from the body and curve superiorly. The inferior and lateral surfaces form the roof of the infratemporal fossa and the medial wall of the temporal fossa, respectively.

The sharply angled boundary between the lateral and inferior surfaces of the greater wing is the **infratemporal crest** (Fig. 8.118).

Two apertures (the foramen ovale and the foramen spinosum) pass through the base of the greater wing and allow the mandibular nerve [V₃] and the middle meningeal artery, respectively, to pass between the middle cranial fossa and infratemporal fossa. In addition, one or more small sphenoidal emissary foramina penetrate the base of the greater wing anteromedial to the foramen ovale and allow emissary veins to pass between the pterygoid plexus of veins in the infratemporal fossa and the cavernous sinus in the middle cranial fossa.

Projecting vertically downward from the greater wing immediately medial to the foramen spinosum is the irregularly shaped **spine of sphenoid,** which is the attachment site for the cranial end of the sphenomandibular ligament (Fig. 8.118).

The lateral plate of the pterygoid process is a vertically oriented sheet of bone that projects posterolaterally from the pterygoid process (Fig. 8.118). Its lateral and medial surfaces provide attachment for the lateral and medial pterygoid muscles, respectively.

Maxilla

The posterior surface of the maxilla contributes to the anterior wall of the infratemporal fossa (Fig. 8.118). This surface is marked by a foramen for the posterior superior alveolar nerve and vessels. The superior margin forms the inferior border of the inferior orbital fissure.

Zygomatic bone

The zygomatic bone is a quadrangular-shaped bone that forms the palpable bony prominence of the cheek (Fig. 8.118):

- A **maxillary process** extends anteromedially to articulate with the zygomatic process of the maxilla.

- A **frontal process** extends superiorly to articulate with the zygomatic process of the frontal bone.
- A **temporal process** extends posteriorly to articulate with the zygomatic process of the temporal bone to complete the zygomatic arch.

A small zygomaticofacial foramen on the lateral surface of the zygomatic bone transmits the zygomaticofacial nerve and vessels onto the cheek (Fig. 8.118).

A thin plate of bone extends posteromedially from the frontal process and contributes to the lateral wall of the orbit on one side and the anterior wall of the temporal fossa on the other. A zygomaticotemporal foramen on the temporal fossa surface of the plate where it attaches to the frontal process is for the zygomaticotemporal nerve.

Ramus of mandible

The **ramus of mandible** is quadrangular in shape and has medial and lateral surfaces and condylar and coronoid processes (Fig. 8.119).

The lateral surface of the ramus of mandible is generally smooth except for the presence of a few obliquely oriented

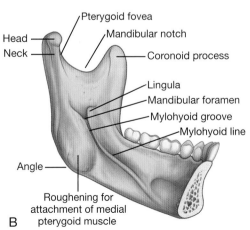

Fig. 8.119 Mandible. **A.** Lateral view of left side. **B.** Medial view of left side.

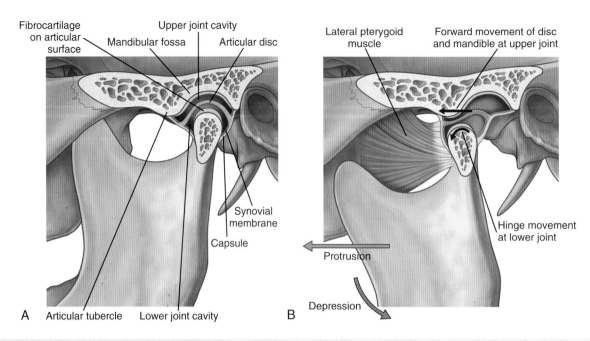

Fig. 8.120 Temporomandibular joint. **A.** Mouth closed. **B.** Mouth open.

ridges. Most of the lateral surface provides attachment for the masseter muscle.

The posterior and inferior borders of the ramus intersect to form the **angle of mandible,** while the superior border is notched to form the **mandibular notch** (Fig. 8.119). The anterior border is sharp and is continuous below with the **oblique line** on the body of mandible.

The **coronoid process** extends superiorly from the junction of the anterior and superior borders of the ramus. It is a flat, triangular process that provides attachment for the temporalis muscle (Fig. 8.119).

The **condylar process** extends superiorly from the posterior and superior borders of the ramus (Fig. 8.119). It consists of:

- the **head of mandible,** which is expanded medially and participates in forming the temporomandibular joint; and
- the **neck of mandible,** which bears a shallow depression (the **pterygoid fovea**) on its anterior surface for attachment of the lateral pterygoid muscle.

The medial surface of the ramus of mandible is the lateral wall of the infratemporal fossa (Fig. 8.119B). Its most distinctive feature is the **mandibular foramen,** which is the superior opening of the mandibular canal. The inferior alveolar nerve and vessels pass through this foramen.

Immediately anterosuperior to the mandibular foramen is a triangular elevation (the **lingula**) for attachment of the mandibular end of the sphenomandibular ligament (see Fig. 8.119).

An elongate groove (the **mylohyoid groove**) extends anteroinferiorly from the mandibular foramen (see Fig. 8.119). The **nerve to mylohyoid** is in this groove.

Posteroinferior to the mylohyoid groove and mandibular foramen, the medial surface of the ramus of mandible is roughened for attachment of the medial pterygoid muscle.

Temporomandibular joints

The temporomandibular joints, one on each side, allow opening and closing of the mouth and complex chewing or side-to-side movements of the lower jaw.

Each joint is synovial and is formed between the head of mandible and the articular fossa and articular tubercle of the temporal bone (see Fig. 8.120A).

Unlike most other synovial joints where the articular surfaces of the bones are covered by a layer of hyaline cartilage, those of the temporomandibular joint are covered by fibrocartilage. In addition, the joint is completely divided by a fibrous **articular disc** into two parts:

- The lower part of the joint allows mainly the hinge-like depression and elevation of the mandible.
- The upper part of the joint allows the head of the mandible to translocate forward (protrusion) onto the articular tubercle and backward (retraction) into the mandibular fossa.

Opening the mouth involves both depression and protrusion (see Fig. 8.120B).

The forward or protrusive movement allows greater depression of the mandible by preventing backward movement of the angle of mandible into structures in the neck.

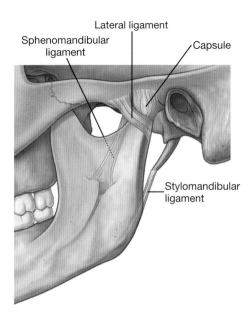

Fig. 8.121 Ligaments associated with the temporomandibular joint.

Joint capsule

The **synovial membrane** of the joint capsule lines all nonarticular surfaces of the upper and lower compartments of the joint and is attached to the margins of the articular disc (see Fig. 8.120B).

The **fibrous membrane** of the joint capsule encloses the temporomandibular joint complex and is attached (see Fig. 8.120B):

- above, along the anterior margin of the articular tubercle;
- laterally and medially along the margins of the articular fossa;
- posteriorly to the region of the tympanosquamous suture; and
- below around the upper part of the neck of mandible.

The articular disc attaches around its periphery to the inner aspect of the fibrous membrane (see Fig. 8.120B).

Extracapsular ligaments

Three extracapsular ligaments are associated with the temporomandibular joint—the lateral, sphenomandibular, and the stylomandibular ligaments (Fig. 8.121):

- The **lateral ligament** is closest to the joint, just lateral to the capsule, and runs diagonally backward from the margin of the articular tubercle to the neck of the mandible.
- The **sphenomandibular ligament** is medial to the temporomandibular joint and runs from the spine of the sphenoid bone at the base of the skull to the lingula on the medial side of the ramus of mandible.

- The **stylomandibular ligament** passes from the styloid process of the temporal bone to the posterior margin and angle of mandible.

Movements of the mandible

A chewing or grinding motion occurs when the movements at the temporomandibular joint on one side are coordinated with a reciprocal set of movements at the joint on the other side. Muscles that generate these movements are the four muscles of mastication (masseter, temporalis, medial pterygoid, and lateral pterygoid) (Table 8.11), and a number of muscles associated with the floor of the oral cavity (geniohyoid, mylohyoid) and anterior triangle of the neck (anterior belly of digastric). Movements of the mandible include depression, elevation, protrusion, and retraction (Fig. 8.122).

Clinical app

Temporomandibular joint disorders

The term *temporomandibular joint disorder* refers to a number of problems in and around the temporomandibular joint. Like other synovial joints, the temporomandibular joint is subject to arthritis, bony fusion, trauma, dislocation and fracture as well as developmental anomalies. Typical symptoms associated with temporomandibular joint problems include eating difficulties, clicking and popping, pain, earache, and headache. The joint and most muscles that move the joint are innervated by the trigeminal nerve. Inflammation of the joint or surrounding tissues can result in reflex muscle spasms that limit movement. "Grinding of the teeth" and malalignment of the occlusal surfaces of the teeth also can result in temporomandibular joint problems.

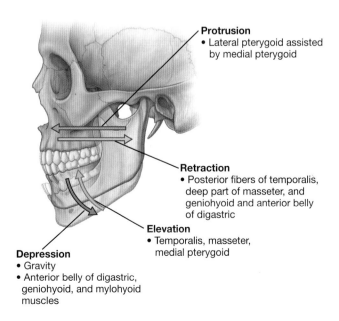

Fig. 8.122 Movements of the temporomandibular joint.

Table 8.11 Muscles of mastication

Muscle	Origin	Insertion	Innervation	Function
Masseter	Superficial part: maxillary process of the zygomatic bone and the anterior two-thirds of the zygomatic process of the maxilla Deep part: medial aspect of the zygomatic arch and posterior part of its inferior margin	Superficial part: angle of the mandible and related posterior part of the lateral surface of the ramus of the mandible Deep part: central and upper part of ramus of mandible as high as the coronoid process	Masseteric nerve from the anterior trunk of the mandibular nerve [V₃]	Elevation of mandible
Temporalis	Bone of temporal fossa and temporal fascia	Coronoid process of mandible and anterior margin of ramus of mandible almost to last molar tooth	Deep temporal nerves from the anterior trunk of the mandibular nerve [V₃]	Elevation and retraction of mandible; also participates in side-to-side movements
Medial pterygoid	Deep head—medial surface of lateral plate of pterygoid process and pyramidal process of palatine bone; superficial head—tuberosity of maxilla and pyramidal process of palatine bone	Medial surface of mandible near angle	Nerve to medial pterygoid from the mandibular nerve [V₃]	Elevation and side-to-side movements of the mandible
Lateral pterygoid	Upper head—roof of infratemporal fossa; lower head—lateral surface of lateral plate of the pterygoid process	Capsule of temporomandibular joint in the region of attachment to the articular disc and to the pterygoid fovea on the neck of mandible	Nerve to lateral pterygoid from the anterior trunk of mandibular nerve [V₃] or from buccal branch	Protrusion and side-to-side movements of the mandible

Masseter muscle

The **masseter** muscle is a powerful muscle of mastication that elevates the mandible (Table 8.11, Fig. 8.123). It overlies the lateral surface of the ramus of mandible.

Temporal fossa

The temporal fossa is a narrow, fan-shaped space that covers the lateral surface of the skull (Fig. 8.124A):

■ Its upper margin is defined by a pair of temporal lines that arch across the skull from the zygomatic process of the frontal bone to the supramastoid crest of the temporal bone.

■ It is limited laterally by the **temporal fascia,** which is a tough, fan-shaped aponeurosis overlying the temporalis muscle and attached by its outer margin to the superior temporal line and by its inferior margin to the zygomatic arch.

■ Anteriorly, it is limited by the posterior surface of the frontal process of the zygomatic bone and the posterior surface of the zygomatic process of the frontal bone, which separate the temporal fossa behind from the orbit in front.

■ Its inferior margin is marked by the zygomatic arch laterally and by the infratemporal crest of the greater wing of the sphenoid medially (Fig. 8.124B)—between these two features, the floor of the temporal fossa is open medially to the infratemporal fossa and laterally to the region containing the masseter muscle.

Contents

The major structure in the temporal fossa is the temporalis muscle (Fig. 8.125).

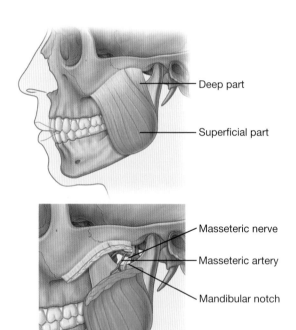

Fig. 8.123 Masseter muscle.

Deep part

Superficial part

Masseteric nerve

Masseteric artery

Mandibular notch

Also passing through the fossa is the zygomaticotemporal branch of the maxillary nerve [V₂], which enters the region through the zygomaticotemporal foramen on the temporal fossa surface of the zygomatic bone (Fig. 8.126).

Temporalis muscle

The **temporalis** muscle is a large, flat muscle that fills much of the temporal fossa (Table 8.11, Fig. 8.125). The more

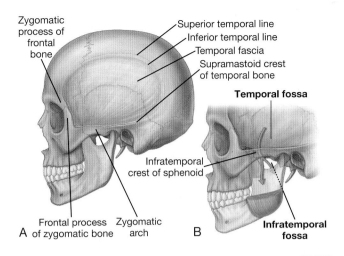

Fig. 8.124 Temporal fossa. **A.** Lateral view. **B.** Lateral view showing the infratemporal fossa.

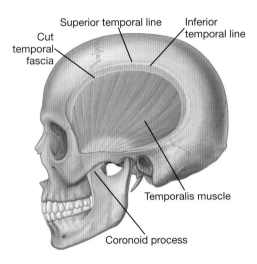

Fig. 8.125 Temporalis muscle. Lateral view.

anterior fibers are oriented vertically, and the more posterior fibers are oriented horizontally.

Deep temporal nerves

The deep temporal nerves, usually two in number, originate from the anterior trunk of the mandibular nerve [V_3] in the infratemporal fossa (Fig. 8.126). They pass superiorly and around the infratemporal crest of the greater wing of the sphenoid to enter the temporal fossa deep to the temporalis muscle, and supply the temporalis muscle.

Zygomaticotemporal nerve

The zygomaticotemporal nerve is a branch of the zygomatic nerve (Fig. 8.126). The zygomatic nerve is a branch of the maxillary nerve [V_2], which originates in the pterygopalatine fossa and passes into the orbit.

The zygomaticotemporal nerve enters the temporal fossa through one or more small foramina on the temporal fossa surface of the zygomatic bone (Fig. 8.126).

Branches of the zygomaticotemporal nerve pass superiorly between the bone and the temporalis muscle to penetrate the temporal fascia and supply the skin of the temple (Fig. 8.126).

Deep temporal arteries

Normally two in number, these vessels originate from the maxillary artery in the infratemporal fossa and travel with the deep temporal nerves around the infratemporal crest of the greater wing of the sphenoid to supply the temporalis muscle (Fig. 8.126). They anastomose with branches of the middle temporal artery.

Middle temporal artery

The middle temporal artery originates from the superficial temporal artery just superior to the root of the zygomatic arch between this structure and the external ear (Fig. 8.126). It penetrates the temporalis fascia, passes under the margin of the temporalis muscle, and travels superiorly on the deep surface of the temporalis muscle.

The middle temporal artery supplies the temporalis and anastomoses with branches of the deep temporal arteries.

Infratemporal fossa

The wedge-shaped infratemporal fossa is inferior to the temporal fossa and between the ramus of mandible laterally and the wall of the pharynx medially. It has a roof, a lateral wall, and a medial wall and is open to the neck posteroinferiorly (Fig. 8.127):

- The **roof** is formed by the inferior surfaces of the greater wing of the sphenoid and the temporal bone; contains the foramen spinosum, foramen ovale, and the petrotympanic fissure; is lateral to the infratemporal crest of the greater wing of the sphenoid; and is open superiorly to the temporal fossa.
- The **lateral wall** is the medial surface of the ramus of mandible, which contains the opening to the mandibular canal.
- The **medial wall** is formed anteriorly by the lateral plate of the pterygoid process and more posteriorly by the pharynx and by two muscles of the soft palate (tensor and levator veli palatini muscles), and contains the pterygomaxillary fissure anteriorly, which allows structures to pass between the infratemporal and pterygopalatine fossae.
- The **anterior wall** is formed by part of the posterior surface of the maxilla and contains the alveolar foramen, and the upper part opens as the inferior orbital fissure into the orbit.

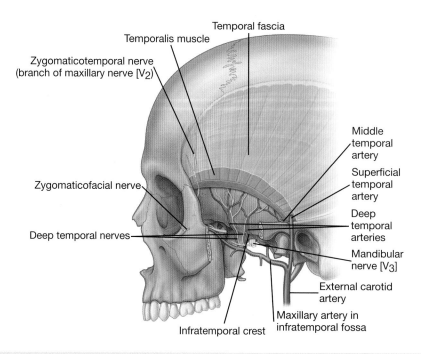

Fig. 8.126 Nerves and arteries of the temporal fossa.

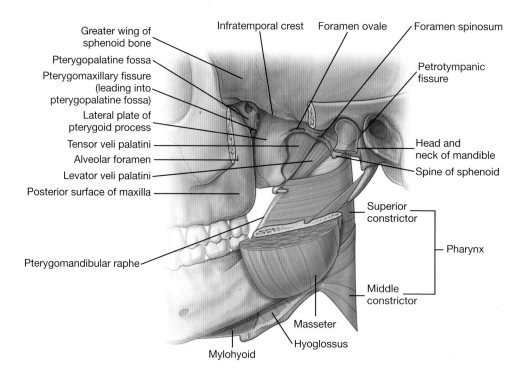

Fig. 8.127 Borders of the infratemporal fossa.

Contents

Major contents of the infratemporal fossa include the sphenomandibular ligament, medial and lateral pterygoid muscles, the maxillary artery, the mandibular nerve [V$_3$], branches of the facial nerve [VII] and the glossopharyngeal nerve [IX], and the pterygoid plexus of veins.

Sphenomandibular ligament

The sphenomandibular ligament is an extracapsular ligament of the temporomandibular joint (Fig. 8.128). It is attached superiorly to the spine of the sphenoid bone and expands inferiorly to attach to the lingula of the mandible and the posterior margin of the mandibular foramen (Fig. 8.128).

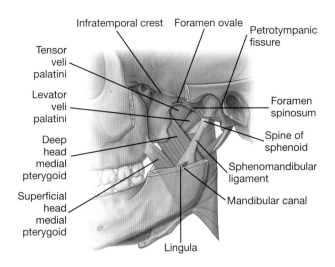

Fig. 8.128 Medial pterygoid muscle.

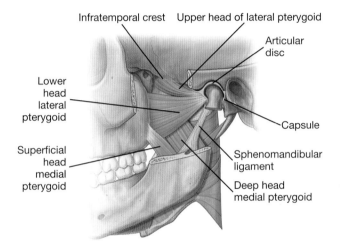

Fig. 8.129 Lateral pterygoid muscle.

Medial and lateral pterygoid muscles

The **medial pterygoid** muscle is quadrangular in shape and has deep and superficial heads (Table 8.11, Fig. 8.128).

The medial pterygoid mainly elevates the mandible. Because it passes obliquely backward to insert into the mandible, it also assists the lateral pterygoid muscle in protruding the lower jaw.

The **lateral pterygoid** is a thick triangular muscle and like the medial pterygoid muscle has two heads (Table 8.11, Fig. 8.129). The fibers from both heads of the lateral pterygoid muscle converge to insert into the pterygoid fovea of the neck of mandible and into the capsule of the temporomandibular joint in the region where the capsule is attached internally to the articular disc.

Unlike the medial pterygoid muscle whose fibers tend to be oriented vertically, those of the lateral pterygoid are oriented almost horizontally. As a result, when the lateral

pterygoid contracts, it pulls the articular disc and head of mandible forward onto the articular tubercle and is therefore the major protruder of the lower jaw.

When the lateral and medial pterygoids contract on only one side, the chin moves to the opposite side. When opposite movements at the two temporomandibular joints are coordinated, a chewing movement results.

Mandibular nerve [V₃]

The mandibular nerve $[V_3]$ is the largest of the three divisions of the trigeminal nerve [V].

Unlike the ophthalmic $[V_1]$ and maxillary $[V_2]$ nerves, which are purely sensory, the mandibular nerve $[V_3]$ is both motor and sensory.

In addition to carrying general sensation from the teeth and gingivae of the mandible, the anterior two-thirds of the tongue, mucosa on the floor of the oral cavity, the lower lip, skin over the temple and lower face, and part of the cranial dura mater, the mandibular nerve $[V_3]$ also carries motor innervation to most of the muscles that move the mandible, one of the muscles (tensor tympani) in the middle ear, and one of the muscles of the soft palate (tensor veli palatini).

All branches of the mandibular nerve $[V_3]$ originate in the infratemporal fossa.

Like the ophthalmic $[V_1]$ and maxillary $[V_2]$ nerves, the sensory part of the mandibular nerve $[V_3]$ originates from the trigeminal ganglion in the middle cranial fossa (Fig. 8.130; also see Fig. 8.36, pg. 477):

- The sensory part of the mandibular nerve $[V_3]$ drops vertically through the foramen ovale and enters the infratemporal fossa between the tensor veli palatini muscle and the upper head of the lateral pterygoid muscle.
- The small motor root of the trigeminal nerve [V] passes medial to the trigeminal ganglion in the cranial cavity, then passes through the foramen ovale and immediately joins the sensory part of the mandibular nerve $[V_3]$.

Branches

Soon after the sensory and motor roots join, the mandibular nerve $[V_3]$ gives rise to a small meningeal branch and to the nerve to the medial pterygoid and then divides into anterior and posterior trunks (Fig. 8.130):

- Branches from the anterior trunk are the buccal, masseteric, and deep temporal nerves and the nerve to lateral pterygoid, all of which, except the buccal nerve (which is predominantly sensory), are motor nerves.
- Branches from the posterior trunk are the auriculotemporal, lingual, and inferior alveolar nerves, all of which, except a small nerve (nerve to mylohyoid) that branches from the inferior alveolar nerve, are sensory nerves.

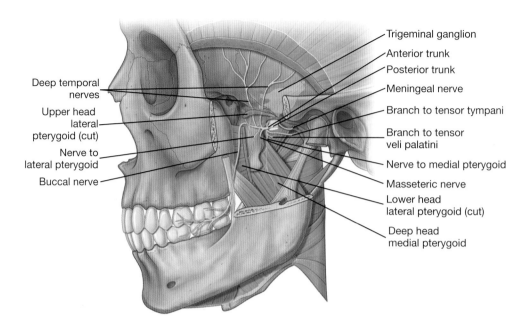

Deep temporal nerves

Upper head lateral pterygoid (cut)

Nerve to lateral pterygoid

Buccal nerve

Trigeminal ganglion

Anterior trunk

Posterior trunk

Meningeal nerve

Branch to tensor tympani

Branch to tensor veli palatini

Nerve to medial pterygoid

Masseteric nerve

Lower head lateral pterygoid (cut)

Deep head medial pterygoid

Fig. 8.130 Mandibular nerve [V₃]—meningeal nerve, nerve to medial pterygoid, and branches of anterior trunk.

Meningeal branch

The meningeal branch originates from the medial side of the mandibular nerve [V₃] and ascends to leave the infratemporal fossa with the middle meningeal artery, and re-enters the cranial cavity through the foramen spinosum (Fig. 8.130). It is sensory for the dura mater, mainly of the middle cranial fossa, and also supplies the mastoid cells that communicate with the middle ear.

Nerve to medial pterygoid

The nerve to medial pterygoid also originates medially from the mandibular nerve [V₃] (Fig. 8.130). It descends to enter and supply the deep surface of the medial pterygoid muscle. Near its origin from the mandibular nerve [V₃], it has two small branches:

- One of these supplies the tensor veli palatini.
- The other ascends to supply the tensor tympani muscle, which occupies a small bony canal above and parallel to the pharyngotympanic tube in the temporal bone.

Buccal nerve

The buccal nerve is a branch of the anterior trunk of the mandibular nerve [V₃] (Fig. 8.130). It is predominantly a sensory nerve, but may also carry the motor innervation to the lateral pterygoid muscle and to part of the temporalis muscle.

The buccal nerve passes laterally between the upper and lower heads of lateral pterygoid and then descends around the anterior margin of the insertion of temporalis muscle to the anterior margin of the ramus of mandible, often slipping through the tendon of temporalis. It continues into the cheek lateral to the buccinator muscle to supply general sensory nerves to the adjacent skin and oral mucosa and the buccal gingivae of the lower molars.

Masseteric nerve

The masseteric nerve is a branch of the anterior trunk of the mandibular nerve [V₃]. It passes laterally over the lateral pterygoid muscle and through the mandibular notch to penetrate and supply the masseter muscle (Fig. 8.130; also see Fig. 8.123).

Deep temporal nerves

The deep temporal nerves, usually two in number, originate from the anterior trunk of the mandibular nerve [V₃] (Fig. 8.130). They pass laterally above the lateral pterygoid muscle and curve around the infratemporal crest to ascend in the temporal fossa and supply the temporalis muscle from its deep surface (Fig. 8.130; also see Fig. 8.126).

Nerve to lateral pterygoid

The nerve to lateral pterygoid may originate directly as a branch from the anterior trunk of the mandibular nerve [V₃] or from its buccal branch (Fig. 8.130). From its origin, it passes directly into the deep surface of the lateral pterygoid muscle.

Auriculotemporal nerve

The auriculotemporal nerve is the first branch of the posterior trunk of the mandibular nerve [V₃] and originates as two roots that pass posteriorly and enclose between them the middle meningeal artery ascending from the maxillary artery to the foramen spinosum (Fig. 8.131A).

After the two roots join, the auriculotemporal nerve passes first between the tensor veli palatini muscle and the upper head of lateral pterygoid muscle and then between the sphenomandibular ligament and the neck of mandible. It curves laterally around the neck of mandible and then ascends deep to the parotid gland between the temporomandibular joint and ear.

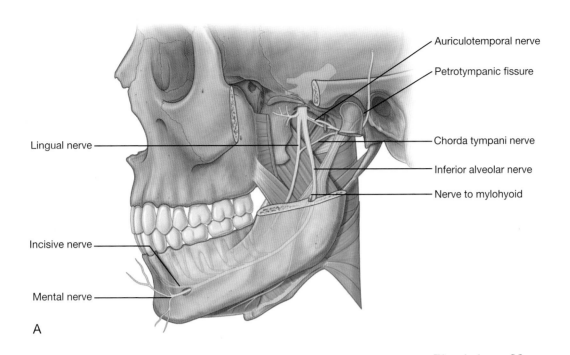

Auriculotemporal nerve

Petrotympanic fissure

Lingual nerve

Chorda tympani nerve

Inferior alveolar nerve

Nerve to mylohyoid

Incisive nerve

Mental nerve

A

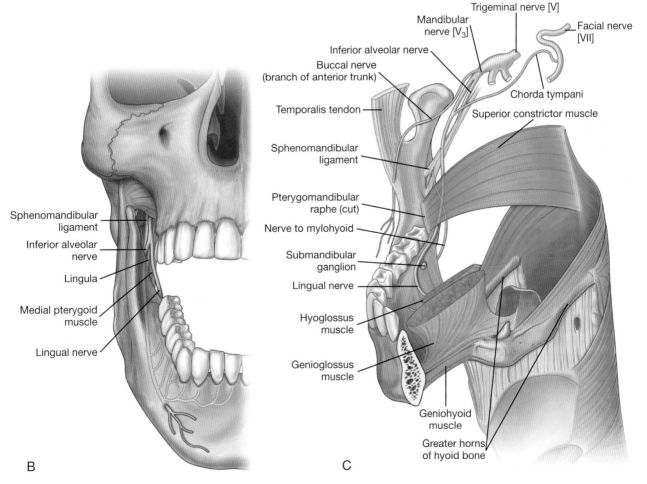

Sphenomandibular ligament

Inferior alveolar nerve

Lingula

Medial pterygoid muscle

Lingual nerve

B

Trigeminal nerve [V]

Mandibular nerve [V₃]

Inferior alveolar nerve

Buccal nerve (branch of anterior trunk)

Temporalis tendon

Sphenomandibular ligament

Pterygomandibular raphe (cut)

Nerve to mylohyoid

Submandibular ganglion

Lingual nerve

Hyoglossus muscle

Genioglossus muscle

Geniohyoid muscle

Greater horns of hyoid bone

Facial nerve [VII]

Chorda tympani

Superior constrictor muscle

C

Fig. 8.131 Mandibular nerve [V₃]—posterior trunk. **A.** Lateral view. **B.** Anterior view. **C.** Anteromedial view.

The terminal branches of the auriculotemporal nerve carry general sensation from skin over a large area of the temple. In addition, the auriculotemporal nerve contributes to sensory innervation of the external ear, the external auditory meatus, tympanic membrane, and temporomandibular joint. It also delivers postganglionic parasympathetic nerves from the glossopharyngeal nerve [IX] to the parotid gland.

Lingual nerve

The **lingual nerve** is a major sensory branch of the posterior trunk of the mandibular nerve [V$_3$] (Fig. 8.131). It carries general sensation from the anterior two-thirds of the tongue, oral mucosa on the floor of the oral cavity, and lingual gingivae associated with the lower teeth.

The lingual nerve is joined high in the infratemporal fossa by the chorda tympani branch of the facial nerve [VII] (Fig. 8.131A,C), which carries:

- taste from the anterior two-thirds of the tongue, and
- parasympathetic fibers to all salivary glands below the level of the oral fissure.

The lingual nerve first descends between the tensor veli palatini muscle and the lateral pterygoid muscle where it is joined by the chorda tympani nerve and then descends across the lateral surface of the medial pterygoid muscle to enter the oral cavity (Fig. 8.131A).

The lingual nerve enters the oral cavity between the posterior attachment of the mylohyoid muscle to the mylohyoid line and the attachment of the superior constrictor of the pharynx to the pterygomandibular raphe. As the lingual nerve enters the floor of the oral cavity, it is in a shallow groove on the medial surface of the mandible immediately inferior to the last molar tooth (Fig. 8.131B,C). In this position, it is palpable through the oral mucosa and in danger when operating on the molar teeth and gingivae.

The lingual nerve passes into the tongue on the lateral surface of the hyoglossus muscle where it is attached to the **submandibular ganglion** (Fig. 8.131C), which contains the cell bodies for the postganglionic parasympathetic fibers of the chorda tympani nerve carried from the infratemporal fossa into the floor of the oral cavity on the lingual nerve.

Inferior alveolar nerve

The **inferior alveolar nerve**, like the lingual nerve, is a major sensory branch of the posterior trunk of the mandibular nerve [V$_3$] (Fig. 8.131). In addition to innervating all lower teeth and much of the associated gingivae, it also supplies the mucosa and skin of the lower lip and skin of the chin. It has one motor branch, which innervates the mylohyoid muscle and the anterior belly of the digastric muscle.

The inferior alveolar nerve originates deep to the lateral pterygoid muscle from the posterior trunk of the mandibular

nerve [V$_3$] in association with the lingual nerve. It descends on the lateral surface of the medial pterygoid muscle, passes between the sphenomandibular ligament and the ramus of mandible, and then enters the mandibular canal through the mandibular foramen. Just before entering the mandibular foramen, it gives origin to the **nerve to mylohyoid** (Fig. 8.131A,C), which lies in the mylohyoid groove inferior to the foramen and continues anteriorly below the floor of the oral cavity to innervate the mylohyoid muscle and the anterior belly of the digastric muscle.

The inferior alveolar nerve passes anteriorly within the mandibular canal of the lower jaw (Fig. 8.131A,B). The mandibular canal and its contents are inferior to the roots of the molar teeth, and the roots can sometimes curve around the canal, making extraction of these teeth difficult.

The inferior alveolar nerve supplies branches to the three molar teeth and the second premolar tooth and associated labial gingivae and then divides into its two terminal branches (Fig. 8.131A):

- the **incisive nerve,** which continues in the mandibular canal to supply the first premolar, incisor, and canine teeth and related gingivae; and
- the **mental nerve,** which exits the mandible through the mental foramen and supplies the lower lip and chin. The mental nerve is palpable and sometimes visible through the oral mucosa adjacent to the roots of the premolar teeth.

Clinical app

Lingual nerve injury

A lingual nerve injury proximal to where the chorda tympani joins it in the infratemporal fossa will produce loss of general sensation from the anterior two-thirds of the tongue, oral mucosa, gingivae, the lower lip, and the chin.

If a lingual nerve lesion is distal to the site where it is joined by the chorda tympani, secretion from the salivary glands below the oral fissure and taste from the anterior two-thirds of the tongue will also be lost.

Clinical app

Anesthesia of the inferior alveolar nerve

Anesthesia of the inferior alveolar nerve is widely practiced by most dentists. To anesthetize this nerve, the needle is placed lateral to the palatoglossal arch in the oral cavity and is advanced along the medial surface of the inferior third of the ramus of the mandible so that the anesthetic can be deposited in the region of the mandibular foramen.

Chorda tympani and the lesser petrosal nerve

Branches of two cranial nerves join branches of the mandibular nerve [V_3] in the infratemporal fossa (Fig. 8.132). These are the chorda tympani branch of the facial nerve [VII] and the lesser petrosal nerve, a branch of the tympanic plexus in the middle ear, which had its origin from a branch of the glossopharyngeal nerve [IX] (see Fig. 8.102, pg. 527).

Chorda tympani

The chorda tympani (Fig. 8.132) carries taste from the anterior two-thirds of the tongue and parasympathetic innervation to all salivary glands below the level of the oral fissure.

The chorda tympani originates from the facial nerve [VII] within the temporal bone and in association with the mastoid wall of the middle ear, passes anteriorly through a small canal, and enters the lateral aspect of the middle ear. As it continues anterosuperiorly across the middle ear, it is separated from the tympanic membrane by the handle of malleus. It leaves the middle ear through the medial end of the petrotympanic fissure, enters the infratemporal fossa, descends medial to the spine of the sphenoid and then to the lateral pterygoid muscle, and joins the lingual nerve.

Preganglionic parasympathetic fibers carried in the chorda tympani synapse with postganglionic parasympathetic fibers in the submandibular ganglion, which "hangs off" the lingual nerve in the floor of the oral cavity (Fig. 8.132).

Postganglionic parasympathetic fibers leave the submandibular ganglion and either (Fig. 8.132):

- re-enter the lingual nerve to travel with its terminal branches to reach target tissues; or
- pass directly from the submandibular ganglion into glands.

The taste (SA) fibers do not pass through the ganglion and are distributed with terminal branches of the lingual nerve.

Lesser petrosal nerve

The lesser petrosal nerve carries mainly parasympathetic fibers destined for the parotid gland (Fig. 8.132B). The preganglionic parasympathetic fibers are located in the glossopharyngeal nerve [IX] as it exits the jugular foramen at the base of the skull (Fig. 8.132B). Branching from the glossopharyngeal nerve [IX] either within or immediately outside the jugular foramen is the tympanic nerve.

The tympanic nerve re-enters the temporal bone through a small foramen on the ridge of bone separating the jugular foramen from the carotid canal and ascends through a small bony canal (inferior tympanic canaliculus) to the promontory located on the labyrinthine (medial) wall of the middle ear. Here it participates in the formation of the tympanic plexus. The lesser petrosal nerve is a branch of this plexus.

The lesser petrosal nerve contains mainly preganglionic parasympathetic fibers. It leaves the middle ear and enters the middle cranial fossa through a small opening on the anterior surface of the petrous part of the temporal bone just lateral and inferior to the opening for the greater petrosal nerve, a branch of the facial nerve [VII]. The lesser petrosal nerve then passes medially and descends through the foramen ovale with the mandibular nerve [V_3].

In the infratemporal fossa, the preganglionic parasympathetic fibers synapse with cell bodies of postganglionic parasympathetic fibers in the otic ganglion located on the medial side of the mandibular nerve [V_3], around the origin of the nerve to the medial pterygoid (Fig. 8.132). Postganglionic parasympathetic fibers leave the otic ganglion and join the auriculotemporal nerve, which carries them to the parotid gland.

Maxillary artery

The maxillary artery is the largest branch of the external carotid artery in the neck and is a major source of blood supply for the nasal cavity, the lateral wall and roof of the oral cavity, all teeth, and the dura mater in the cranial cavity. It passes through and supplies the infratemporal fossa and then enters the pterygopalatine fossa, where it gives origin to terminal branches (Fig. 8.133).

The maxillary artery originates within the substance of the parotid gland and then passes forward, between the neck of mandible and sphenomandibular ligament, into the infratemporal fossa. It ascends obliquely through the infratemporal fossa to enter the pterygopalatine fossa by passing through the pterygomaxillary fissure. This part of the vessel may pass either lateral or medial to the lower head of lateral pterygoid. If it passes medial to the lower head, the maxillary artery then loops laterally between the upper and lower heads of lateral pterygoid to access the **pterygomaxillary fissure**.

Branches

Branches of the maxillary artery are as follows (Fig. 8.133):

- The first part of the maxillary artery (the part between the neck of mandible and the sphenomandibular ligament) gives origin to two major branches (the middle meningeal and inferior alveolar arteries) and a number of smaller branches (deep auricular, anterior tympanic, and accessory meningeal).
- The second part of the maxillary artery (the part related to the lateral pterygoid muscle) gives origin to deep temporal, masseteric, buccal, and pterygoid branches, which course with branches of the mandibular nerve [V_3].
- The third part of the maxillary artery is in the pterygopalatine fossa (see p. 514).

A

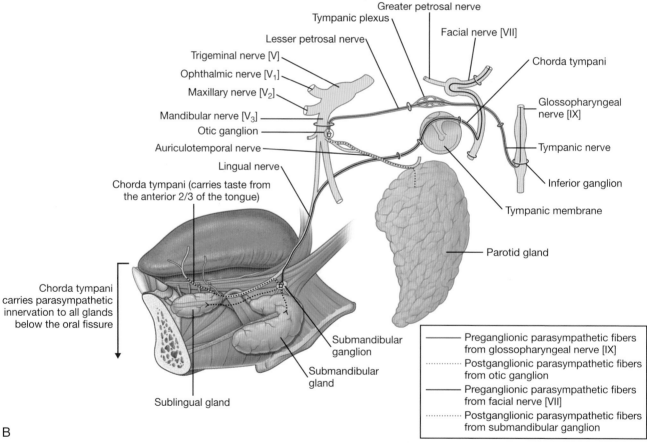

B

Fig. 8.132 Chorda tympani and lesser petrosal nerves. **A.** Course after emerging from the skull. **B.** Course of parasympathetic fibers.

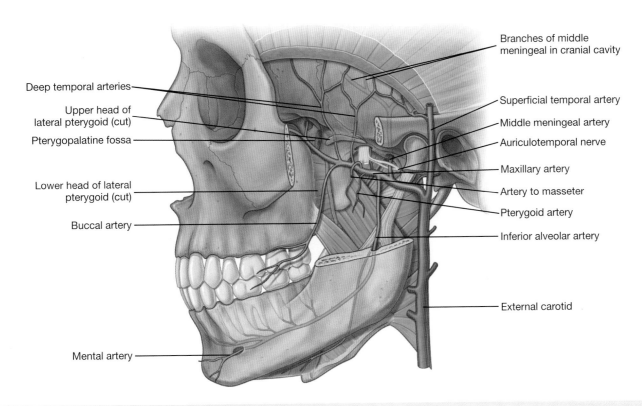

Fig. 8.133 Maxillary artery.

Labels (clockwise from top left):
Deep temporal arteries
Upper head of lateral pterygoid (cut)
Pterygopalatine fossa
Lower head of lateral pterygoid (cut)
Buccal artery
Mental artery
Branches of middle meningeal in cranial cavity
Superficial temporal artery
Middle meningeal artery
Auriculotemporal nerve
Maxillary artery
Artery to masseter
Pterygoid artery
Inferior alveolar artery
External carotid

Middle meningeal artery

The middle meningeal artery ascends vertically from the maxillary artery and passes through the foramen spinosum to enter the cranial cavity (Fig. 8.133). In the infratemporal fossa, it passes superiorly between the sphenomandibular ligament on the medial side and the lateral pterygoid muscle on the lateral side. Just inferior to the foramen spinosum, it passes between the two roots of the auriculotemporal nerve at their origin from the mandibular nerve [V_3].

The middle meningeal artery is the largest of the meningeal vessels and supplies much of the dura mater, bone, and related bone marrow of the cranial cavity walls.

Inferior alveolar artery

The inferior alveolar artery descends from the maxillary artery to enter the mandibular foramen and canal with the inferior alveolar nerve (Fig. 8.133). It is distributed with the inferior alveolar nerve and supplies all lower teeth, and contributes to the supply of the buccal gingivae, chin, and lower lip.

Before entering the mandible, the inferior alveolar artery gives origin to a small mylohyoid branch, which accompanies the nerve to mylohyoid.

Deep auricular, anterior tympanic, and accessory meningeal arteries

The deep auricular, anterior tympanic, and accessory meningeal arteries are small branches from the first part of the maxillary artery and contribute to the blood supply of the external acoustic meatus, deep surface of the tympanic membrane, and cranial dura mater, respectively.

The accessory meningeal branch also contributes small branches to surrounding muscles in the infratemporal fossa before ascending through the foramen ovale into the cranial cavity to supply dura mater.

Branches from the second part

Deep temporal arteries, usually two in number, originate from the second part of the maxillary artery and travel with the deep temporal nerves to supply the temporalis muscle in the temporal fossa (Fig. 8.133).

Numerous pterygoid arteries also originate from the second part of the maxillary artery and supply the pterygoid muscles.

The masseteric artery, also from the second part of the maxillary artery, accompanies the masseteric nerve laterally through the mandibular notch to supply the masseter muscle.

The buccal artery is distributed with the buccal nerve and supplies skin, muscle, and oral mucosa of the cheek.

Pterygoid plexus

The **pterygoid plexus** is a network of veins between the medial and lateral pterygoid muscles and between the lateral pterygoid and temporalis muscles (Fig. 8.134).

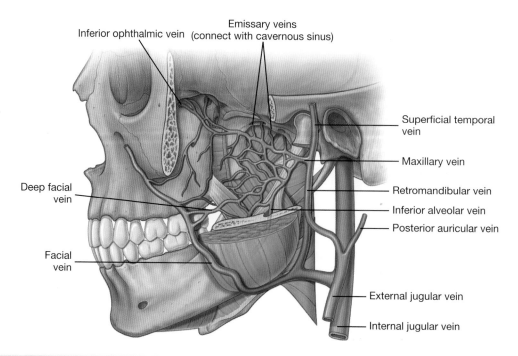

Inferior ophthalmic vein

Emissary veins (connect with cavernous sinus)

Superficial temporal vein

Maxillary vein

Deep facial vein

Retromandibular vein

Inferior alveolar vein

Posterior auricular vein

Facial vein

External jugular vein

Internal jugular vein

Fig. 8.134 Pterygoid plexus of veins.

Veins that drain regions supplied by arteries branching from the maxillary artery in the infratemporal fossa and pterygopalatine fossa connect with the pterygoid plexus. These tributary veins include those that drain the nasal cavity, roof and lateral wall of the oral cavity, all teeth, muscles of the infratemporal fossa, paranasal sinuses, and nasopharynx. In addition, the inferior ophthalmic vein from the orbit can drain through the inferior orbital fissure into the pterygoid plexus.

The pterygoid plexus connects (Fig. 8.134):

- posteriorly, via a short maxillary vein, with the retromandibular vein in the neck; and
- anteriorly, via a deep facial vein, with the facial vein on the face.

Clinical app

Middle meningeal artery and extradural hematoma
Within the cranial cavity, the middle meningeal artery and its branches travel in the periosteal (outer) layer of dura mater, which is tightly adherent to the bony walls. As major branches of the middle meningeal artery pass superiorly up the walls of the cranial cavity in the region of the "pterion," they can be damaged by lateral blows to the head. When the vessels are torn, the leaking blood results in an extradural hematoma.

Clinical app

Spread of infection from the pterygoid plexus into the cranial cavity
Small emissary veins often connect the pterygoid plexus in the infratemporal fossa to the cavernous sinus in the cranial cavity. These emissary veins pass through the foramen ovale, the cartilage that fills the foramen lacerum, and a small sphenoidal foramen on the medial side of the lateral plate of the pterygoid process at the base of the skull. They are a route by which infections can spread into the cranial cavity from structures, such as the teeth, that are drained by the pterygoid plexus. Also, because there are no valves in veins of the head and neck, anesthetic inadvertently injected under pressure into veins of the pterygoid plexus can backflow into tissues or into the cranial cavity.

PTERYGOPALATINE FOSSA

The pterygopalatine fossa is an inverted teardrop-shaped space between bones on the lateral side of the skull immediately posterior to the maxilla (Fig. 8.135).

Although small in size, the pterygopalatine fossa communicates via fissures and foramina in its walls with the:

- middle cranial fossa,
- infratemporal fossa,
- floor of the orbit,

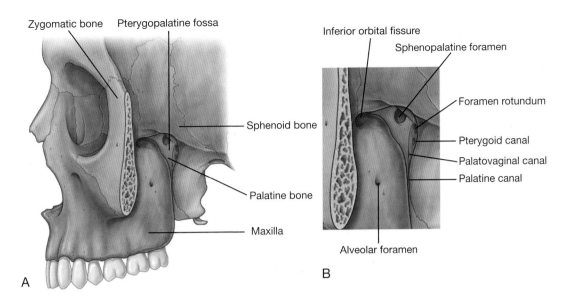

Fig. 8.135 Pterygopalatine fossa. A. Anterolateral view. B. Lateral view.

- lateral wall of the nasal cavity,
- oropharynx, and
- roof of the oral cavity.

Because of its strategic location, the pterygopalatine fossa is a major site of distribution for the maxillary nerve [V₂] and for the terminal part of the maxillary artery. It also contains the pterygopalatine ganglion where preganglionic parasympathetic fibers originating in the facial nerve [VII] synapse with postganglionic parasympathetic fibers and these fibers, along with sympathetic fibers originating from the T1 spinal cord level join branches of the maxillary nerve [V₂].

All the upper teeth receive their innervation and blood supply from the maxillary nerve [V₂] and the terminal part of the maxillary artery, respectively, that pass through the pterygopalatine fossa.

Skeletal framework

The walls of the pterygopalatine fossa are formed by parts of the palatine, maxilla, and sphenoid bones (Fig. 8.135):

- The anterior wall is formed by the posterior surface of the maxilla.
- The medial wall is formed by the lateral surface of the palatine bone.
- The posterior wall and roof are formed by parts of the sphenoid bone.

Sphenoid bone

The part of the sphenoid bone that contributes to the formation of the pterygopalatine fossa is the anterosuperior surface of the pterygoid process (Fig. 8.136). Opening onto this surface are two large foramina:

- The maxillary nerve [V₂] passes through the most lateral and superior of these—**the foramen rotundum**—which communicates posteriorly with the middle cranial fossa (Fig. 8.136B).
- The greater petrosal nerve from the facial nerve [VII] and sympathetic fibers from the internal carotid plexus join to form the nerve of the pterygoid canal that passes forward into the pterygopalatine fossa through the more medial and inferior foramen—**the anterior opening of the pterygoid canal** (Fig. 8.136A).

Pterygoid canal

The pterygoid canal is a bony canal running horizontally through the root of the pterygoid process of the sphenoid bone. It opens anteriorly into the pterygopalatine fossa. Posteriorly it continues through the cartilage filling the foramen lacerum and opens into the middle cranial fossa just anteroinferior to the internal carotid as the vessel enters the cranial cavity through the carotid canal (Fig. 8.136B).

Gateways

Seven foramina and fissures provide apertures through which structures enter and leave the pterygopalatine fossa (Fig. 8.137):

- The **foramen rotundum** and **pterygoid canal** communicate with the middle cranial fossa and open onto the posterior wall.
- A small **palatovaginal canal** opens onto the posterior wall and leads to the nasopharynx.
- The **palatine canal** leads to the roof of the oral cavity (hard palate) and opens inferiorly.
- The **sphenopalatine foramen** opens onto the lateral wall of the nasal cavity and is in the medial wall.

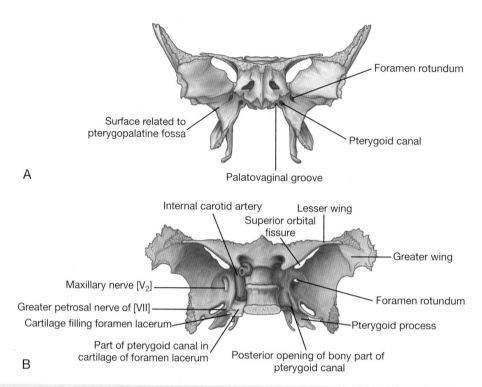

Fig. 8.136 Sphenoid bone. **A.** Anterior view. **B.** Posterosuperior view.

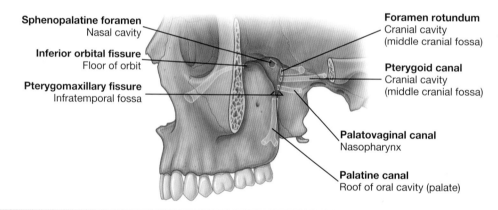

Fig. 8.137 Gateways of the pterygopalatine fossa.

- The lateral aspect of the pterygopalatine fossa is continuous with the infratemporal fossa via a large gap (the **pterygomaxillary fissure**) between the posterior surface of the maxilla and pterygoid process of the sphenoid bone.
- The superior aspect of the anterior wall of the fossa opens into the floor of the orbit via the **inferior orbital fissure.**

Contents

The maxillary nerve [V$_2$] and terminal part of the maxillary artery enter and branch within the pterygopalatine fossa. In addition, the nerve of the pterygoid canal enters the fossa carrying:

- preganglionic parasympathetic fibers from the greater petrosal branch of the facial nerve [VII], and

- postganglionic sympathetic fibers from the deep petrosal branch of the carotid plexus.

The preganglionic parasympathetic fibers synapse in the pterygopalatine ganglion and both the sympathetic and postganglionic parasympathetic fibers pass with branches of the maxillary nerve [V$_2$] out of the fossa and into adjacent regions.

In addition to nerves and arteries, veins and lymphatics also pass through the pterygopalatine fossa.

Maxillary nerve [V$_2$]

The maxillary nerve [V$_2$] is purely sensory. It originates from the trigeminal ganglion in the cranial cavity, exits the middle cranial fossa, and enters the pterygopalatine fossa through the foramen rotundum (Fig. 8.138). It passes anteriorly through the fossa and exits as the infra-orbital nerve through the inferior orbital fissure.

While passing through the pterygopalatine fossa, the maxillary nerve [V₂] gives rise to the zygomatic nerve, the posterior superior alveolar nerve, and two ganglionic branches. The two ganglionic branches originate from its inferior surface and pass to the pterygopalatine ganglion.

Postganglionic parasympathetic fibers, arising in the pterygopalatine ganglion, join the general sensory branches of the maxillary nerve [V₂] in the pterygopalatine ganglion, as do postganglionic sympathetic fibers from the carotid plexus, and the three types of fibers leave the ganglion as orbital, palatine, nasal, and pharyngeal branches.

Branches of maxillary nerve [V₂] or pterygopalatine ganglion

Orbital branches. The **orbital branches** are small and pass through the inferior orbital fissure to contribute to the supply of the orbital wall and of the sphenoidal and ethmoidal sinuses.

Greater and lesser palatine nerves. The **greater** and **lesser palatine nerves** (Fig. 8.138) pass inferiorly from the pterygopalatine ganglion, enter and pass through the palatine canal, and enter the oral surface of the palate through the greater and lesser palatine foramina.

The greater palatine nerve passes forward on the roof of the oral cavity to innervate mucosa and glands of the hard palate and the adjacent gingiva, almost as far forward as the incisor teeth.

In the palatine canal, the greater palatine nerve gives origin to **posterior inferior nasal nerves,** which pass medially through small foramina in the perpendicular plate of the palatine bone and contribute to the innervation of the lateral nasal wall.

After passing through the lesser palatine foramen, the lesser palatine nerve passes posteriorly to supply the soft palate.

Nasal nerves. The nasal nerves (Fig. 8.138), approximately seven in number, pass medially through the sphenopalatine foramen to enter the nasal cavity. Most pass anteriorly to supply the lateral wall of the nasal cavity, while others pass across the roof to supply the medial wall.

One of the nerves passing across the roof to supply the medial wall of the nasal cavity (the **nasopalatine nerve**) is the largest of the nasal nerves and passes anteriorly down the nasal septum, through the incisive canal and fossa in the hard palate to enter the roof of the oral cavity and supply mucosa, gingiva, and glands adjacent to the incisor teeth.

Pharyngeal nerve. The **pharyngeal nerve** passes posteriorly from the pterygopalatine ganglion and leaves the fossa through the palatovaginal canal, which it then exits to supply the mucosa and glands of the nasopharynx (Fig. 8.138).

Zygomatic nerve. The **zygomatic nerve** (Fig. 8.138) originates directly from the maxillary nerve [V₂] in the pterygopalatine fossa, which it leaves to enter the orbit through the inferior orbital fissure. It passes forward on the lateral orbital wall and divides into zygomaticotemporal and zygomaticofacial branches:

- The **zygomaticotemporal branch** continues forward at the base of the lateral orbital wall, passes through a small bony

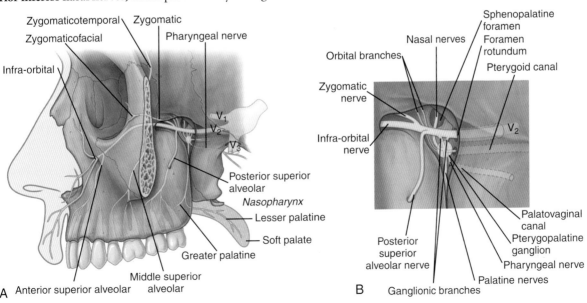

Fig. 8.138 Maxillary nerve [V₂]. A. Terminal branches. B. In relationship to the pterygopalatine ganglion.

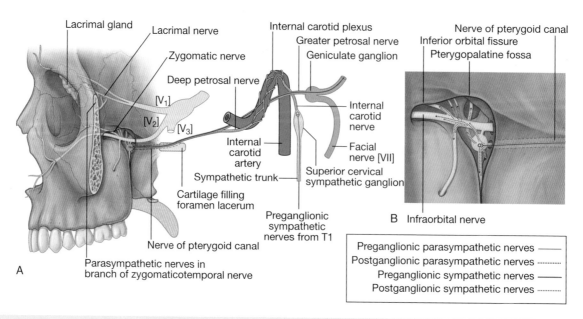

Fig. 8.139 Nerve of the pterygoid canal. A. Overview. B. In relationship to the pterygopalatine ganglion.

canal in the zygomatic bone to enter the temporal fossa through a small foramen in the lateral orbital margin on the posterior surface of the frontal process of the zygomatic bone, and passes superficially to supply skin over the temple.

- The **zygomaticofacial branch** also passes forward at the base of the lateral orbital wall and leaves through a small bony canal in the orbital margin, which opens via multiple small foramina on the anterolateral surface of the zygomatic bone, and its branches supply the adjacent skin.

Posterior superior alveolar nerve. The **posterior superior alveolar nerve** (Fig. 8.138) originates from the maxillary nerve [V_2] in the pterygopalatine fossa and passes laterally out of the fossa through the pterygomaxillary fissure to enter the infratemporal fossa. It continues laterally and inferiorly to enter the posterior surface of the maxilla through a small alveolar foramen approximately midway between the last molar tooth and the inferior orbital fissure. It then passes inferiorly just deep to the mucosa of the maxillary sinus to join the **superior dental plexus**.

The posterior superior alveolar nerve supplies the molar teeth and adjacent buccal gingivae and contributes to the supply of the maxillary sinus.

Infra-orbital nerve. The infra-orbital nerve (Fig. 8.138) is the anterior continuation of the maxillary nerve [V_2] that leaves the pterygopalatine fossa through the inferior orbital fissure. It lies first in the infra-orbital groove in the floor of the orbit and then continues forward in the infra-orbital canal.

While in the infra-orbital groove and canal, the infra-orbital nerve gives origin to **middle** and **anterior superior**

alveolar nerves, respectively, which ultimately join the superior alveolar plexus to supply the upper teeth:

- The middle superior alveolar nerve also supplies the maxillary sinus.
- The anterior superior alveolar nerve also gives origin to a small nasal branch, which passes medially through the lateral wall of the nasal cavity to supply parts of the areas of the nasal floor and walls.

The infra-orbital nerve exits the infra-orbital canal through the infra-orbital foramen inferior to the orbital margin and divides into nasal, palpebral, and superior labial branches:

- Nasal branches supply skin over the lateral aspect of the external nose and part of the nasal septum.
- Palpebral branches supply skin of the lower eyelid.
- Superior labial branches supply skin over the cheek, upper lip, and the related oral mucosa (Fig. 8.138).

Nerve of the pterygoid canal and the pterygopalatine ganglion

The nerve of the pterygoid canal (Fig. 8.139) is formed in the middle cranial fossa by the union of:

- the greater petrosal nerve (a branch of the facial nerve [VII]), and
- the deep petrosal nerve (a branch of the internal carotid plexus).

The nerve of the pterygoid canal passes into the pterygopalatine fossa and joins the pterygopalatine ganglion. It carries mainly preganglionic parasympathetic and postganglionic sympathetic fibers.

Greater petrosal nerve

The greater petrosal nerve, which originates from the geniculate ganglion of the facial nerve [VII] (Fig. 8.139A) in the temporal bone, exits the temporal bone through a small canal that opens via a fissure onto the anterior surface of the petrous part of the temporal bone. It passes anteromedially along the posterior margin of the middle cranial fossa and then under the internal carotid artery to reach the superior surface of the cartilage filling the foramen lacerum.

As the greater petrosal nerve passes under the internal carotid artery, it is joined by the deep petrosal nerve to form the nerve of the pterygoid canal (Fig. 8.139A).

The greater petrosal nerve carries parasympathetic innervation to all glands above the oral fissure, including:

- mucous glands in the nasal cavity;
- salivary glands in the upper half of the oral cavity; and
- the lacrimal gland in the orbit.

The greater petrosal nerve also carries some taste (SA) fibers from the soft palate in the lesser palatine nerve.

Deep petrosal nerve

The **deep petrosal nerve** is formed by postganglionic sympathetic fibers that originate in the **superior cervical sympathetic ganglion** in the neck and leave the ganglion as the **internal carotid nerve** (Fig. 8.139A).

Preganglionic sympathetic fibers that synapse in the ganglion are from the T1 spinal nerve.

The internal carotid nerve forms the internal carotid plexus around the internal carotid artery as the internal carotid artery passes through the skull and into the cranial cavity. Some of the fibers from the internal carotid plexus converge to form the deep petrosal nerve, which leaves the internal carotid plexus in the middle cranial fossa and joins the greater petrosal branch of the facial nerve [VII].

The deep petrosal nerve carries postganglionic sympathetic fibers destined mainly for blood vessels.

Pterygopalatine ganglion

The nerve of the pterygoid canal (preganglionic parasympathetic fibers and postganglionic sympathetic fibers) enters the superior surface of the cartilage that fills the foramen lacerum and passes anteriorly through the cartilage to enter the pterygoid canal in the root of the pterygoid process of the sphenoid bone. It passes through the canal and into the pterygopalatine fossa where it joins the pterygopalatine ganglion formed around the branches of the maxillary nerve [V₂] (see Fig. 8.139).

The **pterygopalatine ganglion** is the largest of the four parasympathetic ganglia in the head and is formed by the cell bodies of the postganglionic neurons associated with preganglionic parasympathetic fibers of the facial nerve [VII] carried by the greater petrosal nerve and the nerve of the pterygoid canal.

The postganglionic parasympathetic fibers that originate in the pterygopalatine ganglion, together with postganglionic sympathetic fibers passing through the ganglion, join fibers from the ganglionic branches of the maxillary nerve [V₂] to form orbital, palatine, nasal, and pharyngeal branches, which leave the ganglion (Fig. 8.140)

Other postganglionic parasympathetic and sympathetic fibers pass superiorly through the ganglionic branches of the maxillary nerve [V₂] to enter the main trunk of the maxillary nerve and be distributed with the zygomatic, posterior superior alveolar, and infra-orbital nerves. Of these, the postganglionic parasympathetic and sympathetic fibers that pass into the orbit with the zygomatic nerve are particularly important because they ultimately innervate the lacrimal gland.

Innervation of the lacrimal gland

Approximately midway along the orbital wall, the postganglionic parasympathetic and sympathetic fibers leave the zygomaticotemporal branch of the zygomatic nerve and form a special autonomic nerve, which travels up the lateral orbital wall to join the lacrimal nerve (Fig. 8.139; also see Fig. 8.70, pg. 508).

The lacrimal nerve is a major general sensory branch of the ophthalmic nerve [V₁], which passes forward in the orbit at the margin between the lateral wall and roof.

The postganglionic parasympathetic and sympathetic fibers pass with the lacrimal nerve to the lacrimal gland.

Clinical app

Dry eye

A lesion anywhere along the course of the parasympathetic fibers that leave the brain as part of the facial nerve [VII] and are ultimately carried to the lacrimal gland along branches of the ophthalmic nerve [V₁] results in "dry eye" and can eventually lead to opacity of the cornea, resulting in loss of vision in the affected eye.

Maxillary artery

The maxillary artery is a major branch of the external carotid artery in the neck. It originates adjacent to the neck of mandible, passes forward through the infratemporal fossa, and then enters the pterygopalatine fossa through the pterygomaxillary fissure (Fig. 8.140).

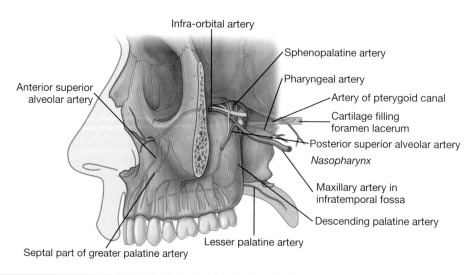

Fig. 8.140 Maxillary artery in the pterygopalatine fossa.

The part of the maxillary artery in the pterygopalatine fossa (the third part) is anterior to the pterygopalatine ganglion and gives origin to branches that accompany branches of the maxillary nerve [V$_2$] and the pterygopalatine ganglion.

Branches of the maxillary artery include the posterior superior alveolar, infra-orbital, greater palatine, pharyngeal, and sphenopalatine arteries and the artery of the pterygoid canal. Collectively, these branches supply much of the nasal cavity, the roof of the oral cavity, and all upper teeth. In addition, they contribute to the blood supply of the sinuses, oropharynx, and floor of the orbit.

Branches

Posterior superior alveolar artery. The **posterior superior alveolar artery** originates from the maxillary artery as it passes through the pterygomaxillary fissure (Fig. 8.140). It meets the posterior superior alveolar nerve, accompanies it through the alveolar foramen on the infratemporal surface of the maxilla, and supplies the molar and premolar teeth, adjacent gingiva, and the maxillary sinus.

Infra-orbital artery. The infra-orbital artery passes forward with the infra-orbital nerve and leaves the pterygopalatine fossa through the inferior orbital fissure (Fig. 8.140). With the infra-orbital nerve, it lies in the infra-orbital groove and infra-orbital canal, and emerges through the infra-orbital foramen to supply parts of the face.

Within the infra-orbital canal, the infra-orbital artery gives origin to:

- branches that contribute to the blood supply of structures near the floor of the orbit—the inferior rectus and inferior oblique muscles and the lacrimal sac; and

- **anterior superior alveolar arteries**, which supply the incisor and canine teeth and the maxillary sinus.

Greater palatine artery. The **greater palatine artery** passes inferiorly with the palatine nerves into the palatine canal (Fig. 8.140). It gives origin to a **lesser palatine branch**, which passes through the lesser palatine foramen to supply the soft palate, and then continues through the greater palatine foramen to supply the hard palate. The latter vessel passes forward on the inferior surface of the palate to enter the incisive fossa and pass superiorly through the incisive canal to supply the anterior aspect of the septal wall of the nasal cavity.

Pharyngeal branch. The **pharyngeal branch** of the maxillary artery travels posteriorly and leaves the pterygopalatine fossa through the palatovaginal canal with the pharyngeal nerve (Fig. 8.140). It supplies the posterior aspect of the roof of the nasal cavity, the sphenoidal sinus, and the pharyngotympanic tube.

Sphenopalatine artery. The **sphenopalatine artery** is the terminal branch of the maxillary artery (Fig. 8.140). It leaves the pterygopalatine fossa medially through the sphenopalatine foramen and accompanies the nasal nerves, giving off:

- posterior lateral nasal arteries, which supply the lateral wall of the nasal cavity and contribute to the supply of the paranasal sinuses; and
- posterior septal branches, which travel medially across the roof to supply the nasal septum—the largest of these branches passes anteriorly down the septum to anastomose with the end of the greater palatine artery.

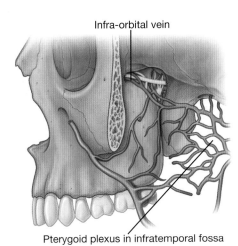

Infra-orbital vein

Pterygoid plexus in infratemporal fossa

Fig. 8.141 Veins of the pterygopalatine fossa.

Artery of pterygoid canal. The **artery of pterygoid canal** passes posteriorly into the pterygoid canal (Fig. 8.140). It supplies surrounding tissues and terminates, after passing inferiorly through cartilage filling the foramen lacerum, in the mucosa of the nasopharynx.

Veins. Veins that drain areas supplied by branches of the terminal part of the maxillary artery generally travel with these branches back into the pterygopalatine fossa.

The veins coalesce in the pterygopalatine fossa and then pass laterally through the pterygomaxillary fissure to join the pterygoid plexus of veins in the infratemporal fossa (Fig. 8.141).

The infra-orbital vein, which drains the inferior aspect of the orbit, may pass directly into the infratemporal fossa through the lateral aspect of the inferior orbital fissure, so bypassing the pterygopalatine fossa.

NECK

The neck is a tube providing continuity from the head to the trunk. It extends anteriorly from the lower border of the mandible to the upper surface of the manubrium of sternum and posteriorly from the superior nuchal line on the occipital bone of the skull to the intervertebral disc between the CVII and TI vertebrae. Within the tube, four compartments provide longitudinal organization (Fig. 8.142):

- The visceral compartment is anterior and contains parts of the digestive and respiratory systems and several endocrine glands.
- The vertebral compartment is posterior and contains the cervical vertebrae, spinal cord, cervical nerves, and muscles associated with the vertebral column.
- The two vascular compartments, one on each side, are lateral and contain the major blood vessels and the vagus nerve [X].

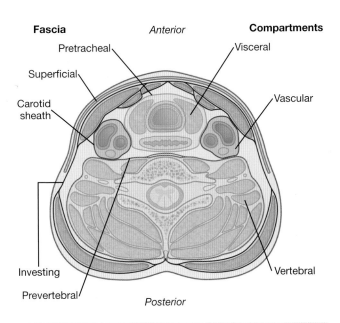

Fascia   *Anterior*   **Compartments**

Pretracheal · · · · · · · · · · · · · · · · · Visceral

Superficial

Carotid sheath · · · · · · · · · · · · · · · · Vascular

Investing

Prevertebral   Vertebral

Posterior

Fig. 8.142 Compartments of the neck.

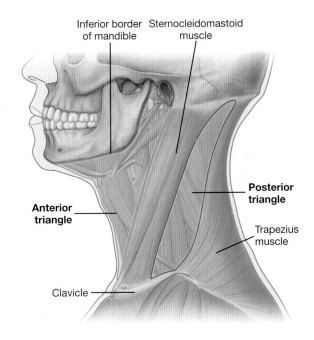

Inferior border of mandible   Sternocleidomastoid muscle

Posterior triangle

Trapezius muscle

Anterior triangle

Clavicle

Fig. 8.143 Anterior and posterior triangles of the neck.

All these compartments are contained within unique layers of cervical fascia.

For descriptive purposes the neck is divided into anterior and posterior triangles (Fig. 8.143):

- The boundaries of the **anterior triangle** are the anterior border of the sternocleidomastoid muscle, the inferior border of the mandible, and the midline of the neck.
- The boundaries of the **posterior triangle** are the posterior border of the sternocleidomastoid muscle, the anterior

The boundaries of the anterior and posterior triangles on each side of the neck are easily established using readily visible bony and muscular landmarks (Fig. 8.144).

The base of each anterior triangle is the inferior margin of the mandible; the anterior margin is the midline of the neck, and the posterior margin is the anterior border of the sternocleidomastoid muscle. The apex of each anterior triangle points inferiorly and is at the suprasternal notch.

The anterior triangles are associated with structures such as the airway and digestive tract and nerves and vessels that pass between the thorax and head. They are also associated with the thyroid and parathyroid glands.

The base of each posterior triangle is the middle one-third of the clavicle. The medial margin is the posterior border of the sternocleidomastoid muscle, and the lateral margin is the anterior border of the trapezius muscle. The apex points superiorly and is immediately posteroinferior to the mastoid process.

The posterior triangles are associated with nerves and vessels that pass into and out of the upper limbs.

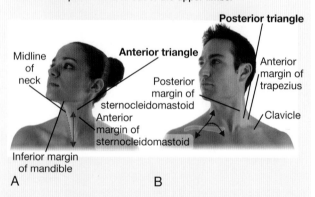

Fig. 8.144 How to outline the anterior and posterior triangles of the neck. **A.** In a woman, anterolateral view. The left anterior triangle is indicated. Structures coursing between head and thorax are associated with the anterior triangles (*arrow in green area*). **B.** In a man, anterior view of the posterior triangles. Structures coursing between thorax/neck and upper limb are associated with the posterior triangles (*blue arrows*).

border of the trapezius muscle, and the middle one-third of the clavicle.

Fascia

The fascia of the neck has a number of unique features.

The **superficial fascia** in the neck contains a thin sheet of muscle (the **platysma,** see Table 8.7, pg. 486), while the deep cervical fascia is organized into several distinct layers, including (Fig. 8.142):

- an investing layer, which surrounds all structures in the neck;
- the prevertebral layer, which surrounds the vertebral column and the deep muscles associated with the back;
- the pretracheal layer, which encloses the viscera of the neck; and
- the carotid sheaths, which receive a contribution from the other three fascial layers and surround the two major neurovascular bundles on either side of the neck.

Investing layer

The **investing layer** completely surrounds the neck (Fig. 8.145).

Attaching posteriorly to the ligamentum nuchae and the spinous process of the CVII vertebra, this fascial layer splits as it passes forward to enclose the trapezius muscle, reunites into a single layer as it forms the roof of the posterior triangle, splits again to surround the sternocleidomastoid muscle, and reunites again to join its twin from the other side.

Anteriorly, the investing fascia surrounds the infrahyoid muscles.

The investing fascia is attached:

- superiorly to the external occipital protuberance and the superior nuchal line,
- laterally to the mastoid process and zygomatic arch, and
- inferiorly to the spine of the scapula, the acromion, the clavicle, and the manubrium of sternum.

The external and anterior jugular veins; the lesser occipital, great auricular, transverse cervical, and supraclavicular nerves; and all branches of the cervical plexus pierce the investing fascia.

Prevertebral layer

The prevertebral layer is a cylindrical layer of fascia that surrounds the vertebral column and the muscles associated with it (Fig. 8.145). Muscles in this group include the prevertebral muscles, the anterior, middle, and posterior scalene muscles, and the deep muscles of the back.

The prevertebral fascia is attached posteriorly along the length of the ligamentum nuchae and superiorly forms a continuous circular line attaching to the base of the skull. This circle:

- begins anteriorly as the fascia attaches to the basilar part of the occipital bone, the area of the jugular foramen, and the carotid canal;
- continues laterally, attaching to the mastoid process; and
- continues posteriorly along the superior nuchal line, ending at the external occipital protuberance where it associates with its partner from the opposite side.

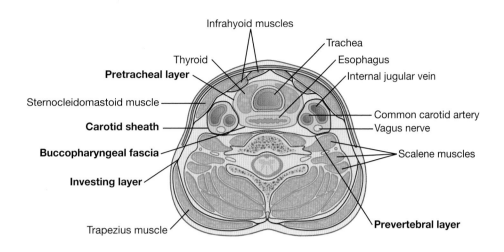

Fig. 8.145 Fascia of neck, transverse view.

Infrahyoid muscles
Trachea
Esophagus
Internal jugular vein
Thyroid
Pretracheal layer
Sternocleidomastoid muscle
Carotid sheath
Common carotid artery
Vagus nerve
Buccopharyngeal fascia
Scalene muscles
Investing layer
Trapezius muscle
Prevertebral layer

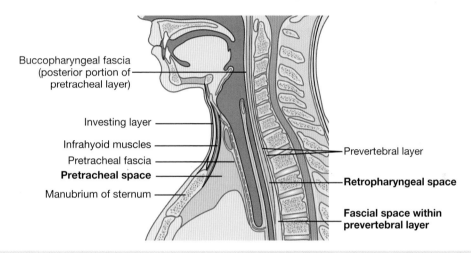

Fig. 8.146 Fascia of the neck, sagittal view.

Buccopharyngeal fascia
(posterior portion of
pretracheal layer)
Investing layer
Infrahyoid muscles
Pretracheal fascia
Pretracheal space
Manubrium of sternum
Prevertebral layer
Retropharyngeal space
**Fascial space within
prevertebral layer**

Anteriorly, the prevertebral fascia is attached to the anterior surfaces of the transverse processes and bodies of vertebrae CI to CVII.

The prevertebral fascia passing between the attachment points on the transverse processes is unique. In this location, it splits into two layers, creating a longitudinal fascial space containing loose connective tissue that extends from the base of the skull through the thorax (Figs. 8.145, 8.146).

There is one additional specialization of the prevertebral fascia in the lower region of the neck. The prevertebral fascia in an anterolateral position extends from the anterior and middle scalene muscles to surround the brachial plexus and subclavian artery as these structures pass into the axilla. This fascial extension is the **axillary sheath**.

Pretracheal layer

The **pretracheal layer** consists of a collection of fascias that surround the trachea, esophagus, and thyroid gland (Fig. 8.145). Anteriorly, it consists of a pretracheal fascia that crosses the neck, just posterior to the infrahyoid muscles, and covers the trachea and the thyroid gland. The pretracheal fascia begins superiorly at the hyoid bone and ends inferiorly in the upper thoracic cavity. Laterally, this fascia continues and covers the thyroid gland and the esophagus.

Posteriorly, the pretracheal layer is referred to as the buccopharyngeal fascia and separates the pharynx and the esophagus from the prevertebral layer (Fig. 8.146).

The buccopharyngeal fascia begins superiorly at the base of the skull and ends inferiorly in the thoracic cavity.

Carotid sheath

Each **carotid sheath** is a column of fascia that surrounds the common carotid artery, the internal carotid artery, the internal jugular vein, and the vagus nerve as these structures pass through the neck (Fig. 8.145).

It receives contributions from the investing, prevertebral, and pretracheal layers, though the extent of each component's contribution varies.

Head and Neck

Fascial compartments

The arrangement of the various layers of cervical fascia organizes the neck into four longitudinal compartments (see Fig. 8.142):

- The first compartment is the largest, includes the other three, and consists of the area surrounded by the investing layer.
- The second compartment (vertebral compartment) consists of the vertebral column, the deep muscles associated with this structure, and is the area contained within the prevertebral layer.
- The third compartment (the visceral compartment) contains the pharynx, the trachea, the esophagus, and the thyroid and parathyroid glands, which are surrounded by the pretracheal layer.
- Finally, there is a compartment (the carotid sheath) consisting of the neurovascular structures that pass from the base of the skull to the thoracic cavity, and the sheath enclosing these structures receives contributions from the other cervical fascias.

Clinical app

Spread of neck infections

Between the fascial layers in the neck are spaces that may provide a conduit for the spread of infections from the neck to the mediastinum.

Three spaces could be involved in this process (Fig. 8.146):

- The first is the **pretracheal space** between the investing layer of cervical fascia (covering the posterior surface of the infrahyoid muscles) and the pretracheal fascia (covering the anterior surface of the trachea and the thyroid gland), which passes between the neck and the anterior part of the superior mediastinum.
- The second is the **retropharyngeal space** between the buccopharyngeal fascia (on the posterior surface of the pharynx and esophagus) and the prevertebral fascia (on the anterior surface of the transverse processes and bodies of the cervical vertebrae), which extends from the base of the skull to the upper part of the posterior mediastinum.
- The **third space** is within the prevertebral layer (covering the anterior surface of the transverse processes and bodies of the cervical vertebrae). This layer splits into two laminae to create a fascial space that begins at the base of the skull and extends through the posterior mediastinum to the diaphragm.

Superficial venous drainage

The external jugular and anterior jugular veins are the primary venous channels for superficial venous drainage of the neck (Fig. 8.147).

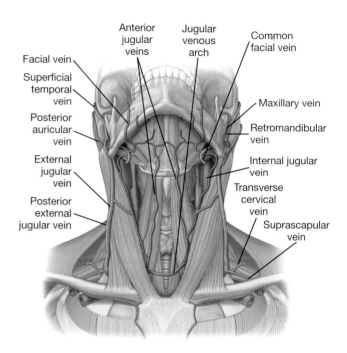

Fig. 8.147 Superficial veins of neck.

External jugular veins

The external jugular vein is formed posterior to the angle of mandible as the **posterior auricular vein** and the **retromandibular vein** join (Fig. 8.147):

- The posterior auricular vein drains the scalp behind and above the ear.
- The retromandibular vein is formed when the **superficial temporal** and **maxillary veins** join in the substance of the parotid gland and descends to the angle of mandible where it divides into an anterior and a posterior division (Fig. 8.147)— the posterior division joins the posterior auricular vein to form the external jugular vein, and the anterior division joins the **facial vein** to form the common facial vein, which passes deep and becomes a tributary to the internal jugular vein.

Once formed, the external jugular vein passes straight down the neck in the superficial fascia and is superficial to the sternocleidomastoid muscle throughout its course, crossing it diagonally as it descends.

Reaching the lower part of the neck, just superior to the clavicle and immediately posterior to the sternocleidomastoid muscle, the external jugular vein pierces the investing layer of cervical fascia, passes deep to the clavicle, and enters the **subclavian vein**.

Tributaries received by the external jugular vein along its course include the **posterior external jugular vein** (draining superficial areas of the back of the neck) and the **transverse cervical** and **suprascapular veins** (draining the posterior scapular region).

560

Clinical app

Central venous access

In most instances, access to peripheral veins of the arm and the leg will suffice for administering intravenous drugs and fluids and for obtaining blood for analysis; however, in certain circumstances it is necessary to place larger-bore catheters in the central veins, for example for dialysis, parenteral nutrition, or the administration of drugs that have a tendency to produce phlebitis.

"Blind puncture" of the subclavian and jugular veins to obtain central venous access used to be standard practice. However, subclavian vein puncture is not without complications. As the subclavian vein passes inferiorly, posterior to the clavicle, it passes over the apex of the lung. Any misplacement of a needle into or through this structure may puncture the apical pleura, producing a pneumothorax. Inadvertent arterial puncture and vein laceration may also produce a hemopneumothorax.

Placing a catheter in the internal jugular vein (Fig. 8.148) carries fewer risks, but local hematoma and damage to the carotid artery are again important complications.

Current practice is to identify major vessels using ultrasound and to obtain central venous access under direct vision to avoid any significant complication.

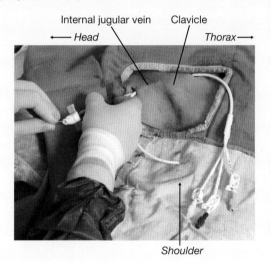

Fig. 8.148 Placing a central venous catheter in the neck.

Anterior jugular veins

The **anterior jugular veins,** although variable and inconsistent, are usually described as draining the anterior aspect of the neck (Fig. 8.147). These paired venous channels, which begin as small veins, come together at or just superior to the hyoid bone. Once formed, each anterior jugular vein descends on either side of the midline of the neck.

Inferiorly, near the medial attachment of the sterno-cleidomastoid muscle, each anterior jugular vein pierces the

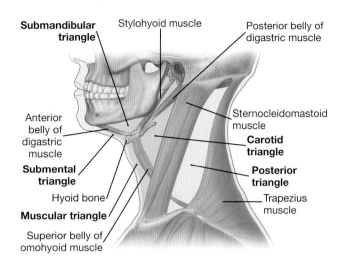

Fig. 8.149 Borders and subdivisions of the anterior triangle of the neck.

investing layer of cervical fascia to enter the subclavian vein. Occasionally, the anterior jugular vein may enter the external jugular vein immediately before the external jugular vein enters the subclavian vein.

Often, the right and left anterior jugular veins communicate with each other, being connected by a **jugular venous arch** in the area of the suprasternal notch.

Anterior triangle of the neck

The anterior triangle of the neck is outlined by the anterior border of the sternocleidomastoid muscle laterally, the inferior border of the mandible superiorly, and the midline of the neck medially (Fig. 8.149). It is further subdivided into several smaller triangles as follows:

- The **submandibular triangle** is outlined by the inferior border of the mandible superiorly and the anterior and posterior bellies of the digastric muscle inferiorly.
- The single **submental triangle** is outlined by the body of the hyoid bone inferiorly, the anterior belly of the digastric muscle laterally on each side, and the mandibular symphysis superiorly in the midline.
- The **muscular triangle** is outlined by the hyoid bone superiorly, the superior belly of the omohyoid muscles and the anterior border of the sternocleidomastoid muscle laterally, and the mandibular symphysis.
- The **carotid triangle** is outlined by the superior belly of the omohyoid muscle anteroinferiorly, the stylohyoid muscle and posterior belly of the digastric superiorly, and the anterior border of the sternocleidomastoid muscle posteriorly.

Each of these triangles contains numerous structures that can be identified as being within a specific triangle, passing into a specific triangle from outside the area, originating

Table 8.12   Muscles in the anterior triangle of the neck

Muscle	Origin	Insertion	Innervation	Function
Stylohyoid	Base of styloid process	Lateral area of body of hyoid bone	Facial nerve [VII]	Pulls hyoid bone upward in a posterosuperior direction
Digastric —Anterior belly	Digastric fossa on lower inside of mandible	Attachment of tendon between two bellies to body of hyoid bone	Mylohyoid nerve from inferior alveolar branch of mandibular nerve [V₃]	Opens mouth by lowering mandible; raises hyoid bone
—Posterior belly	Mastoid notch on medial side of mastoid process of temporal bone	Attachment of tendon between two bellies to body of hyoid bone	Facial nerve [VII]	Pulls hyoid bone upward and back
Mylohyoid	Mylohyoid line on mandible	Body of hyoid bone and fibers from muscle on opposite side	Mylohyoid nerve from inferior alveolar branch of mandibular nerve [V₃]	Support and elevation of floor of mouth; elevation of hyoid
Geniohyoid	Inferior mental spine on inner surface of mandible	Anterior surface of body of hyoid bone	Branch from anterior ramus of C1 (carried along the hypoglossal nerve [XII])	Fixed mandible elevates and pulls hyoid bone forward; fixed hyoid bone pulls mandible downward and inward
Sternohyoid	Posterior aspect of sternoclavicular joint and adjacent manubrium of sternum	Body of hyoid bone medial to attachment of omohyoid muscle	Anterior rami of C1 to C3 through the ansa cervicalis	Depresses hyoid bone after swallowing
Omohyoid	Superior border of scapula medial to suprascapular notch	Lower border of body of hyoid bone just lateral to attachment of sternohyoid	Anterior rami of C1 to C3 through the ansa cervicalis	Depresses and fixes hyoid bone
Thyrohyoid	Oblique line on lamina of thyroid cartilage	Greater horn and adjacent aspect of body of hyoid bone	Fibers from anterior ramus of C1 carried along hypoglossal nerve [XII]	Depresses hyoid bone, but when hyoid bone is fixed, it raises larynx
Sternothyroid	Posterior surface of manubrium of sternum	Oblique line on lamina of thyroid cartilage	Anterior rami of C1 to C3 through the ansa cervicalis	Draws larynx (thyroid cartilage) downward

in one triangle and passing to another triangle, or passing through several triangles while passing through the region.

A discussion of the anterior triangle of the neck must therefore combine a systemic approach describing the muscles, vessels, and nerves in the area with a regional approach describing the contents of each triangle.

Muscles

The muscles in the anterior triangle of the neck (Table 8.12) can be grouped according to their location relative to the hyoid bone:

- Muscles superior to the hyoid are classified as **suprahyoid muscles** and include the stylohyoid, digastric, mylohyoid, and geniohyoid.
- Muscles inferior to the hyoid are **infrahyoid muscles** and include the omohyoid, sternohyoid, thyrohyoid, and sternothyroid.

Suprahyoid muscles

The four pairs of suprahyoid muscles are in the submental and submandibular triangles (Table 8.12, Fig. 8.149). They pass in a superior direction from the hyoid bone to the skull or mandible and raise the hyoid, as occurs during swallowing.

The **stylohyoid** muscle arises from the base of the styloid process and passes anteroinferiorly to attach to the lateral area of the body of the hyoid bone (Table 8.12, Fig. 8.150).

The **digastric** muscle has anterior and posterior bellies connected by a tendon, which attaches to the body of the hyoid bone (Table 8.12, Fig. 8.150). Because of this arrangement, the muscle has multiple actions depending on which bone is fixed. The innervation of the posterior belly of the digastric muscle is by the facial nerve [VII], whereas the anterior belly of the muscle is innervated by the mandibular division [V₃] of the trigeminal nerve [V].

The **mylohyoid** muscle is superior to the anterior belly of the digastric and, with its partner from the opposite side, forms the floor of the mouth (Table 8.12, Fig. 8.150). The mylohyoid muscle supports and elevates the floor of the mouth and elevates the hyoid bone.

The **geniohyoid** muscle is superior to the floor of the oral cavity and is not generally considered a muscle of the anterior triangle of the neck; however, it can be regarded as a suprahyoid muscle. It is the final muscle in the suprahyoid group (Table 8.12, Fig. 8.150). A narrow muscle, it is superior to the medial part of each mylohyoid muscle. The muscles from each side are next to each other in the midline.

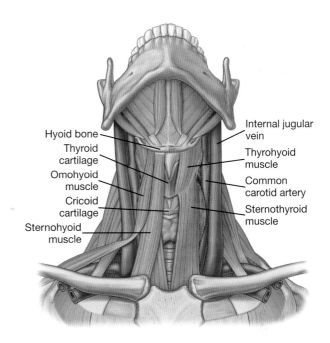

Fig. 8.151 Infrahyoid muscles.

Fig. 8.150 Suprahyoid muscles. **A.** Lateral view. **B.** Inferior view.

Infrahyoid muscles

The four infrahyoid muscles are in the muscular triangle (Table 8.12, Fig. 8.151). They attach the hyoid bone to inferior structures and depress the hyoid bone. They also provide a stable point of attachment for the suprahyoid muscles. Because of their appearance, they are sometimes referred to as the **"strap muscles."**

The **sternohyoid** muscle is a long, thin muscle that depresses the hyoid bone (Table 8.12, Fig. 8.152).

Lateral to the sternohyoid muscle is the **omohyoid** muscle (Table 8.12, Fig. 8.151). This muscle consists of two bellies with an intermediate tendon and is in both the posterior and anterior triangles of the neck. The omohyoid depresses and fixes the hyoid bone. It is innervated by the anterior rami of C1 to C3 through the ansa cervicalis.

The **thyrohyoid** muscle is deep to the superior parts of the omohyoid and sternohyoid (Table 8.12, Fig. 8.151). The thyrohyoid muscle depresses the hyoid, but when the hyoid is fixed it raises the larynx (e.g., when high notes are sung).

Lying beneath the sternohyoid and, in continuity with the thyrohyoid, the **sternothyroid** is the last muscle in the infrahyoid group (Table 8.12, Fig. 8.151) and draws the larynx (thyroid cartilage) downward.

Vessels

Passing through the anterior triangle of the neck are the common carotid arteries and their branches and the external and internal carotid arteries. These vessels supply all structures of the head and neck.

Associated with this arterial system are the internal jugular vein and its tributaries. These vessels receive blood from all structures of the head and neck.

Carotid system

Common carotid arteries

The **common carotid arteries** are the beginning of the carotid system (Fig. 8.152):

- The **right common carotid artery** originates from the brachiocephalic trunk immediately posterior to the right sternoclavicular joint and is entirely in the neck throughout its course.
- The **left common carotid artery** begins in the thorax as a direct branch of the arch of the aorta and passes superiorly to enter the neck near the left sternoclavicular joint.

Both right and left common carotid arteries ascend through the neck, just lateral to the trachea and esophagus, within a fascial compartment (the carotid sheath). They give off no branches as they pass through the neck.

Near the superior edge of the thyroid cartilage each common carotid artery divides into its two terminal branches—the **external** and **internal carotid arteries** (Fig. 8.153).

The superior part of each common carotid artery and its division into external and internal carotid arteries occurs in

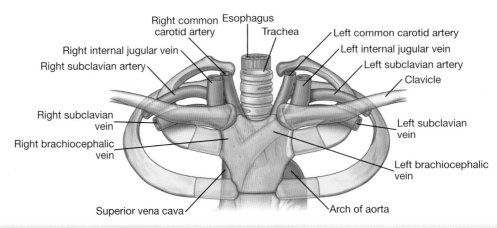

Fig. 8.152 Origin of common carotid arteries.

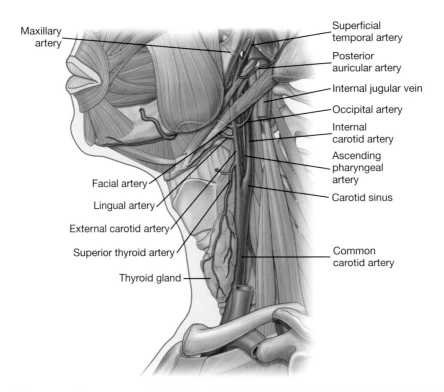

Fig. 8.153 Carotid system.

the carotid triangle, which is a subdivision of the anterior triangle of the neck (see Fig. 8.149).

At the bifurcation, the common carotid artery and the beginning of the internal carotid artery are dilated. This dilation is the **carotid sinus** and contains receptors that monitor changes in blood pressure and are innervated by a branch of the glossopharyngeal nerve [IX].

Another accumulation of receptors in the area of the bifurcation is responsible for detecting changes in blood chemistry, primarily oxygen content. This is the **carotid body** and is innervated by branches from both the glossopharyngeal [IX] and vagus [X] nerves.

Internal carotid arteries

After its origin, the internal carotid artery ascends toward the base of the skull (Fig. 8.153). It gives off no branches in the neck and enters the cranial cavity through the carotid canal in the petrous part of the temporal bone.

The internal carotid arteries supply the cerebral hemispheres, the eyes and the contents of the orbits, and the forehead.

External carotid arteries

The external carotid arteries begin giving off branches immediately after the bifurcation of the common carotid arteries (Table 8.13, Fig. 8.153) as follows:

Table 8.13 Branches of the external carotid artery

Branch	Supplies
Superior thyroid artery	Thyrohyoid muscle, internal structures of the larynx, sternocleidomastoid and cricothyroid muscles, thyroid gland
Ascending pharyngeal artery	Pharyngeal constrictors and stylopharyngeus muscle, palate, palatine, tonsil, pharyngotympanic tube, meninges in posterior cranial fossa
Lingual artery	Muscles of the tongue, palatine tonsil, soft palate, epiglottis, floor of mouth, sublingual gland
Facial artery	All structures in the face from the inferior border of the mandible anterior to the masseter muscle to the medial corner of the eye, the soft palate, palatine tonsil, pharyngotympanic tube, submandibular gland
Occipital artery	Sternocleidomastoid muscle, meninges in posterior cranial fossa, mastoid cells, deep muscles of the back, posterior scalp
Posterior auricular artery	Parotid gland and nearby muscles, external ear and scalp posterior to ear, middle and inner ear structures
Superficial temporal artery	Parotid gland and duct, masseter muscle, lateral face, anterior part of external ear, temporalis muscle, parietal and temporal fossae
Maxillary artery	External acoustic meatus, lateral and medial surface of tympanic membrane, temporomandibular joint, dura mater on lateral wall of skull and inner table of cranial bones, trigeminal ganglion and dura in vicinity, mylohyoid muscle, mandibular teeth, skin on chin, temporalis muscle, outer table of bones of skull in temporal fossa, structures in infratemporal fossa, maxillary sinus, upper teeth and gingivae, infra-orbital skin, palate, roof of pharynx, nasal cavity

- The **superior thyroid artery** is the first branch, arises from the anterior surface near or at the bifurcation, and passes in a downward and forward direction to reach the superior pole of the thyroid gland.

- The **ascending pharyngeal artery** is the second and smallest branch—it arises from the posterior aspect of the external carotid artery and ascends between the internal carotid artery and the pharynx.

- The **lingual artery** arises from the anterior surface of the external carotid artery just above the superior thyroid artery at the level of the hyoid bone, passes deep to the hypoglossal nerve [XII], and passes between the middle constrictor of the pharynx and hyoglossus muscles.

- The **facial artery** is the third anterior branch of the external carotid artery, arises just above the lingual artery, passes deep to the stylohyoid and posterior belly of the digastric muscles, continues deep between the submandibular gland and mandible, and emerges over the edge of the mandible just anterior to the masseter muscle, to enter the face.

- The **occipital artery** arises from the posterior surface of the external carotid artery, near the level of origin of the facial artery, passes upward and posteriorly deep to the posterior belly of the digastric muscle, and emerges on the posterior aspect of the scalp.

- The **posterior auricular artery** is a small branch arising from the posterior surface of the external carotid artery; it passes upward and posteriorly.

- The **superficial temporal artery** is one of the terminal branches and appears as an upward continuation of the external carotid artery; beginning posterior to the neck of mandible, it passes anterior to the ear, crosses the zygomatic process of the temporal bone, and above this point divides into anterior and posterior branches.

- The **maxillary artery** is the larger of the two terminal branches of the external carotid artery—arising posterior to the neck of mandible, it passes through the parotid gland, continues medial to the neck of mandible and into the infratemporal fossa, and continues through this area into the pterygopalatine fossa.

Veins

Collecting blood from the skull, brain, superficial face, and parts of the neck, the **internal jugular vein** (Fig. 8.153) begins as a dilated continuation of the **sigmoid sinus,** which is a dural venous sinus. This initial dilated part is referred to as the **superior bulb of jugular vein** and receives another dural venous sinus (the **inferior petrosal sinus**) soon after it is formed. It exits the skull through the jugular foramen associated with the glossopharyngeal [IX], vagus [X], and accessory [XI] nerves, and enters the carotid sheath.

The internal jugular vein traverses the neck within the carotid sheath, initially posterior to the internal carotid artery, but passes to a more lateral position farther down. It remains lateral to the common carotid artery through the rest of the neck with the vagus nerve [X] posterior and partially between the two vessels.

The paired internal jugular veins join with the subclavian veins posterior to the sternal end of the clavicle to form the right and left **brachiocephalic veins** (see Fig. 8.152).

Tributaries to each internal jugular vein include the inferior petrosal sinus, and the **facial, lingual, pharyngeal, occipital, superior thyroid,** and **middle thyroid veins.**

Nerves

Numerous cranial and peripheral nerves:

- pass through the anterior triangle of the neck as they continue to their final destination;

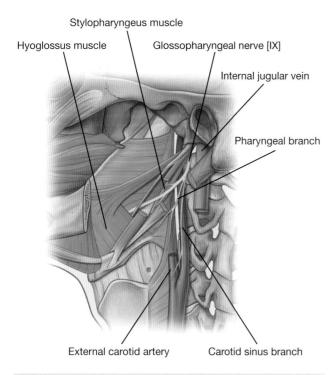

Fig. 8.154 Glossopharyngeal nerve [IX] in the anterior triangle of the neck.

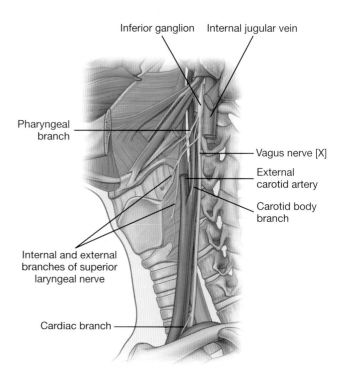

Fig. 8.155 Vagus nerve [X] in the anterior triangle of the neck.

- send branches to structures in or forming boundaries of the anterior triangle of the neck; and
- while in the anterior triangle of the neck, send branches to nearby structures.

The cranial nerves in these categories include the facial [VII], glossopharyngeal [IX], vagus [X], accessory [XI], and hypoglossal [XII].

Branches of spinal nerves in these categories include the transverse cervical nerve from the cervical plexus and the upper and lower roots of the ansa cervicalis.

Facial nerve [VII]

After emerging from the stylomastoid foramen, the facial nerve [VII] gives off branches that innervate the posterior belly of the digastric and the stylohyoid in the anterior triangle of the neck (see Fig. 8.47, pg. 493). The facial nerve [VII] also innervates platysma muscle that overlies the anterior triangle and part of the posterior triangle of the neck.

Glossopharyngeal nerve [IX]

The glossopharyngeal nerve [IX] leaves the cranial cavity through the jugular foramen. It begins its descent between the internal carotid artery and the internal jugular vein, lying deep to the styloid process and the muscles associated with the styloid process. As the glossopharyngeal nerve [IX] completes its descent, it passes forward between the internal and external carotid arteries, and curves around the lateral

border of the stylopharyngeus muscle (Fig. 8.154). At this point, it continues in an anterior direction, deep to the hyoglossus muscle, to reach the base of the tongue and the area of the palatine tonsil.

As the glossopharyngeal nerve [IX] passes through the area of the anterior triangle of the neck, it innervates the stylopharyngeus muscle, sends a branch to the carotid sinus, and supplies sensory branches to the pharynx.

Vagus nerve [X]

The vagus nerve [X] exits the cranial cavity through the jugular foramen between the glossopharyngeal [IX] and accessory [XI] nerves.

Outside the skull the vagus nerve [X] enters the carotid sheath and descends through the neck enclosed in this structure medial to the internal jugular vein and posterior to the internal carotid and common carotid arteries (Fig. 8.155).

Branches of the vagus nerve [X] as it passes through the anterior triangle of the neck include a motor branch to the pharynx, a branch to the carotid body, the superior laryngeal nerve (which divides into external and internal laryngeal branches), and possibly a cardiac branch (Fig. 8.155).

Accessory nerve [XI]

The accessory nerve [XI] is the most posterior of the three cranial nerves exiting the cranial cavity through the jugular foramen. It begins its descent medial to the internal jugular vein, emerging from between the internal jugular vein

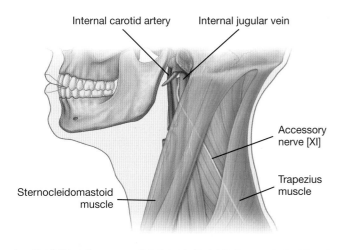

Fig. 8.156 Accessory nerve [XI] in the neck.

Hypoglossal nerve [XII]

The hypoglossal nerve [XII] leaves the cranial cavity through the hypoglossal canal and is medial to the internal jugular vein and internal carotid artery immediately outside the skull. As it descends, it passes outward between the internal jugular vein and internal carotid artery (Fig. 8.157). At this point it passes forward, hooking around the occipital artery, across the lateral surfaces of the internal and external carotid arteries and the lingual artery, and then continues deep to the posterior belly of the digastric and stylohyoid muscles. It passes over the surface of the hyoglossus muscle and disappears deep to the mylohyoid muscle.

The hypoglossal nerve [XII], which supplies the tongue, does not give off any branches as it passes through the anterior triangle of the neck.

Transverse cervical nerve

The transverse cervical nerve is a branch of the cervical plexus arising from the anterior rami of cervical nerves C2 and C3. It emerges from beneath the posterior border of the sternocleidomastoid muscle, near the middle of the muscle, and loops around the sternocleidomastoid to cross its

and internal carotid artery to cross the lateral surface of the internal jugular vein as it passes downward and backward to disappear either into or beneath the anterior border of the sternocleidomastoid muscle (Fig. 8.156).

The accessory nerve gives off no branches as it passes through the anterior triangle of the neck.

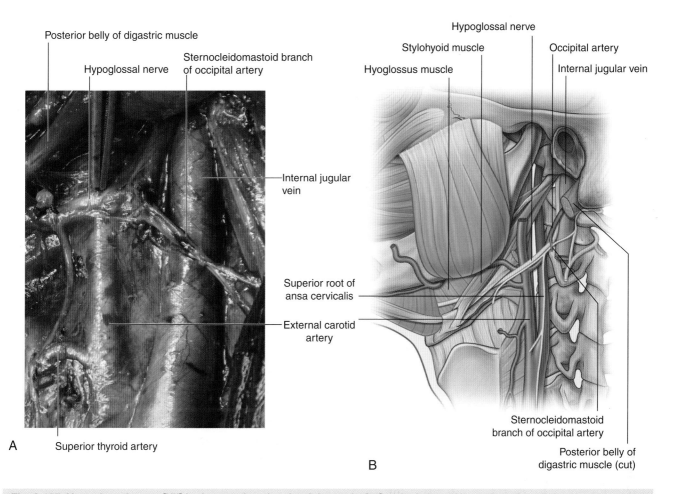

Fig. 8.157 Hypoglossal nerve [XII] in the anterior triangle of the neck. **A.** Surgical view of hypoglossal nerve in anterior triangle. **B.** Diagram.

anterior surface in a transverse direction (Fig. 8.158). It continues across the neck and provides cutaneous innervation to this area.

Ansa cervicalis

The ansa cervicalis is a loop of nerve fibers from cervical nerves C1 to C3 that innervate the "strap muscles" in the anterior triangle of the neck (Fig. 8.159). It begins as branches from the cervical nerve C1 join the hypoglossal nerve [XII] soon after it leaves the skull.

Transverse cervical nerve

Sternocleidomastoid muscle   Trapezius muscle

Fig. 8.158 Transverse cervical nerve in the anterior triangle of the neck.

As the hypoglossal nerve [XII] completes its descent and begins to pass forward across the internal and external carotid arteries, some of the cervical nerve fibers leave it and descend between the internal jugular vein and the internal, and then common, carotid arteries. These nerve fibers are the **superior root** of the ansa cervicalis and innervate the superior belly of the omohyoid muscle, and the upper parts of the sternohyoid and sternothyroid muscles.

Completing the loop is a direct branch from the cervical plexus containing nerve fibers from the second and third cervical nerves C2 and C3 (Fig. 8.159). This is the **inferior root** of the ansa cervicalis. It descends either medial or lateral to the internal jugular vein before turning medially to join the superior root. At this location, the ansa cervicalis gives off branches that innervate the inferior belly of the omohyoid, and the lower parts of the sternohyoid and sternothyroid muscles.

Elements of the gastrointestinal and respiratory systems

The esophagus, trachea, pharynx, and larynx lie in the neck and are related to the anterior triangles.

Esophagus

The esophagus is part of the gastrointestinal system and has only a short course in the lower neck. It begins at vertebral level CVI where it is continuous with the pharynx above and courses inferiorly to pass through the thoracic inlet. It lies directly anterior to the vertebral column (Fig. 8.160A).

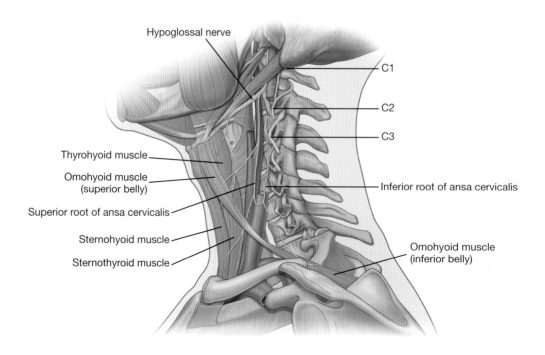

Hypoglossal nerve

C1

C2

C3

Thyrohyoid muscle

Omohyoid muscle (superior belly)

Superior root of ansa cervicalis

Sternohyoid muscle

Sternothyroid muscle

Inferior root of ansa cervicalis

Omohyoid muscle (inferior belly)

Fig. 8.159 Ansa cervicalis.

Trachea

The trachea is part of the lower airway and, like the esophagus, begins at vertebral level CVI, where it is continuous with the larynx above (Fig. 8.160A). The trachea lies directly anterior to the esophagus and passes inferiorly in the midline to enter the thorax.

Clinical app

Tracheobronchial injury

Tracheobronchial injuries rarely occur in isolation and are most often associated with other significant injuries to the neck and chest.

Penetrating injuries occur most frequently in the mid and upper thirds of the trachea whereas injuries involving blunt trauma (e.g., road traffic accidents) occur more frequently at the level of the carina. It is important to remember that all sites of the tracheobronchial tree may be involved in the traumatized patient.

There are no specific signs or symptoms attributable to tracheobronchial injury. These injuries are often associated with other significant chest injuries, including pneumothorax, esophageal rupture, cardiac injury, and spinal injury. The diagnosis is usually obtained by performing a CT scan of the chest (this would be part of a trauma series including the head, neck, chest, abdomen, and pelvis). Direct visualization of the tracheobronchial tree can be performed using a flexible bronchoscope, and, if necessary, surgery may be required to deal with ruptures or strictures.

The surgical mortality rate for treatment on tracheobronchial injuries is relatively low; however, many of these do not occur in isolation, and in many instances, due to the severity of the injury, death occurs at the time of the injury.

Pharynx and Larynx

The pharynx is a common pathway for air and food, and it connects respiratory and digestive compartments in the head with similar compartments in the lower neck (see pp. 584-592).

The larynx is the upper end of the lower airway. It is continuous with the trachea below and the pharynx posterosuperiorly (see pp. 592-604).

Thyroid and parathyroid glands

The thyroid and parathyroid glands are endocrine glands positioned anteriorly in the neck (Fig. 8.160).

Both glands begin as pharyngeal outgrowths that migrate caudally to their final position as development continues.

The thyroid gland is a large, unpaired gland, while the parathyroid glands, usually four in number, are small and are on the posterior surface of the thyroid gland.

Thyroid gland

The thyroid gland is anterior in the neck below and lateral to the thyroid cartilage (Fig. 8.160). It consists of two lateral **lobes** (which cover the anterolateral surfaces of the trachea, the cricoid cartilage, and the lower part of the thyroid cartilage) with an **isthmus** that connects the lateral lobes and crosses the anterior surfaces of the second and third tracheal cartilages.

Lying deep to the sternohyoid, sternothyroid, and omohyoid muscles, the thyroid gland is in the visceral compartment of the neck (Fig. 8.160A). This compartment also includes the pharynx, trachea, and esophagus and is surrounded by the pretracheal layers of fascia.

The thyroid gland arises as a median outgrowth from the floor of the pharynx near the base of the tongue. The foramen cecum of the tongue indicates the site of origin and the thyroglossal duct marks the path of migration of the thyroid gland to its final adult location. The thyroglossal duct usually disappears early in development, but remnants may persist as a cyst or as a connection to the foramen cecum (i.e., a fistula).

There may also be a functional thyroid gland:

- associated with the tongue (a lingual thyroid);
- anywhere along the path of migration of the thyroid gland; or
- extending upward from the gland along the path of the thyroglossal duct (a pyramidal lobe).

Arterial supply

Two major arteries supply the thyroid gland.

Superior thyroid artery. The superior thyroid artery is the first branch of the external carotid artery (Fig. 8.161). It descends, passing along the lateral margin of the thyrohyoid muscle, to reach the superior pole of the lateral lobe of the gland where it divides into anterior and posterior glandular branches:

- The **anterior glandular branch** passes along the superior border of the thyroid gland and anastomoses with its twin from the opposite side across the isthmus (Fig. 8.161).
- The **posterior glandular branch** passes to the posterior side of the gland and may anastomose with the inferior thyroid artery (Fig. 8.162).

Inferior thyroid artery. The **inferior thyroid artery** is a branch of the **thyrocervical trunk,** which arises from the first part of the subclavian artery (Figs. 8.161, 8.162). It ascends along the medial edge of the anterior scalene muscle, passes posteriorly to the carotid sheath, and reaches the inferior pole of the lateral lobe of the thyroid gland.

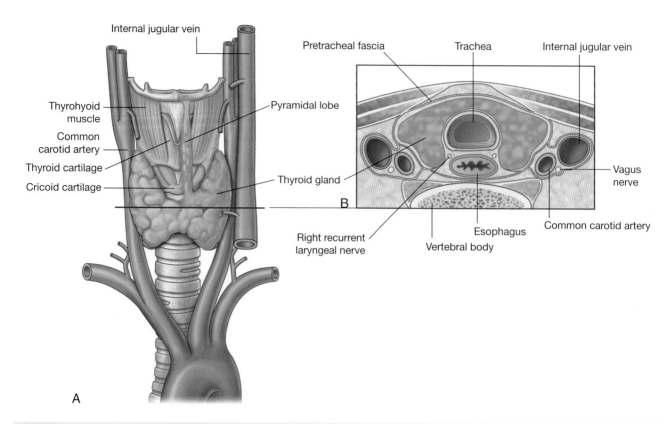

Fig. 8.160 Thyroid gland in the anterior triangle of neck. **A.** Anterior view. **B.** Transverse view showing trachea and esophagus below vertebral level CVI.

At the thyroid gland the inferior thyroid artery divides into an:

- inferior branch, which supplies the lower part of the thyroid gland and anastomoses with the posterior branch of the superior thyroid artery; and
- an ascending branch, which supplies the parathyroid glands.

Occasionally, a small **thyroid ima artery** arises from the brachiocephalic trunk or the arch of the aorta and ascends on the anterior surface of the trachea to supply the thyroid gland.

Venous and lymphatic drainage

Three veins drain the thyroid gland (Fig. 8.161):

- The **superior thyroid vein** primarily drains the area supplied by the superior thyroid artery.
- The **middle** and **inferior thyroid veins** drain the rest of the thyroid gland.

The superior and middle thyroid veins drain into the internal jugular vein, and the inferior thyroid veins empty into the right and left brachiocephalic veins, respectively.

Lymphatic drainage of the thyroid gland is into nodes beside the trachea (paratracheal nodes) and to deep cervical nodes inferior to the omohyoid muscle along the internal jugular vein.

Recurrent laryngeal nerves

The thyroid gland is closely related to the recurrent laryngeal nerves. After branching from the vagus nerve [X] and looping around the subclavian artery on the right and the arch of the aorta on the left, the **recurrent laryngeal nerves** ascend in a groove on each side between the trachea and esophagus (Fig. 8.162). They pass deep to the posteromedial surface of the lateral lobes of the thyroid gland and enter the larynx by passing deep to the lower margin of the inferior constrictor of the pharynx.

Together with branches of the inferior thyroid arteries, the recurrent laryngeal nerves are clearly related to and may pass through ligaments, one on each side, that bind the thyroid gland to the trachea and to the cricoid cartilage of the larynx. These relationships need to be considered when surgically removing or manipulating the thyroid gland.

Parathyroid glands

The parathyroid glands are two pairs of small, ovoid, yellowish structures on the deep surface of the lateral lobes of the

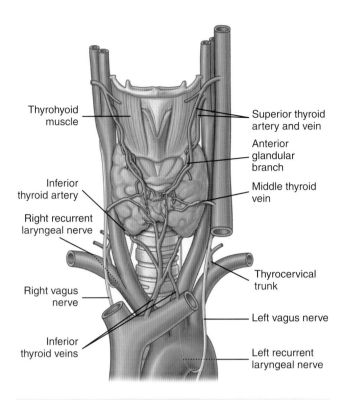

Thyrohyoid muscle

Superior thyroid artery and vein

Anterior glandular branch

Inferior thyroid artery

Middle thyroid vein

Right recurrent laryngeal nerve

Right vagus nerve

Thyrocervical trunk

Left vagus nerve

Inferior thyroid veins

Left recurrent laryngeal nerve

Fig. 8.161 Vasculature of the thyroid: anterior view.

thyroid gland. They are designated as the superior and inferior parathyroid glands (Fig. 8.162). However, their position is quite variable and they may be anywhere from the carotid bifurcation superiorly to the mediastinum inferiorly.

Derived from the third (the inferior parathyroid glands) and fourth (the superior parathyroid glands) pharyngeal pouches, these paired structures migrate to their final adult position and are named accordingly.

The arteries supplying the parathyroid glands are usually the inferior thyroid arteries, and venous and lymphatic drainage follows that described for the thyroid gland.

Clinical app

Thyroidectomy

A thyroidectomy is a relatively common surgical procedure. In most cases it involves excision of part or most of the thyroid gland, leaving some gland behind. This surgical procedure is usually carried out for benign diseases, such as multinodular goiter. However, thyroid carcinoma, albeit rare, is also an indication for thyroidectomy.

Given the location of the thyroid gland, there is a possibility of damaging other structures when carrying out a thyroidectomy, namely the parathyroid glands (which may be excised en masse with the thyroid gland), the recurrent laryngeal nerve, and the sympathetic trunk.

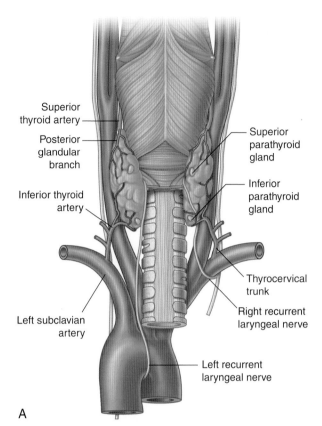

Superior thyroid artery

Posterior glandular branch

Inferior thyroid artery

Superior parathyroid gland

Inferior parathyroid gland

Thyrocervical trunk

Right recurrent laryngeal nerve

Left subclavian artery

Left recurrent laryngeal nerve

A

Left lobe of thyroid gland

Parathyroid gland

B

Fig. 8.162 Superior and inferior thyroid arteries and left and right recurrent laryngeal nerves. **A.** Posterior view. **B.** Surgical (anterolateral) view of parathyroid gland with left lobe of thyroid retracted.

Location of structures in subdivisions of the anterior triangle of the neck

The regional location of major structures in the anterior triangle of the neck is summarized in Table 8.14. Structures can be identified as being within a specific subdivision, passing into a specific subdivision from outside the area, originating in one subdivision and passing to another subdivision, or passing through several subdivisions while traversing the region.

Clinical app

Goiter

One of the commonest disorders of the thyroid gland is a **multinodular goiter,** which is a diffuse irregular enlargement of the thyroid gland with areas of thyroid hypertrophy and colloid cyst formation. Most patients are euthyroid (i.e., have normal serum thyroxine levels). The typical symptom is a diffuse mass in the neck, which may be managed medically or may need surgical excision if the mass is large enough to affect the patient's life or cause respiratory problems.

Surface anatomy
How to find the thyroid gland

The left and right lobes of the thyroid gland are in the anterior triangles in the lower neck on either side of the airway and digestive tract inferior to the position of the oblique line of the thyroid cartilage (Fig. 8.163). In fact, the sternothyroid muscles, which attach superiorly to the oblique lines, lie anterior to the lobes of the thyroid gland and prevent the lobes from moving upward in the neck.

The lobes of the thyroid gland can be most easily palpated by finding the thyroid prominence and arch of the cricoid cartilage and then feeling posterolateral to the larynx.

The isthmus of the thyroid gland crosses anterior to the upper end of the trachea and can be easily palpated in the midline inferior to the arch of the cricoid.

The presence of the isthmus of the thyroid gland makes palpating the tracheal cartilages difficult in the neck. Also, the presence of the isthmus of the thyroid gland and the associated vessels found in and crossing the midline makes it difficult to artificially enter the airway anteriorly through the trachea. This procedure, a tracheostomy, is a surgical procedure.

Position of oblique line on thyroid cartilage

Hyoid bone
Thyroid notch
Laryngeal prominence
Median cricothyroid ligament
Arch of cricoid

A   B

Right lobe of thyroid gland   Left lobe of thyroid gland
Isthmus of thyroid gland

Fig. 8.163 How to find the thyroid gland. **A.** In a woman, anterior view of Neck. **B.** In a man, anterior view of neck.

Clinical app

Hyperparathyroidism

Hyperparathyroidism involves the excess production of parathyroid hormone, which may be in response to a tumor within a parathyroid gland or as a secondary response due to low calcium levels.

Clinical app

Ectopic parathyroid glands

The parathyroid glands develop from the third and fourth pharyngeal pouches and translocate to their more adult locations during development. The position of the glands can be highly variable, sometimes being situated high in the neck or in the thorax.

Posterior triangle of the neck

The posterior triangle of the neck is on the lateral aspect of the neck in direct continuity with the upper limb. It is bordered:

- anteriorly by the posterior edge of the sternocleidomastoid muscle;
- posteriorly by the anterior edge of the trapezius muscle;
- basally by the middle one-third of the clavicle; and
- apically by the occipital bone just posterior to the mastoid process where the attachments of the trapezius and sternocleidomastoid come together (Fig. 8.164).

The roof of the posterior triangle consists of an investing layer of cervical fascia that surrounds the sternocleidomastoid and trapezius muscles as it passes through the region.

The muscular floor of the posterior triangle is covered by the prevertebral layer of cervical fascia and, from superior to inferior, consists of the splenius capitis, levator scapulae, and the posterior, middle, and anterior scalene muscles.

Muscles

Numerous muscles participate in forming the borders and floor of the posterior triangle of the neck (Table 8.15).

In addition, the **omohyoid** muscle passes across the inferior part of the posterior triangle before disappearing under the sternocleidomastoid muscle and emerging in the anterior triangle (Table 8.15, Fig. 8.165). It is enclosed in the investing layer of cervical fascia and crosses the posterior triangle from lateral to medial as it continues in a superior direction. It has two bellies connected by a tendon, which is anchored by a fascial sling to the clavicle:

Table 8.14 Subdivisions of the anterior triangle of the neck—a regional approach

Subdivision	Boundaries	Contents
Submental triangle (unpaired)	Mandibular symphysis; anterior belly of digastric muscle; body of hyoid bone	Submental lymph nodes; tributaries forming the anterior jugular vein
Submandibular triangle (paired)	Lower border of mandible; anterior belly of digastric muscle; posterior belly of digastric muscle	Submandibular gland; submandibular lymph nodes; hypoglossal nerve [XII]; mylohyoid nerve; facial artery and vein
Carotid triangle (paired)	Posterior belly of digastric muscle; superior belly of omohyoid muscle; anterior border of sternocleidomastoid muscle	Tributaries to common facial vein; cervical branch of facial nerve [VII]; common carotid artery; external and internal carotid arteries; superior thyroid; ascending pharyngeal; lingual, facial, and occipital arteries; internal jugular vein; vagus [X], accessory [XI], and hypoglossal [XII] nerves; superior and inferior roots of ansa cervicalis; transverse cervical nerve
Muscular triangle (paired)	Midline of neck; superior belly of omohyoid muscle; anterior border of sternocleidomastoid muscle	Sternohyoid, omohyoid, sternothyroid, and thyrohyoid muscles; thyroid and parathyroid glands; pharynx

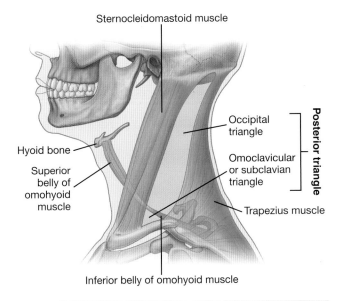

Fig. 8.164 Borders of the posterior triangle of the neck.

- The **superior belly** is in the anterior triangle.
- The **inferior belly** crosses the posterior triangle, subdividing it into a small, **omoclavicular or subclavian triangle** inferiorly and a much larger **occipital triangle** superiorly.

Vessels

External jugular vein

One of the most superficial structures passing through the posterior triangle of the neck is the external jugular vein (Fig. 8.166). This large vein forms near the angle of mandible, when the posterior branch of the retromandibular and posterior auricular veins join, and descends through the neck in the superficial fascia.

After crossing the sternocleidomastoid muscle, the external jugular vein enters the posterior triangle and continues its vertical descent.

In the lower part of the posterior triangle, the external jugular vein pierces the investing layer of cervical fascia and ends in the subclavian vein.

Tributaries to the external jugular vein, while it traverses the posterior triangle of the neck, include the transverse cervical, suprascapular, and anterior jugular veins.

Subclavian artery and its branches

Several arteries are found within the boundaries of the posterior triangle of the neck. The largest is the third part of the subclavian artery as it crosses the base of the posterior triangle (Fig. 8.167).

The **first part of the subclavian artery** ascends to the medial border of the anterior scalene muscle from either the brachiocephalic trunk on the right side or directly from the arch of the aorta on the left side. It has numerous branches.

The **second part of the subclavian artery** passes laterally between the anterior and middle scalene muscles, and one branch may arise from it.

The **third part of the subclavian artery** emerges from between the anterior and middle scalene muscles to cross the base of the posterior triangle (see Fig. 8.167). It extends from the lateral border of the anterior scalene muscle to the lateral border of rib I where it becomes the **axillary artery** and continues into the upper limb.

A single branch (the **dorsal scapular artery**) may arise from the third part of the subclavian artery. This branch passes posterolaterally to reach the superior angle of the scapula where it descends along the medial border of the scapula posterior to the rhomboid muscles.

Transverse cervical and suprascapular arteries

Two other small arteries also cross the base of the posterior triangle. These are the transverse cervical and the suprascapular arteries (see Fig. 8.167). They are both branches of the thyrocervical trunk, which arises from the first part of the subclavian artery.

After branching from the thyrocervical trunk, the **transverse cervical artery** passes laterally and slightly posteriorly across the base of the posterior triangle anterior to the anterior scalene muscle and the brachial plexus. Reaching the

Table 8.15 Muscles associated with the posterior triangle of the neck (parentheses indicate possible involvement)

Muscle	Origin	Insertion	Innervation	Function
Sternocleidomastoid —Sternal head	Upper part of anterior surface of manubrium of sternum	Lateral one-half of superior nuchal line	Accessory nerve [XI] and branches from anterior rami of C2 to C3 (C4)	Individually—will tilt head toward shoulder on same side, rotating head to turn face to opposite side; acting together, draw head forward
—Clavicular head	Superior surface of medial one-third of clavicle	Lateral surface of mastoid process		
Trapezius	Superior nuchal line; external occipital protuberance; ligamentum nuchae; spinous processes of vertebrae CVII to TXII	Lateral one-third of clavicle; acromion; spine of scapula	Motor—accessory nerve [XI]; proprioception—C3 and C4	Assists in rotating the scapula during abduction of humerus above horizontal; upper fibers—elevate, middle fibers—adduct, lower fibers—depress scapula
Splenius capitis	Lower half of ligamentum nuchae; spinous processes of vertebrae CVII to TIV	Mastoid process; skull below lateral one-third of superior nuchal line	Posterior rami of middle cervical nerves	Together, draw head backward; individually, draw and rotate head to one side (turn face to same side)
Levator scapulae	Transverse processes of CI to CIV	Upper part of medial border of scapula	C3, C4, and dorsal scapular nerve (C4, C5)	Elevates scapula
Posterior scalene	Posterior tubercles of transverse processes of vertebrae CIV to CVI	Upper surface of rib II	Anterior rami of C5 to C7	Elevation of rib II
Middle scalene	Transverse processes of vertebrae CII to CVII	Upper surface of rib I posterior to the groove for the subclavian artery	Anterior rami of C3 to C7	Elevation of rib I
Anterior scalene	Anterior tubercles of the transverse processes of vertebrae CIII to CVI	Scalene tubercle and upper surface of rib I	Anterior rami of C4 to C7	Elevation of rib I
Omohyoid	Superior border of scapula medial to scapular notch	Inferior border of body of hyoid bone	Ansa cervicalis; anterior rami of C1 to C3	Depress the hyoid bone

Fig. 8.165 Muscles of the posterior triangle of the neck.

Sternocleidomastoid muscle
Splenius capitis muscle
Levator scapulae muscle
Anterior scalene muscle
Posterior scalene muscle
Middle scalene muscle
Trapezius muscle
Clavicle
Acromion of scapula
Inferior belly of omohyoid muscle

Fig. 8.166 External jugular vein in the posterior triangle of the neck.

Posterior auricular vein
Retromandibular vein
External jugular vein
Posterior external jugular vein
Anterior jugular vein
Trapezius muscle
Transverse cervical vein
Sternocleidomastoid muscle

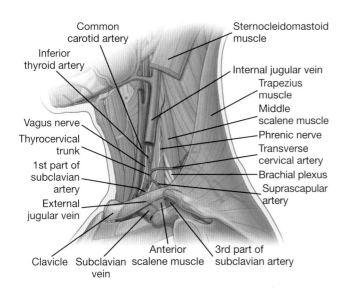

Common carotid artery
Inferior thyroid artery
Vagus nerve
Thyrocervical trunk
1st part of subclavian artery
External jugular vein
Clavicle   Subclavian vein
Anterior scalene muscle
3rd part of subclavian artery
Sternocleidomastoid muscle
Internal jugular vein
Trapezius muscle
Middle scalene muscle
Phrenic nerve
Transverse cervical artery
Brachial plexus
Suprascapular artery

Fig. 8.167 Arteries in the posterior triangle of the neck.

deep surface of the trapezius muscle, it divides into superficial and deep branches:

- The **superficial branch** continues on the deep surface of the trapezius muscle.
- The **deep branch** continues on the deep surface of the rhomboid muscles near the medial border of the scapula.

The **suprascapular artery,** also a branch of the thyrocervical trunk, passes laterally, in a slightly downward direction across the lowest part of the posterior triangle, and ends up posterior to the clavicle (see Fig. 8.167). Approaching the scapula, it passes over the superior transverse scapular ligament and distributes branches to muscles on the posterior surface of the scapula.

Veins

Veins accompany all the arteries described previously.

The **subclavian vein** is a continuation of the axillary vein and begins at the lateral border of rib I. It crosses the base of the posterior triangle, and the external jugular and possibly the suprascapular and transverse cervical veins enter it. It ends by joining with the internal jugular vein to form the brachiocephalic vein near the sternoclavicular joint. In the posterior triangle it is anterior to, and slightly lower than, the subclavian artery and passes anterior to the anterior scalene muscle.

Transverse cervical and suprascapular veins travel with each of the similarly named arteries. These veins become tributaries to either the external jugular vein or the initial part of the subclavian vein.

Nerves

A variety of nerves pass through or are within the posterior triangle (Fig. 8.168). These include the accessory nerve [XI], branches of the cervical plexus, components forming the brachial plexus, and branches of the brachial plexus.

Accessory nerve

The accessory nerve [XI] exits the cranial cavity through the jugular foramen. It descends through the neck in a posterior direction to reach the anterior border of the sternocleidomastoid muscle. Passing either deep to or through and innervating the sternocleidomastoid muscle, the accessory nerve [XI] continues to descend and enters the posterior triangle (Fig. 8.168). It crosses the posterior triangle, still in an obliquely downward direction, within the investing layer of cervical fascia as this fascia crosses between the sternocleidomastoid and trapezius muscles. When the accessory nerve [XI] reaches the anterior border of the trapezius muscle, it

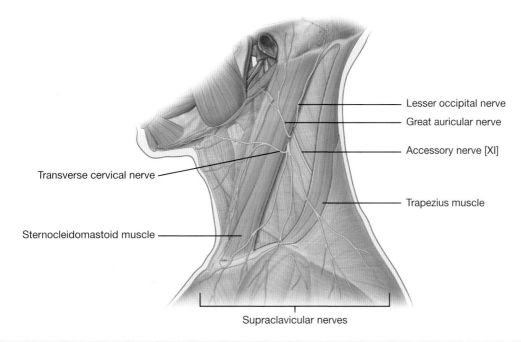

Transverse cervical nerve
Sternocleidomastoid muscle
Lesser occipital nerve
Great auricular nerve
Accessory nerve [XI]
Trapezius muscle
Supraclavicular nerves

Fig. 8.168 Accessory nerve in the posterior triangle of the neck.

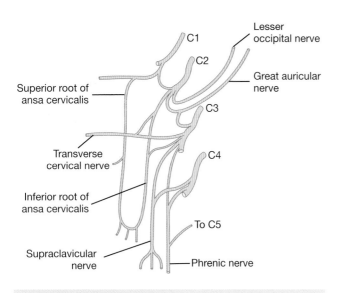

Superior root of ansa cervicalis

Transverse cervical nerve

Inferior root of ansa cervicalis

Supraclavicular nerve

C1

C2

C3

C4

To C5

Lesser occipital nerve

Great auricular nerve

Phrenic nerve

Fig. 8.169 Cervical plexus.

continues on the deep surface of the trapezius and innervates it. The superficial location of the accessory nerve as it crosses the posterior triangle makes it susceptible to injury.

Cervical plexus

The cervical plexus is formed by the anterior rami of cervical nerves C1 to C4 (Figs. 8.168, 8.169).

The cervical plexus forms in the substance of the muscles, making up the floor of the posterior triangle within the prevertebral layer of cervical fascia, and consists of muscular (or deep) and cutaneous (or superficial) branches.

Muscular branches

Muscular (deep) branches of the cervical plexus distribute to several groups of muscles. A major branch is the **phrenic nerve**, which supplies the diaphragm with both sensory and motor

innervation (Fig. 8.169). It arises from the anterior rami of cervical nerves C3 to C5. Hooking around the upper lateral border of the anterior scalene muscle, the nerve continues inferiorly across the anterior surface of the anterior scalene within the prevertebral fascia to enter the thorax (see Fig. 8.167). As the nerve descends in the neck, it is "pinned" to the anterior scalene muscle by the transverse cervical and suprascapular arteries.

Several muscular branches of the cervical plexus supply prevertebral and lateral vertebral muscles, including the rectus capitis anterior, rectus capitis lateralis, longus colli, and longus capitis (Table 8.16, Fig. 8.170).

The cervical plexus also contributes to the formation of the superior and inferior roots of the ansa cervicalis (Fig. 8.169). This loop of nerves receives contributions from the anterior rami of the cervical nerves C1 to C3 and innervates the infrahyoid muscles.

Cutaneous branches

Cutaneous (superficial) branches of the cervical plexus are visible in the posterior triangle as they pass outward from the posterior border of the sternocleidomastoid muscle (Figs. 8.168, 8.169):

- The **lesser occipital nerve** consists of contributions from cervical nerve C2, ascends along the posterior border of the sternocleidomastoid muscle, and distributes to the skin of the neck and scalp posterior to the ear.
- The **great auricular nerve** consists of branches from cervical nerves C2 and C3 (see Fig. 8.169), emerges from the posterior border of the sternocleidomastoid muscle, and ascends across the muscle to the base of the ear, supplying the skin of the parotid region, the ear, and the mastoid area.

Muscle	Origin	Insertion	Innervation	Function
Rectus capitis anterior	Anterior surface of lateral part of atlas and its transverse process	Inferior surface of basilar part of occipital bone	Branches from anterior rami of C1, C2	Flexes head at atlanto-occipital joint
Rectus capitis lateralis	Superior surface of transverse process of atlas	Inferior surface of jugular process of occipital bone	Branches from anterior rami of C1, C2	Flexes head laterally to same side
Longus colli —Superior oblique part	Anterior tubercles of transverse processes of vertebrae CIII to CV	Tubercle of anterior arch of atlas	Branches from anterior rami of C2 to C6	Flexes neck anteriorly and laterally and slight rotation to opposite side
—Inferior oblique part	Anterior surface of bodies of vertebrae TI, TII, and maybe TIII	Anterior tubercles of transverse processes of vertebrae CV and CVI		
—Vertical part	Anterior surface of bodies of TI to TIII and CV to CVII	Anterior surface of bodies of vertebrae CII to CIV		
Longus capitis	Tendinous slips to transverse processes of vertebrae CIII to CVI	Inferior surface of basilar part of occipital bone	Branches from anterior rami of C1 to C3	Flexes the head

Table 8.16 Prevertebral and lateral muscles

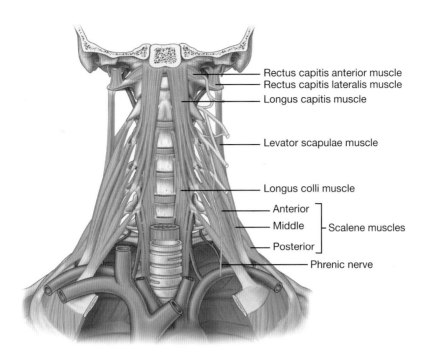

Fig. 8.170 Prevertebral and lateral vertebral muscles supplied by cervical plexus.

Rectus capitis anterior muscle
Rectus capitis lateralis muscle
Longus capitis muscle
Levator scapulae muscle
Longus colli muscle
Anterior ⎤
Middle ⎬ Scalene muscles
Posterior ⎦
Phrenic nerve

- The **transverse cervical nerve** consists of branches from the cervical nerves C2 and C3 (see Fig. 8.169), passes around the midpart of the sternocleidomastoid muscle, and continues horizontally across the muscle to supply the lateral and anterior parts of the neck.
- The **supraclavicular nerves** are a group of cutaneous nerves from cervical nerves C3 and C4 (see Fig. 8.169) that, after emerging from beneath the posterior border of the sternocleidomastoid muscle, descend and supply the skin over the clavicle and shoulder as far inferiorly as rib II.

Brachial plexus

The brachial plexus forms from the anterior rami of cervical nerves C5 to C8 and thoracic nerve T1. The contributions of each of these nerves, which are between the anterior and middle scalene muscles, are the **roots** of the brachial plexus. As the roots emerge from between these muscles, they form the next component of the brachial plexus (the **trunks**). The anterior rami of C5 and C6 form the upper trunk; the anterior ramus of C7 forms the middle trunk; and the anterior rami of C8 and T1 form the lower trunk.

The trunks cross the base of the posterior triangle (Fig. 8.167). Several branches of the brachial plexus may be visible in the posterior triangle. These include the:

- **dorsal scapular nerve** to the rhomboid muscles,
- **long thoracic nerve** to the serratus anterior muscle,
- nerve to the subclavius muscle, and
- **suprascapular nerve** to the supraspinatus and infraspinatus muscles.

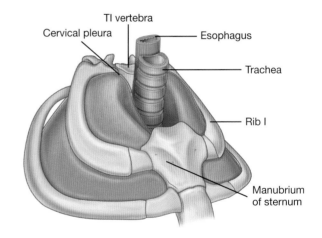

TI vertebra
Cervical pleura
Esophagus
Trachea
Rib I
Manubrium of sternum

Fig. 8.171 Root of the neck.

Root of the neck

The root of the neck (Fig. 8.171) is the area immediately superior to the superior thoracic aperture and axillary inlets. It is bounded by:

- the top of the manubrium of sternum and superior margin of the clavicle anteriorly, and
- the top of the thoracic vertebra TI and the superior margin of the scapula to the coracoid process posteriorly.

It contains structures passing between the neck, thorax, and upper limb. There is also an extension of the thoracic cavity projecting into the root of the neck. This consists of an

577

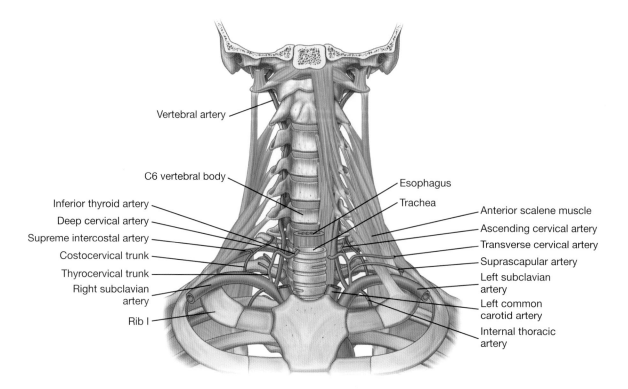

Vertebral artery

C6 vertebral body

Inferior thyroid artery
Deep cervical artery
Supreme intercostal artery
Costocervical trunk
Thyrocervical trunk
Right subclavian artery
Rib I

Esophagus
Trachea
Anterior scalene muscle
Ascending cervical artery
Transverse cervical artery
Suprascapular artery
Left subclavian artery
Left common carotid artery
Internal thoracic artery

Fig. 8.172 Vasculature of the root of the neck.

upward projection of the pleural cavity, on both sides, and includes the cervical part of the parietal pleura (cupula) and the apical part of the superior lobe of each lung.

Anteriorly, the pleural cavity extends above the top of the manubrium of sternum and superior border of rib I, while posteriorly, due to the downward slope of the superior thoracic aperture, the pleural cavity remains below the top of vertebra TI.

Vessels

Subclavian arteries

The subclavian arteries on both sides arch upward out of the thorax to enter the root of the neck (Fig. 8.172).

The **right subclavian artery** begins posterior to the sternoclavicular joint as one of two terminal branches of the brachiocephalic trunk. It arches superiorly and laterally to pass anterior to the extension of the pleural cavity in the root of the neck and posterior to the anterior scalene muscle. Continuing laterally across rib I, it becomes the **axillary artery** as it crosses its lateral border.

The **left subclavian artery** begins lower in the thorax than the right subclavian artery as a direct branch of the arch of the aorta. Lying posterior to the left common carotid artery and lateral to the trachea, it ascends and arches laterally, passing anterior to the extension of the pleural cavity and posterior to the anterior scalene muscle. It continues laterally over rib I, and becomes the axillary artery as it crosses the lateral border of rib I.

Both subclavian arteries are divided into three parts by the anterior scalene muscle (Fig. 8.172):

- The first part extends from the origin of the artery to the anterior scalene muscle.
- The second part is the part of the artery posterior to the anterior scalene muscle.
- The third part is the part lateral to the anterior scalene muscle before the artery reaches the lateral border of rib I.

All branches from the right and left subclavian arteries arise from the first part of the artery, except in the case of one branch (the costocervical trunk) on the right side (Fig. 8.172). The branches include the vertebral artery, the thyrocervical trunk, the internal thoracic artery, and the costocervical trunk.

Vertebral artery

The **vertebral artery** is the first branch of the subclavian artery as it enters the root of the neck (Fig. 8.172). A large branch, arising from the first part of the subclavian artery medial to the anterior scalene muscle, it ascends and enters the foramen in the transverse process of vertebra CVI. Continuing to pass superiorly, the vertebral artery passes through the foramina of vertebrae CV to CI. At the superior border of vertebra CI, the artery turns medially and crosses the posterior arch of vertebra CI. From here it passes through the foramen magnum to enter the posterior cranial fossa.

Thyrocervical trunk

The second branch of the subclavian artery is the **thyrocervical trunk** (Fig. 8.172). It arises from the first part of the subclavian artery medial to the anterior scalene muscle and divides into three branches—the inferior thyroid, the transverse cervical, and the suprascapular arteries.

Inferior thyroid artery. The **inferior thyroid artery** (Fig. 8.172) is the superior continuation of the thyrocervical trunk. It ascends, anterior to the anterior scalene muscle, and eventually turns medially, crossing posterior to the carotid sheath and its contents, and anterior to the vertebral artery. Reaching the posterior surface of the thyroid gland, it supplies the thyroid gland.

When the inferior thyroid artery turns medially, it gives off an important branch (the **ascending cervical artery,** Fig. 8.172), which continues to ascend on the anterior surface of the prevertebral muscles, supplying these muscles and sending branches to the spinal cord.

Transverse cervical artery. The middle branch of the thyrocervical trunk is the **transverse cervical artery** (see Fig. 8.172). This branch passes laterally, across the anterior surface of the anterior scalene muscle and the phrenic nerve, and enters and crosses the base of the posterior triangle of the neck. It continues to the deep surface of the trapezius muscle, where it divides into superficial and deep branches:

- The **superficial branch** continues on the deep surface of the trapezius muscle.
- The **deep branch** continues on the deep surface of the rhomboid muscles near the medial border of the scapula.

Suprascapular artery. The lowest branch of the thyrocervical trunk is the **suprascapular artery** (see Fig. 8.172). This branch passes laterally, crossing anterior to the anterior scalene muscle, the phrenic nerve, the third part of the subclavian artery, and the trunks of the brachial plexus. At the superior border of the scapula, it crosses over the superior transverse scapular ligament and enters the supraspinatus fossa.

Internal thoracic artery

The third branch of the subclavian artery is the **internal thoracic artery** (see Fig. 8.172). This artery branches from the inferior edge of the subclavian artery and descends.

It passes posterior to the clavicle and the large veins in the region and anterior to the pleural cavity. It enters the thoracic cavity posterior to the ribs and anterior to the transversus thoracis muscle and continues to descend, giving off numerous branches.

Costocervical trunk

The final branch of the subclavian artery in the root of the neck is the **costocervical trunk** (see Fig. 8.172). It arises in a slightly different position, depending on the side:

- On the left, it arises from the first part of the subclavian artery, just medial to the anterior scalene muscle.
- On the right, it arises from the second part of the subclavian artery.

On both sides, the costocervical trunk ascends and passes posteriorly over the dome of the pleural cavity and continues in a posterior direction behind the anterior scalene muscle. Eventually it divides into two branches—the deep cervical and the supreme intercostal arteries:

- The **deep cervical artery** ascends in the back of the neck and anastomoses with the descending branch of the occipital artery.
- The **supreme intercostal artery** descends anterior to rib I and divides to form the posterior intercostal arteries for the first two intercostal spaces.

Veins

Numerous veins pass through the root of the neck. Small veins accompany each of the arteries described previously, and large veins form major drainage channels.

The **subclavian veins** begin at the lateral margin of rib I as continuations of the **axillary veins.** Passing medially on each side, just anterior to the anterior scalene muscles, each subclavian vein is joined by the internal jugular vein to form the brachiocephalic veins.

The only tributary to the subclavian veins are the external jugular veins.

The veins accompanying the numerous arteries in this region empty into other veins.

Nerves

Several nerves and components of the nervous system pass through the root of the neck.

Phrenic nerves

The phrenic nerves are branches of the cervical plexus and arise on each side as contributions from the anterior rami of cervical nerves C3 to C5 come together. Passing around the upper lateral border of each anterior scalene muscle, the phrenic nerves continue inferiorly across the anterior surface of each anterior scalene muscle within the prevertebral layer of cervical fascia (Fig. 8.173). Leaving the lower edge of the anterior scalene muscle, each phrenic nerve passes between the subclavian vein and artery to enter the thorax and continue to the diaphragm.

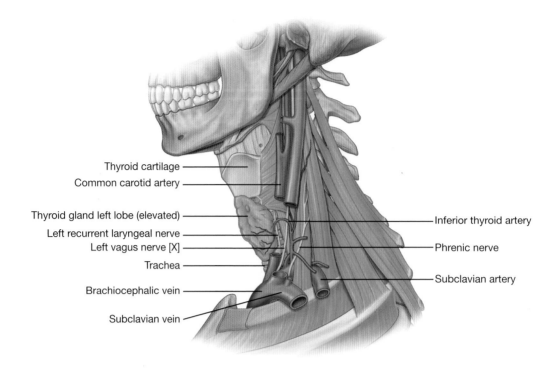

Thyroid cartilage
Common carotid artery

Thyroid gland left lobe (elevated)
Left recurrent laryngeal nerve
Left vagus nerve [X]
Trachea
Brachiocephalic vein
Subclavian vein

Inferior thyroid artery
Phrenic nerve
Subclavian artery

Fig. 8.173 Nerves in the root of the neck.

Vagus nerves [X]

The vagus nerves [X] descend through the neck within the carotid sheath, posterior to and just between the common carotid artery and the internal jugular vein.

In the lower part of the neck, the vagus nerves [X] give off cardiac branches, which continue downward and medially, passing posterior to the subclavian arteries to disappear into the thorax.

In the root of the neck, each vagus nerve [X] passes anterior to the subclavian artery and posterior to the subclavian vein as it enters the thorax (Fig. 8.173).

Recurrent laryngeal nerves

The right and left recurrent laryngeal nerves are visible as they originate in (the right recurrent laryngeal nerve), or pass through (the left recurrent laryngeal nerve), the root of the neck.

The **right recurrent laryngeal nerve** is a branch of the right vagus nerve [X] as it reaches the lower edge of the first part of the subclavian artery in the root of the neck. It passes around the subclavian artery and upward and medially in a groove between the trachea and the esophagus as it heads to the larynx.

The **left recurrent laryngeal nerve** is a branch of the left vagus nerve [X] as it crosses the arch of the aorta in the superior mediastinum. It passes below and behind the arch of the aorta and ascends beside the trachea to the larynx.

Clinical app

Recurrent laryngeal nerve palsy

Damage to either the right or left recurrent laryngeal nerves may lead initially to a hoarse voice and finally to an inability to speak. Recurrent laryngeal nerve palsy can occur from disruption of the nerves anywhere along their course. Furthermore, interruption of the vagus nerves before the division of the recurrent laryngeal nerves can also produce vocal symptoms.

Lung cancer in the apex of the right lung can affect the right recurrent laryngeal nerve, whereas cancers that infiltrate into the area between the pulmonary artery and aorta, an area known clinically as the "aortopulmonary window," can affect the left recurrent laryngeal nerve.

Assessment of the vocal cords is necessary before and after thyroid surgery because the recurrent laryngeal nerves are closely related to ligaments that bind the gland to the larynx and can be easily traumatized during surgical procedures.

Sympathetic nervous system

Various components of the sympathetic nervous system are visible as they pass through the root of the neck (Fig. 8.174). These include:

- the cervical part of the sympathetic trunk,
- the ganglia associated with the cervical part of the sympathetic trunk, and

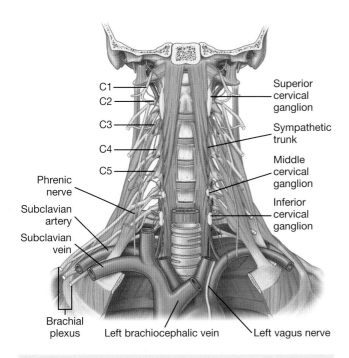

Fig. 8.174 Cervical part of the sympathetic trunk.

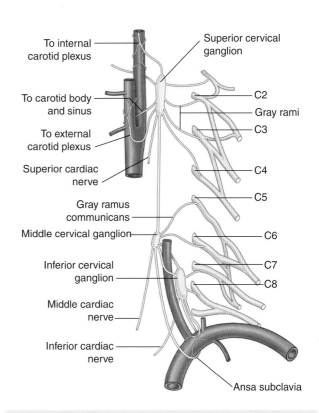

Fig. 8.175 Components of the sympathetic nervous system in the root of the neck.

▨ cardiac nerves branching from the cervical part of the sympathetic trunk (Fig. 8.174).

The sympathetic trunks are two parallel cords that run from the base of the skull to the coccyx. Along the way they are punctuated by ganglia, which are collections of neuronal cell bodies outside the CNS.

Cervical part of the sympathetic trunk

The **cervical part of the sympathetic trunk** is anterior to the longus colli and longus capitis muscles, and posterior to the common carotid artery in the carotid sheath and the internal carotid artery. It is connected to each cervical spinal nerve by a gray ramus communicans (Fig. 8.174). There are no white rami communicantes in the cervical region.

Ganglia

Three ganglia are usually described along the course of the sympathetic trunk in the cervical region, and in these ganglia ascending preganglionic sympathetic fibers from the upper thoracic spinal cord levels synapse with postganglionic sympathetic fibers. The postganglionic sympathetic fibers are distributed in branches from these ganglia.

Superior cervical ganglion. A very large **superior cervical ganglion** in the area of cervical vertebrae CI and CII marks the superior extent of the sympathetic trunk (Figs. 8.174, 8.175). Its branches pass to:

▨ the internal carotid and external carotid arteries, forming plexuses around these vessels,

▨ cervical spinal nerves C1 to C4 through gray rami communicantes,

▨ the pharynx, and

▨ the heart as **superior cardiac nerves**.

Middle cervical ganglion. A second ganglion inferior to the superior cervical ganglion along the course of the sympathetic trunk (the **middle cervical ganglion**) is encountered at about the level of cervical vertebra CVI (Figs. 8.174, 8.175). Branches from this ganglion pass to:

▨ cervical spinal nerves C5 and C6 through gray rami communicantes, and

▨ the heart as **middle cardiac nerves.**

Inferior cervical ganglion. At the lower end of the cervical part of the sympathetic trunk is another ganglion (the inferior cervical ganglion), which becomes very large when it combines with the first thoracic ganglion and forms the **cervicothoracic ganglion (stellate ganglion).** The inferior cervical ganglion (Figs. 8.174, 8.175) is anterior to the neck of rib I and the transverse process of cervical vertebra CVII, and posterior to the first part of the subclavian artery and the origin of the vertebral artery.

Branches from this ganglion pass to:

▨ spinal nerves C7 to T1 through gray rami communicantes,

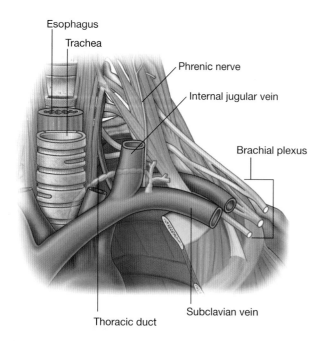

Fig. 8.176 Thoracic duct in the root of the neck.

- the vertebral artery, forming a plexus associated with this vessel, and
- the heart as **inferior cardiac nerves.**

This ganglion may also receive white rami communicantes from thoracic spinal nerve T1 and occasionally from T2.

Lymphatics

Thoracic duct

The **thoracic duct** is a major lymphatic channel that begins in the abdomen, passes superiorly through the thorax, and ends in the venous channels in the neck. It passes through the lower thoracic cavity in the midline with:

- the thoracic aorta on the left,
- the azygos vein on the right, and
- the esophagus anteriorly.

At about the level of thoracic vertebra TV the thoracic duct passes to the left and continues to ascend just to the left of the esophagus. It passes through the superior mediastinum and enters the root of the neck to the left of the esophagus (Fig. 8.176). Arching laterally, it passes posterior to the carotid sheath and turns inferiorly in front of the thyrocervical trunk, the phrenic nerve, and the vertebral artery.

The thoracic duct terminates in the junction between the left internal jugular and the left subclavian veins. Near its junction with the venous system it is joined by (Fig. 8.177):

- the **left jugular trunk,** which drains lymph from the left side of the head and neck;

- the **left subclavian trunk,** which drains lymph from the left upper limb; and
- occasionally, the **left bronchomediastinal trunk,** which drains lymph from the left half of the thoracic structures.

A similar confluence of three lymphatic trunks occurs on the right side of the body. Emptying into the junction between the right internal jugular and right subclavian veins are (Fig. 8.177):

- the **right jugular trunk** from the head and neck,
- the **right subclavian trunk** from the right upper limb, and
- occasionally, the **right bronchomediastinal trunk** carrying lymph from the structures in the right half of the thoracic cavity and the right upper intercostal spaces.

There is variability in how these trunks enter the veins. They may combine into a single right lymphatic duct to enter the venous system or enter as three separate trunks.

Lymphatics of the neck

A description of the organization of the lymphatic system in the neck becomes a summary of the lymphatic system in the head and neck. It is impossible to separate the two regions. The components of this system include superficial nodes around the head, superficial cervical nodes along the external jugular vein, and deep cervical nodes forming a chain along the internal jugular vein (Fig. 8.178).

The basic pattern of drainage is for superficial lymphatic vessels to drain to the superficial nodes. Some of these drain to the superficial cervical nodes on their way to the deep cervical nodes, and others drain directly to the deep cervical nodes.

Superficial lymph nodes

Five groups of superficial lymph nodes form a ring around the head and are primarily responsible for the lymphatic drainage of the face and scalp. Their pattern of drainage is very similar to the area of distribution of the arteries near their location.

Beginning posteriorly these groups are (Fig. 8.178):

- **occipital nodes** near the attachment of the trapezius muscle to the skull and associated with the occipital artery—lymphatic drainage is from the posterior scalp and neck;
- **mastoid nodes (retroauricular/posterior auricular nodes)** posterior to the ear near the attachment of the sternocleidomastoid muscle and associated with the posterior auricular artery—lymphatic drainage is from the posterolateral half of the scalp;
- **pre-auricular and parotid nodes** anterior to the ear and associated with the superficial temporal and transverse

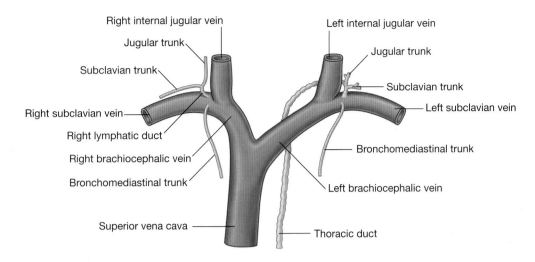

Fig. 8.177 Termination of lymphatic trunks in the root of the neck.

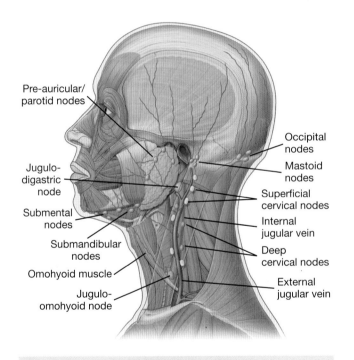

Fig. 8.178 Lymphatic system in the neck.

facial arteries—lymphatic drainage is from the anterior surface of the auricle, the anterolateral scalp, the upper half of the face, the eyelids, and the cheeks;

■ **submandibular nodes** inferior to the body of mandible and associated with the facial artery—lymphatic drainage is from structures along the path of the facial artery as high as the forehead, as well as the gingivae, the teeth, and the tongue; and

■ **submental nodes** inferior and posterior to the chin—lymphatic drainage is from the center part of the lower lip, the chin, the floor of the mouth, the tip of the tongue, and the lower incisor teeth.

Lymphatic flow from these superficial lymph nodes passes in several directions:

■ Drainage from the occipital and mastoid nodes passes to the superficial cervical nodes along the external jugular vein.
■ Drainage from the pre-auricular and parotid nodes, the submandibular nodes, and the submental nodes passes to the deep cervical nodes.

Superficial cervical lymph nodes

The **superficial cervical nodes** are a collection of lymph nodes along the external jugular vein on the superficial surface of the sternocleidomastoid muscle (see Fig. 8.178). They primarily receive lymphatic drainage from the posterior and posterolateral regions of the scalp through the occipital and mastoid nodes, and send lymphatic vessels in the direction of the deep cervical nodes.

Deep cervical lymph nodes

The **deep cervical nodes** are a collection of lymph nodes that form a chain along the internal jugular vein (see Fig. 8.178). They are divided into upper and lower groups where the intermediate tendon of the omohyoid muscle crosses the common carotid artery and the internal jugular vein.

The most superior node in the upper deep cervical group is the **jugulodigastric node** (see Fig. 8.178). This large node is where the posterior belly of the digastric muscle crosses the internal jugular vein and receives lymphatic drainage from the tonsils and tonsillar region.

Another large node, usually associated with the lower deep cervical group because it is at or just inferior to the intermediate tendon of the omohyoid muscle, is the **jugulo-omohyoid node** (see Fig. 8.178). This node receives lymphatic drainage from the tongue.

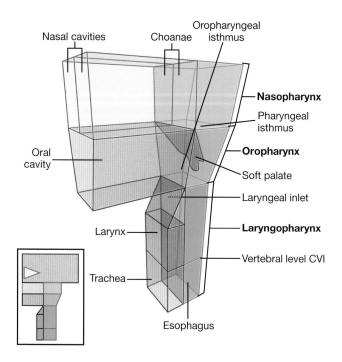

Fig. 8.179 Pharynx.

The deep cervical nodes eventually receive all lymphatic drainage from the head and neck either directly or through regional groups of nodes.

From the deep cervical nodes, lymphatic vessels form the right and left jugular trunks, which empty into the right lymphatic duct on the right side or the thoracic duct on the left side.

Clinical app

Clinical lymphatic drainage of the head and neck

Enlargement of the neck lymph nodes (cervical lymphadenopathy) is a common manifestation of disease processes that occur in the head and neck. Evaluation of cervical lymph nodes is extremely important in determining the nature and etiology of the primary disease process that has produced nodal enlargement. Examination of the lymph nodes often gives the clinician a clue as to the nature of the pathological process.

- Soft, tender, and inflamed lymph nodes suggest an acute inflammatory process, which is most likely to be infective.
- Firm, multinodular, large-volume rubbery nodes often suggest a diagnosis of lymphoma. Most cervical lymph nodes are easily palpable and suitable for biopsy to establish a tissue diagnosis.

A relatively simple "level" system of nodal enlargement has been designed that is extremely helpful in evaluating

---

Clinical app—cont'd

lymph node spread of primary head and neck tumors. Once the number of levels of nodes are determined, as well as the size of the lymph nodes, the best mode of treatment can be instituted. The lymph node level also enables a prognosis to be made. The levels are as follows:

- Level I—from the midline of the submental triangle up to the level of the submandibular gland.
- Level II—from the skull base to the level of the hyoid bone anteriorly to the posterior border of the sternocleidomastoid muscle.
- Level III—the inferior aspect of the hyoid bone to the bottom cricoid arch and anterior to the posterior border of the sternocleidomastoid up to the midline.
- Level IV—from the inferior aspect of the cricoid to the top of the manubrium of sternum and anterior to the posterior border of the sternocleidomastoid muscle.
- Level V—posterior to the sternocleidomastoid muscle and anterior to the trapezius muscle above the level of the clavicle.
- Level VI—below the hyoid bone and above the jugular (sternal) notch in the midline.
- Level VII—below the level of the jugular (sternal) notch.

PHARYNX

The pharynx is a musculofascial half-cylinder that links the oral and nasal cavities in the head to the larynx and esophagus in the neck (Fig. 8.179). The pharyngeal cavity is a common pathway for air and food.

The pharynx is attached above to the base of the skull and is continuous below, approximately at the level of vertebra CVI, with the top of the esophagus. The walls of the pharynx are attached anteriorly to the margins of the nasal cavities, oral cavity, and larynx. Based on these anterior relationships, the pharynx is subdivided into three regions—the nasopharynx, oropharynx, and laryngopharynx:

- The posterior apertures (choanae) of the nasal cavities open into the nasopharynx.
- The posterior opening of the oral cavity (oropharyngeal isthmus) opens into the oropharynx.
- The superior aperture of the larynx (laryngeal inlet) opens into the laryngopharynx.

In addition to these openings, the pharyngeal cavity is related anteriorly to the posterior one-third of the tongue and to the posterior aspect of the larynx. The pharyngotympanic tubes open into the lateral walls of the nasopharynx.

Lingual, pharyngeal, and palatine tonsils are on the deep surface of the pharyngeal walls.

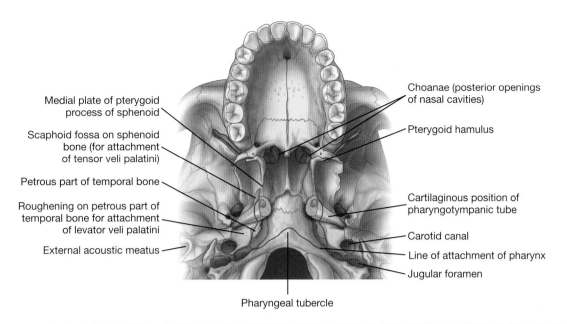

Medial plate of pterygoid process of sphenoid

Scaphoid fossa on sphenoid bone (for attachment of tensor veli palatini)

Petrous part of temporal bone

Roughening on petrous part of temporal bone for attachment of levator veli palatini

External acoustic meatus

Choanae (posterior openings of nasal cavities)

Pterygoid hamulus

Cartilaginous position of pharyngotympanic tube

Carotid canal

Line of attachment of pharynx

Jugular foramen

Pharyngeal tubercle

Fig. 8.180 Line of attachment of the pharynx to the base of the skull.

The pharynx is separated from the posteriorly positioned vertebral column by a thin retropharyngeal space containing loose connective tissue.

Although the soft palate is generally considered part of the roof of the oral cavity, it is also related to the pharynx. The soft palate is attached to the posterior margin of the hard palate and is a type of "flutter valve" that can:

- swing up (elevate) to close the pharyngeal isthmus and seal off the nasopharynx from the oropharynx; and
- swing down (depress) to close the oropharyngeal isthmus and seal off the oral cavity from the oropharynx.

Skeletal framework

The superior and anterior margins of the pharyngeal wall are attached to bone and cartilage, and to ligaments. The two sides of the pharyngeal wall are welded together posteriorly in the midline by a vertically oriented cord-like ligament (the pharyngeal raphe). This connective tissue structure descends from the pharyngeal tubercle on the base of the skull to the level of cervical vertebra CVI where the raphe blends with connective tissue in the posterior wall of the esophagus.

There is an irregular C-shaped line of pharyngeal wall attachment on the base of the skull (Fig. 8.180). The open part of the C faces the nasal cavities. Each arm of the C begins at the posterior margin of the medial plate of the pterygoid process of the sphenoid bone, just inferior to the cartilaginous part of the pharyngotympanic tube. The line crosses inferior to the pharyngotympanic tube and then passes onto the petrous part of the temporal bone where it is just medial to the roughening for the attachment of one of the muscles (levator veli palatini) of the soft palate. From

here, the line swings medially onto the occipital bone and joins the line from the other side at a prominent elevation of bone in the midline (the pharyngeal tubercle).

Anterior vertical line of attachment for the lateral pharyngeal walls

The vertical line of attachment for the lateral pharyngeal walls to structures related to the nasal and oral cavities and larynx is discontinuous and in three parts.

First part

On each side, the anterior line of attachment of the lateral pharyngeal wall begins superiorly on the posterior edge of the medial pterygoid plate of the sphenoid bone just inferior to where the pharyngotympanic tube lies against this plate (Fig. 8.181). It continues inferiorly along the edge of the medial plate of the pterygoid process and onto the pterygoid hamulus. From this point, the line descends along the pterygomandibular raphe to the mandible where this part of the line terminates.

The **pterygomandibular raphe** is a linear cord-like connective tissue ligament that spans the distance between the tip of the pterygoid hamulus and a triangular roughening immediately posterior to the third molar on the mandible (Fig. 8.181). It joins a muscle of the lateral pharyngeal wall (superior constrictor) with a muscle of the lateral wall of the oral cavity (buccinator).

Second part

The second part of the line of attachment of the lateral pharyngeal wall is related to the hyoid bone (Fig. 8.181). It begins on the lower aspect of the stylohyoid ligament, which connects

Fig. 8.181 Attachments of the lateral pharyngeal wall.

the tip of the styloid process of the temporal bone to the lesser horn of the hyoid bone. The line continues onto the lesser horn and then turns and runs posteriorly along the entire upper surface of the greater horn of the hyoid where it terminates.

Third part

The most inferior and third part of the line of attachment of the lateral pharyngeal wall begins superiorly on the superior tubercle of the thyroid cartilage, and descends along the oblique line to the inferior tubercle.

From the inferior tubercle, the line of attachment continues over the cricothyroid muscle along a tendinous thickening of fascia to the cricoid cartilage where it terminates.

Pharyngeal wall

The pharyngeal wall is formed by skeletal muscles and by fascia. Gaps between the muscles are reinforced by the fascia and provide routes for structures to pass through the wall.

Muscles

The muscles of the pharynx are organized into two groups based on the orientation of muscle fibers.

The constrictor muscles have fibers oriented in a circular direction relative to the pharyngeal wall, whereas the longitudinal muscles have fibers oriented vertically.

Constrictor muscles

The three constrictor muscles on each side are major contributors to the structure of the pharyngeal wall (Table 8.17, Fig. 8.182), and their names indicate their position—**superior, middle,** and **inferior constrictor muscles.** Posteriorly, the muscles from each side are joined together by the pharyngeal raphe (Fig. 8.182B). Anteriorly, these muscles attach to bones, cartilages, and ligaments related to the lateral margins of the nasal and oral cavities and the larynx.

The constrictor muscles overlap each other in a fashion resembling the walls of three flower pots stacked one on the other (Fig. 8.182A). The inferior constrictors overlap the lower margins of the middle constrictors and, in the same way, the middle constrictors overlap the superior constrictors.

Collectively, the muscles constrict or narrow the pharyngeal cavity.

When the constrictor muscles contract sequentially from top to bottom, as in swallowing, they move a bolus of food through the pharynx and into the esophagus.

All of the constrictors are innervated by the pharyngeal branch of the vagus nerve [X].

Longitudinal muscles

The three longitudinal muscles of the pharyngeal wall (Table 8.18, Fig. 8.183) are named according to their origins—**stylopharyngeus,** from the styloid process of the temporal bone; **salpingopharyngeus,** from the cartilaginous part of the pharyngotympanic tube (*salpinx* is Greek for "tube"); and **palatopharyngeus** from the soft palate. From their sites of origin, these muscles descend and attach into the pharyngeal wall.

Table 8.17 Constrictor muscles of the pharynx

Muscle	Posterior attachment	Anterior attachment	Innervation	Function
Superior constrictor	Pharyngeal raphe	Pterygomandibular raphe and adjacent bone on the mandible and pterygoid hamulus	Vagus nerve [X]	Constriction of pharynx
Middle constrictor	Pharyngeal raphe	Upper margin of greater horn of hyoid bone and adjacent margins of lesser horn and stylohyoid ligament	Vagus nerve [X]	Constriction of pharynx
Inferior constrictor	Pharyngeal raphe	Cricoid cartilage, oblique line of thyroid cartilage, and a ligament that spans between these attachments and crosses the cricothyroid muscle	Vagus nerve [X]	Constriction of pharynx

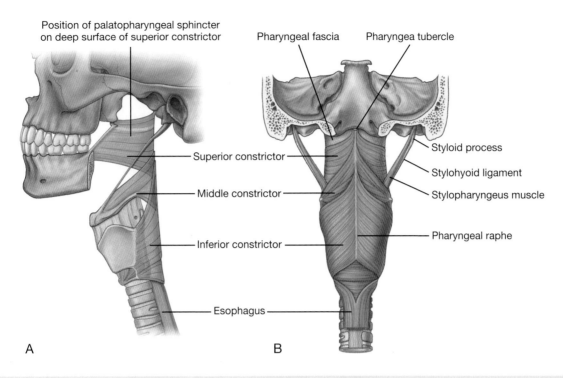

Position of palatopharyngeal sphincter on deep surface of superior constrictor

Pharyngeal fascia

Pharyngea tubercle

Superior constrictor

Middle constrictor

Inferior constrictor

Esophagus

Styloid process

Stylohyoid ligament

Stylopharyngeus muscle

Pharyngeal raphe

A

B

Fig. 8.182 Constrictor muscles of the pharynx. **A.** Lateral view. **B.** Posterior view.

Table 8.18 Longitudinal muscles of the pharynx

Muscle	Origin	Insertion	Innervation	Function
Stylopharyngeus	Medial side of base of styloid process	Pharyngeal wall	Glossopharyngeal nerve [IX]	Elevation of the pharynx
Salpingopharyngeus	Inferior aspect of pharyngeal end of pharyngotympanic tube	Pharyngeal wall	Vagus nerve [X]	Elevation of the pharynx
Palatopharyngeus	Upper surface of palatine aponeurosis	Pharyngeal wall	Vagus nerve [X]	Elevation of the pharynx; closure of the oropharyngeal isthmus

The longitudinal muscles elevate the pharyngeal wall or, during swallowing, pull the pharyngeal wall up and over a bolus of food being moved through the pharynx and into the esophagus.

Fascia

The pharyngeal fascia is separated into two layers, which sandwich the pharyngeal muscles between them:

- A thin layer (**buccopharyngeal fascia**) coats the outside of the muscular part of the wall and is a component of the pretracheal layer of cervical fascia (see p. 559).
- A much thicker layer (**pharyngobasilar fascia**) lines the inner surface.

The fascia reinforces the pharyngeal wall where muscle is deficient. This is particularly evident above the level of the superior constrictor where the pharyngeal wall is formed almost entirely of fascia (Fig. 8.184). This part of the wall is reinforced externally by muscles of the soft palate (tensor and levator veli palatini).

Gaps in the pharyngeal wall and structures passing through them

Gaps between muscles of the pharyngeal wall provide important routes for muscles and neurovascular tissues (Fig. 8.184).

Above the margin of superior constrictor, the pharyngeal wall is deficient in muscle and completed by pharyngeal fascia.

The tensor and levator veli palatini muscles of the soft palate initially descend from the base of the skull and are lateral to the pharyngeal fascia. In this position, they reinforce the pharyngeal wall:

- Levator veli palatini passes through the pharyngeal fascia inferior to the pharyngotympanic tube and enters the soft palate.

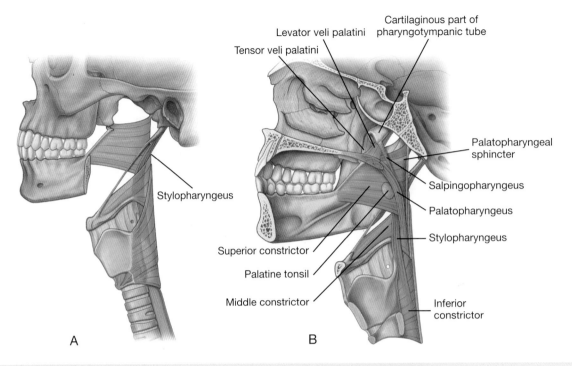

Fig. 8.183 Longitudinal muscles of the pharynx. **A.** Stylopharyngeus muscle. **B.** Medial view.

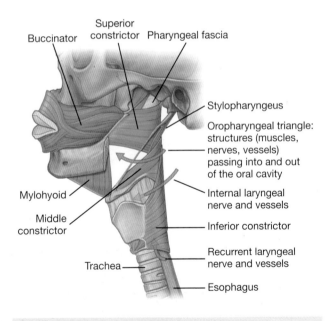

Fig. 8.184 Gaps between muscles in the pharyngeal wall.

■ The tendon of tensor veli palatini turns medially around the pterygoid hamulus and passes through the origin of the buccinator muscle to enter the soft palate.

One of the largest and most important apertures in the pharyngeal wall is between the superior and middle constrictor muscles of the pharynx and the posterior border of the mylohyoid muscle, which forms the floor of the mouth (Fig. 8.184). This triangular-shaped gap (**oropharyngeal**

triangle) not only enables stylopharyngeus to slip into the pharyngeal wall, but also allows muscles, nerves, and vessels to pass between regions lateral to the pharyngeal wall and the oral cavity, particularly to the tongue.

The gap between the middle and inferior constrictor muscles allows the internal laryngeal vessels and nerve access to the aperture in the thyrohyoid membrane to enter the larynx (Fig. 8.184).

The recurrent laryngeal nerves and accompanying inferior laryngeal vessels enter the larynx posterior to the inferior horn of the thyroid cartilage deep to the inferior margin of the inferior constrictor muscle (Fig. 8.184).

Nasopharynx

The nasopharynx is behind the posterior apertures (choanae) of the nasal cavities and above the level of the soft palate (Fig. 8.185). Its ceiling is formed by the sloping base of the skull and consists of the posterior part of the body of the sphenoid bone and the basal part of the occipital bone. The ceiling and lateral walls of the nasopharynx form a domed vault at the top of the pharyngeal cavity that is always open.

The cavity of the nasopharynx is continuous below with the cavity of the oropharynx at the pharyngeal isthmus (Fig. 8.185A). The position of the pharyngeal isthmus is marked on the pharyngeal wall by a mucosal fold caused by the underlying **palatopharyngeal sphincter,** which is part of the superior constrictor muscle.

Elevation of the soft palate and constriction of the palatopharyngeal sphincter closes the pharyngeal isthmus

Fig. 8.185 Mucosal features of the pharynx. **A.** Lateral view. **B.** Posterior view with the pharyngeal wall opened. **C.** Superior view.

during swallowing and separates the nasopharynx from the oropharynx.

There is a large collection of lymphoid tissue (the **pharyngeal tonsil**) in the mucosa covering the roof of the nasopharynx (Fig. 8.185A). Enlargement of this tonsil, known then as adenoids, can occlude the nasopharynx so that breathing is only possible through the oral cavity.

The most prominent features on each lateral wall of the nasopharynx are (Fig. 8.185A):

- the pharyngeal opening of the pharyngotympanic tube, and
- mucosal elevations and folds covering the end of the pharyngotympanic tube and the adjacent muscles.

The opening of the pharyngotympanic tube is posterior to and slightly above the level of the hard palate and lateral to the top of the soft palate.

Because the pharyngotympanic tube projects into the nasopharynx from a posterolateral direction, its posterior rim forms an elevation or bulge on the pharyngeal wall. Posterior to this tubal elevation (**torus tubarius**) is a deep recess (**pharyngeal recess**) (Fig. 8.185A,B).

Mucosal folds related to the pharyngotympanic tube include (Fig. 8.185A):

- the small vertical **salpingopharyngeal fold**, which descends from the tubal elevation and overlies **salpingopharyngeus muscle**; and
- a broad fold or elevation (**torus levatorius**) that appears to emerge from just under the opening of the pharyngotympanic tube, continues medially onto the upper surface of the soft palate, and overlies the levator veli palatini muscle.

Oropharynx

The oropharynx is posterior to the oral cavity, inferior to the level of the soft palate, and superior to the upper margin of the epiglottis (Fig. 8.185). The **palatoglossal folds** (arches), one on each side, that cover the **palatoglossal muscles,** mark the boundary between the oral cavity and the oropharynx. The arched opening between the two folds is the **oropharyngeal isthmus.** Just posterior and medial to these folds are another pair of folds (arches), the **palatopharyngeal folds,** one on each side, that overlie the **palatopharyngeus muscles** (see Fig. 8.185A).

The anterior wall of the oropharynx inferior to the oropharyngeal isthmus is formed by the upper part of the posterior one-third or pharyngeal part of the tongue. When holding liquid or solids in the oral cavity, the oropharyngeal isthmus is closed by depression of the soft palate, elevation of the back of the tongue, and movement toward the midline of the palatoglossal and palatopharyngeal folds. This allows

a person to breathe while chewing or manipulating material in the oral cavity.

On swallowing, the oropharyngeal isthmus is opened, the palate is elevated, the laryngeal cavity is closed, and the food or liquid is directed into the esophagus. A person cannot breathe and swallow at the same time because the airway is closed at two sites, the pharyngeal isthmus and the larynx.

Laryngopharynx

The laryngopharynx extends from the superior margin of the epiglottis to the top of the esophagus at the level of vertebra CVI (Fig. 8.185).

The laryngeal inlet opens into the anterior wall of the laryngopharynx. Inferior to the laryngeal inlet, the anterior wall consists of the posterior aspect of the larynx.

The cavity of the laryngopharynx is related anteriorly to a pair of mucosal pouches (**valleculae**), one on each side of the midline, between the base of the tongue and epiglottis (see Fig. 8.185C). The valleculae are depressions formed between a midline mucosal fold and two lateral folds that connect the tongue to the epiglottis.

There is another pair of mucosal recesses (**piriform fossae**) between the central part of the larynx and the more lateral lamina of the thyroid cartilage (see Fig. 8.185B,C). The piriform fossae form channels that direct solids and liquids from the oral cavity around the raised laryngeal inlet and into the esophagus.

Tonsils

Collections of lymphoid tissue in the mucosa of the pharynx surrounding the openings of the nasal and oral cavities (Waldeyer's tonsillar ring) are part of the body's defense system. The largest of these collections form distinct masses (**tonsils**). Tonsils occur mainly in three areas (Fig. 8.185):

- The pharyngeal tonsil, known as adenoids when enlarged, is in the midline on the roof of the nasopharynx.
- The palatine tonsils are on each side of the oropharynx between the palatoglossal and palatopharyngeal arches just posterior to the oropharyngeal isthmus. (The palatine tonsils are visible through the open mouth of a patient when the tongue is depressed.)
- The lingual tonsil refers collectively to numerous lymphoid nodules on the posterior one-third of the tongue.

Small lymphoid nodules also occur in the pharyngotympanic tube near its opening into the nasopharynx and on the upper surface of the soft palate.

Vessels

Arteries

Numerous vessels supply the pharyngeal wall (Fig. 8.186).

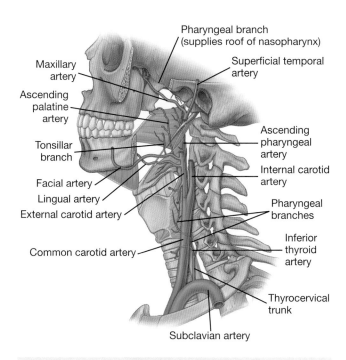

Fig. 8.186 Arterial supply of the pharynx.

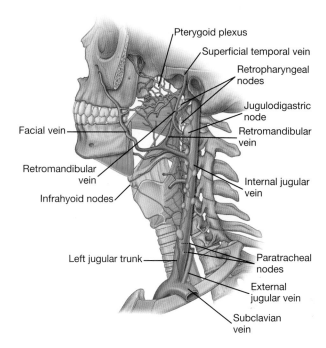

Fig. 8.187 Venous and lymphatic drainage of the pharynx.

Arteries that supply upper parts of the pharynx include:

- the ascending pharyngeal artery,
- the ascending palatine and tonsillar branches of the facial artery, and
- numerous branches of the maxillary and the lingual arteries.

All these vessels are from the external carotid artery.

Arteries that supply the lower parts of the pharynx include pharyngeal branches from the inferior thyroid artery, which originates from the thyrocervical trunk of the subclavian artery.

The major blood supply to the palatine tonsil is from the tonsillar branch of the facial artery, which penetrates the superior constrictor muscle.

Veins

Veins of the pharynx form a plexus, which drains superiorly into the pterygoid plexus in the infratemporal fossa and inferiorly into the facial and internal jugular veins (Fig. 8.187).

Lymphatics

Lymphatic vessels from the pharynx drain into the deep cervical nodes and include **retropharyngeal** (between nasopharynx and vertebral column), **paratracheal**, and **infrahyoid nodes** (Fig. 8.187).

The palatine tonsils drain through the pharyngeal wall into the jugulodigastric nodes in the region where the facial

vein drains into the internal jugular vein (and inferior to the posterior belly of the digastric muscle).

Nerves

Motor and most sensory innervation (except for the nasal region) of the pharynx is mainly through branches of the vagus [X] and glossopharyngeal [IX] nerves, which form a plexus in the outer fascia of the pharyngeal wall (Fig. 8.188).

The **pharyngeal plexus** is formed by:

- the pharyngeal branch of the vagus nerve [X],
- branches from the **external laryngeal nerve** from the **superior laryngeal branch** of the vagus nerve [X], and
- pharyngeal branches of the glossopharyngeal nerve [IX].

The **pharyngeal branch of the vagus nerve [X]** originates from the upper part of its **inferior ganglion** above the origin of the superior laryngeal nerve and is the major motor nerve of the pharynx (Fig. 8.188).

All muscles of the pharynx are innervated by the vagus nerve [X] mainly through the pharyngeal plexus, except for the stylopharyngeus, which is innervated directly by a branch of the glossopharyngeal nerve [IX].

Each subdivision of the pharynx has a different sensory innervation:

- The nasopharynx is innervated by a pharyngeal branch of the maxillary nerve $[V_2]$ that originates in the pterygopalatine fossa and passes through the palatovaginal

Fig. 8.188 Innervation of the pharynx. **A.** Lateral view. **B.** Posterior view showing innervation of stylopharyngeus.

canal in the sphenoid bone to reach the roof of the pharynx (see Fig. 8.138A, pg. 553).

- The oropharynx is innervated by the glossopharyngeal nerve [IX] via the pharyngeal plexus.
- The laryngopharynx is innervated by the vagus nerve [X] via the internal branch of the superior laryngeal nerve.

Glossopharyngeal nerve [IX]

The glossopharyngeal nerve [IX] is related to the pharynx throughout most of its course outside the cranial cavity.

After exiting the skull through the jugular foramen, the glossopharyngeal nerve [IX] descends on the posterior surface of the stylopharyngeus muscle, passes onto the lateral surface of the stylopharyngeus, and then passes anteriorly through the gap between the superior and middle constrictors to eventually reach the posterior aspect of the tongue (see Fig. 8.188B).

As the glossopharyngeal nerve [IX] passes under the free edge of the superior constrictor, it is just inferior to the palatine tonsil lying on the deep surface of the superior constrictor.

Pharyngeal branches to the pharyngeal plexus and a motor branch to the stylopharyngeus muscle are among branches that originate from the glossopharyngeal nerve [IX] in the neck. Because sensory innervation of the

oropharynx is by the glossopharyngeal nerve [IX], this nerve carries sensory innervation from the palatine tonsil and is also the afferent limb of the gag reflex.

LARYNX

The larynx is a hollow musculoligamentous structure with a cartilaginous framework that caps the lower respiratory tract.

The cavity of the larynx is continuous below with the trachea and, above, opens into the pharynx immediately posterior and slightly inferior to the tongue and the posterior opening (oropharyngeal isthmus) of the oral cavity (Fig. 8.189).

The larynx is both a valve (or sphincter) to close the lower respiratory tract and an instrument to produce sound. It is composed of:

- three large unpaired cartilages (cricoid, thyroid, and epiglottis),
- three pairs of smaller cartilages (arytenoid, corniculate, and cuneiform), and
- a fibro-elastic membrane and numerous intrinsic muscles.

The larynx is suspended from the hyoid bone above and attached to the trachea below by membranes and ligaments. It

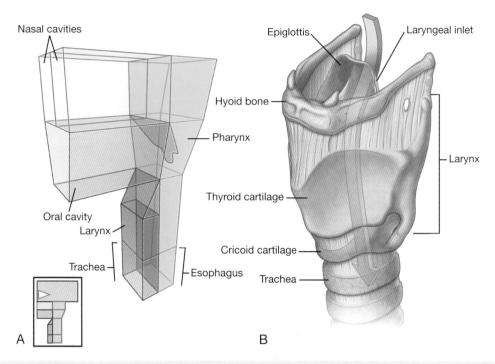

Fig. 8.189 Larynx. **A.** Relationship to other cavities. **B.** Lateral view.

is highly mobile in the neck and can be moved up and down and forward and backward by the action of extrinsic muscles that attach either to the larynx itself or to the hyoid bone.

During swallowing, the dramatic upward and forward movements of the larynx facilitate closing the laryngeal inlet and opening the esophagus.

Motor and sensory innervation of the larynx is provided by the vagus nerve [X].

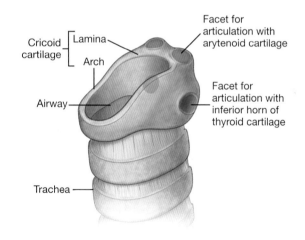

Fig. 8.190 Cricoid cartilage.

Laryngeal cartilages

Cricoid cartilage

The cricoid cartilage is the most inferior of the laryngeal cartilages and completely encircles the airway (Fig. 8.190). It is shaped like a signet ring with a broad **lamina of cricoid cartilage** posterior to the airway and a much narrower **arch of cricoid cartilage** circling anteriorly.

The cricoid cartilage has two articular facets on each side for articulation with other laryngeal cartilages:

■ One facet is on the sloping superolateral surface of the lamina and articulates with the base of an arytenoid cartilage.

593

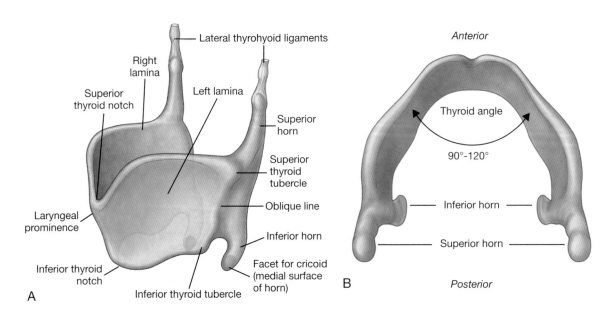

Fig. 8.191 Thyroid cartilage. **A.** Anterolateral view. **B.** Superior view.

■ The other facet is on the lateral surface of the lamina near its base and is for articulation with the medial surface of the inferior horn of the thyroid cartilage.

Thyroid cartilage

The thyroid cartilage (Fig. 8.191) is the largest of the laryngeal cartilages. It is formed by a right and a left lamina, which are widely separated posteriorly, but converge and join anteriorly. The most superior point of the site of fusion between the two broad flat laminae projects forward as the **laryngeal prominence** (Adam's apple). The angle between the two laminae is more acute in men (90°) than in women (120°) so the laryngeal prominence is more apparent in men than women.

Just superior to the laryngeal prominence, the **superior thyroid notch** separates the two laminae as they diverge laterally. Both the superior thyroid notch and the laryngeal prominence are palpable landmarks in the neck. There is a less distinct **inferior thyroid notch** in the midline along the base of the thyroid cartilage.

The posterior margin of each lamina of the thyroid cartilage is elongated to form a **superior horn** and an **inferior horn**:

■ The medial surface of the inferior horn has a facet for articulation with the cricoid cartilage.
■ The superior horn is connected by a **lateral thyrohyoid ligament** to the posterior end of the greater horn of the hyoid bone.

The lateral surface of each thyroid lamina is marked by a ridge (the **oblique line**), which curves anteriorly from the base of the superior horn to a little short of midway along the inferior margin of the lamina (Fig. 8.191). The oblique line is a site of attachment for the extrinsic muscles of the larynx (sternothyroid, thyrohyoid, and inferior constrictor).

The ends of the oblique line are expanded to form **superior** and **inferior thyroid tubercles**.

Epiglottis

The epiglottis is a leaf-shaped cartilage attached by its stem to the posterior aspect of the thyroid cartilage at the angle (Fig. 8.192) and projects posterosuperiorly from its attachment to the thyroid cartilage. The attachment is via the **thyro-epiglottic ligament** in the midline approximately midway between the laryngeal prominence and the inferior thyroid notch. The upper margin of the epiglottis is behind the pharyngeal part of the tongue.

The inferior half of the posterior surface of the epiglottis is raised slightly to form an epiglottic tubercle.

Arytenoid cartilages

The two arytenoid cartilages are pyramid-shaped cartilages with three surfaces, a **base of arytenoid cartilage** and an **apex of arytenoid cartilage** (Fig. 8.193):

■ The base is concave and articulates with the sloping articular facet on the superolateral surface of the lamina of cricoid cartilage.
■ The apex articulates with a corniculate cartilage.
■ The **medial surface** of each cartilage faces the other.
■ The **anterolateral surface** has two depressions separated by a ridge for muscle (vocalis) and ligament (vestibular ligament) attachment.
■ The **posterior surface** is covered by the transverse arytenoid muscles (see Fig. 8.204).

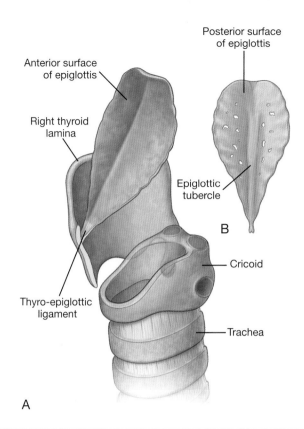

Anterior surface of epiglottis

Right thyroid lamina

Thyro-epiglottic ligament

A

Posterior surface of epiglottis

Epiglottic tubercle

B

Cricoid

Trachea

Fig. 8.192 Epiglottis. **A.** Anterolateral view. **B.** Posterior surface.

The anterior angle of the base is elongated into a **vocal process** to which the vocal ligament is attached. The lateral angle is similarly elongated into a muscular process for attachment of the posterior and lateral crico-arytenoid muscles.

Corniculate

The corniculate cartilages (Fig. 8.194) are two small conical cartilages whose bases articulate with the apices of the arytenoid cartilages. Their apices project posteromedially toward each other.

Cuneiform

These two small club-shaped cartilages (Fig. 8.194) lie anterior to the corniculate cartilages and are suspended in the part of the fibro-elastic membrane of the larynx that attaches the arytenoid cartilages to the lateral margin of the epiglottis.

Extrinsic ligaments

Thyrohyoid membrane

The thyrohyoid membrane is a tough fibro-elastic ligament that spans between the superior margin of the thyroid cartilage below and the hyoid bone above (Fig. 8.195).

An aperture in the lateral part of the thyrohyoid membrane on each side is for the superior laryngeal artery, the internal branch of the superior laryngeal nerve and lymphatics.

The posterior borders of the thyrohyoid membrane are thickened to form the **lateral thyrohyoid ligaments.** The membrane is also thickened anteriorly in the midline to form the **median thyrohyoid ligament.**

Occasionally, there is a small cartilage (**triticeal cartilage**) in each lateral thyrohyoid ligament.

Hyo-epiglottic ligament

The hyo-epiglottic ligament (Fig. 8.195) extends from the midline of the epiglottis anterosuperiorly to the body of the hyoid bone.

Cricotracheal ligament

The cricotracheal ligament (Fig. 8.195) runs from the lower border of the cricoid cartilage to the adjacent upper border of the first tracheal cartilage.

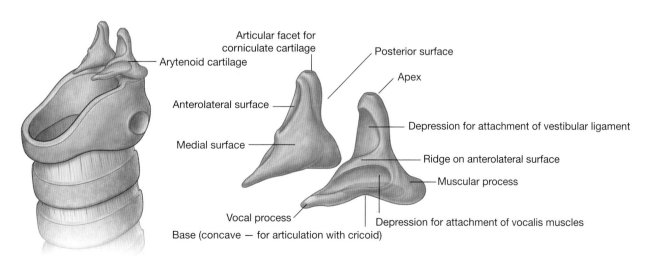

Arytenoid cartilage

Articular facet for corniculate cartilage

Anterolateral surface

Medial surface

Vocal process

Base (concave — for articulation with cricoid)

Posterior surface

Apex

Depression for attachment of vestibular ligament

Ridge on anterolateral surface

Muscular process

Depression for attachment of vocalis muscles

Fig. 8.193 Arytenoid cartilages.

595

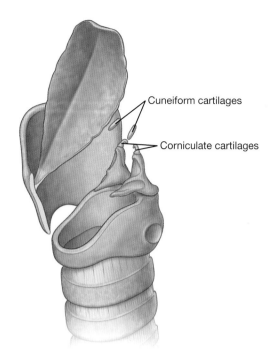

Fig. 8.194 Corniculate and cuneiform cartilages.

Cuneiform cartilages

Corniculate cartilages

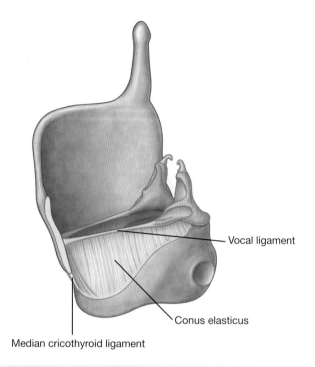

Fig. 8.196 Cricothyroid ligament.

Vocal ligament

Conus elasticus

Median cricothyroid ligament

Fig. 8.195 Extrinsic ligaments of the larynx.

Hyo-epiglottic ligament

Hyoid bone

Lateral thyrohyoid ligaments

Triticeal cartilage

Aperture for internal branch of superior laryngeal nerve and associated artery

Thyrohyoid membrane

Median thyrohyoid ligament

Cricotracheal ligament

Intrinsic ligaments

Fibro-elastic membrane of the larynx

The fibro-elastic membrane of the larynx links together the laryngeal cartilages and completes the architectural framework of the laryngeal cavity. It is composed of two parts—a lower cricothyroid ligament and an upper quadrangular membrane.

Conus elasticus (cricovocal membrane)

The conus elasticus (Fig. 8.196) is attached to the arch of cricoid cartilage and extends superiorly to end in a free upper margin within the space enclosed by the thyroid cartilage. On each side, this upper free margin attaches:

- anteriorly to the thyroid cartilage, and
- posteriorly to the vocal processes of the arytenoid cartilages.

The free margin between these two points of attachment is thickened to form the **vocal ligament**, which is under the **vocal fold (true vocal cord)** of the larynx.

The conus elasticus is also thickened anteriorly in the midline to form a distinct **median cricothyroid ligament**, which spans the distance between the arch of cricoid cartilage and the inferior thyroid notch and adjacent deep surface of the thyroid cartilage up to the attachment of the vocal ligaments.

Quadrangular membrane

The quadrangular membrane on each side runs between the lateral margin of the epiglottis and the anterolateral surface of the arytenoid cartilage on the same side (Fig. 8.198). It is also attached to the corniculate cartilage, which articulates with the apex of arytenoid cartilage.

Surface anatomy
How to locate the cricothyroid ligament

The median cricothyroid ligament (Fig. 8.197) can be easily found using palpable features of the larynx as landmarks.

Using a finger to gently feel laryngeal structures in the midline, first find the thyroid notch in the superior margin of the thyroid cartilage and then move the finger inferiorly over the laryngeal prominence and down the anterior surface of the thyroid angle. As the finger crosses the inferior margin of the thyroid cartilage in the midline, a soft depression is felt before the finger slides onto the arch of the cricoid cartilage, which is hard.

The soft depression between the lower margin of the thyroid cartilage and the arch of the cricoid is the position of the cricothyroid ligament.

A tube passed through the median cricothyroid ligament enters the airway just inferior to the position of the vocal folds of the larynx.

Structures that may occur in or cross the midline between the skin and the median cricothyroid ligament include the pyramidal lobe of the thyroid gland and small vessels, respectively.

Inferior to the cricoid cartilage, the upper cartilage of the trachea can sometimes be palpated above the level of the isthmus of the thyroid gland that crosses the trachea anteriorly.

The landmarks used for finding the median cricothyroid ligament are similar in men and women; however, because the laminae of the thyroid cartilage meet at a more acute angle in men, the structures are more prominent in men than in women.

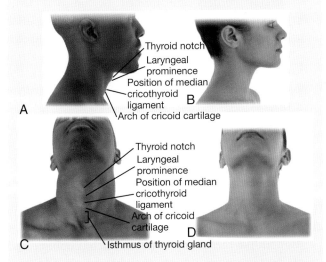

Fig. 8.197 How to locate the median cricothyroid ligament. **A.** In a man, lateral view of head and neck. **B.** In a woman, lateral view of head and neck. **C.** In a man, anterior neck with the chin elevated. **D.** In a woman, anterior neck with the chin elevated.

Each quadrangular membrane has a free upper margin between the top of the epiglottis and the corniculate cartilage and a free lower margin. The free lower margin is

Clinical app

Cricothyrotomy

In emergency situations, when the airway is blocked above the level of the vocal folds, the median cricothyroid ligament can be perforated and a small tube inserted through the incision to establish an airway. Except for small vessels and the occasional presence of a pyramidal lobe of the thyroid gland, normally there are few structures between the median cricothyroid ligament and skin.

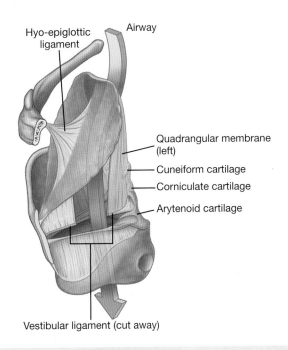

Fig. 8.198 Quadrangular membrane.

thickened to form the **vestibular ligament** under the **vestibular fold (false vocal cord)** of the larynx.

On each side, the vestibular ligament of the quadrangular membrane is separated from the vocal ligament of the cricothyroid ligament below by a gap. Because the vestibular ligament attaches to the anterolateral surface of the arytenoid cartilage and the vocal ligament attaches to the vocal process of the same cartilage, the vestibular ligament is lateral to the vocal ligament when viewed from above (Fig. 8.199).

Laryngeal joints

Cricothyroid joints

The joints between the inferior horns of the thyroid cartilage and the cricoid cartilage, and between the cricoid cartilage and arytenoid cartilages are synovial. Each is surrounded by a capsule and is reinforced by associated ligaments. The cricothyroid joints enable the thyroid cartilage to move forward and tilt downward on the cricoid cartilage (Fig. 8.200).

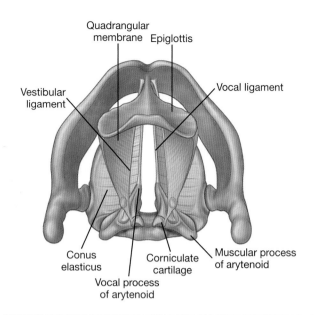

Fig. 8.199 Fibro-elastic membrane of the larynx (superior view).

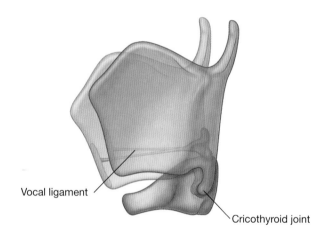

Fig. 8.200 Movements of the cricothyroid joints.

Because the vocal ligaments pass between the posterior aspect of the thyroid angle and the arytenoid cartilages sit on the lamina of cricoid cartilage, forward movement and downward rotation of the thyroid cartilage on the cricoid cartilage effectively lengthens and puts tension on the vocal ligaments (Fig. 8.200).

Crico-arytenoid joints

The crico-arytenoid joints between articular facets on the superolateral surfaces of the cricoid cartilage and the bases of the arytenoid cartilages enable the arytenoid cartilages to slide away or toward each other and to rotate so that the vocal processes pivot either toward or away from the midline. These movements abduct and adduct the vocal ligaments (Fig. 8.201).

Fig. 8.201 Movements of the crico-arytenoid joints.

Cavity of the larynx

The central cavity of the larynx (Fig. 8.202) is tubular and lined by mucosa. Its architectural support is provided by the fibro-elastic membrane of the larynx and by the laryngeal cartilages to which it is attached.

The superior aperture of the cavity (laryngeal inlet) opens into the anterior aspect of the pharynx just below and posterior to the tongue (Fig. 8.202A):

- Its anterior border is formed by mucosa covering the superior margin of the epiglottis.
- Its lateral borders are formed by mucosal folds (**aryepiglottic folds**), which enclose the superior margins of the quadrangular membranes and adjacent soft tissues, and two tubercles on the more posterolateral margin of the laryngeal inlet on each side mark the positions of the underlying cuneiform and corniculate cartilages.
- Its posterior border in the midline is formed by a mucosal fold that forms a depression (**interarytenoid notch**) between the two corniculate tubercles.

The inferior opening of the laryngeal cavity is continuous with the lumen of the trachea, is completely encircled by the cricoid cartilage, and is horizontal in position unlike the laryngeal inlet, which is oblique and points posterosuperiorly into the pharynx. In addition, the inferior opening is continuously open, whereas the laryngeal inlet can be closed by downward movement of the epiglottis.

Division into three major regions

Two pairs of mucosal folds, the vestibular and vocal folds, which project medially from the lateral walls of the laryngeal cavity, constrict it and divide it into three major

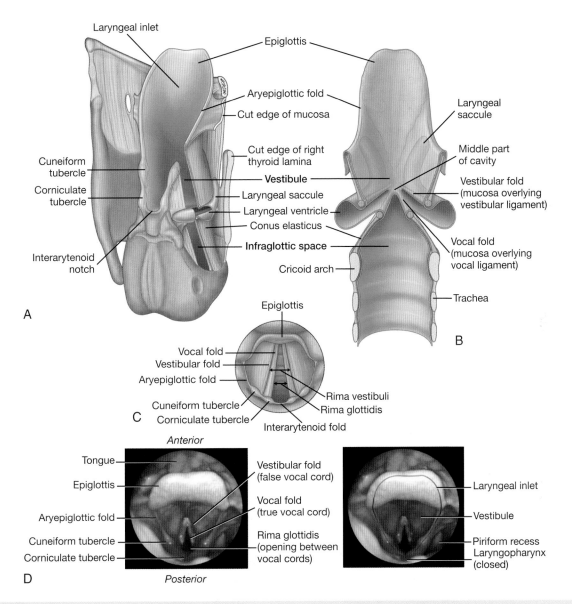

Fig. 8.202 Laryngeal cavity. **A.** Posterolateral view. **B.** Posterior view (cutaway). **C.** Superior view through the laryngeal inlet. **D.** Labeled photographs of the larynx, superior view.

regions—the vestibule, a middle chamber, and the infraglottic cavity (Fig. 8.202B):

- The **vestibule** is the upper chamber of the laryngeal cavity between the laryngeal inlet and the vestibular folds, which enclose the vestibular ligaments and associated soft tissues.

- The middle part of the laryngeal cavity is very thin and is between the vestibular folds above and the vocal folds below.

- The **infraglottic space** is the most inferior chamber of the laryngeal cavity and is between the vocal folds (which enclose the vocal ligaments and related soft tissues) and the inferior opening of the larynx.

Laryngeal ventricles and saccules

On each side, the mucosa of the middle cavity bulges laterally through the gap between the vestibular and vocal ligaments to produce an expanded trough-shaped space (a **laryngeal ventricle**) (Fig. 8.202A,B). An elongate tubular extension of each ventricle (**laryngeal saccule**) projects anterosuperiorly between the vestibular fold and thyroid cartilage and may reach as high as the top of the thyroid cartilage (Fig. 8.202A). Within the walls of these laryngeal saccules are numerous mucous glands. Mucus secreted into the saccules lubricates the vocal folds.

Rima vestibuli and rima glottidis

When viewed from above (Fig. 8.202C,D), there is a triangular opening (the **rima vestibuli**) between the two adjacent vestibular folds at the entrance to the middle chamber of the laryngeal cavity. The apex of the opening is anterior, and its base is formed by the posterior wall of the laryngeal cavity.

Inferior to the vestibular folds, the vocal folds (true vocal cords) and adjacent mucosa-covered parts of the arytenoid cartilages form the lateral walls of a similar, but narrower triangular opening (the **rima glottidis** between the two adjacent vocal folds) (Fig. 8.202C,D). This opening separates the middle chamber above from the infraglottic cavity below. The base of this triangular opening is formed by the fold of mucosa (**interarytenoid fold**) at the bottom of the interarytenoid notch.

Both the rima glottidis and the rima vestibuli can be opened and closed by movement of the arytenoid cartilages and associated fibro-elastic membranes.

Intrinsic muscles

The intrinsic muscles of the larynx (Table 8.19, Figs. 8.203, 8.204, 8.205) adjust tension in the vocal ligaments, open and close the rima glottidis, control the inner dimensions of the vestibule, close the rima vestibuli, and facilitate closing of the laryngeal inlet. They do this mainly by:

- acting on the cricothyroid and cricoarytenoid joints,
- adjusting the distance between the epiglottis and arytenoid cartilages,

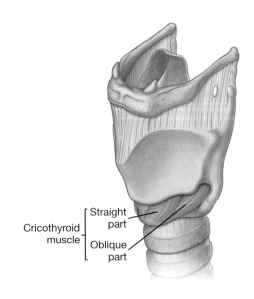

Fig. 8.203 Cricothyroid muscle.

- pulling directly on the vocal ligaments, and
- forcing soft tissues associated with the quadrangular membranes and vestibular ligaments toward the midline.

The **cricothyroid muscles** are the only intrinsic muscles of the larynx innervated by the superior laryngeal branches of the vagus nerves [X] (see Fig. 8.203). All other intrinsic

Table 8.19	Intrinsic muscles of the larynx			
Muscle	**Origin**	**Insertion**	**Innervation**	**Function**
Cricothyroid	Anterolateral aspect of arch of cricoid cartilage	Oblique part—inferior horn of the thyroid cartilage; straight part—inferior margin of thyroid cartilage	External branch of superior laryngeal nerve from the vagus nerve [X]	Forward and downward rotation of the thyroid cartilage at the cricothyroid joint
Posterior crico-arytenoid	Oval depression on posterior surface of lamina of cricoid cartilage	Posterior surface of muscular process of arytenoid cartilage	Recurrent laryngeal branch of the vagus nerve [X]	Abduction and external rotation of the arytenoid cartilage. The posterior crico-arytenoid muscles are the primary abductors of the vocal folds. In other words, they are the primary openers of the rima glottidis.
Lateral crico-arytenoid	Superior surface of arch of cricoid cartilage	Anterior surface of muscular process of arytenoid cartilage	Recurrent laryngeal branch of the vagus nerve [X]	Internal rotation of the arytenoid cartilage and adduction of vocal folds
Transverse arytenoid	Lateral border of posterior surface of arytenoid cartilage	Lateral border of posterior surface of opposite arytenoid cartilage	Recurrent laryngeal branch of the vagus nerve [X]	Adduction of arytenoid cartilages
Oblique arytenoid	Posterior surface of muscular process of arytenoid cartilage	Posterior surface of apex of adjacent arytenoid cartilage; extends into aryepiglottic fold	Recurrent laryngeal branch of the vagus nerve [X]	Sphincter of the laryngeal inlet
Thyro-arytenoid	Thyroid angle and adjacent cricothyroid ligament	Anterolateral surface of arytenoid cartilage; some fibers continue in aryepiglottic folds to the lateral margin of the epiglottis	Recurrent laryngeal branch of the vagus nerve [X]	Sphincter of vestibule and of laryngeal inlet
Vocalis	Lateral surface of vocal process of arytenoid cartilage	Vocal ligament and thyroid angle	Recurrent laryngeal branch of the vagus nerve [X]	Adjusts tension in vocal folds

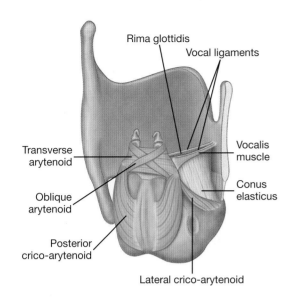

Fig. 8.204 Crico-arytenoid, oblique and transverse arytenoids, and vocalis muscles.

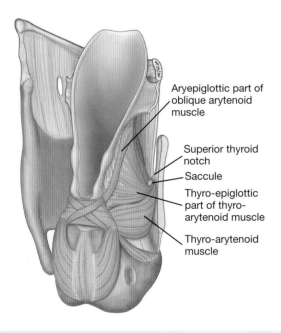

Fig. 8.205 Thyro-arytenoid muscle.

muscles are innervated by the recurrent laryngeal branches of the vagus nerves [X] (Figs. 8.204, 8.205).

Function of the larynx

The larynx is an elaborate sphincter for the lower respiratory tract and provides a mechanism for producing sounds. Adjustments of the size of the central cavity of the larynx result from changes in the dimensions of the rima glottidis, the rima vestibuli, the vestibule, and the laryngeal inlet (Fig. 8.206). These changes result from muscle actions and laryngeal mechanics.

Respiration

During quiet respiration, the laryngeal inlet, vestibule, rima vestibuli, and rima glottidis are open. The arytenoid cartilages are abducted and the rima glottidis is triangular shaped (Fig. 8.206A). During forced inspiration (Fig. 8.206B), the arytenoid cartilages are rotated laterally, mainly by the action of the **posterior cricoarytenoid muscles.** As a result, the vocal folds are abducted, and the rima glottidis widens into a rhomboid shape, which effectively increases the diameter of the laryngeal airway.

Phonation

When phonating, the arytenoid cartilages and vocal folds are adducted and air is forced through the closed rima glottidis (Fig. 8.206C). This action causes the vocal folds to vibrate against each other and produce sounds, which can then be modified by the upper parts of the airway and oral cavity. Tension in the vocal folds can be adjusted by the **vocalis and cricothyroid muscles.**

Effort closure

Effort closure of the larynx (Fig. 8.206D) occurs when air is retained in the thoracic cavity to stabilize the trunk (e.g., during heavy lifting) or as part of the mechanism for increasing intra-abdominal pressure. During effort closure, the rima glottidis is completely closed, as is the rima vestibuli and lower parts of the vestibule. The result is to completely and forcefully shut the airway.

Swallowing

During swallowing, the rima glottidis, the rima vestibuli, and vestibule are closed and the laryngeal inlet is narrowed. In addition, the larynx moves up and forward. This action causes the epiglottis to swing downward toward the arytenoid cartilages and to effectively narrow or close the laryngeal inlet (Fig. 8.206E). The up and forward movement of the larynx also opens the esophagus, which is attached to the posterior aspect of the lamina of cricoid cartilage. All these actions together prevent solids and liquids from entry into the airway and facilitate their movement through the piriform fossae into the esophagus.

Clinical app

Exogenous Testosterone and Vocal Cord Mass
In individuals receiving testosterone as part of masculinizing hormone therapy (e.g., transgender men), the vocal cords will lengthen and thicken, causing the fundamental frequency and pitch to decrease, producing a more masculine voice.

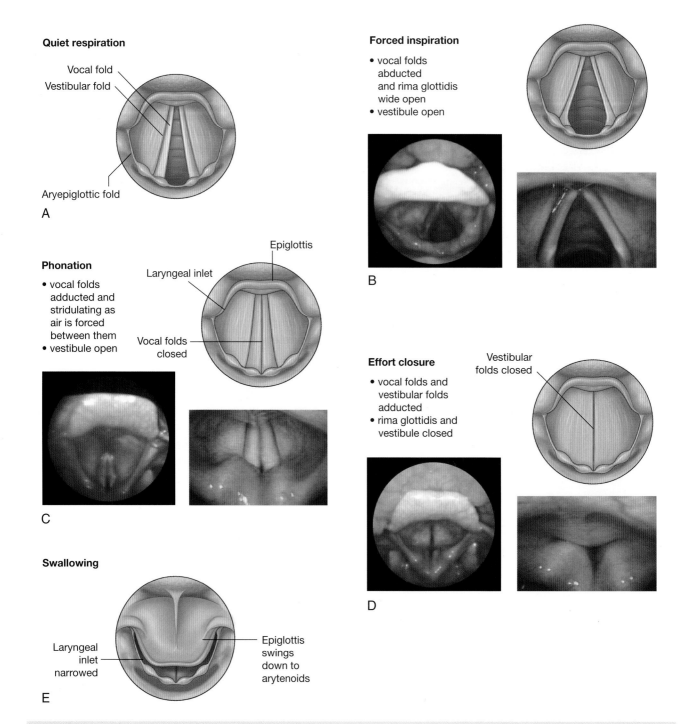

Quiet respiration

- Vocal fold
- Vestibular fold
- Aryepiglottic fold

A

Forced inspiration

- vocal folds abducted and rima glottidis wide open
- vestibule open

B

Phonation

- vocal folds adducted and stridulating as air is forced between them
- vestibule open

- Epiglottis
- Laryngeal inlet
- Vocal folds closed

C

Effort closure

- vocal folds and vestibular folds adducted
- rima glottidis and vestibule closed

- Vestibular folds closed

D

Swallowing

- Laryngeal inlet narrowed
- Epiglottis swings down to arytenoids

E

Fig. 8.206 Laryngeal function. **A.** Quiet respiration. **B.** Forced inspiration. **C.** Phonation. **D.** Effort closure. **E.** Swallowing.

Vessels

Arteries

The major blood supply to the larynx is by the superior and inferior laryngeal arteries (Fig. 8.207):

- The **superior laryngeal artery** originates near the upper margin of the thyroid cartilage from the superior thyroid branch of the external carotid artery and accompanies the internal branch of the superior laryngeal nerve through the thyrohyoid membrane to reach the larynx.

- The **inferior laryngeal artery** originates from the inferior thyroid branch of the thyrocervical trunk of the subclavian artery low in the neck and, together with the recurrent laryngeal nerve, ascends in the groove between the esophagus and trachea—it enters the larynx by passing deep to the margin of the inferior constrictor muscle of the pharynx.

Clinical app

Tracheostomy

A tracheostomy is a surgical procedure in which a hole is made in the trachea and a tube is inserted to enable ventilation.

The typical situation in which a tracheostomy is performed is in the calm atmosphere of an operating theater. A small transverse incision is placed in the lower third of the neck anteriorly. The strap muscles are retracted laterally and the trachea can be easily visualized. Occasionally, it is necessary to divide the isthmus of thyroid gland. An incision is made in the second and third tracheal rings and a small tracheostomy tube inserted.

After the tracheostomy has been in situ for the required length of time, it is simply removed. The hole through which it was inserted almost inevitably closes without any intervention.

Patients with long-term tracheostomies are unable to vocalize because no air is passing through the vocal cords.

Veins

Veins draining the larynx accompany the arteries (Fig. 8.208):

- **Superior laryngeal veins** drain into superior thyroid veins, which, in turn, drain into the internal jugular veins.
- **Inferior laryngeal veins** drain into inferior thyroid veins, which drain into the left brachiocephalic vein.

Lymphatics

Lymphatics drain regions above and below the vocal folds:

- Those above the vocal folds follow the superior laryngeal artery and terminate in deep cervical nodes associated with the bifurcation of the common carotid artery.
- Those below the vocal folds drain into deep nodes associated with the inferior thyroid artery or with nodes associated with the front of the cricothyroid ligament or upper trachea.

Nerves

Sensory and motor innervation of the larynx is by two branches of the vagus nerves [X]—the superior laryngeal nerves and the recurrent laryngeal nerves (Fig. 8.209).

Superior laryngeal nerves

The **superior laryngeal nerves** originate from the inferior vagal ganglia high in the neck (Fig. 8.209). On each side, they descend medial to the internal carotid artery and divide into internal and external branches just above the level of the superior horn of the hyoid bone:

- The external branch (**external laryngeal nerve**) descends along the lateral wall of the pharynx to supply and penetrate the inferior constrictor of the pharynx and ends by supplying the cricothyroid muscle.

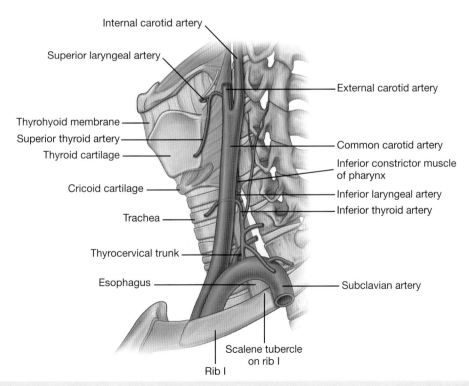

Fig. 8.207 Arterial supply of the larynx, left lateral view.

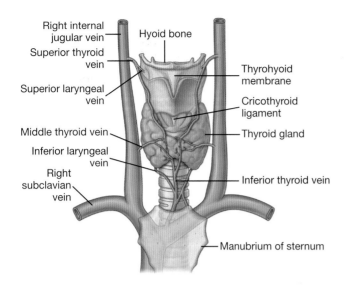

Fig. 8.208 Venous drainage of the larynx, anterior view.

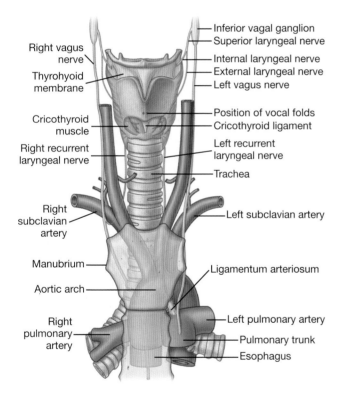

Fig. 8.209 Innervation of the larynx.

- The internal branch (**internal laryngeal nerve**) passes anteroinferiorly to penetrate the thyrohyoid membrane—it is mainly sensory and supplies the laryngeal cavity down to the level of the vocal folds.

Recurrent laryngeal nerves

The recurrent laryngeal nerves are (Fig. 8.209):

- sensory to the laryngeal cavity below the level of the vocal folds, and

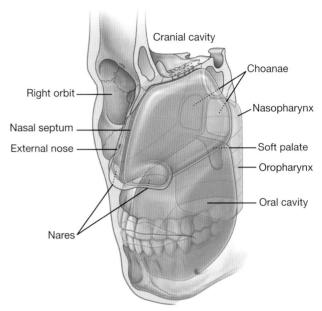

Fig. 8.210 Nasal cavities (anterolateral view). Relationship to other cavities.

- motor to all intrinsic muscles of the larynx except for the cricothyroid.

The left recurrent laryngeal nerve originates in the thorax, whereas the right recurrent laryngeal nerve originates in the root of the neck. Both nerves generally ascend in the neck in the groove between the esophagus and trachea and enter the larynx deep to the margin of the inferior constrictor. They may pass medial, lateral, or through the lateral ligament of the thyroid gland, which attaches the thyroid gland to the trachea and lower part of the cricoid cartilage on each side.

NASAL CAVITIES

The two nasal cavities are the uppermost parts of the respiratory tract and contain the olfactory receptors. They are elongated wedge-shaped spaces with a large inferior base and a narrow superior apex (Fig. 8.210), and are held open by a skeletal framework consisting mainly of bone and cartilage.

The smaller anterior regions of the cavities are enclosed by the external nose, whereas the larger posterior regions are more central within the skull. The anterior apertures of the nasal cavities are the nares, which open onto the inferior surface of the nose (Fig. 8.210). The posterior apertures are the choanae, which open into the nasopharynx.

The nasal cavities are separated:

- from each other by a midline nasal septum,
- from the oral cavity below by the hard palate, and

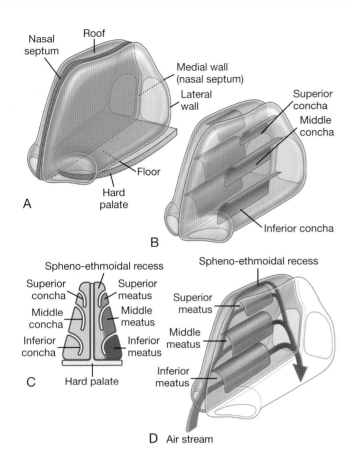

Fig. 8.211 Nasal cavities. A. Floor, roof, and lateral walls. B. Conchae on lateral walls. C. Coronal section. D. Air channels in right nasal cavity.

- from the cranial cavity above by parts of the frontal, ethmoid, and sphenoid bones.

Lateral to the nasal cavities are the orbits.

Each nasal cavity has a floor, roof, medial wall, and lateral wall.

Lateral wall

The lateral wall is characterized by three curved shelves of bone (conchae), which are one above the other and project medially and inferiorly across the nasal cavity (Fig. 8.211B). The medial, anterior, and posterior margins of the conchae are free.

The conchae divide each nasal cavity into four air channels (Fig. 8.211C,D):

- an **inferior nasal meatus** between the **inferior concha** and the nasal floor;
- a **middle nasal meatus** between the inferior and **middle concha**;
- a **superior nasal meatus** between the middle and **superior concha**; and
- a **spheno-ethmoidal recess** between the superior concha and the nasal roof.

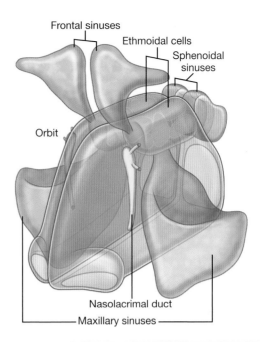

Fig. 8.212 Paranasal sinuses and nasolacrimal duct.

These conchae increase the surface area of contact between tissues of the lateral wall and the respired air.

The openings of the paranasal sinuses, which are extensions of the nasal cavity that erode into the surrounding bones during childhood and early adulthood, are on the lateral wall and roof of the nasal cavities (Fig. 8.212). In addition, the lateral wall also contains the opening of the nasolacrimal duct, which drains tears from the eye into the nasal cavity.

Regions

Each nasal cavity consists of three general regions—the nasal vestibule, the respiratory region, and the olfactory region (Fig. 8.213):

- The **nasal vestibule** is a small dilated space just internal to the naris that is lined by skin and contains hair follicles.
- The **respiratory region** is the largest part of the nasal cavity, has a rich neurovascular supply, and is lined by respiratory epithelium composed mainly of ciliated and mucous cells.
- The **olfactory region** is small, is at the apex of each nasal cavity, is lined by olfactory epithelium, and contains the olfactory receptors.

In addition to housing receptors for the sense of smell (olfaction), the nasal cavities adjust the temperature and humidity of respired air by the action of a rich blood supply, and trap and remove particulate matter from the airway by filtering the air through hair in the vestibule and by capturing foreign material in abundant mucus. The mucus normally is moved posteriorly by cilia on epithelial cells in the nasal cavities and is swallowed.

605

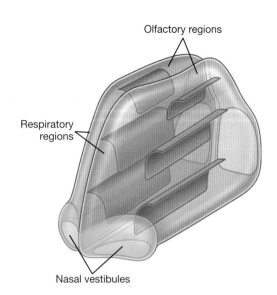

Fig. 8.213 Regions of the nasal cavities.

Skeletal framework

Bones that contribute to the skeletal framework of the nasal cavities include the:

- unpaired ethmoid, sphenoid, frontal bone, and vomer; and
- paired nasal, maxillary, palatine and lacrimal bones and the inferior conchae bone.

Of all the bones associated with the nasal cavities, the ethmoid is a key element.

Ethmoid bone

The single ethmoid bone is one of the most complex bones in the skull. It contributes to the roof, lateral wall, and medial wall of both nasal cavities, and contains the ethmoidal cells (ethmoidal sinuses).

The ethmoid bone is cuboidal in overall shape (Fig. 8.214A) and is composed of two rectangular box-shaped **ethmoidal labyrinths,** one on each side, united superiorly across the midline by a perforated sheet of bone (the **cribriform plate**). A second sheet of bone (the **perpendicular plate**) descends vertically in the median sagittal plane from the cribriform plate to form part of the nasal septum.

Each ethmoidal labyrinth is composed of two delicate sheets of bone, which sandwich between the ethmoidal cells.

The cribriform plate is at the apex of the nasal cavities and fills the **ethmoidal notch** in the frontal bone (Fig. 8.214B) and separates the nasal cavities below from the cranial cavity above. Small perforations in the bone allow the fibers of the olfactory nerve [I] to pass between the two regions.

A large triangular process (the **crista galli**) at the midline on the superior surface of the cribriform plate anchors a fold (falx cerebri) of dura mater in the cranial cavity.

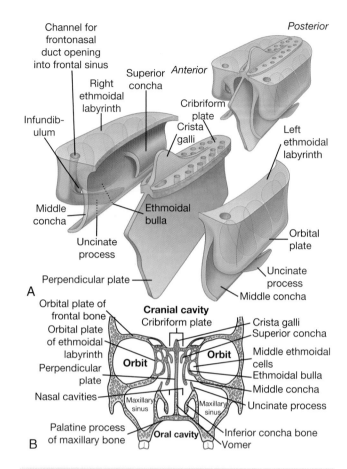

Fig. 8.214 Ethmoid bone. A. Overall shape. B. Coronal section through skull.

The perpendicular plate of the ethmoid bone is quadrangular in shape, descends in the midline from the cribriform plate, and forms the upper part of the median nasal septum (Fig. 8.214).

Clinical app

Deviated nasal septum

The nasal septum is typically situated in the midline; however, septal deviation to one side or the other is not uncommon and in many cases is secondary to direct trauma. Extreme septal deviation can produce nasal occlusion. The deviation can be corrected surgically.

External nose

The external nose extends the nasal cavities onto the front of the face and positions the nares so that they point downward (Fig. 8.215). It is pyramidal in shape with its apex anterior in position. The upper angle of the nose between the openings of the orbits is continuous with the forehead.

Like posterior regions, the anterior parts of the nasal cavities found within the nose are held open by a skeletal

Fig. 8.215 External nose.

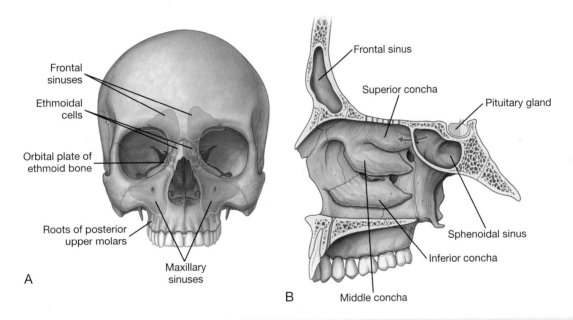

Fig. 8.216 Paranasal sinuses. A. Anterior view. B. Paramedian view of right nasal cavity.

framework, which is composed partly of bone and mainly of cartilage (Fig. 8.215):

- The bony parts are where the nose is continuous with the skull—here the nasal bones and parts of the maxillae and frontal bones provide support.
- Anteriorly and on each side, support is provided by **lateral** processes of the septal cartilage, **major alar,** three or four **minor alar cartilages,** and a single septal cartilage in the midline that forms the anterior part of the nasal septum.

Paranasal sinuses

There are four paranasal air sinuses—the ethmoidal cells and the sphenoidal, maxillary, and frontal sinuses (Figs. 8.216, 8.217). Each is named according to the bone in which it is found.

The paranasal sinuses develop as outgrowths from the nasal cavities and erode into the surrounding bones. All are:

- lined by respiratory mucosa, which is ciliated and mucus secreting;
- open into the nasal cavities; and
- innervated by branches of the trigeminal nerve [V].

Imaging app

Visualizing the nasal cavities and paranasal sinuses

Fig. 8.217 A. Anterior view (posteroanterior skull radiograph). **B.** Lateral view (skull radiograph). **C.** CT image in coronal plane.

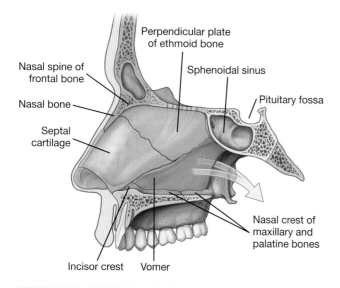

Fig. 8.218 Medial wall of the nasal cavity—the nasal septum.

Frontal sinuses

The frontal sinuses, one on each side, are variable in size and are the most superior of the sinuses (Figs. 8.216A,B, 8.217A). Each is triangular in shape and is in the part of the frontal bone under the forehead. The base of each triangular sinus is oriented vertically in the bone at the midline above the bridge of the nose and the apex is laterally approximately one-third of the way along the upper margin of the orbit.

Each frontal sinus drains onto the lateral wall of the middle meatus via the frontonasal duct, which penetrates the ethmoidal labyrinth and continues as the ethmoidal infundibulum at the front end of the **semilunar hiatus.**

Ethmoidal cells

The ethmoidal cells on each side fill the ethmoidal labyrinth (Figs. 8.216A,B; 8.217A,C). Each cluster of cells is separated from the orbit by the thin orbital plate of the ethmoidal labyrinth and from the nasal cavity by the medial wall of the ethmoidal labyrinth.

The ethmoidal cells are formed by a variable number of individual air chambers, which are divided into anterior, middle, and posterior ethmoidal cells based on the location of their apertures on the lateral wall of the nasal cavity.

Maxillary sinuses

The maxillary sinuses, one on each side, are the largest of the paranasal sinuses and completely fill the bodies of the maxillae (Figs. 8.216B, 8.217A,C). Each is pyramidal in shape with the apex directed laterally and the base deep to the lateral wall of the adjacent nasal cavity. The medial wall or base of the maxillary sinus is formed by the maxilla, and by parts of the inferior concha and palatine bone that overlie the maxillary hiatus.

The opening of the maxillary sinus is near the top of the base, in the center of the semilunar hiatus, which grooves the lateral wall of the middle nasal meatus.

Sphenoidal sinuses

The sphenoidal sinuses, one on either side within the body of the sphenoid, open into the roof of the nasal cavity via apertures on the posterior wall of the spheno-ethmoidal recess (Figs. 8.216C, 8.217C). The apertures are high on the anterior walls of the sphenoidal sinuses.

The sphenoidal sinuses are related:

- above to the cranial cavity, particularly to the pituitary gland and to the optic chiasm;
- laterally, to the cranial cavity, particularly to the cavernous sinuses; and
- below and in front, to the nasal cavities.

Clinical app

Surgical approach to the pituitary gland

Because only thin shelves of bone separate the sphenoidal sinuses from the nasal cavities below and hypophyseal fossa above, the pituitary gland can be surgically approached through the roof of the nasal cavities by passing first through the anteroinferior aspect of the sphenoid bone and into the sphenoidal sinuses and then through the top of the sphenoid bone into the hypophyseal fossa.

Walls, floor, and roof

Medial wall

The medial wall of each nasal cavity is the mucosa-covered surface of the thin nasal septum, which is oriented vertically

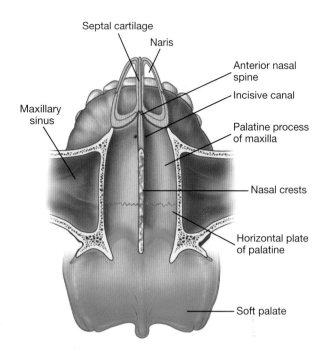

Fig. 8.219 Floor of the nasal cavity (superior view).

in the median sagittal plane and separates the right and left nasal cavities from each other.

The nasal septum (Fig. 8.218) consists of:

- the **septal nasal cartilage** anteriorly;
- posteriorly, mainly the vomer and the perpendicular plate of the ethmoid bone;
- small contributions by the nasal bones where they meet in the midline and the nasal spine of the frontal bone; and
- contributions by the nasal crests of the maxillary and palatine bones, rostrum of the sphenoid bone, and the incisor crest of the maxilla.

Floor

The floor of each nasal cavity (Fig. 8.219) is smooth, concave, and much wider than the roof. It consists of:

- soft tissues of the external nose, and
- the upper surface of the palatine process of the maxilla and the horizontal plate of the palatine bone, which together form the hard palate.

The naris opens anteriorly into the floor, and the superior aperture of the incisive canal is deep to the mucosa immediately lateral to the nasal septum near the front of the hard palate.

Roof

The roof of the nasal cavity is narrow and is highest in central regions where it is formed by the cribriform plate of the ethmoid bone (Fig. 8.220).

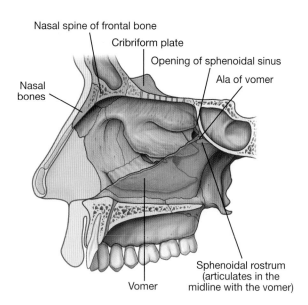

Nasal spine of frontal bone
Cribriform plate
Opening of sphenoidal sinus
Ala of vomer
Nasal bones
Sphenoidal rostrum (articulates in the midline with the vomer)
Vomer

Fig. 8.220 Roof of the nasal cavity.

Anterior to the cribriform plate, the roof slopes inferiorly to the nares and is formed by:

- the nasal spine of the frontal bone and the nasal bones, and
- the lateral processes of the septal cartilage and major alar cartilages of the external nose.

Posteriorly, the roof of each cavity slopes inferiorly to the choana and is formed by:

- the anterior surface of the sphenoid bone,
- the ala of the vomer and adjacent sphenoidal process of the palatine bone, and
- the vaginal process of the medial plate of the pterygoid process.

Underlying the mucosa, the roof is perforated superiorly by openings in the cribriform plate and, anterior to these openings, by a separate foramen for the anterior ethmoidal nerve and vessels.

The opening between the sphenoidal sinus and the spheno-ethmoidal recess is on the posterior slope of the roof.

Lateral wall

The lateral wall of each nasal cavity is complex and is formed by bone, cartilage, and soft tissues.

Bony support for the lateral wall (Fig. 8.221A) is provided by:

- the ethmoidal labyrinth and uncinate process,
- the perpendicular plate of the palatine bone,
- the medial plate of the pterygoid process of the sphenoid bone,

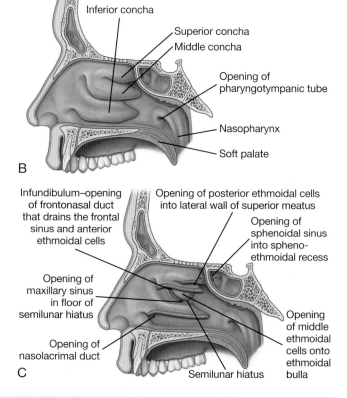

Frontal process of maxilla
Lacrimal bone
Nasal bone
Superior concha
Middle concha
Lateral process of septal cartilage
Uncinate process of ethmoid
Major alar cartilage
Medial pterygoid plate of sphenoid bone
Minor alar cartilage
Inferior concha
Perpendicular plate of palatine bone
A

Inferior concha
Superior concha
Middle concha
Opening of pharyngotympanic tube
Nasopharynx
Soft palate
B

Infundibulum–opening of frontonasal duct that drains the frontal sinus and anterior ethmoidal cells
Opening of posterior ethmoidal cells into lateral wall of superior meatus
Opening of sphenoidal sinus into spheno-ethmoidal recess
Opening of maxillary sinus in floor of semilunar hiatus
Opening of nasolacrimal duct
Opening of middle ethmoidal cells onto ethmoidal bulla
Semilunar hiatus
C

Fig. 8.221 Lateral wall of the nasal cavity. **A.** Bones. **B.** Covered with mucosa. **C.** Conchae broken away at attachment to lateral wall.

- the medial surfaces of the lacrimal bones and maxillae, and
- the inferior concha bone.

In the external nose, the lateral wall of the cavity is supported by cartilage (lateral process of the septal cartilage and major and minor alar cartilages) and by soft tissues. The surface of the lateral wall is irregular in contour and is interrupted by the three nasal conchae.

The inferior, middle, and superior conchae (Fig. 8.221B) extend medially across the nasal cavity, separating it into four air channels, an inferior, middle, and superior meatus, and a spheno-ethmoidal recess (see Fig. 8.211C,D). The conchae do not extend forward into the external nose. The anterior end of each concha curves inferiorly to form a lip that overlies the end of the related meatus.

Immediately inferior to the attachment of the middle concha and just anterior to the midpoint of the concha, the lateral wall of the middle meatus elevates to form the dome-shaped **ethmoidal bulla** (Fig. 8.221C). This is formed by the underlying middle ethmoidal cells, which expand the medial wall of the ethmoidal labyrinth.

Inferior to the ethmoidal bulla is a curved gutter (the **semilunar hiatus**), which is formed by the mucosa covering the lateral wall as it spans a defect in the bony wall between the ethmoidal bulla above and the uncinate process below.

The anterior end of the semilunar hiatus forms a channel (the **ethmoidal infundibulum**), which curves upward and continues as the **frontonasal duct** through the anterior part of the ethmoidal labyrinth to open into the frontal sinus.

The **nasolacrimal duct** and most of the paranasal sinuses open onto the lateral wall of the nasal cavity (Fig. 8.221C):

- The nasolacrimal duct opens onto the lateral wall of the inferior nasal meatus under the anterior lip of the inferior concha—it drains tears from the conjunctival sac of the eye into the nasal cavity and originates at the inferior end of the lacrimal sac on the anteromedial wall of the orbit.
- The frontal sinus drains via the frontonasal duct and ethmoidal infundibulum into the anterior end of the semilunar hiatus on the lateral wall of the middle nasal meatus—the anterior ethmoidal cells drain into the frontonasal duct or ethmoidal infundibulum (in some cases, the frontal sinus drains directly into the anterior end of the middle nasal meatus and the frontonasal duct ends blindly in the anterior ethmoidal cells).
- The middle ethmoidal cells open onto or just above the ethmoidal bulla.
- The posterior ethmoidal cells usually open onto the lateral wall of the superior nasal meatus.
- The large maxillary sinus opens into the semilunar hiatus, usually just inferior to the center of the ethmoidal bulla. This opening is near the roof of the maxillary sinus.

The only paranasal sinus that does not drain onto the lateral wall of the nasal cavity is the sphenoidal sinus, which usually opens onto the sloping posterior roof of the nasal cavity.

Nares

The nares are oval apertures on the inferior aspect of the external nose and are the anterior openings of the nasal cavities (Fig. 8.222A). They are held open by the surrounding alar cartilages and septal cartilage and by the inferior nasal spine and adjacent margins of the maxillae.

Although the nares are continuously open, they can be widened further by the action of the related muscles of facial expression (nasalis, depressor septi nasi, and levator labii superioris alaeque nasi muscles; Fig. 8.222B).

Choanae

The choanae are the oval-shaped openings between the nasal cavities and the nasopharynx (Fig. 8.223). Unlike the nares, which have flexible borders of cartilage and soft tissues, the choanae are rigid openings completely surrounded by bone, and their margins are formed:

- inferiorly, by the posterior border of the horizontal plate of the palatine bone;
- laterally, by the posterior margin of the medial plate of the pterygoid process; and
- medially, by the posterior border of the vomer.

The roof of the choanae is formed:

- anteriorly, by the ala of the vomer and the vaginal process of the medial plate of the pterygoid process; and
- posteriorly, by the body of the sphenoid bone.

Gateways

There are a number of routes by which nerves and vessels enter and leave the soft tissues lining each nasal cavity (Fig. 8.224), and these include the cribriform plate, sphenopalatine foramen, the incisive canal, small foramina in the lateral wall, and around the margin of the nares.

Cribriform plate

The fibers of the olfactory nerve [I] exit the nasal cavity and enter the cranial cavity through perforations in the cribriform plate (Fig. 8.224). In addition, small foramina between the cribriform plate and surrounding bone allow the anterior ethmoidal nerve, a branch of the ophthalmic nerve [V_1], and accompanying vessels to pass from the orbit into the cranial cavity and then down into the nasal cavity.

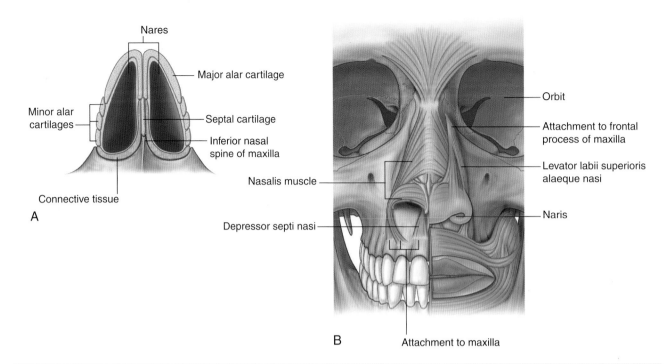

Fig. 8.222 Nares. **A.** Inferior view. **B.** Associated muscles.

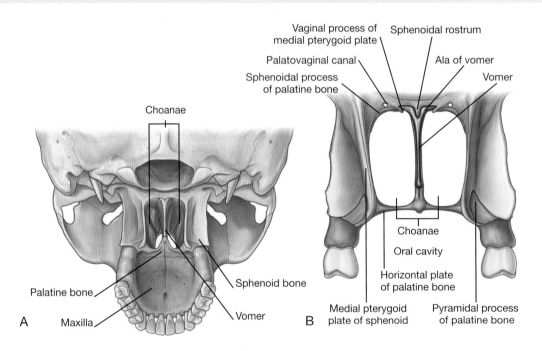

Fig. 8.223 Choanae (posterior view). **A.** Overview. **B.** Magnified view.

In addition, there is a connection in some individuals between nasal veins and the superior sagittal sinus of the cranial cavity through a prominent foramen (the foramen cecum) in the midline between the crista galli and frontal bone.

Sphenopalatine foramen

One of the most important routes by which nerves and vessels enter and leave the nasal cavity is the sphenopalatine foramen in the posterolateral wall of the superior nasal meatus (Fig. 8.224). This foramen is just superior to the attachment of the posterior end of the middle nasal concha and is formed by the sphenopalatine notch in the palatine bone and the body of the sphenoid bone.

The sphenopalatine foramen is a route of communication between the nasal cavity and the pterygopalatine fossa. Major structures passing through the foramen are:

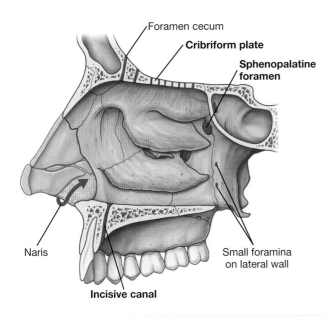

Foramen cecum
Cribriform plate
Sphenopalatine foramen
Naris
Small foramina on lateral wall
Incisive canal

Fig. 8.224 Gateways to the nasal cavities.

- the sphenopalatine branch of the maxillary artery,
- the nasopalatine branch of the maxillary nerve [V_2], and
- superior nasal branches of the maxillary nerve [V_2].

Incisive canal

Another route by which structures enter and leave the nasal cavities is through the **incisive canal** in the floor of each nasal cavity (Fig. 8.224). This canal is immediately lateral to the nasal septum and just posterosuperior to the root of the central incisor in the maxilla. The two incisive canals, one on each side, both open into the single unpaired incisive fossa in the roof of the oral cavity and transmits:

- the nasopalatine nerve from the nasal cavity into the oral cavity, and
- the terminal end of the greater palatine artery from the oral cavity into the nasal cavity.

Small foramina in the lateral wall

Other routes by which vessels and nerves get into and out of the nasal cavity include the nares and small foramina in the lateral wall (Fig. 8.224):

- Internal nasal branches of the infra-orbital nerve of the maxillary nerve [V_2] and alar branches of the nasal artery from the facial artery loop around the margin of the naris to gain entry to the lateral wall of the nasal cavity from the face.
- Inferior nasal branches from the greater palatine branch of the maxillary nerve [V_2] enter the lateral wall of the nasal cavity from the palatine canal by passing through small foramina on the lateral wall.

Vessels

The nasal cavities have a rich vascular supply for altering the humidity and temperature of respired air. In fact, the submucosa of the respiratory region, particularly that related to the conchae and septum, is often described as "erectile" or "cavernous" because the tissue enlarges or shrinks depending on the amount of blood flowing into the system.

Arteries

Arteries that supply the nasal cavity include vessels that originate from both the internal and external carotid arteries (Fig. 8.225):

- Vessels that originate from branches of the external carotid artery include the sphenopalatine, greater palatine, superior labial, and lateral nasal arteries.
- Vessels that originate from branches of the internal carotid artery are the anterior and posterior ethmoidal arteries.

Sphenopalatine artery

The largest vessel supplying the nasal cavity is the **sphenopalatine artery** (Fig. 8.225), which is the terminal branch of the maxillary artery in the pterygopalatine fossa. It leaves the pterygopalatine fossa and enters the nasal cavity by passing medially through the sphenopalatine foramen and onto the lateral wall of the nasal cavity.

Greater palatine artery

The terminal end of the **greater palatine artery** enters the anterior aspect of the floor of the nasal cavity by passing up through the incisive canal from the roof of the oral cavity (Fig. 8.225).

Like the sphenopalatine artery, the greater palatine artery arises in the pterygopalatine fossa as a branch of the maxillary artery. It passes first onto the roof of the oral cavity by passing down through the palatine canal and greater palatine foramen to the posterior aspect of the palate, then passes forward on the undersurface of the palate, and up through the incisive fossa and canal to reach the floor of the nasal cavity. The greater palatine artery supplies anterior regions of the medial wall and adjacent floor of the nasal cavity, and anastomoses with the septal branch of the sphenopalatine artery.

Superior labial and lateral nasal arteries

The superior labial artery and the lateral nasal artery originate from the facial artery on the front of the face (Fig. 8.225).

The **superior labial artery** originates from the facial artery near the lateral end of the oral fissure and passes medially in the lip, supplying the lip and giving rise to branches that supply the nose and nasal cavity. An alar branch supplies the region around the lateral aspect of the naris, and a septal branch passes into the nasal cavity and supplies anterior regions of the nasal septum.

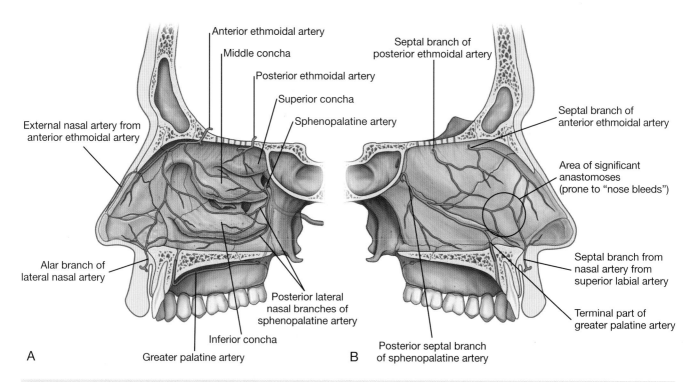

Fig. 8.225 Arterial supply of the nasal cavities. **A.** Lateral wall of the right nasal cavity. **B.** Septum (medial wall of right nasal cavity).

The **lateral nasal artery** originates from the facial artery in association with the margin of the external nose and contributes to the blood supply of the external nose. Alar branches pass around the lateral margin of the naris and supply the nasal vestibule.

Anterior and posterior ethmoidal arteries

The anterior and posterior ethmoidal arteries (Fig. 8.225) originate in the orbit from the ophthalmic artery, which originates in the cranial cavity as a major branch of the internal carotid artery. They pass through canals in the medial wall of the orbit between the ethmoidal labyrinth and frontal bone, supply the adjacent paranasal sinuses, and then enter the cranial cavity immediately lateral and superior to the cribriform plate.

Clinical app

Epistaxis
Vessels that supply the nasal cavities form extensive anastomoses with each other. This is particularly evident in the anterior region of the medial wall where there are anastomoses between branches of the greater palatine, sphenopalatine, superior labial, and anterior ethmoidal arteries and where the vessels are relatively close to the surface (Fig. 8.225C). This area is the major site of nosebleeds, or epistaxis.

The **posterior ethmoidal artery** descends into the nasal cavity through the cribriform plate and has branches to the upper parts of the medial and lateral walls.

The **anterior ethmoidal artery** passes forward, with the accompanying anterior ethmoidal nerve, in a groove on the cribriform plate and enters the nasal cavity by descending through a slit-like foramen immediately lateral to the crista galli.

Veins

Veins draining the nasal cavities generally follow the arteries (Fig. 8.226):

- Veins that pass with branches that ultimately originate from the maxillary artery drain into the pterygoid plexus of veins in the infratemporal fossa.
- Veins from anterior regions of the nasal cavities join the facial vein.

Innervation

Nerves that innervate the nasal cavities are (Fig. 8.227):

- the olfactory nerve [I] for olfaction, and
- branches of the ophthalmic [V_1] and maxillary [V_2] nerves for general sensation.

Secretomotor innervation of mucous glands in the nasal cavities and paranasal sinuses is by parasympathetic fibers

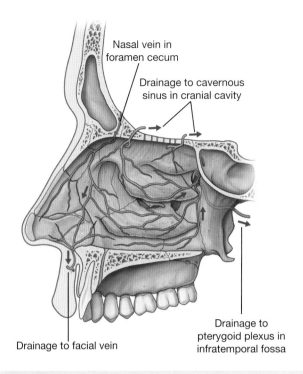

Fig. 8.226 Venous drainage of the nasal cavities.

Bundles of these axons pass superiorly through perforations in the cribriform plate to synapse with neurons in the olfactory bulb of the brain (Fig. 8.227).

Branches from the ophthalmic nerve [V₁]

Branches from the ophthalmic nerve $[V_1]$ that innervate the nasal cavity are the anterior and posterior ethmoidal nerves, which originate from the nasociliary nerve in the orbit (Fig. 8.227).

Anterior and posterior ethmoidal nerves

The anterior ethmoidal nerve (Fig. 8.227) travels with the anterior ethmoidal artery and leaves the orbit through a canal between the ethmoidal labyrinth and the frontal bone. It passes through and supplies the adjacent ethmoidal cells and frontal sinus, and then enters the cranial cavity immediately lateral and superior to the cribriform plate.

The anterior ethmoidal nerve travels forward in a groove on the cribriform plate and then enters the nasal cavity by descending through a slit-like foramen immediately lateral to the crista galli. It has branches to the medial and lateral wall of the nasal cavity and then continues forward on the undersurface of the nasal bone. It passes onto the external surface of the nose by traveling between the nasal bone and lateral nasal cartilage, and then terminates as the **external nasal nerve,** which supplies skin around the naris, in the nasal vestibule, and on the tip of the nose.

Like the anterior ethmoidal nerve, the posterior ethmoidal nerve leaves the orbit through a similar canal in the

from the facial nerve [VII], which mainly join branches of the maxillary nerve $[V_2]$ in the pterygopalatine fossa.

Olfactory nerve [I]

The olfactory nerve [I] is composed of axons from receptors in the olfactory epithelium at the top of each nasal cavity.

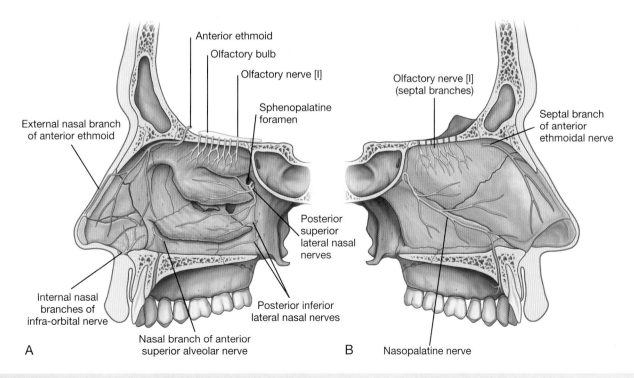

Fig. 8.227 Innervation of the nasal cavities. **A.** Lateral wall of right nasal cavity. **B.** Medial wall of right nasal cavity.

medial wall of the orbit. It terminates by supplying the mucosa of the ethmoidal cells and sphenoidal sinus and normally does not extend into the nasal cavity itself.

Branches from the maxillary nerve [V₂]

A number of nasal branches from the maxillary nerve [V₂] innervate the nasal cavity. Many of these nasal branches (Fig. 8.227) originate in the pterygopalatine fossa, which is just lateral to the lateral wall of the nasal cavity, and leave the fossa to enter the nasal cavity by passing medially through the sphenopalatine foramen:

- A number of these nerves (**posterior superior lateral nasal nerves**) pass forward on and supply the lateral wall of the nasal cavity.
- Others (**posterior superior medial nasal nerves**) cross the roof to the nasal septum and supply both these regions.
- The largest of these nerves is the **nasopalatine nerve**, which passes forward and down the medial wall of the nasal cavity to pass through the incisive canal onto the roof of the oral cavity and terminates by supplying the oral mucosa posterior to the incisor teeth.
- Other nasal nerves (**posterior inferior nasal nerves**) originate from the greater palatine nerve, descending from the pterygopalatine fossa in the palatine canal just lateral to the nasal cavity, and pass through small bony foramina to innervate the lateral wall of the nasal cavity.
- A small nasal nerve also originates from the anterior superior alveolar branch of the infra-orbital nerve and passes medially through the maxilla to supply the lateral wall near the anterior end of the inferior concha.

Parasympathetic innervation

Secretomotor innervation of glands in the mucosa of the nasal cavity and paranasal sinuses is by preganglionic parasympathetic fibers carried in the greater petrosal branch of the facial nerve [VII]. These fibers enter the pterygopalatine fossa and synapse in the pterygopalatine ganglion (see Fig. 8.139). Postganglionic parasympathetic fibers then join branches of the maxillary nerve [V₂] to leave the fossa and ultimately reach target glands.

Sympathetic innervation

Sympathetic innervation, mainly involved with regulating blood flow in the nasal mucosa, is from the spinal cord level T1. Preganglionic sympathetic fibers enter the sympathetic trunk and ascend to synapse in the superior cervical sympathetic ganglion. Postganglionic sympathetic fibers pass onto the internal carotid artery, enter the cranial cavity, and then leave the internal carotid artery to form the deep petrosal nerve, which joins the greater petrosal nerve of the

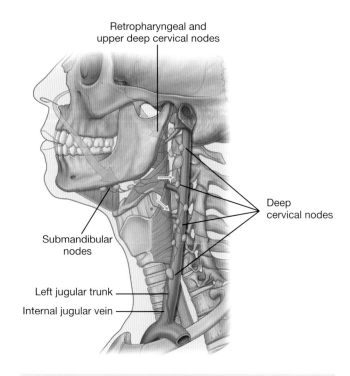

Fig. 8.228 Lymphatic drainage of the nasal cavities.

facial nerve [VII] and enters the pterygopalatine fossa (see Fig. 8.139, pg. 554).

Like the parasympathetic fibers, the sympathetic fibers follow branches of the maxillary nerve [V₂] into the nasal cavity.

Lymphatics

Lymph from anterior regions of the nasal cavities drains forward onto the face by passing around the margins of the nares (Fig. 8.228). These lymphatics ultimately connect with the submandibular nodes.

Lymph from posterior regions of the nasal cavity and the paranasal sinuses drains into upper deep cervical nodes. Some of this lymph passes first through the retropharyngeal nodes.

ORAL CAVITY

The oral cavity is inferior to the nasal cavities (Fig. 8.229A). It has a roof and floor, and lateral walls, opens onto the face through the oral fissure, and is continuous with the cavity of the pharynx at the oropharyngeal isthmus.

The roof of the oral cavity consists of the hard and soft palates. The floor is formed mainly of soft tissues, which include a muscular diaphragm and the tongue. The lateral walls (cheeks) are muscular and merge anteriorly with the lips surrounding the **oral fissure** (the anterior opening of the oral cavity).

The posterior aperture of the oral cavity is the oropharyngeal isthmus, which opens into the oral part of the pharynx.

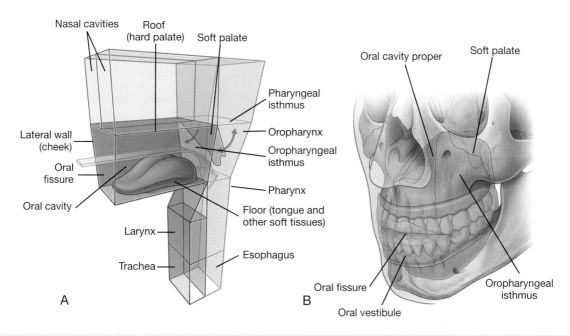

Fig. 8.229 Oral cavity. A. Relationship to other cavities. B. Oral vestibule and oral cavity proper.

The oral cavity is separated into two regions by the upper and lower dental arches consisting of the teeth and alveolar bone that supports them (Fig. 8.229B):

- The outer **oral vestibule,** which is horseshoe-shaped, is between the dental arches and the deep surfaces of the cheeks and lips—the oral fissure opens into it and can be opened and closed by muscles of facial expression, and by movements of the lower jaw.
- The inner **oral cavity proper** is enclosed by the dental arches.

The degree of separation between the upper and lower dental arches is established by elevating or depressing the lower jaw (mandible) at the temporomandibular joint.

The oropharyngeal isthmus at the back of the oral cavity proper can be opened and closed by surrounding soft tissues, which include the soft palate and tongue.

The oral cavity has multiple functions:

- It is the inlet for the digestive system involved with the initial processing of food, which is aided by secretions from salivary glands;
- It manipulates sounds produced by the larynx, and one outcome of this is speech; and
- It can be used for breathing because it opens into the pharynx, which is a common pathway for food and air.

Skeletal framework

Bones that contribute to the skeletal framework of the oral cavity or are related to the anatomy of structures in the oral cavity include:

Clinical app

Oral cancer

Oral cancer is a subtype of head and neck malignancy. Malignant tissue may grow anywhere in the oral cavity including the lips, tongue, mandible, and maxilla. Typically, oral cancers are squamous; however, malignancies may also occur within the salivary glands and lymph nodes. Oral cancers can spread relatively rapidly to local lymph node groups and to the lungs. The early signs and symptoms include; white or red patches of mucosal change within the mouth (leukoplakia or erythroplakia), which are usually painless. Ulceration may occur within these plaques exposing the malignant tissue. Although some patients may have a genetic predisposition to oral cancer, the three commonest risk factors include tobacco smoking, alcohol abuse, and human papillomavirus.

- the paired maxillae, palatine, and temporal bones; and
- the unpaired mandible, sphenoid, and hyoid bones.

In addition, the cartilaginous parts of the pharyngotympanic tubes on the inferior aspect of the base of the skull are related to the attachment of muscles of the soft palate.

Maxillae

The two maxillae contribute substantially to the architecture of the roof of the oral cavity. The parts involved are the alveolar and palatine processes (Fig. 8.230A).

The palatine process is a horizontal shelf that projects from the medial surface of each maxilla. It originates just

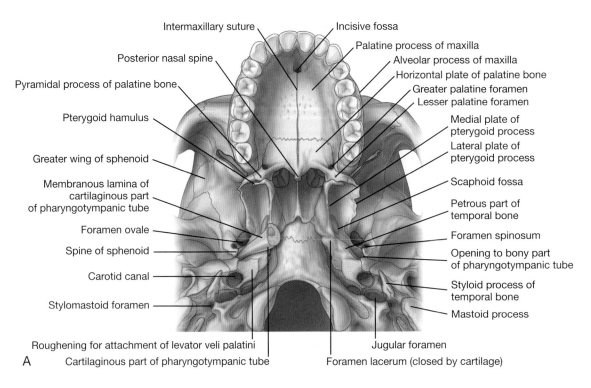

Intermaxillary suture
Incisive fossa
Posterior nasal spine
Palatine process of maxilla
Pyramidal process of palatine bone
Alveolar process of maxilla
Horizontal plate of palatine bone
Greater palatine foramen
Lesser palatine foramen
Pterygoid hamulus
Medial plate of pterygoid process
Lateral plate of pterygoid process
Greater wing of sphenoid
Scaphoid fossa
Membranous lamina of cartilaginous part of pharyngotympanic tube
Petrous part of temporal bone
Foramen ovale
Foramen spinosum
Spine of sphenoid
Opening to bony part of pharyngotympanic tube
Carotid canal
Styloid process of temporal bone
Stylomastoid foramen
Mastoid process
Roughening for attachment of levator veli palatini
Jugular foramen
A   Cartilaginous part of pharyngotympanic tube
Foramen lacerum (closed by cartilage)

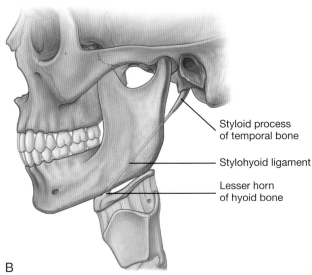

Styloid process of temporal bone

Stylohyoid ligament

Lesser horn of hyoid bone

B

Fig. 8.230 Base and lateral aspects of the skull. **A.** Features in the base of the skull related to structures associated with the oral cavity. **B.** Styloid process of the temporal bone.

superior to the medial aspect of the alveolar process and extends to the midline where it is joined, at a suture, with the palatine process from the other side. Together, the two palatine processes form the anterior two-thirds of the hard palate.

In the midline on the inferior surface of the hard palate and at the anterior end of the intermaxillary suture is a single small fossa (incisive fossa) just behind the incisor teeth. Two incisive canals, one on each side, extend posterosuperiorly from the roof of this fossa to open onto the floor of the nasal cavity. The canals and fossae allow

passage of the greater palatine vessels and the nasopalatine nerves.

Palatine bones

The parts of each L-shaped palatine bone that contribute to the roof of the oral cavity are the horizontal plate and the pyramidal process (Fig. 8.230A).

The horizontal plate projects medially from the inferior aspect of the palatine bone and is joined by sutures to its partner in the midline and, on the same side, with the palatine process of the maxilla anteriorly.

A single **posterior nasal spine** is formed at the midline where the two horizontal plates join and projects backward from the margin of the hard palate. The posterior margin of the horizontal plates and the posterior nasal spine are associated with attachment of the soft palate.

The greater palatine foramen, formed mainly by the horizontal plate of the palatine bone and completed laterally by the adjacent part of the maxilla, opens onto the posterolateral aspect of the horizontal plate (Fig. 8.230A). This foramen is the inferior opening of the palatine canal, which continues superiorly into the pterygopalatine fossa and transmits the greater palatine nerve and vessels to the palate.

Also opening onto the palatine bone is the lesser palatine foramen (Fig. 8.230A). This foramen is the inferior opening of the lesser palatine canal, which branches from the greater palatine canal and transmits the lesser palatine nerve and vessels to the soft palate.

The pyramidal process projects posteriorly and fills the space between the inferior ends of the medial and lateral plates of the pterygoid process of the sphenoid bone (Fig. 8.230A).

Sphenoid bone

The pterygoid processes and spines of the sphenoid bone are associated with structures related to the soft palate, which forms part of the roof of the oral cavity (Fig. 8.230A).

The pterygoid processes descend, one on each side, from the lateral aspect of the body of the sphenoid bone. Each process has a medial and a lateral plate. These two vertically oriented plates project from the posterior aspect of the process. The V-shaped gap that occurs inferiorly between the two plates is filled by the pyramidal process of the palatine bone.

Projecting posterolaterally from the inferior margin of the medial plate of the pterygoid process is an elongate hook-shaped structure (the pterygoid hamulus) (Fig. 8.230A). This hamulus is immediately behind the alveolar arch and inferior to the posterior margin of the hard palate. It is:

- a "pulley" for one of the muscles (tensor veli palatini) of the soft palate, and
- the attachment site for the upper end of the pterygomandibular raphe, which is attached below to the mandible and joins together the superior constrictor of the pharynx and the buccinator muscle of the cheek.

At the root of the medial plate of the pterygoid process on the base of the skull is a small canoe-shaped fossa **(scaphoid fossa),** which begins just medial to the foramen ovale and descends anteriorly and medially to the root of the medial plate of the pterygoid process (Fig. 8.230A). This fossa is for the attachment of one of the muscles of the soft palate (tensor veli palatini).

The spines of the sphenoid, one on each side, are vertical projections from the inferior surfaces of the greater wings of the sphenoid bone (Fig. 8.230A). Each spine is immediately posteromedial to the foramen spinosum.

The medial aspect of the spine provides attachment for the most lateral part of the tensor veli palatini muscle of the soft palate.

Temporal bone

The styloid process and inferior aspect of the petrous part of the temporal bone provide attachment for muscles associated with the tongue and soft palate, respectively.

The styloid process projects anteroinferiorly from the underside of the temporal bone. It can be as long as 1 inch (2.5 cm) and points toward the lesser horn of the hyoid bone to which it is attached by the stylohyoid ligament (Fig. 8.230B). The root of the styloid process is immediately anterior to the stylomastoid foramen and lateral to the jugular foramen. The styloglossus muscle of the tongue attaches to the anterolateral surface of the styloid process.

The inferior aspect of the temporal bone has a triangular roughened area immediately anteromedial to the opening of the carotid canal (Fig. 8.230A). The levator veli palatini muscle of the soft palate is attached here.

Cartilaginous part of the pharyngotympanic tube

The trumpet-shaped cartilaginous part of the pharyngotympanic tube is in a groove between the anterior margin of the petrous part of the temporal bone and the posterior margin of the greater wing of the sphenoid (Fig. 8.230A).

The medial and lateral walls of the cartilaginous part of the pharyngotympanic tube are formed mainly of cartilage, whereas the more inferolateral wall is more fibrous and is known as the **membranous lamina.**

The apex of the cartilaginous part of the pharyngotympanic tube connects laterally to the opening of the bony part in the temporal bone.

The expanded medial end of the cartilaginous part of the pharyngotympanic tube is immediately posterior to the upper margin of the medial plate of the pterygoid process and opens into the nasopharynx.

The cartilaginous part of the pharyngotympanic tube is lateral to the attachment of the levator veli palatini muscle to the petrous part of the temporal bone and medial to the spine of the sphenoid. The tensor veli palatini muscle is attached, in part, to the membranous lamina.

Mandible

The mandible is the bone of the lower jaw (Fig. 8.231). It consists of a body of right and left parts, which are fused anteriorly in the midline **(mandibular symphysis),** and two rami.

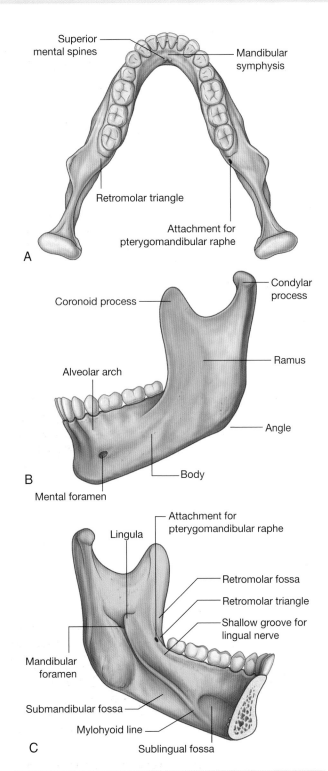

Fig. 8.231 Mandible. **A.** Superior view. **B.** Lateral view. **C.** Medial view.

Posterior to the mandibular symphysis on the internal surface of the mandible are two pairs of small spines, one pair immediately above the other pair. These are the **superior** and **inferior mental spines (superior** and **inferior genial spines),** and are attachment sites for a pair of muscles that pass into the tongue and a pair of muscles that connect the mandible to the hyoid bone (Fig. 8.231A; also see Fig. 8.234A).

Extending from the midline and originating inferior to the mental spines is a raised line or ridge (the **mylohyoid line**), which runs posteriorly and superiorly along the internal surface of each side of the body of the mandible to end just below the level of the last molar tooth (Fig. 8.231C).

Above the anterior one-third of the mylohyoid line is a shallow depression (the **sublingual fossa**), and below the posterior two-thirds of the mylohyoid line is another depression (the **submandibular fossa**).

Between the last molar tooth and the mylohyoid line is a shallow groove for the lingual nerve.

Immediately posterior to the last molar tooth on the medial upper surface of the body of mandible is a small triangular depression **(retromolar triangle)** (Fig. 8.231C). The pterygomandibular raphe attaches just medial to the apex of this triangle and extends from here to the tip of the pterygoid hamulus above.

The ramus of mandible, one on each side, is quadrangular shaped and oriented in the sagittal plane. On the medial surface of the ramus is a large **mandibular foramen** for transmission of the inferior alveolar nerve and vessels (Fig. 8.231C).

Hyoid bone

The hyoid bone is a small U-shaped bone in the neck between the larynx and the mandible. It has an anterior body of hyoid bone and two large greater horns, one on each side, which project posteriorly and superiorly from the body (Fig. 8.232). There are two small conical lesser horns on the superior surface where the greater horns join with the body. The stylohyoid ligaments attach to the apices of the lesser horns.

The hyoid bone is a key bone in the neck because it connects the floor of the oral cavity in front with the pharynx behind and the larynx below.

Walls: the cheeks

The walls of the oral cavity are formed by the cheeks.

Each cheek consists of fascia and a layer of skeletal muscle sandwiched between skin externally and oral mucosa internally. The thin layer of skeletal muscle within the cheeks is principally the buccinator muscle, which is a muscle of facial expression (Table 8.20, Fig. 8.233).

The site of fusion is particularly visible on the external surface of the bone as a small vertical ridge in the midline.

The upper surface of the body of mandible bears the alveolar arch, which anchors the lower teeth, and on its external surface on each side is a small mental foramen (Fig. 8.231B).

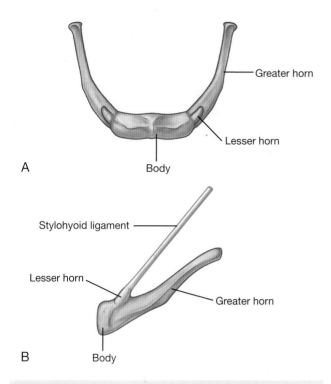

Fig. 8.232 Hyoid bone. A. Anterior view. B. Lateral view.

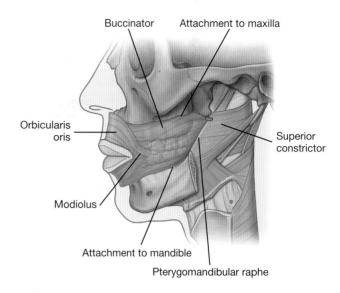

Fig. 8.233 Buccinator muscle.

Floor

The floor of the oral cavity proper is formed mainly by three structures:

- a muscular diaphragm, which fills the U-shaped gap between the left and right sides of the body of the mandible and is composed of the paired mylohyoid muscles (Table 8.21, Fig. 8.234A);
- two cord-like geniohyoid muscles above the diaphragm, which run from the mandible in front to the hyoid bone behind (Fig. 8.234B,C); and
- the tongue, which is superior to the geniohyoid muscles.

Also present in the floor of the oral cavity proper are salivary glands and their ducts. The largest of these glands, on each side, are the sublingual gland and the oral part of the submandibular gland.

Tongue

The tongue is a muscular structure that forms part of the floor of the oral cavity and part of the anterior wall of the oropharynx (Fig. 8.235A). Its anterior (oral) part is in the oral cavity and is somewhat triangular in shape with a blunt **apex of tongue.** The apex is directed anteriorly and sits immediately behind the incisor teeth. The **root of tongue** is attached to the mandible and the hyoid bone.

The superior surface of the oral or anterior two-thirds of the tongue is oriented in the horizontal plane.

The pharyngeal surface or posterior one-third of the tongue curves inferiorly and becomes oriented more in the vertical plane. The oral and pharyngeal surfaces are separated by a V-shaped **terminal sulcus of tongue.** This terminal sulcus forms the inferior margin of the oropharyngeal isthmus between the oral and pharyngeal cavities. At the apex of the V-shaped sulcus is a small depression (the **foramen cecum of tongue**), which marks the site in the embryo where the epithelium invaginated to form the thyroid gland. In some people a thyroglossal duct persists and connects the foramen cecum on the tongue with the thyroid gland in the neck.

Papillae

The superior surface of the oral part of the tongue is covered by hundreds of papillae (Fig. 8.235B):

- **Filiform papillae** are small cone-shaped projections of the mucosa that end in one or more points.

Muscle	Origin	Insertion	Innervation	Function
Table 8.20	General sensation from the skin and oral mucosa of the cheeks is carried by the buccal branch of the mandibular nerve [V$_3$]			
Buccinator	Pterygomandibular raphe, alveolar part of mandible, alveolar process of maxilla	Blends with fibers of orbicularis oris muscle; modiolus (button-shaped nodule of connective tissue at the interface between the muscles of the lips and cheeks)	Buccal branch of VII	Holds the cheeks against the alveolar arches; keeps food between the teeth when chewing

Table 8.21   Muscles in the floor of the oral cavity

Muscle	Origin	Insertion	Innervation	Function
Mylohyoid	Mylohyoid line of mandible	Median fibrous raphe and adjacent part of hyoid bone	Nerve to mylohyoid from the inferior alveolar branch of mandibular nerve [V₃]	Supports and elevates floor of oral cavity; elevates and pulls forward hyoid bone, and therefore attached larynx, during initial stages of swallowing; depresses mandible when hyoid is fixed.
Geniohyoid	Inferior mental spines of mandible	Body of hyoid bone	C1	Depresses mandible when hyoid is fixed; elevates and pulls hyoid forward when mandible is fixed

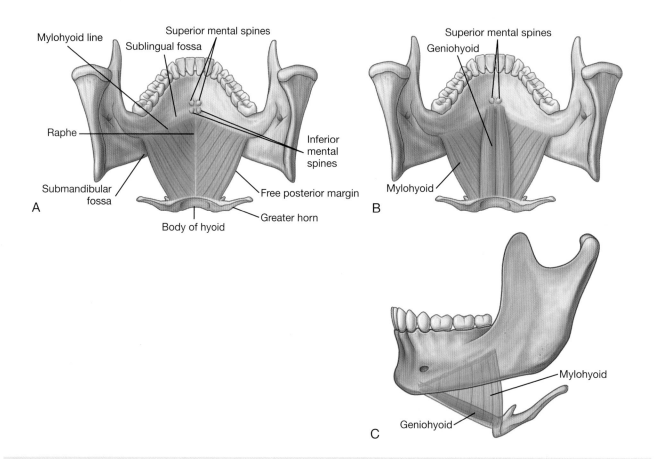

Fig. 8.234 A. Mylohyoid muscles. **B.** Geniohyoid muscles. **C.** Lateral view.

- **Fungiform papillae** are rounder in shape and larger than the filiform papillae and tend to be concentrated along the margins of the tongue.
- The largest of the papillae are the **vallate papillae,** which are blunt-ended cylindrical papillae invaginations in the tongue's surface—there are only about 8 to 12 vallate papillae in a single V-shaped line immediately anterior to the terminal sulcus of tongue.
- **Foliate papillae** are linear folds of mucosa on the sides of the tongue near the terminal sulcus of tongue.

The papillae in general increase the area of contact between the surface of the tongue and the contents of the oral cavity. All except the filiform papillae have taste buds on their surfaces.

Inferior surface of tongue

The undersurface of the oral part of the tongue lacks papillae, but does have a number of linear mucosal folds (Fig. 8.236C,D). A single median fold (the **frenulum of tongue**) is continuous with the mucosa covering the floor of the oral cavity, and overlies the lower margin of a mid-line sagittal septum, which internally separates the right and left sides of the tongue. On each side of the frenulum is a lingual vein, and lateral to each vein is a rough **fimbriated fold.**

Pharyngeal surface

The mucosa covering the pharyngeal surface of the tongue is irregular in contour because of the many small nodules

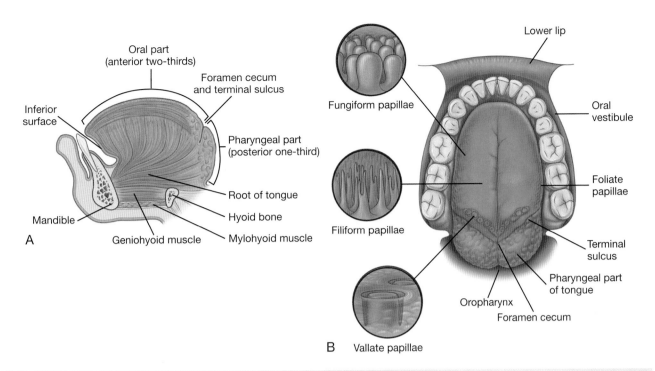

Fig. 8.235 Tongue. **A.** Paramedian sagittal section. **B.** Superior view.

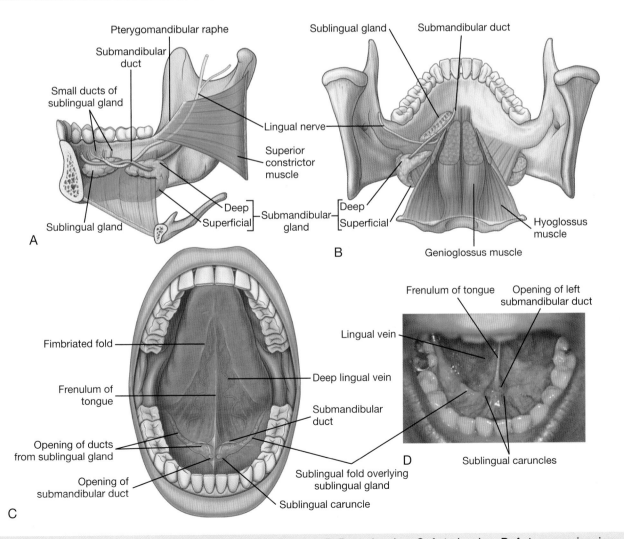

Fig. 8.236 Submandibular and sublingual glands. **A.** Medial view. **B.** Posterior view. **C.** Anterior view. **D.** Anterosuperior view.

Table 8.22 Muscles of the tongue

Muscle	Origin	Insertion	Innervation	Function
Intrinsic				
Superior longitudinal (just deep to surface of tongue)	Submucosal connective tissue at the back of the tongue and from the median septum of the tongue	Muscle fibers pass forward and obliquely to submucosal connective tissue and mucosa on margins of tongue	Hypoglossal nerve [XII]	Shortens tongue; curls apex and sides of tongue
Inferior longitudinal (between genioglossus and hyoglossus muscles)	Root of tongue (some fibers from hyoid)	Apex of tongue	Hypoglossal nerve [XII]	Shortens tongue; uncurls apex and turns it downward
Transverse	Median septum of the tongue	Submucosal connective tissue on lateral margins of tongue	Hypoglossal nerve [XII]	Narrows and elongates tongue
Vertical	Submucosal connective tissue on dorsum of tongue	Connective tissue in more ventral regions of tongue	Hypoglossal nerve [XII]	Flattens and widens tongue
Extrinsic				
Genioglossus	Superior mental spines	Body of hyoid; entire length of tongue	Hypoglossal nerve [XII]	Protrudes tongue; depresses center of tongue
Hyoglossus	Greater horn and adjacent part of body of hyoid bone	Lateral surface of tongue	Hypoglossal nerve [XII]	Depresses tongue
Styloglossus	Styloid process (anterolateral surface)	Lateral surface of tongue	Hypoglossal nerve [XII]	Elevates and retracts tongue
Palatoglossus	Inferior surface of palatine aponeurosis	Lateral margin of tongue	Vagus nerve [X] (via pharyngeal branch to pharyngeal plexus)	Depresses palate; moves palatoglossal fold toward midline; elevates back of the tongue

of lymphoid tissue in the submucosa. These nodules are collectively the **lingual tonsil**.

There are no papillae on the pharyngeal surface.

Muscles

The bulk of the tongue is composed of muscle (Table 8.22, Fig. 8.235A).

The tongue is completely divided into a left and right half by a median sagittal septum composed of connective tissue. This means that all muscles of the tongue are paired. There are intrinsic and extrinsic lingual muscles.

Intrinsic muscles of the tongue (Fig. 8.237) originate and insert within the substance of the tongue. They are divided into **superior longitudinal, inferior longitudinal, transverse,** and **vertical muscles,** and they alter the shape of the tongue.

Extrinsic muscles of the tongue (Table 8.22, Fig. 8.237) originate from structures outside the tongue and insert into the tongue. There are four major extrinsic muscles on each side, the **genioglossus, hyoglossus, styloglossus,** and **palatoglossus.** These muscles protrude, retract, depress, and elevate the tongue.

Except for the palatoglossus, which is innervated by the vagus nerve [X], all muscles of the tongue are innervated by the hypoglossal nerve [XII].

Clinical app

Test for cranial nerve XII

Asking a patient to "stick your tongue out" can be used as a test for the hypoglossal nerves [XII] (genioglossus muscle). If the nerves are functioning normally, the tongue should protrude evenly in the midline. If the nerve on one side is not fully functional, the tip of the tongue will point to that side when protruded.

Vessels

Arteries

The major artery of the tongue is the **lingual artery** (Fig. 8.238).

On each side, the lingual artery originates from the external carotid artery in the neck adjacent to the tip of the greater horn of the hyoid bone. It forms an upward bend and then loops downward and forward to pass deep to the hyoglossus muscle; accompanies the muscle through the aperture formed by the margins of the mylohyoid, superior constrictor, and middle constrictor muscles; and enters the floor of the oral cavity.

The lingual artery then travels forward in the plane between the hyoglossus and genioglossus muscles to the apex of the tongue.

Extrinsic muscles

Palatoglossus

Styloglossus

Hyoglossus

Genioglossus

Intrinsic muscles

Superior longitudinal

Vertical

Transverse

Inferior longitudinal

Septum

Fig. 8.237 Muscles of the tongue.

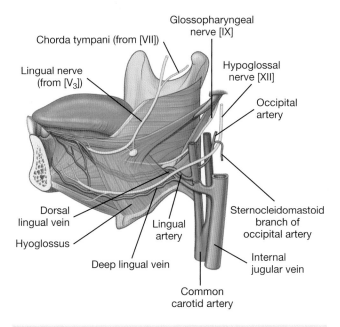

Chorda tympani (from [VII])

Glossopharyngeal nerve [IX]

Lingual nerve (from [V₃])

Hypoglossal nerve [XII]

Occipital artery

Dorsal lingual vein

Hyoglossus

Lingual artery

Deep lingual vein

Sternocleidomastoid branch of occipital artery

Internal jugular vein

Common carotid artery

Fig. 8.238 Arteries, veins, and nerves of the tongue.

In addition to the tongue, the lingual artery supplies the sublingual gland, gingiva, and oral mucosa in the floor of the oral cavity.

Veins

The tongue is drained by dorsal lingual and deep lingual veins (Fig. 8.238).

The **deep lingual veins** are visible through the mucosa on the undersurface of the tongue. Although they accompany the lingual arteries in anterior parts of the tongue, they become separated from the arteries posteriorly by the hyoglossus muscles. On each side, the deep lingual vein travels with the hypoglossal nerve [XII] on the external surface of the hyoglossus muscle and passes out of the floor of the oral cavity through the aperture (oropharyngeal triangle) formed by the margins of the mylohyoid, superior constrictor, and middle constrictor muscles. It joins the internal jugular vein in the neck.

The **dorsal lingual vein** follows the lingual artery between the hyoglossus and genioglossus muscles and, like

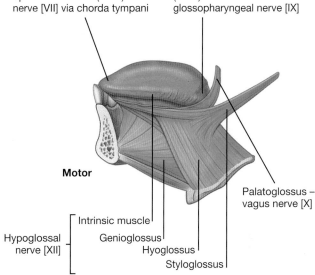

Sensory

Anterior two-thirds (oral)
- General sensation: mandibular nerve [V₃] via lingual nerve
- Special sensation (taste): facial nerve [VII] via chorda tympani

Posterior one-third (pharyngeal)
- General and special (taste) sensation via glossopharyngeal nerve [IX]

Motor

Hypoglossal nerve [XII]

Intrinsic muscle

Genioglossus

Hyoglossus

Styloglossus

Palatoglossus – vagus nerve [X]

Fig. 8.239 Innervation of the tongue.

the deep lingual vein, drains into the internal jugular vein in the neck.

Innervation

Innervation of the tongue is complex and involves a number of nerves (Figs. 8.238 and 8.239).

Glossopharyngeal nerve [IX]

Taste (SA) and general sensation from the pharyngeal part of the tongue are carried by the glossopharyngeal nerve [IX].

The glossopharyngeal nerve [IX] leaves the skull through the jugular foramen and descends along the posterior surface of the stylopharyngeus muscle. It passes around the lateral surface of the stylopharyngeus and then slips through the posterior aspect of the gap (oropharyngeal triangle) between the superior constrictor, middle constrictor, and mylohyoid muscles. The nerve then passes forward on the oropharyngeal wall just below the inferior pole of the palatine tonsil and enters the pharyngeal part of the tongue deep to the styloglossus and hyoglossus muscles. In addition to taste and general sensation on the posterior one-third of the tongue, branches creep anterior to the terminal sulcus of tongue to carry taste (SA) and general sensation from the vallate papillae.

Lingual nerve

General sensory innervation from the anterior two-thirds or oral part of the tongue is carried by the **lingual nerve,** which is a major branch of the mandibular nerve [V₃]. It originates

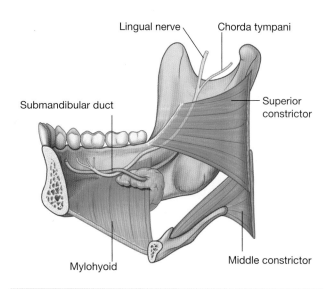

Fig. 8.240 Lingual nerve in the floor of the oral cavity (medial view).

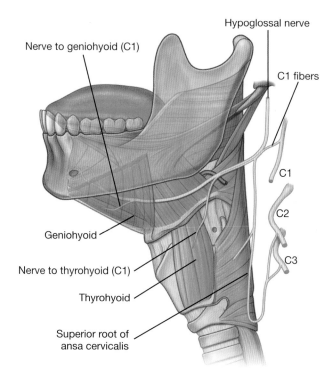

Fig. 8.241 Hypoglossal nerve and C1 fibers.

in the infratemporal fossa and passes anteriorly into the floor of the oral cavity by passing through the gap (oropharyngeal triangle) between the mylohyoid, superior constrictor, and middle constrictor muscles (Fig. 8.240).

The lingual nerve then continues anteromedially across the floor of the oral cavity, loops under the submandibular duct, and ascends into the tongue on the external and superior surface of the hyoglossus muscle (Fig. 8.240).

In addition to general sensation from the oral part of the tongue, the lingual nerve also carries general sensation from the mucosa on the floor of the oral cavity and gingiva associated with the lower teeth. The lingual nerve also carries parasympathetic and taste fibers from the oral part of the tongue that are part of the facial nerve [VII].

Facial nerve [VII]

Taste (SA) from the oral part of the tongue is carried into the CNS by the facial nerve [VII]. Special sensory (SA) fibers of the facial nerve [VII] leave the tongue and oral cavity as part of the lingual nerve. The fibers then enter the chorda tympani nerve, which is a branch of the facial nerve [VII] that joins the lingual nerve in the infratemporal fossa (see Fig. 8.240).

Hypoglossal nerve [XII]

All muscles of the tongue are innervated by the hypoglossal nerve [XII] except for the palatoglossus muscle, which is innervated by the vagus nerve [X].

The hypoglossal nerve [XII] leaves the skull through the hypoglossal canal and descends almost vertically in the neck to a level just below the angle of mandible (Fig. 8.241). Here it angles sharply forward around the sternocleidomastoid branch of the occipital artery, crosses the external carotid

artery, and continues forward, crossing the loop of the lingual artery to reach the external surface of the lower one-third of the hyoglossus muscle.

The hypoglossal nerve [XII] follows the hyoglossus muscle through the gap (oropharyngeal triangle) between the superior constrictor, middle constrictor, and mylohyoid muscles to reach the tongue.

In the upper neck, a branch from the anterior ramus of C1 joins the hypoglossal nerve [XII]. Most of these C1 fibers leave the hypoglossal nerve [XII] as the superior root of the ansa cervicalis (Fig. 8.241). Near the posterior border of the hyoglossus muscle, the remaining fibers leave the hypoglossal nerve [XII] and form two nerves:

- the thyrohyoid branch, which remains in the neck to innervate the thyrohyoid muscle; and
- the branch to the geniohyoid, which passes into the floor of the oral cavity to innervate the geniohyoid.

Lymphatics

All lymphatic vessels from the tongue ultimately drain into the deep cervical chain of nodes along the internal jugular vein:

- The pharyngeal part of the tongue drains through the pharyngeal wall directly into mainly the jugulodigastric node of the deep cervical chain.
- The oral part of the tongue drains both directly into the deep cervical nodes and indirectly into these nodes by

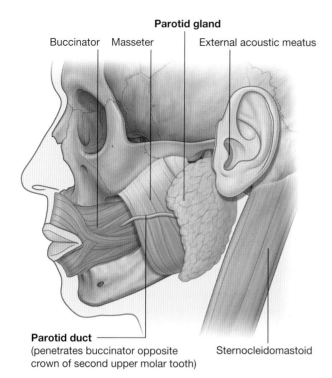

Parotid gland

Buccinator   Masseter   External acoustic meatus

Parotid duct
(penetrates buccinator opposite
crown of second upper molar tooth)

Sternocleidomastoid

Fig. 8.242 Parotid gland.

passing first through the mylohyoid muscle and into submental and submandibular nodes.

The submental nodes are inferior to the mylohyoid muscles and between the digastric muscles, while the submandibular nodes are below the floor of the oral cavity along the inner aspect of the inferior margins of the mandible.

The tip of the tongue drains through the mylohyoid muscle into the submental nodes and then into mainly the jugulo-omohyoid node of the deep cervical chain.

Salivary glands

Salivary glands are glands that open or secrete into the oral cavity. Most are small glands in the submucosa or mucosa of the oral epithelium lining the tongue, palate, cheeks, and lips, and open into the oral cavity directly or via small ducts. In addition to these small glands are much larger glands, which include the paired parotid, submandibular, and sublingual glands.

Parotid gland

The parotid gland (also see pp. 487-490) on each side is entirely outside the boundaries of the oral cavity in a shallow triangular-shaped trench (Fig. 8.242) formed by:

- the sternocleidomastoid muscle behind;
- the ramus of mandible in front; and
- the external acoustic meatus and the posterior aspect of the zygomatic arch superiorly.

The gland normally extends anteriorly over the masseter muscle and inferiorly over the posterior belly of the digastric muscle.

The parotid duct passes anteriorly across the external surface of the masseter muscle and then turns medially to penetrate the buccinator muscle of the cheek and open into the oral cavity adjacent to the crown of the second upper molar tooth (Fig. 8.242).

The parotid gland encloses the external carotid artery, the retromandibular vein, and the origin of the extracranial part of the facial nerve [VII].

Submandibular glands

The elongate **submandibular glands** are smaller than the parotid glands but larger than the sublingual glands. Each is hook shaped (Fig. 8.243, Fig. 8.44):

- The larger arm of the hook is directed forward in the horizontal plane below the mylohyoid muscle and is therefore outside the boundaries of the oral cavity. This larger superficial part of the gland is directly against a shallow impression on the medial side of the mandible (submandibular fossa) inferior to the mylohyoid line.
- The smaller arm of the hook (or deep part) of the gland loops around the posterior margin of the mylohyoid muscle to enter and lie within the floor of the oral cavity where it is lateral to the root of the tongue on the lateral surface of the hyoglossus muscle.

The **submandibular duct** emerges from the medial side of the deep part of the gland in the oral cavity and passes forward to open on the summit of a small **sublingual caruncle** (papilla) beside the base of frenulum of the tongue (see Fig. 8.236C,D).

The lingual nerve loops under the submandibular duct, crossing first the lateral side and then the medial side of the duct, as the nerve descends anteromedially through the floor of the oral cavity and then ascends into the tongue.

Sublingual glands

The sublingual glands are the smallest of the three major paired salivary glands. Each is almond shaped and is immediately lateral to the submandibular duct and associated lingual nerve in the floor of the oral cavity (see Fig. 8.236A,B).

Each sublingual gland lies directly against the medial surface of the mandible where it forms a shallow groove (sublingual fossa) superior to the anterior one-third of the mylohyoid line.

The superior margin of the sublingual gland raises an elongate fold of mucosa **(sublingual fold),** which extends from the posterolateral aspect of the floor of the oral cavity to the sublingual papilla beside the base of the frenulum of the tongue at the midline anteriorly (see Fig. 8.236C,D).

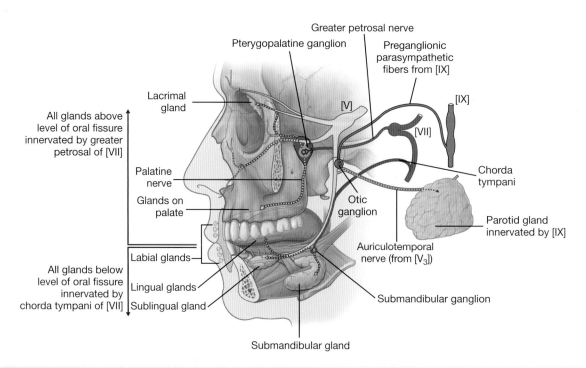

Fig. 8.243 Summary of parasympathetic (secretomotor) innervation of glands in the head.

The sublingual gland drains into the oral cavity via numerous small ducts (minor sublingual ducts), which open onto the crest of the sublingual fold. Occasionally, the more anterior part of the gland is drained by a duct (major sublingual duct) that opens together with the submandibular duct on the sublingual caruncle.

Vessels

Vessels that supply the parotid gland originate from the external carotid artery and from its branches that are adjacent to the gland. The submandibular and sublingual glands are supplied by branches of the facial and lingual arteries.

Veins from the parotid gland drain into the external jugular vein, and those from the submandibular and sublingual glands drain into lingual and facial veins.

Lymphatic vessels from the parotid gland drain into nodes that are on or in the gland. These parotid nodes then drain into superficial and deep cervical nodes.

Lymphatics from the submandibular and sublingual glands drain mainly into submandibular nodes and then into deep cervical nodes, particularly the jugulo-omohyoid node.

Innervation

Parasympathetic

Parasympathetic innervation to all salivary glands in the oral cavity is by branches of the facial nerve [VII], which join branches of the maxillary [V_2] and mandibular [V_3] nerves to reach their target destinations (Fig. 8.243).

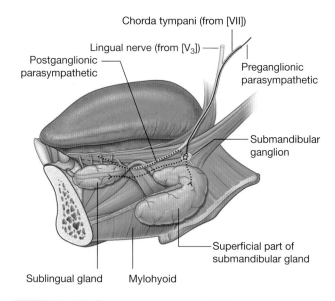

Fig. 8.244 Course of parasympathetic fibers carried in the chorda tympani nerve.

The parotid gland receives its parasympathetic innervation from fibers that initially traveled in the glossopharyngeal nerve [IX], which eventually joins a branch of the mandibular nerve [V_3] in the infratemporal fossa (Fig. 8.243).

Greater petrosal nerve

All salivary glands above the level of the oral fissure, as well as all mucous glands in the nose and the lacrimal gland in the orbit, are innervated by parasympathetic fibers carried in the greater petrosal branch of the facial nerve [VII] (Fig. 8.243).

Preganglionic parasympathetic fibers carried in this nerve enter the pterygopalatine fossa and synapse with postganglionic parasympathetic fibers in the pterygopalatine ganglion formed around branches of the maxillary nerve [V_2]. Postganglionic parasympathetic fibers join general sensory branches of the maxillary nerve, such as the palatine nerves, destined for the roof of the oral cavity, to reach their target glands.

Chorda tympani

All glands below the level of the oral fissure, which include those small glands in the floor of the oral cavity, in the lower lip, and in the tongue, and the larger submandibular and sublingual glands, are innervated by parasympathetic fibers carried in the chorda tympani branch of the facial nerve [VII] (Fig. 8.243-8.244).

The chorda tympani joins the lingual nerve of the mandibular nerve [V_3] in the infratemporal fossa and passes with it into the oral cavity. On the external surface of the hyoglossus muscle, preganglionic parasympathetic fibers leave the inferior aspect of the lingual nerve to synapse with postganglionic parasympathetic fibers in the submandibular ganglion, which appears to hang off the lingual nerve (Fig. 8.243-8.244). Postganglionic parasympathetic fibers leave the ganglion and pass directly to the submandibular and sublingual glands while others hop back onto the lingual nerve and travel with branches of the lingual nerve to target glands.

Sympathetic

Sympathetic innervation to the salivary glands is from spinal cord level T1. Preganglionic sympathetic fibers enter the sympathetic trunk and ascend to synapse in the superior cervical sympathetic ganglion (Fig. 8.245). Postganglionic fibers hop onto adjacent blood vessels and nerves to reach the glands.

Roof—palate

The roof of the oral cavity consists of the palate, which has two parts—an anterior hard palate and a posterior soft palate (Fig. 8.246).

Hard palate

The hard palate separates the oral cavity from the nasal cavities. It consists of a bony plate covered above and below by mucosa (Fig. 8.246):

- Above, it is covered by respiratory mucosa and forms the floor of the nasal cavities.
- Below, it is covered by a tightly bound layer of oral mucosa and forms much of the roof of the oral cavity.

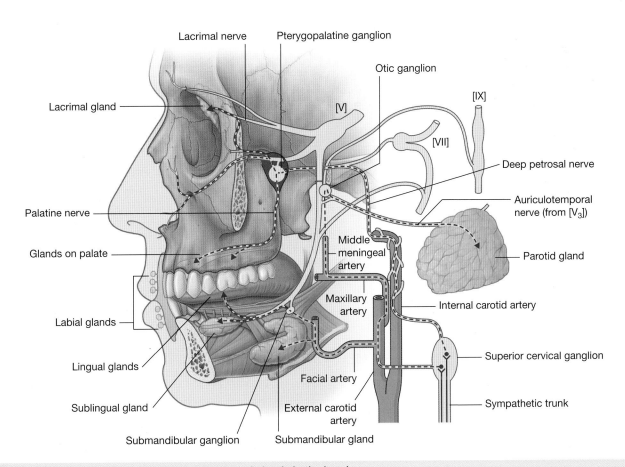

Fig. 8.245 Summary of sympathetic innervation of glands in the head.

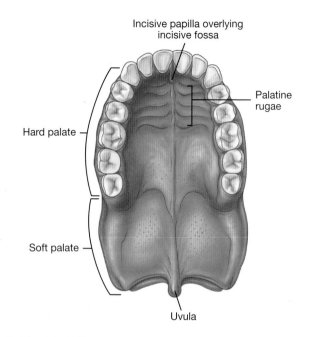

Incisive papilla overlying incisive fossa

Palatine rugae

Hard palate

Soft palate

Uvula

Fig. 8.246 Palate.

The palatine processes of the maxillae form the anterior three-quarters of the hard palate. The horizontal plates of the palatine bones form the posterior one-quarter. In the oral cavity, the upper alveolar arch borders the hard palate anteriorly and laterally. Posteriorly, the hard palate is continuous with the soft palate.

The mucosa of the hard palate in the oral cavity possesses numerous **transverse palatine folds (palatine rugae)** and a median longitudinal ridge **(palatine raphe),** which ends anteriorly in a small oval elevation **(incisive papilla)** (Fig. 8.246).

The incisive papilla overlies the incisive fossa formed between the horizontal plates of the maxillae immediately behind the incisor teeth.

Soft palate

The soft palate (Fig. 8.246) continues posteriorly from the hard palate and acts as a valve that can be:

- depressed to help close the oropharyngeal isthmus; or
- elevated to separate the nasopharynx from the oropharynx.

The soft palate is formed and moved by four muscles and is covered by mucosa that is continuous with the mucosa lining the pharynx and oral and nasal cavities.

The small tear-shaped muscular projection that hangs from the posterior free margin of the soft palate is the **uvula.**

Muscles of the soft palate

Five muscles (Table 8.23, Figs. 8.247, 8.248) on each side contribute to the formation and movement of the soft palate. Two of these, the **tensor veli palatini** and **levator veli palatini**, descend into the palate from the base of the skull. Two others, the **palatoglossus** and **palatopharyngeus,** ascend into the palate from the tongue and pharynx, respectively. The palatine tonsils are placed on each side between mucosal folds over the palatoglossus and palatopharyngeus muscles. The last muscle, the **musculus uvulae,** is associated with the uvula.

All muscles of the palate are innervated by the vagus nerve [X] except for the tensor veli palatini, which is innervated by the mandibular nerve [V$_3$] (via the nerve to medial pterygoid).

Table 8.23 Muscles of the soft palate

Muscle	Origin	Insertion	Innervation	Function
Tensor veli palatini	Scaphoid fossa of sphenoid bone; fibrous part of pharyngotympanic tube; spine of sphenoid	Palatine aponeurosis	Mandibular nerve [V$_3$] via the branch to medial pterygoid muscle	Tenses the soft palate; opens the pharyngotympanic tube
Levator veli palatini	Petrous part of temporal bone anterior to opening for carotid canal	Superior surface of palatine aponeurosis	Vagus nerve [X] via pharyngeal branch to pharyngeal plexus	Only muscle to elevate the soft palate above the neutral position
Palatopharyngeus	Superior surface of palatine aponeurosis	Pharyngeal wall	Vagus nerve [X] via pharyngeal branch to pharyngeal plexus	Depresses soft palate; moves palatopharyngeal arch toward midline, thereby helping to close the oropharyngeal isthmus; elevates pharynx
Palatoglossus	Inferior surface of palatine aponeurosis	Lateral margin of tongue	Vagus nerve [X] via pharyngeal branch to pharyngeal plexus	Depresses palate; moves palatoglossal arch toward midline, thereby helping to close the oropharyngeal isthmus; elevates back of the tongue
Musculus uvulae	Posterior nasal spine of hard palate	Connective tissue of uvula	Vagus nerve [X] via pharyngeal branch to pharyngeal plexus	Elevates and retracts uvula; thickens central region of soft palate

Clinical app

Test for cranial nerve X

Clinically, the levator veli palatini, which is innervated by cranial nerve X, can be tested by asking a patient to say "ah." If the muscle on each side is functioning normally, the palate elevates evenly in the midline. If one side is not functioning, the palate deviates away from the abnormal side.

A

B Levator veli palatini

C Palatopharyngeus

Fig. 8.247 A. Tensor veli palatini muscles and the palatine aponeurosis. **B.** Levator veli palatini muscles. **C.** Palatopharyngeus muscles.

Vessels

Arteries

Arteries of the palate include the greater palatine branch of the maxillary artery, the ascending palatine branch of the facial artery, and the palatine branch of the ascending

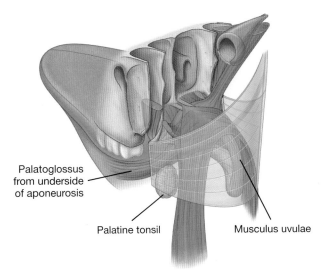

Fig. 8.248 Palatoglossus muscles and musculus uvulae.

pharyngeal artery. The maxillary, facial, and ascending pharyngeal arteries are all branches that arise in the neck from the external carotid artery (Fig. 8.249).

Ascending palatine artery and palatine branch

The **ascending palatine artery** of the facial artery ascends along the external surface of the pharynx. The palatine branch loops medially over the top of the superior constrictor muscle of the pharynx to penetrate the pharyngeal fascia with the levator veli palatini muscle and follows the levator veli palatini to the soft palate.

The **palatine branch** of the ascending pharyngeal artery follows the same course as the palatine branch of the ascending palatine artery from the facial artery and may replace the vessel.

Greater palatine artery

The **greater palatine artery** originates from the maxillary artery in the pterygopalatine fossa. It descends into the palatine canal, where it gives origin to a small **lesser palatine branch,** and then continues through the greater palatine foramen onto the inferior surface of the hard palate (Figs. 8.249, 8.250). The greater palatine artery passes forward on the hard palate and then leaves the palate superiorly through the incisive canal to enter the medial wall of the nasal cavity where it terminates. The greater palatine artery is the major artery of the hard palate. It also supplies palatal gingiva. The lesser palatine branch passes through the lesser palatine foramen just posterior to the greater palatine foramen, and contributes to the vascular supply of the soft palate (Figs. 8.249, 8.250).

Veins

Veins from the palate generally follow the arteries and ultimately drain into the pterygoid plexus of veins in the

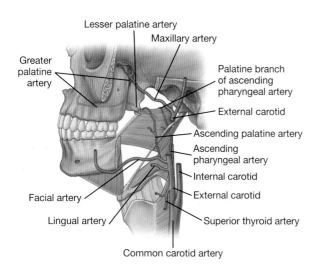

Fig. 8.249 Arteries of the palate.

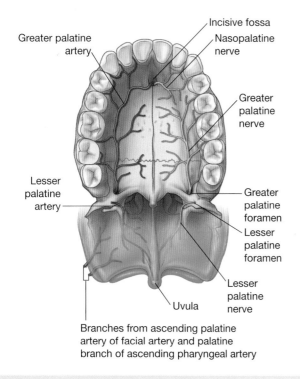

Fig. 8.250 Palatine nerves and arteries.

infratemporal fossa (Fig. 8.251) or into a network of veins associated with the palatine tonsil, which drain into the pharyngeal plexus of veins or directly into the facial vein.

Lymphatics

Lymphatic vessels from the palate drain into deep cervical nodes (Fig. 8.251).

Innervation

The palate is supplied by the greater and lesser palatine nerves and the nasopalatine nerve (Figs. 8.250).

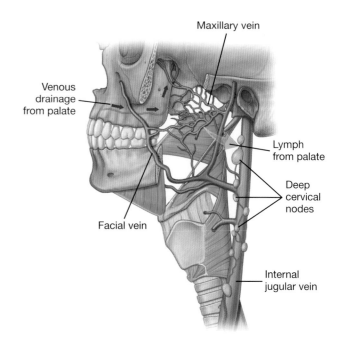

Fig. 8.251 Venous and lymphatic drainage of the palate.

General sensory fibers carried in all these nerves originate in the pterygopalatine fossa from the maxillary nerve [V₂].

Parasympathetic (to glands) and SA (taste on soft palate) fibers from a branch of the facial nerve [VII] join the nerves in the pterygopalatine fossa as do the sympathetics (mainly to blood vessels) ultimately derived from the T1 spinal cord level (Fig. 8.252).

Greater and lesser palatine nerves

The greater and lesser palatine nerves descend through the pterygopalatine fossa and palatine canal to reach the palate (Figs. 8.250, 8.252):

- The greater palatine nerve travels through the greater palatine foramen and turns anteriorly to supply the hard palate and gingiva as far as the first premolar.
- The lesser palatine nerve passes posteromedially to supply the soft palate.

Nasopalatine nerve

The nasopalatine nerve also originates in the pterygopalatine fossa, but passes medially into the nasal cavity. It continues medially over the roof of the nasal cavity to reach the medial wall, then anteriorly and obliquely down the wall to reach the incisive canal in the anterior floor, and descends through the incisive canal and fossa to reach the inferior surface of the hard palate.

The nasopalatine nerve supplies gingiva and mucosa adjacent to the incisors and canine.

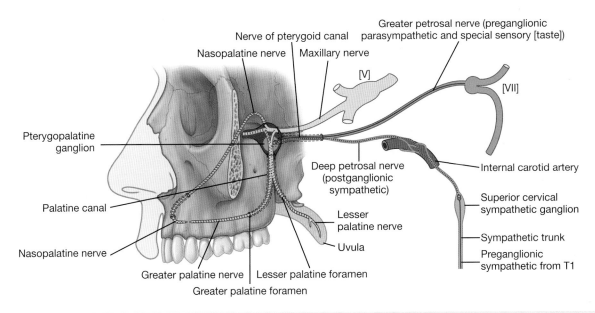

Fig. 8.252 Innervation of the palate.

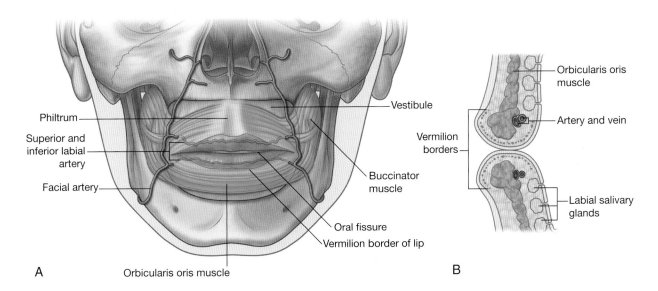

Fig. 8.253 Oral fissure and lips. **A.** Anterior view. **B.** Lateral view.

Oral fissure and lips

The oral fissure is the slit-like opening between the lips that connects the oral vestibule to the outside (Fig. 8.253). It can be opened and closed, and altered in shape by the movements of the muscles of facial expression associated with the lips and surrounding regions, and by movements of the lower jaw (mandible).

The **lips** are entirely composed of soft tissues (Fig. 8.253B). They are lined internally by oral mucosa and covered externally by skin (Fig. 8.253A). Externally, there is an area of transition from the thicker skin that covers the face to the thinner skin that overlies the margins of the lips and continues as oral mucosa onto the deep surfaces of the lips.

Blood vessels are closer to the surface in areas where the skin is thin and as a consequence there is a vermilion border that covers the margins of the lips.

The upper lip has a shallow vertical groove on its external surface (the **philtrum**) sandwiched between two elevated ridges of skin (Fig. 8.253A). The philtrum and ridges are formed embryologically by fusion of the medial nasal processes.

On the inner surface of both lips, a fold of mucosa (the **median labial frenulum**) connects the lip to the adjacent gum.

The lips enclose the orbicularis oris muscle, neurovascular tissues, and labial glands. The small pea-shaped labial

633

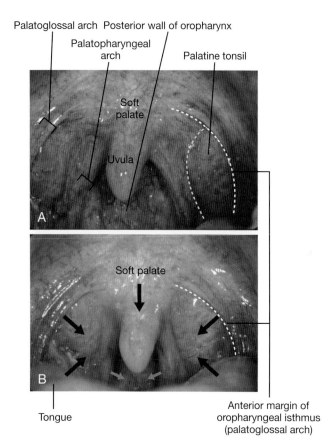

Palatoglossal arch Posterior wall of oropharynx

Palatopharyngeal arch

Palatine tonsil

Soft palate

Uvula

A

Soft palate

B

Tongue

Anterior margin of oropharyngeal isthmus (palatoglossal arch)

Closure of oropharyngeal isthmus
• Medial and downward movement of palatoglossal arches
• Medial and downward movement of palatopharyngeal arches
• Upward movement of tongue
• Downward and forward movement of soft palate

Fig. 8.254 Open mouth with soft palate. **A.** Oropharyngeal isthmus opened. **B.** Oropharyngeal isthmus closed.

glands are between the muscle tissue and the oral mucosa and open into the oral vestibule (Fig. 8.253B).

A number of muscles of facial expression control the shape and size of the oral fissure. The most important of these is the orbicularis oris muscle, which encircles the orifice and acts as a sphincter. A number of other muscles of facial expression blend into the orbicularis oris or other tissues of the lips and open or adjust the contours of the oral fissure. These include the buccinator, levator labii superioris, zygomaticus major and minor, levator anguli oris, depressor labii inferioris, depressor anguli oris, and platysma (see pp. 484–486).

Oropharyngeal isthmus

The oropharyngeal isthmus is the opening between the oral cavity and the oropharynx (Fig. 8.254). It is formed:

- laterally by the palatoglossal arches,
- superiorly by the soft palate, and

- inferiorly by the sulcus terminalis of the tongue that divides the oral surface of the tongue (anterior two-thirds) from the pharyngeal surface (posterior one-third).

The oropharyngeal isthmus can be closed by elevation of the posterior aspect of the tongue, depression of the palate, and medial movement of the palatoglossal arches toward the midline (Fig. 8.254B).

Medial movement of the palatopharyngeal arches medial and posterior to the palatoglossal arches is also involved in closing the oropharyngeal isthmus. By closing the oropharyngeal isthmus, food or liquid can be held in the oral cavity while breathing.

Teeth and gingivae

The **teeth** are attached to sockets (alveoli) in two elevated arches of bone on the mandible below and the maxillae above (alveolar arches). If the teeth are removed, the alveolar bone is resorbed and the arches disappear.

The **gingivae** (**gums**) are specialized regions of the oral mucosa that surround the teeth and cover adjacent regions of the alveolar bone.

The different types of teeth are distinguished on the basis of morphology, position, and function (Fig. 8.255A).

In adults, there are 32 teeth: 16 in the upper jaw and 16 in the lower jaw. On each side in both maxillary and mandibular arches are two incisor, one canine, two premolar, and three molar teeth (Fig. 8.255A).

- The **incisor teeth** are the "front teeth" and have one root and a chisel-shaped crown, which "cuts."
- The **canine teeth** are posterior to the incisors, are the longest teeth, have a crown with a single pointed cusp, and "grasp."
- The **premolar teeth** (bicuspids) have a crown with two pointed cusps, one on the buccal (cheek) side of the tooth and the other on the lingual (tongue) or palatal (palate) side, generally have one root (but the upper first premolar next to the canine may have two), and "grind."
- The **molar teeth** are behind the premolar teeth, have three roots and crowns with three to five cusps, and "grind."

Two successive sets of teeth develop in humans, deciduous teeth ("baby" teeth) (Fig. 8.255B) and permanent teeth ("adult" teeth). The deciduous teeth emerge from the gingivae at between 6 months and 2 years of age. Permanent teeth begin to emerge and replace the deciduous teeth at around age 6 years, and can continue to emerge into adulthood.

The 20 deciduous teeth consist of two incisor, one canine, and two molar teeth on each side of the upper and lower jaws. These teeth are replaced by the incisor, canine, and premolar teeth of the permanent teeth. The permanent molar

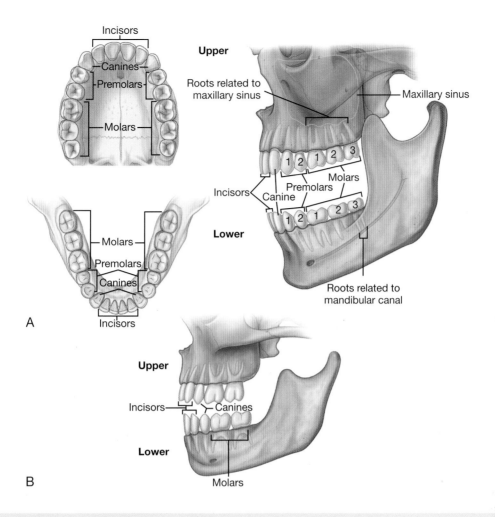

Fig. 8.255 Teeth. A. Adult upper and lower permanent teeth. **B.** Deciduous ("baby") teeth.

teeth erupt posterior to the deciduous molars and require the jaws to elongate forward to accommodate them.

Vessels

Arteries

All teeth are supplied by vessels that branch either directly or indirectly from the maxillary artery (Fig. 8.256).

Inferior alveolar artery

All lower teeth are supplied by the **inferior alveolar artery** (Fig. 8.256), which originates from the maxillary artery in the infratemporal fossa. The vessel enters the mandibular canal of the mandible, passes anteriorly in bone supplying vessels to the more posterior teeth, and divides opposite the first premolar into **incisor** and **mental branches.** The mental branch leaves the mental foramen to supply the chin, while the incisor branch continues in bone to supply the anterior teeth and adjacent structures.

Anterior and posterior superior alveolar arteries

All upper teeth are supplied by anterior and posterior superior alveolar arteries (Fig. 8.256).

The **posterior superior alveolar artery** originates from the maxillary artery just after the maxillary artery enters the pterygopalatine fossa and it leaves the fossa through the pterygomaxillary fissure. It descends on the posterolateral surface of the maxilla, branches, and enters small canals in the bone to supply the molar and premolar teeth.

The **anterior superior alveolar artery** originates from the infra-orbital artery, which arises from the maxillary artery in the pterygopalatine fossa. The infra-orbital artery leaves the pterygopalatine fossa through the inferior orbital fissure and enters the inferior orbital groove and canal in the floor of the orbit. The anterior superior alveolar artery originates from the infra-orbital artery in the infra-orbital canal. It passes through bone and branches to supply the incisor and canine teeth.

Gingival supply

The gingivae are supplied by multiple vessels and the source depends on which side of each tooth the gingiva is—the side facing the oral vestibule or cheek (vestibular or buccal side) or the side facing the tongue or palate (lingual or palatal side):

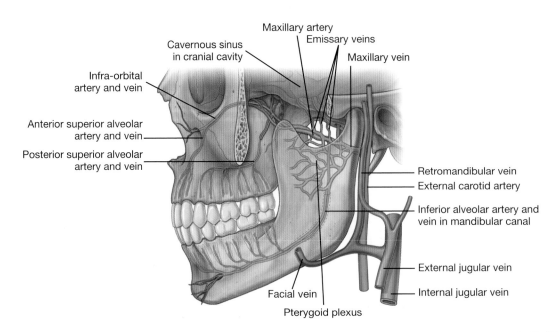

Fig. 8.256 Arteries and veins of the teeth.

- Buccal gingiva of the lower teeth is supplied by branches from the inferior alveolar artery, whereas the lingual side is supplied by branches from the lingual artery of the tongue.
- Buccal gingiva of the upper teeth is supplied by branches of the anterior and posterior superior alveolar arteries.
- Palatal gingiva of the upper teeth is supplied by branches from the nasopalatine (incisor and canine teeth) and greater palatine (premolar and molar teeth) arteries.

Veins

Veins from the upper and lower teeth generally follow the arteries (Fig. 8.256).

Inferior alveolar veins from the lower teeth and superior alveolar veins from the upper teeth drain mainly into the pterygoid plexus of veins in the infratemporal fossa, although some drainage from the anterior teeth may be via tributaries of the facial vein.

The pterygoid plexus drains mainly into the maxillary vein and ultimately into the retromandibular vein and jugular system of veins. In addition, small communicating vessels pass superiorly, from the plexus, and pass through small emissary foramina in the base of the skull to connect with the cavernous sinus in the cranial cavity. Infection originating in the teeth can track into the cranial cavity through these small emissary veins.

Venous drainage from the teeth can also be via vessels that pass through the mental foramen to connect with the facial vein.

Veins from the gingivae also follow the arteries and ultimately drain into the facial vein or into the pterygoid plexus of veins.

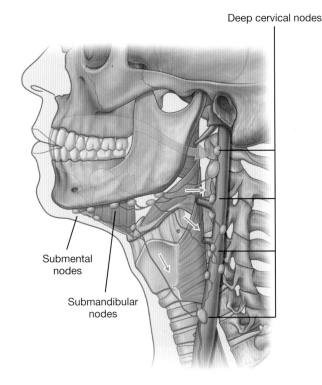

Fig. 8.257 Lymphatic drainage of the teeth and gums.

Lymphatics

Lymphatic vessels from the teeth and gingivae drain mainly into submandibular, submental, and deep cervical nodes (Fig. 8.257).

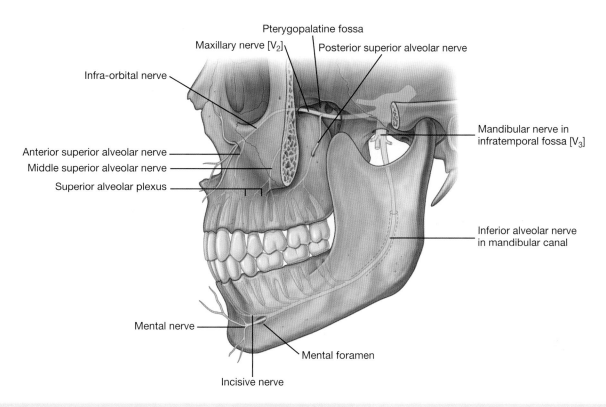

Pterygopalatine fossa
Maxillary nerve [V₂]
Posterior superior alveolar nerve
Infra-orbital nerve
Mandibular nerve in infratemporal fossa [V₃]
Anterior superior alveolar nerve
Middle superior alveolar nerve
Superior alveolar plexus
Inferior alveolar nerve in mandibular canal
Mental nerve
Mental foramen
Incisive nerve

Fig. 8.258 Innervation of the teeth.

Innervation

All nerves that innervate the teeth and gingivae are branches of the trigeminal nerve [V] (Figs. 8.258, 8.259).

Inferior alveolar nerve

The lower teeth are all innervated by branches from the inferior alveolar nerve, which originates in the infratemporal fossa from the mandibular nerve [V₃] (Figs. 8.258, 8.259). The inferior alveolar nerve and its accompanying vessels enter the mandibular foramen on the medial surface of the ramus of mandible and travel anteriorly through the bone in the mandibular canal. Branches to the back teeth originate directly from the inferior alveolar nerve.

Adjacent to the first premolar tooth, the inferior alveolar nerve divides into incisive and mental branches:

- The **incisive branch** innervates the first premolar, the canine, and the incisor teeth, together with the associated vestibular (buccal) gingiva.
- The **mental nerve** exits the mandible through the mental foramen and innervates the chin and lower lip.

Anterior, middle, and posterior superior alveolar nerves

All upper teeth are innervated by the anterior, middle, and posterior superior alveolar nerves, which originate directly

or indirectly from the maxillary nerve [V₂] (Figs. 8.258, 8.259).

The posterior superior alveolar nerve originates directly from the maxillary nerve [V₂] in the pterygopalatine fossa, exits the pterygopalatine fossa through the pterygomaxillary fissure, and descends on the posterolateral surface of the maxilla. It enters the maxilla through a small foramen approximately midway between the pterygomaxillary fissure and the last molar tooth and passes through the bone in the wall of the maxillary sinus. The posterior superior alveolar nerve then innervates the molar teeth through the superior alveolar plexus formed by the posterior, middle, and anterior alveolar nerves.

The middle and anterior superior alveolar nerves originate from the infra-orbital branch of the maxillary nerve [V₂] in the floor of the orbit:

- The middle superior alveolar nerve arises from the infra-orbital nerve in the infra-orbital groove, passes through the bone in the lateral wall of the maxillary sinus, and innervates the premolar teeth via the superior alveolar plexus.
- The anterior superior alveolar nerve originates from the infra-orbital nerve in the infra-orbital canal, passes through the maxilla in the anterior wall of the maxillary sinus, and, via the superior alveolar plexus, supplies the canine and incisor teeth.

637

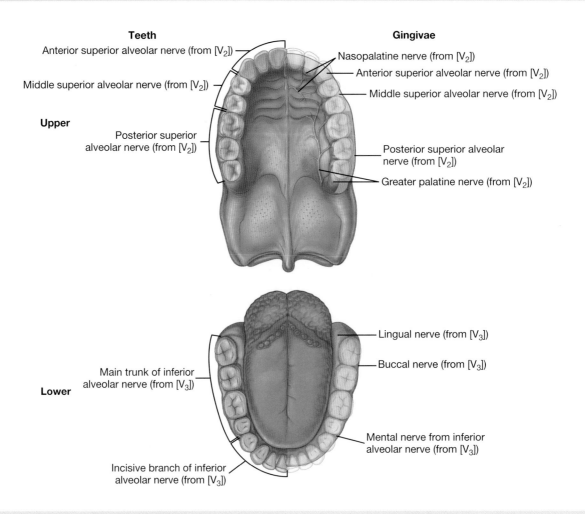

Teeth

Anterior superior alveolar nerve (from [V₂])

Middle superior alveolar nerve (from [V₂])

Upper

Posterior superior alveolar nerve (from [V₂])

Gingivae

Nasopalatine nerve (from [V₂])

Anterior superior alveolar nerve (from [V₂])

Middle superior alveolar nerve (from [V₂])

Posterior superior alveolar nerve (from [V₂])

Greater palatine nerve (from [V₂])

Lingual nerve (from [V₃])

Buccal nerve (from [V₃])

Main trunk of inferior alveolar nerve (from [V₃])

Lower

Mental nerve from inferior alveolar nerve (from [V₃])

Incisive branch of inferior alveolar nerve (from [V₃])

Fig. 8.259 Innervation of the teeth and gums.

Innervation of gingivae

Like the teeth, the gingivae are innervated by nerves that ultimately originate from the trigeminal nerve [V] (Fig. 8.259):

- Gingiva associated with the upper teeth is innervated by branches derived from the maxillary nerve [V₂].
- Gingiva associated with the lower teeth is innervated by branches of the mandibular nerve [V₃].

The gingiva on the buccal side of the upper teeth is innervated by the anterior, middle, and superior alveolar nerves, which also innervate the adjacent teeth. Gingiva on the palatal (lingual) side of the same teeth is innervated by the nasopalatine and the greater palatine nerves:

- The nasopalatine nerve innervates gingiva associated with the incisor and canine teeth.
- The greater palatine nerve supplies gingiva associated with the remaining teeth.

The gingiva associated with the buccal side of the mandibular incisor, canine, and premolar teeth is innervated by the mental branch of the inferior alveolar nerve. Gingiva on the buccal side of the mandibular molar teeth is innervated by the buccal nerve, which originates in the infratemporal fossa from the mandibular nerve [V₃]. Gingiva adjacent to the lingual surface of all lower teeth is innervated by the lingual nerve.

Surface anatomy
Pulse points

Arterial pulses can be felt at four locations in the head and neck (Fig. 8.260).

- Carotid pulse—the common or external carotid artery can be palpated in the anterior triangle of the neck. This is one of the strongest pulses in the body. The pulse can be obtained by palpating either the common carotid artery posterolateral to the larynx or the external carotid artery immediately lateral to the pharynx midway between the superior margin of the thyroid cartilage below and the greater horn of the hyoid bone above.

- Facial pulse—the facial artery can be palpated as it crosses the inferior border of the mandible immediately adjacent to the anterior margin of masseter muscle.
- Temporal pulse—the superficial temporal artery can be palpated anterior to the ear and immediately posterosuperior to the position of the temporomandibular joint.
- Temporal pulse—the anterior branch of the superficial temporal artery can be palpated posterior to the zygomatic process of the frontal bone as it passes lateral to the temporal fascia and into anterolateral regions of the scalp. In some individuals pulsations of the superficial temporal artery can be seen through the skin.

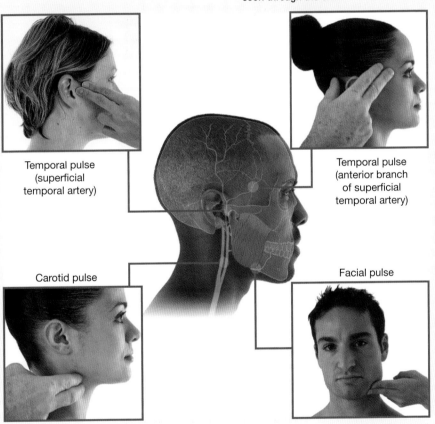

Temporal pulse
(superficial
temporal artery)

Temporal pulse
(anterior branch
of superficial
temporal artery)

Carotid pulse

Facial pulse

Fig. 8.260 Where to take arterial pulses in the head and neck.

Index

Page numbers followed by "*f*" indicate figures, "*t*" indicate tables, and "*b*" indicate boxes.

A

Abdomen, 145–222
  groin of, 156–160
  posterior abdominal region of, 201–222, 201f
  regional anatomy of, 146–222, 146f
  surface topography of, 146–147
  sympathetic innervation of, 28–29, 29f
Abdominal aorta
  anterior branches of, 187–193, 188f
  branches of, 213t
  posterior branches of, 213
  visceral branches of, 213
Abdominal aortic plexus, 217
Abdominal esophagus, 167–168, 168f
Abdominal prevertebral plexus, 198–199, 199f
Abdominal radiograph, image interpretation, 8
Abdominal viscera, 163–201
  innervation of, 196–201
  lymphatics of, 196
  organs of, 167–187
  peritoneal cavity of, 164–167
  peritoneum of, 163–164, 163f, 164b
  venous drainage of, 193–196
Abdominal wall, 147–155
  anterolateral muscles of, 149–152, 150t
  arterial supply and venous drainage of, 155, 155f–156f
  extraperitoneal fascia of, 152–153, 153f
  innervation of, 153–155, 154f
  layers of, 148f, 153f
  lymphatic drainage of, 155, 155f
  peritoneum of, 153
  posterior, 201–205, 201f
    bones of, 201–205
    diaphragm of, 202–205, 203f–204f
    muscles of, 202, 202f, 203t
    ribs of, 202
  superficial fascia of, 148–149, 148f–149f
Abdominopelvic cavity hernias, 163b
Abducent nerve, 477f, 479, 516
Abduction
  of thumb, 421b–422b
  of ulna during pronation, 413–414, 413f
Abductor digiti minimi, 355, 356t
Abductor hallucis, 355, 356t
Abscesses, in ischio-anal fossae, 265b
Accessory hemiazygos vein, 139
Accessory meningeal artery, 463, 549
Accessory nerves (XI), 480–484, 566–567, 575–576
  cranial root of, 480–484
  in neck, 567f
    posterior triangle of, 575f

Acetabular labrum, 293, 293f–294f
Acetabulum, 224f, 225, 288–290, 290f
Achilles tendon, 342
  rupture of, 343b
Acromioclavicular joint, 373, 374f, 374b
  right, 374b
Adductor canal, 302
Adductor hallucis, 357, 358t
Adductor hiatus, 316, 316f, 337f
Adductor magnus, 316, 316f
Adductor pollicis, 432f
Adductor tubercle, 310
Adrenals, sympathetic innervation of, 28–29
Ala, 226–227, 227f
Alar cartilages, 607
Alar fold, 324
Alar ligaments, 38
Allen's test, 435b
Alveolar nerves, 637
Alveolar processes, 447, 452
Ampulla, 246, 246f, 531
Anal canal, 176, 177f, 237, 238f
Anal columns, 237, 238f
Anal sinus, 237, 238f
Anal triangle, 265, 265f, 265t
Anal valves, 237, 238f
Anastomoses
  around knee, 329f
  arterial, around shoulder, 381f
  of gluteal artery, 308f
  portosystemic, 195b
Anatomical position, of head and major landmarks, 450b
Anatomical snuffbox, 421b–422b, 428–429, 428f
Anatomy, 2–3
  terms relating to
    location, 3
    planes, 2–3, 2f
    position, 2
    trans/non-binary terms related, 3
Anesthesia
  of inferior alveolar nerve, 546b
  pudendal block, 254b
Aneurysm
  abdominal aortic, 213b–214b
  intracerebral, 468b
Angiography
  digital subtraction, 4–5, 5f
  magnetic resonance, normal carotid and vertebral arteries, 468b
Angular incisure, 169
Ankle joint, 344–346, 345f
  bracket-shaped socket, 344–345
  dorsiflexion and plantarflexion, 288f
  intertarsal, 346f

Ankle joint (*Continued*)
  lateral ligament, 346, 346f
  medial ligament, 345–346, 345f
Anular pancreas, 184b
Anococcygeal ligament (anococcygeal body), 233f, 234
Anococcygeal nerves, 251f, 254–255
Ansa cervicalis, 568, 568f
Anterior arch, atlas and axis, 38
Anterior cardiac veins, 120
Anterior chamber, of eyeball, 519–520
Anterior circumflex humeral artery, 388, 388f
Anterior compartment
  of forearm
    arteries and veins, 414–417, 416f
    muscles, 414
    nerves, 417–418
  of leg, 338–340
    arteries in, 338–340
    muscles in, 338, 339f, 339t
    nerves in, 340
    veins in, 340
  of thigh, 313–315, 314f, 315t
Anterior cranial fossa, 455–457, 456f, 456t
Anterior cutaneous branches, 81
Anterior (ventral), describing anatomical location, 2f, 3
Anterior divisions, of brachial plexus, 390
Anterior drawer test, 328b
Anterior inferior iliac spine, 224f–225f, 225–226
Anterior intercostal arteries, 79–80, 80f
Anterior interosseous artery, 419, 420f
Anterior interventricular branch, 118
Anterior interventricular sulci, 106
Anterior interventricular vein, 120
Anterior jugular veins, 561
Anterior median fissure, 55, 55f
Anterior mediastinum, 102
Anterior papillary muscle, 111
Anterior rami, 59
Anterior root, of spinal nerves, 59
Anterior sacro-iliac ligament, 228, 228f
Anterior spinal artery, 56, 467
Anterior superior alveolar artery, 635
Anterior superior iliac spine, 224f–225f, 225–226
Anterior surface, of heart, 105, 107f
Anterior talofibular ligament, 346
Anterior tibial artery, 335, 336f, 339f
Anterior triangle, of neck, 557, 558f, 558b, 561–571
Anterior trunk, of internal iliac artery, 258–260, 259f
Anterior tympanic artery, 549
Anterior vagal trunk, 137, 167

Anterior view, of skull, 446–448, 447f
  frontal bone, 446
  mandible, 447–448
  maxillae, 447
  zygomatic and nasal bones, 446
Anterior wall
  of axilla, 382–383
  of infratemporal fossa, 541
  of middle ear, 526–527
Anterolateral muscles, of abdominal wall, 149–152, 150t
Anulus fibrosus, 43
Aorta
  abdominal, 187–193, 188f, 212–213, 212f
  arch and branches of, 130–131
    anomalies in, 132b
  coarctation of, 131b
  traumatic injury to, 131b
Aortic dissection, 132b
Aortic plexus, 199
Aortic valve, 114, 115f
Aortic valve disease, 116b
Apertures
  in pelvic wall, 230–232, 232f
  piriform, 446
Apex
  of the bladder, 237, 239f
  of heart, 105, 107f
  of sacrum, 40
  of tongue, 621
Aponeurosis
  external oblique muscle and, 150f
  internal oblique muscle and, 151f
  palatine, 631f
  palmar, 427–428, 428f
  plantar, 353, 354f
  transversus abdominis muscle and, 151f
Aponeurotic layers, of scalp, 496–498
Appendicitis, 175b
Appendicular group, of back muscles, 48, 49t
Appendicular skeleton, 9, 9f
Appendix, 174, 174f
Aqueous humor, 520
Arachnoid mater, 21, 465
Arachnoid trabeculae, 57
Arches
  of foot, 352–353, 353f
  superciliary, 446
Arcuate eminence, 458
Arcuate ligament, 203–204
Arcuate line, 152, 225f, 226
Areola, 64
Arm
  arteries and veins, 403–404, 404f
  bones, 398–401
  medial cutaneous nerve of, 393f, 394–395
  muscles, 401
  nerves, 401–403
Arterial supply
  of abdominal esophagus, 168f
  of abdominal wall, 155, 155f
  of auricle, 523
  of brain, 467, 467f
  of breast, 65–66
  of cecum and appendix, 175, 175f
  of colon, 177f
  of cranial dura mater, 463–464, 464f

Arterial supply (Continued)
  of diaphragm, 83
  of duodenum, 170, 171f
  of esophagus, 136
  of eyeball, 514f, 520
  of eyelids, 504
  of face, 492
  of gastrointestinal tract, 187–193
  of hand, 433f
  to ileum and jejunum, 170, 171f
  of intercostal spaces, 77f, 78–80
  of internal ear, 534
  of liver and gallbladder, 182f
  of nasal cavities, 613–614, 614f
  of pancreas, 184, 185f
  of parotid glands, 489
  of pharynx, 590–591, 591f
  of rectum and anal canal, 177f
  of scalp, 499
  of small intestine, 171f
  of spleen, 187f
  of suprarenal glands, 211f
  of teeth and gingivae, 635–636
  of thyroid gland, 569–570
Arteria radicularis magna, 56–57
Arteries, 16
  of anterior compartment of leg, 338–340
  associated with posterior scapular region, 380f
  of foot, 357–359, 357f
  of gluteal region, 308, 308f
  of hip, 297–298
  of larynx, 602, 603f
  of lateral compartment of leg, 337, 338f
  of lower limb, 298f
  of palate, 631, 632f
  palatine, 632f
  of pelvis, 258–260, 258f–259f
  of perineum, 272–274, 273f
  of posterior compartment of leg, 335–336, 336f
  of posterior triangle of the neck, 575f
  of pterygoid canal, 557
  of spinal cord, 56–57, 56f
  of temporal fossa, 542f
  of thigh, 317–320
  of tongue, 624–625, 625f
Artery of Adamkiewicz, 56–57, 56f
Arthroscopy, 328b
Articular discs, 12
Articular facets, superior and inferior, 38
Articular processes, superior and inferior, 38
Articular surfaces
  of carpal bones, 424
  of glenohumeral joint, 373, 374f
  of knee joint, 323, 324f
  of talus, 341
Aryepiglottic folds, 598
Arytenoid cartilage, 594–595, 595f
Ascending aorta, 125–126, 126f
Ascending lumbar veins, 215
Ascending palatine artery, 631
Ascending part of duodenum, 169
Ascending pharyngeal artery, 528, 565, 565t
Atheromatous plaques, 468b
Atherosclerosis, 17b

Atlanto-occipital joint, 38
Atlas (CI vertebra), 38, 39f–40f
  articulation between axis and, 40b
  transverse ligament of, 38
Atrial septal defect (ASD), 117b
Atrioventricular bundle, 122–123, 122f
Atrioventricular node, 121–122, 122f
Atrium proper, 110
Atrophy, muscle, 16b
Auditory ossicles, 528–529, 529f
  muscles associated with, 530f
Auricle, 522–524, 523f
  innervation, 522–523
  muscles, 522–524, 523f
  sensory innervation of, 524f
  vessels, 523–524
Auriculotemporal nerve, 489, 498, 544–546
Avascular necrosis, 11b
Axial plane
  female pelvic cavity and perineum in, 282b
  male pelvic cavity and perineum in, 276b
Axial skeleton, 9, 9f
Axilla
  anterior wall, 382–383
  axillary inlet, 382, 382f
  contents of
    axillary artery, 386–389
    axillary vein, 389
    brachial plexus, 389–396
    lymphatics, 396–397, 397f
  floor of, 386f
  lateral wall of, 384, 385f, 385t
  medial wall of, 383, 384f, 384t
  posterior wall of, 384–386, 385f, 385t
  gateways in, 386
Axillary artery, 386–389, 387f
Axillary inlet, 382, 382f
Axillary nerve, 381, 396
Axillary nodes, 66, 155
Axillary process, of breast, 65b
Axillary vein, 389, 389f
Axis
  CII vertebra, 38, 39f–40f
  of eyeball and orbit, 511, 511f
Azygos system, of veins, in posterior mediastinum, 137–139, 139f
Azygos vein, 138

B

Back, 35–62
Back pain, 45b
Balance, organs of, 533
Ball-and-socket joints, 12, 13f
Barium sulfate
  follow-through, 4f
  suspension, 4
Bartholin's glands, 267b–268b
Base
  of bladder, 237–238, 239f
  of brain, arteries on, 469f
  of cochlea, 531–532
  of heart, 105, 106f
  of skull
    anterior part, 452
    middle part, 452
    posterior part, 454

Basilar artery, 467
Basilic vein, 404, 435
Bell's palsy, 496b
Benign prostatic hypertrophy, 244b
Biceps brachii, 387t, 401t
Bicondylar joints, 12
Bile, duct system, 185–186, 185f
Biopsy, bone marrow, 226b
Bladder, 237–239, 239f
  cancer, 239b
  infection, 241b
Bladder stones, 240b
Block, pudendal, 254b
Blood pressure measurement, 409b–410b
Blood supply
  of diaphragm, 205
  of hip joint, 295, 295f
Blood vessels, 16
  of anterior abdominal region, 215b
  of pelvis, 258–262
  of perineum, 272–274
Body, 1–34
  of clitoris, 265f, 266
  of epididymis, 242f, 243
  of penis, 265f, 266
  of pubis, 225f, 226
  of sphenoid, 453
  of stomach, 168
  systems of, 9–33
Bone marrow
  biopsy, 226b
  transplants, 10b
Bones, 9–10
  of arm, 398–401
  classification of, 9
  of foot, 340–344, 340f–341f, 344b
  fractures of, 11b
  function, 9
  of hand, 423–425, 423f
  innervation of, 10
  of lower limb, 287f
  of orbit, 501f
  palatine, 618–619
  of pelvis, 224–227
  of shoulder, 370–372
  of thigh, 309–313
  of wrist, 423f
Bony labyrinth, 531–532, 531f
  cochlea, 531–532, 532f
  semicircular canals, 531
Bony orbit, 501–502, 508f
  floor, 502
  lateral wall, 502
  medial wall, 501–502
  roof, 501
Bony pelvis, 287–290, 289f
  acetabulum, 288–290, 290f
  ilium, 287
  ischial tuberosity, 287, 289f
  ischiopubic ramus and pubic bone, 288
Borders
  of anterior triangle of neck, 561f
  of heart, 106
  of infratemporal fossa, 542f
  of perineum, 263–264, 263f
  of posterior triangle of neck, 573f

Boundaries
  of femoral triangle, 302f
  of middle ear, 526–528, 527f
  of perineum, 263f
  of popliteal fossa, 330f
  of posterior cranial fossa, 458
Bowel lumen, 172b
Bowel obstruction, 178b
Brachial artery, 403–404, 403f–404f, 404b
Brachialis, 401t
Brachial plexus, 577
  branches, 389–396, 390f, 391t–392t, 393f–396f
  cords, 390, 390f
  divisions, 390
  injuries to, 397b
  roots, 389–390
  trunks, 390
Brachiocephalic trunk, 131
Brain, 466–467
  blood supply, 467–468, 467f
  lateral view of, 466f
  MRI in coronal plane, 7f
  parts of, 20
  sagittal section of, 467f
  venous drainage, 469–472
Branches
  of anterior trunk of internal iliac artery, 258f
  axillary artery of, 388f
  brachial artery, 403f, 404
  brachial plexus
    lateral cord, 394
    medial cord, 394–396
    posterior cord, 396
    roots, 390–393
    trunks, 393–394
  external carotid artery, 499, 565t
  facial nerve, 491
  of lumbosacral plexus, 297f, 300t
  mandibular nerve, 543–546
  maxillary nerve, 553–554
  nasociliary nerve, 517
  of ophthalmic artery, 495, 499
  ophthalmic nerve, 615–616
  perforating, 435
  of posterior trunk of internal iliac artery, 258f
  radial artery, 415
  of sacral and coccygeal plexuses, 252t–253t
  subclavian artery, 573
    costocervical trunk, 579
    internal thoracic artery, 579
    thyrocervical trunk, 579
    ulnar nerve, 436f
    vertebral artery, 578
  ulnar artery, 415–417
Breast, 64–66, 65f
  arterial supply of, 65–66
  axillary process of, 65b, 397f
  innervation of, 66
  lymphatic drainage of, 66
  in men, 66
  suspensory ligaments of, 64–65
  venous drainage of, 66
  in women, 67b

Breast cancer, 66b
Bregma, 452
Broad ligament, 249–250, 249f
Bronchial arteries, 96f, 97
Bronchial tree, 90–94, 94f
Bronchial veins, 96f, 97
Bronchomediastinal trunks, 80
Bronchopulmonary segments, 94–95, 95f
Bronchoscopy, 98b–99b
Buccal artery, 494
Buccal nerve, 491, 544
Buccinator, 484, 485t–486t, 488f, 621f, 621t
Buccopharyngeal fascia, 587
Bulb
  of penis, 266
    artery of, 273, 273f
  of vestibule, 265f, 266, 267b–268b
    arteries to, 273
Bulbourethral glands, 242f, 244
Bunions, 350b
Bursa
  of glenohumeral joint, 374, 375f
  suprapatellar, 324

C

Calcaneocuboid joint, 349–350
Calcaneofibular ligament, 346
Calcaneus, 342–343, 343f
Calculi, in bladder, 240b
Calvaria, 446, 452f
  lateral portion of, 448–449
Camper's fascia, 148, 148f
Cancer
  affecting recurrent laryngeal nerve, 580b
  bladder, 239b
  breast, lymphatic drainage and, 398b
  esophageal, 137b
  oral, 617b
  ovarian, 245b
  pancreatic, 185b
  urinary tract, 210b
  vertebrae and, 44b
Canine teeth, 634
Capitate, 424
Capitulum of humerus, 399
Carcinoma
  of the cervix and uterus, 247b
  of colon and rectum, 237b
  of stomach, 172b–173b
Cardia, of stomach, 168
Cardiac auscultation, 117b
Cardiac chambers, 106–114, 109f
  aortic valve, 114, 115f
  left atrium, 113, 114f
  left ventricle, 113–114, 115f
  mitral valve, 114
  pulmonary valve, 113, 113f
  right atrium, 109–111, 111f
  right ventricle, 111–112, 112f
  tricuspid valve, 112–113
  visualizing, 110b
Cardiac conduction system, 120–123, 121b, 122f
  atrioventricular bundle in, 122–123
  atrioventricular node in, 121–122
  sino-atrial node in, 121

Cardiac innervation, 123–124, 123f
  parasympathetic, 124
  sympathetic, 124
  visceral afferents, 124
Cardiac muscle, 16
Cardiac orientation, 105–106, 105f
  base and apex, 105, 106f
  external sulci, 106
  margins and borders, 106
  surfaces, 105, 107f–108f
Cardiac skeleton, 117, 118f
Cardiac veins, 120, 121f
Cardial notch, 169
Cardiovascular system, 16–17
Carotid arteries, 468b
  branches, 488, 499
  carotid system, 563–564
Carotid pulse, 639b
Carotid sheath, of neck fascia, 559
Carotid system, 563–565, 564f
Carotid triangle, 561
Carpal bones, 423–424
  articular surface, 424
  carpal arch, 424
  distal row, 423–424
  proximal row, 423
Carpal joints, 425
Carpal tunnel, and structures at wrist, 427f
Carpal tunnel syndrome, 428b
Carpometacarpal joints, 425–426
Cartilage, 9
  function of, 9
  laryngeal, 593–595
  types of, 9
Cartilaginous joints, 13, 14f
Cataracts, 520b
Catheterization
  of femoral artery, 303b
  suprapubic, 240b
  urethral, 241b
Cathode ray tube, 3, 4f
Cauda equina, 59, 60f
Caudal, describing anatomical location, 3
Caudate lobe, of liver, 181
Cavernous nerves, 255, 256f–257f
Cavernous sinuses, 471, 471f
Cavity
  cranial, 454–459
  of larynx, 598–600, 599f
Cecum, 174, 174f
Ceiling of perineum, 263–264, 263f
Celiac plexus, 198–199, 217
Celiac trunk, 188–190, 189f
Central canal, 55f, 56
Central nervous system (CNS), 20–21, 20f
  subdivisions of, 21–32
Central retinal artery, 513–514, 520
Central venous access
  in neck, 561f, 561b
  via subclavian/axillary vein, 389b
Cephalic vein, 404, 408f, 435
Cerebellum, 20
Cerebral arterial circle, 467
Cerebrospinal fluid
  leakage, 466b
  lumbar tap, 59b–60b
  returns to the venous system, 466

Cerebrum, 466
Cervical enlargement, 55
Cervical lymph nodes
  deep, 583–584
  superficial, 583
Cervical part, of sympathetic trunk, 581, 581f
Cervical pleura, 85
Cervical plexus, 576–577, 576f
  cutaneous branches, 576–577
  muscular branches, 576
Cervical ribs, 72b
Cervical vertebrae, 36, 36f, 36b, 38
  atlas and axis, 38
  typical, 36b
  variations in number of, 44b
Cervical viscera, sympathetic innervation of, 28, 28f
Cervix, 246–247, 247f, 267b–268b
Chalazion, 504
Chambers, of eyeball, 519–520
Check ligaments, 510, 510f
Cheek, 620
Chest
  flail, 72b
  surgical access to, 82b
Chest radiograph, image interpret, 7
Chest tube insertion, 82b
Choanae, 611, 612f
Cholecystectomy, 186b
Cholecystitis, 186b
Chorda tympani, 547, 548f, 629
  nerve to, 534
  parasympathetic fibers, course of, 628f
  in temporal bone, 535f
Choroid, 520–521
Chronic leg ischemia, 320b
Chyle, 18
Chylomicrons, 18
Ciliary arteries, 520
Ciliary body, 521, 521f
Ciliary ganglion, 518–519, 518f
Ciliary muscle, 521, 522t
Ciliary processes, 521
Circumflex branch, 118
Circumflex fibular artery, 336, 336f
Circumflex iliac artery, 155
Circumflex scapular artery, 381
Cirrhosis, hepatic, 195b
Cisterna chyli, 139
Clavicle, 370
  fractures of, 376b–377b
  right, 370f
Clavipectoral fascia, 66, 68f, 382, 383f
"Clawing," of hand, 436b–437b
Clitoris, 265f, 266
  deep dorsal vein of, 274
  dorsal nerve of, 271
  erectile tissues of, 265f
  glans, 266
CNS. See Central nervous system (CNS)
Coccygeal plexus, 250f–251f, 252t–253t, 254–255
Coccygeus muscles, 232
Coccygeus, nerves to, 251f
Coccyx, 36f, 37, 39f–40f, 40, 227, 227f
Cochlea, 527, 530–532, 532f

Colic flexure, 176, 177f
Collateral ligaments, of knee joint, 326–327, 326f
Colles' fascia, 149, 149f, 270
Colon, 176, 176f
  rectum and, carcinoma of, 237b
Colonoscopy, of gastrointestinal tract, 179b
Columns, anal, 237, 238f
Common carotid arteries, 563–564, 564f
Common fibular nerve, 323, 329, 337f–338f
Common fibular part, sciatic nerve to, 251f
Common hepatic artery, 190, 190f
Compact bone, 9
Compartment syndrome, 317b
Compound fractures, 461b
Compressor urethrae, 235, 236f
Computed tomography (CT), 5
  abdominal, 6f
  of head, 461b
  high-resolution, in lung, 98b–99b
  image interpretation, 8
  in pulmonary trunk, 96b
  scanner, 5, 6f
  of urinary tract, 211b
Concha, of auricle, 522
Concussion, 472b
Condylar (ellipsoid) joints, 12, 13f
Condylar process, 451, 538
Condyle
  of humerus, 399, 399f
  occipital, 38, 454
Cones, 522
Confluence of sinuses, 471
Congenital heart defects, 117b
Conjoint tendon, 157–158
Conjunctiva, 504
Connective tissue layer, of scalp, 496
Constrictive pericarditis, 105b
Constrictor muscles, of pharynx, 586, 586t, 587f
Contrast agents, 4
  urological, 8
Conus medullaris, 55
Cooper's ligament, 150, 151f
Coracobrachialis, 387t, 401t
Cords of brachial plexus, 390, 390f
Cornea, 521
Corniculate cartilage, 595, 596f
Cornua, 227, 227f
Coronal planes, 2, 2f
  computed tomography image of hip joint in, 296b
  female pelvic cavity and perineum in, 281b
  MRI of brain in, 7f
Coronal suture, 448
Coronary arteries, 117–120, 119f
  clinical terminology for, 120b
Coronary artery bypass grafts, 124b
Coronary artery disease, 124b
Coronary lymphatics, 120
Coronary sulcus, 106, 109f
Coronary vasculature, 117–120
  cardiac veins, 120, 121f
  coronary arteries, 117–120, 119f, 120b
  coronary lymphatics, 120

Coronoid fossa, 399
Coronoid process, 451, 538
Corpora cavernosa, 265f, 266
Corpus spongiosum, 240, 265f, 266, 269b–270b
Costal groove, 69
Costal part, of parietal pleura, 85
Costocervical trunk, 78, 579
Costodiaphragmatic recesses, 87, 88f
Costomediastinal recesses, 87, 88f
Costotransverse joints, 73, 74f
Costotransverse ligament, 73
Costovertebral joints, 73, 74f
Couinaud's segments, of liver, 182b
Cranial cavity, 454–459
    floor, 455
    infections from pterygoid plexus spreading into, 550b
    roof, 455, 455f
Cranial, describing anatomical location, 3
Cranial dura mater, 462–465
Cranial nerve preganglionic parasympathetic fibers, 30–31
Cranial nerves, 475–484, 475t–476t, 477f
    abducent, 479
    accessory, 480–484
    facial, 479
    glossopharyngeal, 480
    hypoglossal, 484
    lesions, 481b
    mandibular, 479
    maxillary, 479
    oculomotor, 477–478, 478t
    olfactory, 475, 477f
    ophthalmic, 478
    optic, 475, 477f
    overview of, 481b
    test for, 631b
Cremasteric arteries, 274
Cremasteric reflex, 157, 161b
Crest, of ribs, 69
Cribriform plate, 456, 606, 611–612
Crico-arytenoid joints, 598
    movements of, 598f
Crico-arytenoid muscle, 601f
Cricoid cartilage, 593–594, 593f
Cricothyroid joint, 597–598
Cricothyroid ligament, 596, 596f
    how to locate, 597f, 597b
Cricothyroid muscle, 600–601, 600f
Cricothyrotomy, 597b
Cricotracheal ligament, 595
Crista galli, 606
Critical limb ischemia, 320b
Cruciate ligaments, 327, 327f
    clinical tests for, 328b
Crura, 266
    of clitoris, 266, 267b–268b
    of diaphragm, 203, 204f
    of penis, 266, 269b–270b
Cubital fossa, 408–409, 408f–409f
Cuboid, 343
Cuneiform, 343, 595, 596f
Curvatures, of vertebral column, 41, 43f
Cutaneous branches, of cervical plexus, 576–577

D

Dartos fascia, 149, 149f
Deep artery
    of clitoris, 274
    of penis, 273, 273f
    of thigh, 317–320, 319f
Deep auricular artery, 549
Deep cervical artery, 579
Deep cervical lymph nodes, 583–584
Deep, describing anatomical location, 3
Deep dorsal vein, 261
Deep fascia, 15
    of hip, 300–301
Deep fibular nerve, 339f, 340, 361–362, 361f
Deep group of muscles
    in back, 51–53, 51f
    in posterior compartment of leg, 334–335, 335f, 335t
Deep inguinal nodes, 275, 275f, 299
Deep inguinal ring, 157, 157f
Deep layer of forearm muscles
    anterior compartment, 414, 416f, 416t
    posterior compartment, 418, 420f, 420t
Deep palmar arch, 434–435, 434f
Deep perineal pouch (deep perineal space), 232, 234, 235f–236f, 235t, 263–264, 263f
Deep petrosal nerve, 555
Deep temporal arteries, 541
Deep temporal nerves, 541, 544
Deep transverse metacarpal ligaments, 425, 425f
Deep transverse metatarsal ligaments, 350f, 351
Deep transverse perineal muscle, 235, 236f
Deep vein thrombosis, 215b, 298b
Defecation, 234b
Deltoid ligament, 345–346
Deltoid muscle, 377, 378f
Dens, 38, 39f–40f
Dense connective tissue layer, of scalp, 496
Denticulate ligament, 58
Depressed skull fractures, 461b
Depressor anguli oris, 484
Depressor labii inferioris, 484
De Quervain syndrome, 427b
Dermatomes, 22–23, 22f, 23b
    anterior view, 23f
    of anterolateral abdominal wall, 154f
    in lower limb, 362b–363b
    in upper limb, 439b
Dermatomyotomes, 21
Dermis, 15
Descending part, of duodenum, 169
Developmental changes in elbow joint, 406b
Deviated nasal septum, 606b
Dialysis fistula, construction of, 409b
Diaphragm, 81–84, 83f–84f, 202–205, 203f–204f
    arterial supply in, 83
    movement of, during breathing, 84
    pelvic, 233–234, 233f, 233t
Diaphragma sellae, 463
Diaphragmatic hernias, 205b
Diaphragmatic nodes, 80
Diaphragmatic part, of parietal pleura, 85
Diaphragmatic surface, of heart, 105, 108f
Diencephalon, 466–467

Digastric muscle, 562
Digital rectal examination, 237b
Digital subtraction angiography, 4–5, 5f
Dilator pupillae, 521
Diploë, 452
Discectomy, 48b
Disease
    of joints, 46b
    peripheral vascular, 320b
    peritoneal spread of, 164b
Dislocations
    acromioclavicular and sternoclavicular joints, 376b–377b
    anterior, of humeral head, 389b
    of glenohumeral joint, 377b
Distal, describing anatomical location, 3
Distal end
    of femur, 310, 310f
    of fibula, 332–333, 332f
    of humerus, 398–400
    of tibia, 331–332
Distal group, of tarsal bones, 341f, 343
Distal radioulnar joint, 412–414, 412f
Distal row, of carpal bones, 423–424
Distribution pattern, of facial nerve, 492
Diverticular disease, 178b
Domes, of diaphragm, 204
Doppler ultrasound, 5
Dorsal artery
    of clitoris, 274
    of penis, 273, 273f
Dorsal digital nerves, 362
Dorsal interossei, 358t, 431, 432f
Dorsal lingual vein, 625
Dorsal nasal artery, 495, 514
Dorsal nerve, of penis and clitoris, 271
Dorsal scapular nerve, 393, 393f
Dorsal venous arch, of hand, 435f
Dorsalis pedis artery, 358–359, 359f
    finding, 359b
Dorsalis pedis pulse, 365b
Double jointed, 426b
Ducts
    lymphatic, 19, 19f
    nasolacrimal, 505, 605f, 611
    parotid, 487
    submandibular, 627
Ductus arteriosus, 117b, 131
Ductus deferens, 242f, 243
Duodenal ulceration, 172b
Duodenojejunal flexure, 169
Duodenum, 169–170, 170f
Dura mater, 20
    cranial, 462–465
    spinal, 57, 57f
Dural innervation, 464, 464f
Dural partitions, 462–463, 463f
Dural venous sinuses, 469–472, 469f, 470t
    and veins, 470f

E

Ears, 522–535
    external, 522–525
    innervation of scalp
        anterior to, 498
        posterior to, 498

Ears (Continued)
internal, 522, 530–535, 531f
middle, 522, 526–530
Ectopic parathyroid glands, 572b
in thymus, 127b
Efferent ductules, 242–243, 242f
Effort closure, of larynx, 601, 602f
Ejaculatory duct, 242f, 243
Elastic cartilage, 9
Elbow joint, 405–406, 405f–406f, 406b–407b
Emissary veins, 472b
Endarterectomy, 468b
Endolymphatic duct, 533
Endopelvic fascia, 151
Endoscopy, of gastrointestinal tract, 179b
Endothoracic fascia, 15, 78
Enteric system, 31–32, 31f, 200, 200f
Epaxial muscles, 21
Epicondyles, of humerus, 399
Epicondylitis, 407b
Epicranial aponeurosis, 496–497
Epidermis, 15
Epididymis, 242f, 243
Epigastric artery, 155, 156f
Epiglottis, 594, 595f
Epiphyseal fractures, 11b
Episiotomy, 236b
Epistaxis, 614b
Erectile tissues, 265f, 266–267
Erection, 267
Erector spinae muscles, 51, 52f, 52t
Esophageal cancer, 137b
Esophageal plexus, 136–137, 137f
Esophageal rupture, 137b
Esophagus, 568
abdominal, 167–168, 168f
constrictions in, 136b
in posterior mediastinum, 135–137, 135f
arterial supply in, 136
important structures of, relationship to,
135–136
innervation in, 136
venous and lymphatic drainage in, 136
in superior mediastinum, 131
Ethmoid bone, 606, 606f
Ethmoidal artery, 514, 614
Ethmoidal cells, 608–609
Ethmoidal foramina, 502
Exogenous testosterone, 601b
Extension elbow joint, 405f
Extension, knee, 288f
Extensor carpi ulnaris tendon, 421b–422b
Extensor digitorum brevis, 355, 355f, 355t
Extensor digitorum tendon, 421b–422b
Extensor hallucis brevis, 355, 355t
Extensor hoods, 354–355, 355f, 429–430, 430f
Extensor retinacula, 352, 352f
External acoustic meatus, 524, 524f
External anal sphincter, 265
nerves to, 251f
External carotid artery, 563
branches of, 565t
External ear, 522–525
auricle, 522–524, 523f
examination of, 525b–526b
external acoustic meatus, 524, 524f
tympanic membrane, 524–525

External genitalia
of men, 269b–270b
of women, 267b–268b
External iliac nodes, 275, 275f
External intercostal muscle, of thoracic wall,
78, 78t
External jugular veins, 560, 573, 574f
External laryngeal nerve, 603
External nasal nerves, 490, 615
External nose, 606–607, 607f
External oblique, 149–150, 150f, 150t
External os, 246–247, 247f
External pudendal arteries, 274
External rectal venous plexus, 260–261, 261f
External spermatic fascia, 157
External sulci, 106
External urethral sphincter, 235, 236f, 240,
241f
Extracapsular ligaments, 539
Extradural hematoma, 473b, 550b
Extradural space, 465, 465f
Extraperitoneal fascia, 15, 152–153, 153f
Extrinsic ligaments, of larynx, 595, 596f
Extrinsic muscles
of auricle, 522
extra-ocular, 511t
eyeball movements and, 513
orbital, 510–513
of tongue, 4490
Eye
dry, 555b
and lacrimal apparatus, 506b, 507f
Eyeball, 519–522, 519f
actions of muscles of, 513f
anterior and posterior chamber, 519–520
arterial supply, 520
fascial sheath of, 509–510, 510f
fibrous layer of, 520–521
inner layer of, 521–522
innervation, 515f
lens and vitreous humor, 520
movements of, 511f, 513
muscles, 512f, 512b
vascular layer of, 521
venous drainage, 520
walls of, 520
Eyelids, 502–505, 502f
conjunctiva, 504
glands, 504
innervation, 504–505, 504f
orbicularis oculi, 502–503
orbital septum, 503
skin and subcutaneous tissue, 502
tarsus and levator palpebrae superioris,
503–504
vessels, 504

F

Face
major features of, 497f, 497b
motor innervation of, 491–492
muscles, 484–487, 485t–486t, 486f
nasal group of, 487f
orbital group of, 487f
parotid glands, 487–489, 489f
Facial artery, 565

Facial nerve (VII), 477f, 479, 487, 493f, 566,
626
branches, 492, 534
palsy, 496b
in temporal bone, 534, 535f
Facial pulse, 639b
Facial skeleton, visible part of, 450–451
Facial vein, 495, 565
Falciform ligament, 180
False pelvis (greater pelvis), 224, 224f
False ribs, 69
Falx cerebelli, 463
Falx cerebri, 462–463
Fascia, 15
deep, 15
extraperitoneal, 152–153, 153f
importance of, 15b
neck, 558–560, 559f
compartments of, 560
of pectoral region, 68f
of pelvis, 247–248, 248f
pharyngeal, 587
renal, 206–207, 208f
specializations, orbital, 509–510
superficial, 15
abdominal, 148–149, 148f–149f
of urogenital triangle, 270, 271f
Fascia lata, 149, 149f, 300–301, 301f
Fascial sheath, of eyeball, 509–510, 510f
Fat pad
infrapatellar, 324
synovial joint, 12
Fat, renal, 206–207, 208f
Femoral artery, 155, 297, 303b, 317–320, 318f
Femoral hernias, 162b
Femoral neck fractures, 292b
Femoral nerve, 222, 321, 321f, 363b
Femoral pulse, 365b
Femoral sheath, 302–303
Femoral triangle, 301
boundaries of, 302f
contents of, 302f
Femur
proximal, 290–292, 291f
shaft and distal end of, 292f, 310, 310f
Fibrocartilage, 9
Fibro-elastic membrane, of larynx, 596–597,
598f
Fibrous joints, 13, 14f
Fibrous layer, of eyeball, 520–521
Fibrous membrane, 12
of elbow joint, 405
of hip joint, 294, 295f
of joint capsule, 374
of knee joint, 325f, 326
of temporomandibular joint capsule, 539
Fibrous pericardium, 103, 103f
Fibrous sheaths
digital, 429, 429f
of toes, 353–354, 354f
Fibula, 332f
proximal end of, 313, 313f
shaft and distal end of, 332–333
Fibular artery, 336, 336f
Fibular retinacula, 352, 353f
Fibularis brevis, 338t
Fibularis longus, 338t

Filiform papillae, 621
Filum terminale, 55
Fimbriae, 246, 246f
Fingers, 422f
Fissures
  middle cranial fossa, 458
  oral, 633–634, 633f
  orbital, 507–508
  palpebral, 497b, 502
  pterygopalatine fossa, 551
Flail chest, 72b
Flat bones, 10
Flat muscle, of abdomen, 149–151
Flexion
  elbow joint, 405f
  knee joint, 288f
Flexor carpi ulnaris tendon, 421b–422b
Flexor digiti minimi brevis, 357, 358t
Flexor digitorum brevis, 357, 358t
Flexor digitorum profundus, 416t
Flexor digitorum superficialis, 414, 415f–416f,
  415t
Flexor pollicis longus, 416t
Flexor retinaculum, 427b
  of foot, 351–352, 351f
Floating ribs, 69
Floor
  of axilla, 386, 386f
  of bony orbit, 502
  of cranial cavity, 455
  of middle ear, 526
  of nasal cavity, 609, 609f
  of oral cavity, 621–627, 622t
Fluorodeoxyglucose (FDG), labeled with
  fluorine-18, 7
Fluoroscopy unit, 4f
Foliate papillae, 622
Foot, 286, 340–362
  arches of, 352–353, 353f
  arteries in, 357–359, 357f
    dorsalis pedis artery, 358–359, 359f,
      359b
    posterior tibial artery and plantar arch,
      357–358
  bones of, 340–344, 340f–341f, 344b
    metatarsals, 343–344, 344f, 344b
    phalanges, 344, 344f, 344b
    tarsal, 343
  extensor hoods, 354–355, 355f
  extensor retinacula, 352, 352f
  fibrous sheaths of toes, 353–354, 354f
  fibular retinacula, 352, 353f
  flexor retinaculum, 351–352, 351f
  intrinsic muscles of, 355–357,
    355f, 355t
    first layer of, 355, 356f, 356t
    fourth layer, 357, 357f, 358t
    second layer, 355, 356f, 356t
    third layer, 355–357, 357f, 358t
  joints of, 344–351
    ankle, 344–346, 345f
    deep transverse metatarsal ligaments,
      350f, 351
    interphalangeal, 350f, 351
    intertarsal, 346–350
    metatarsophalangeal, 350, 350f
    tarsometatarsal, 350, 350f

Foot (Continued)
  nerves in, 359–362
  plantar aponeurosis, 353, 354f
  tarsal tunnel, 351–352, 351f, 352b
  veins in, 359, 360f
Foot drop, 340b
Foramen
  greater sciatic, 295
  lesser sciatic, 295–297
Foramen cecum, 455–456, 456t
  of tongue, 621
Foramen magnum, 454, 458–459
Foramen ovale, 111
Foramen rotundum, 551
Foramen transversarium, 38
Foramina
  internal, of skull, 456t
  intervertebral, 40, 42f
  middle cranial fossa, 458
  orbital, 507–508
  posterior cranial fossa, 459
  pterygopalatine fossa, 551
  sacral, 226–227, 227f
  sciatic, 230b
  small, in nasal cavity lateral wall, 613
Forearm, 411b
  anterior compartment
    arteries and veins, 414–417, 416f
    muscles, 414
    nerves, 417–418
  bones, 410–412
  joints, 412–414
  medial cutaneous nerve of, 394–395
  movements of, 369f
  posterior compartment of, 418–421
    arteries and veins, 418–419
    nerves, 421
  radiograph of, 411f
Foregut, 188, 188f
Fornix, vaginal, 247, 247f–248f
Fourchette, 267b–268b
Four-quadrant pattern, of abdomen, 146,
  146f
Fovea centralis, 522
Fracture
  across waist of scaphoid bone, 426b
  bone, 11b
  of clavicle, 376b–377b
  epiphyseal, 11b
  femoral neck, 292b
  femoral shaft, 293b
  of head of radius, 407b
  intertrochanteric, 293b
  orbital, 502b
  pars interarticularis, 48b
  pelvic, 230b, 290b
  of proximal humerus, 372b
  of radius and ulna, 412b
  rib, 72b, 389b
  skull vault, 461b
  supracondylar, of humerus, 407b
  of talus, 342b
  vertebral, 47b
Frenulum
  of clitoris, 267b–268b
  of glans, 269b–270b
Frontal bone, 446

Frontal nerve, 517
Frontal sinuses, 608
Fundiform ligament, of penis, 149, 266, 267f
Fundus
  of stomach, 168
  of uterus, 246, 246f
Fungiform papillae, 622
Fusion
  of cervical vertebrae, 44b
  spinal, 48b

G

Gait, 364b
Gallbladder, 183
Gallstones, 186b
Ganglia, 198–199, 199f
  abdominal prevertebral, 217–219, 218f,
    219t
  branches from, 140–141
  ciliary, 518–519, 518f
  pterygopalatine, 555
  in root of neck, 581–582
  spiral, 532f, 534
  superior cervical, 516, 581
Ganglion, 24
Ganglion impar, 197, 255, 256f–257f
Gaps, in pharyngeal wall, 587–588, 588f
Gastroduodenal artery, 189f, 190
Gastroesophageal junction, 171b–172b
Gastrointestinal contrast examinations, 8
Gastrointestinal system, pelvic viscera and,
  236–237, 238f
Gastrointestinal tract
  abdominal
    endoscopy of, 179b
    lymphatic drainage of, 196, 196f
    venous drainage of, 194f
  arterial supply to, 187–193
  congenital disorders of, 178b
  elements in neck, 568–569
  vascular supply to, 193b
Gastrostomy, 182b
Gender differences
  in pelvis, 229–230, 229f
  in urethra, 240, 241f
General somatic afferents (GSAs), 22
General somatic efferents (GSEs), 22, 477
General visceral afferent fibers (GVAs), 24
General visceral efferent fibers (GVEs), 24,
  477
Geniculate ganglion, 479, 534
  lesions, 496b
Geniohyoid muscle, 562, 622f
Genitalia, external
  of men, 269b–270b
  of women, 267b–268b
Genitofemoral nerve, 221
Gingivae, 634–638
  arterial supply, 635–636
  innervation of, 637–638
  lymphatics, 636
  veins, 636
Ginglymus, 13f
Glabella, 446
Glandular branches, of superior thyroid artery,
  569

Index

Glans clitoris, 265f, 266
Glans penis, 265f, 267, 269b–270b
Glaucoma, 520b
Glenohumeral joint, 368, 373–376, 374f–376f, 375b–376b
  dislocations of, 377b
  movements of arm at, 369f
Gliding joint, 13f
Glossopharyngeal nerves (IX), 480, 566, 566f, 592, 625
Gluteal nerve
  inferior, 251f, 254
  superior, 251f, 254
Gluteal region, 286, 303–308, 304f
  arteries of, 308, 308f
  lymphatics of, 308
  muscles of, 303–305, 304f–305f, 306t
  nerves of, 305–308, 306f
  veins of, 308
Gluteal surface, 225f, 226
Gluteus maximus, 305f
Gluteus medius, 304
Gluteus minimus, 304
Gluteus muscle, 301
Goiter, 572b
Golfer's elbow, 407b
Gomphoses, 13, 14f
Grafts, vein harvesting for, 299b
Gray matter, 20, 55f, 56
Gray rami communicantes, 251, 251f
Gray ramus communicans, 25–26
Great auricular nerve, 498, 576
Great cardiac vein, 120
Greater occipital nerve, 498
Greater omentum, 165–166, 166f, 166b
Greater palatine artery, 556, 613
Greater palatine foramen, 619
Greater palatine nerve, 632
Greater petrosal nerve, 555, 628–629
Greater sac, of peritoneal cavity, 164, 165f
Greater sciatic foramen, 230–231, 231f–232f
Greater sciatic notch, 224f, 225
Greater splanchnic nerve, 141
Greater trochanter, 290–292, 291f
Greater tubercle, 372
Greater vestibular glands, 244, 265f, 267, 267b–268b
Greater wing, of sphenoid, 453
Great saphenous vein, 298, 321, 359
Great vessels, abnormal origin of, 133b
Groin, 156–160
  masses around, 161b
Grooves
  for greater and lesser petrosal nerves, 530f
  mylohyoid, 538
  posterior cranial fossa, 459
  superior sagittal sinus, 455
Gubernaculum, 156–157
Gums, 634–638

H

Hamate, 424
Hamstring, 316
  injury to, 317b
Hand
  anatomical snuffbox, 428–429, 428f

Hand (Continued)
  arteries and veins, 432–435
  bones of, 423–425
  extensor hoods, 429–430, 430f
  fibrous digital sheaths, 429, 429f
  joints, 425–426
  muscles, 430–432, 431t
  nerves, 435–438
  palmar aponeurosis, 427–428, 428f
  and wrist joint, 424b
Hard palate, 452, 629–630
Haustra of colon, 174
Head, 443–640
  anatomical position and major landmarks, 450b
  of epididymis, 242f, 243
  of fibula, 331b
  injury to, 472b
  of mandible, 538
  medical imaging of, 461b
  overall design of, 445f
  parasympathetic ganglia of, 478t
  of ribs, 69
Heart, 105–124
  cardiac chambers in, 106–114, 109f, 110b
  cardiac conduction system in, 120–123, 121b, 122f
  cardiac orientation in, 105–106, 105f
  cardiac skeleton in, 117, 118f
  coronary vasculature in, 117–120
  innervation in, 123–124, 123f
  sympathetic nerves to, 28f
  visualizing, 108b
Heart attack, 124b
  symptoms of, 124b
    in men and women, 125b
Heart sounds, 116b
Helicotrema, 532
Helix, 522
Hematoma, extradural, 473b, 550b
Hemiazygos vein, 138–139, 139f
Hemodialysis, 164b
Hemorrhage, subarachnoid, 473f, 473b
Hemorrhoids, 262b
Hepatic cirrhosis, 195b
Hepatic duct, 185, 185f
Hepatopancreatic ampulla, 184
Hepatorenal recess, 180
Hernias
  abdominopelvic cavity, 163b
  diaphragmatic, 205b
  femoral, 162b
  hiatal, 206b
  incisional, 163b
  inguinal, 162b
  potential problem of, 163b
  umbilical, 163b
Herniation, of intervertebral discs, 45b–46b
Herpes zoster, 60b
Hiatal hernia, 206b
High-resolution computed tomography (HRCT), lung, 98b–99b
Hilum
  of kidney, 207
  of lungs, 85, 89, 90f
  splenic, 186

Hindgut, 188, 188f
Hinge joints, 12, 13f
Hip, 287–303
  arteries, 297–298, 298f
  bony pelvis, 287–290, 289f
  deep fascia and saphenous opening of, 300–301, 301f
  femoral triangle, 301, 302f
  gateways to lower limb, 295–297, 296f
  hip joint, 292–295, 293f–295f, 296b
  lymphatics, 299–300, 300f
  movements of, 288f
  nerves, 297, 297f
  proximal femur, 290–292, 291f
  veins, 298, 299f
Hoarseness, 134b–135b
Horizontal plane, 2f, 3
Horner's syndrome, 505b
Humeral head, anterior dislocation, 389b
Humerus
  proximal, 371–372
  proximal end of right, 372f
  shaft and distal end, 398–400, 399f
  supracondylar fracture, 407b
Hyaline cartilage, 9, 11
Hydrocele, of the testis, 243b
Hydrocephalus, 466b
Hymen, 267b–268b
Hyo-epiglottic ligament, 595
Hyoid bone, 585–586, 620, 621f
Hypaxial muscles, 21
Hyperextension, of thumb, 421b–422b
Hyperparathyroidism, 572b
Hypogastric nerves, 199, 255, 256f–257f
Hypoglossal canal, 454, 460f
Hypoglossal nerves (XII), 476t, 477f, 484, 567, 567f, 626, 626f
  test for, 624b
Hypothenar muscles, 431–432, 433f
Hysterectomy, 246b

I

Ileal arteries, 190–192
Ileocecal fold, 172f, 173
Ileocolic artery, 192
Ileum, 170–173, 171f, 171b
Ilia, 202
Iliac crest, 225f, 226
Iliac fossa, 225f, 226
Iliac tuberosity, 225f, 226
Iliacus, 202, 315f
Iliococcygeus, 233f, 234
Iliocostalis, 51
Iliofemoral ligament, 294
Iliohypogastric nerve, 153–154, 220
Ilio-inguinal nerve, 153–154, 220–221
Iliolumbar artery, 258, 258f
Iliolumbar ligaments, 38–40
Iliolumbar vein, 214
Iliopsoas muscle, 202
Iliopubic eminence, 287
Iliotibial tract, 301
Ilium, 225–226, 225f, 287, 289f
Imaging, 3–9
  diagnostic techniques for, 3–7
  image interpretation in, 7–8

Imaging (Continued)
  medical imaging of head, 461b
  safety in, 8–9, 8t
Impotence, prostatectomy and, 258b
Incisional hernias, 163b
Incisive canal, 613
Incisive nerve, 546
Incisor teeth, 634
Incus, 529, 529f
Infections
  of bladder, 241b
  neck, spread of, 560b
  pterygoid plexus, spreading into cranial
    cavity, 550b
Inferior alveolar artery, 549, 635
Inferior alveolar nerve, 546
  anesthesia of, 546b
  innervation, 637
Inferior articular processes, 68
Inferior cervical ganglion, 581–582
Inferior costal facet, 68
Inferior, describing anatomical location, 2f, 3
Inferior gluteal artery, 259, 259f, 297–298,
    308
Inferior gluteal nerve, 251f, 254, 307
Inferior hypogastric plexuses, 255, 256f–257f
Inferior laryngeal artery, 602
Inferior laryngeal veins, 603
Inferior margin, of heart, 106
Inferior mesenteric artery, 192–193, 192f
Inferior mesenteric vein, 196
Inferior oblique, 511t, 513
Inferior ophthalmic vein, 514
Inferior orbital fissure, 508
Inferior part, of duodenum, 169
Inferior petrosal sinuses, 471–472
Inferior phrenic arteries, 83
Inferior pubic ligament, 229, 229f
Inferior ramus, 225f, 226
Inferior rectal arteries, 272–273, 273f
Inferior rectal nerve, 271, 272f
Inferior rectus, 511–512, 511t
Inferior sagittal sinus, 469–471
Inferior subscapular nerve, 393f
Inferior thoracic aperture, 67, 70f
Inferior thyroid artery, 569–570, 579
Inferior vena cava, 130b, 214–215, 214f
  filter, 215b
Inferior vesical artery, 259, 259f
Inferior view, of skull, 452, 453f
  anterior part, 452
  middle part, 452–454
  posterior part, 454
Inferolateral surfaces, of bladder, 238,
    239f
Infraglottic space, 599
Infrahyoid muscle, 562–563, 563f
Infra-orbital artery, 494, 556
Infra-orbital foramen, 508
Infra-orbital nerve, 490, 554
Infrapatellar fat pad, 324
Infrapatellar synovial fold, 324
Infraspinatus muscle, 380
Infratemporal fossa, 541–550, 542f
Infratrochlear nerves, 490, 517
Infundibulopelvic ligament, 250, 260
Infundibulum, 246, 246f

Inguinal canal, 157–160, 157f
  anterior wall of, 157
  contents of, 158
  floor of, 158
  posterior wall of, 157–158
  roof of, 158
Inguinal hernias, 162b
  direct, 162b
  indirect, 162b
Inguinal ligament, 150
  pelvic bone and, gap between, 297
Inhaled objects, 94b
Injections, intramuscular, to gluteal region,
    307b
Injury
  ankle, 348b
  to hamstring, 317b
  head, 472b
  quadriceps, 315b
  soft tissue, to knee, 328b
  tracheobronchial, 569b
Inner layer, of eyeball, 521–522
Innervation
  of abdominal wall, 153–155, 154f
  of bone, 10
  of breast, 66
  cranial dura mater, 464–465
  of diaphragm, 205
  dural, 464f
  external acoustic meatus, 524
  of eyelids, 504–505, 504f
  of hip joint, 295, 295f
  internal ear, 534
  of knee joint, 328
  lacrimal gland, 506, 508f, 555
  of larynx, 603, 604f
  lungs, 97, 97f
  of middle ear, 530, 530f
  nasal cavities, 614–616, 615f
  orbit, 506, 515–519
  of palate, 632, 633f
  parotid gland, 489
  pericardial, 104b
  peripheral sympathetic, 26–28, 27f
  of peritoneum, 164b
  of pharynx, 592f
  salivary gland, 628–629
  of scalp, 498, 499f
  sensory, testing in upper limb, 440b
  suprarenal, 212
  teeth and gingivae, 637–638
  of thoracic wall, by intercostal nerves, 81,
    82f
  of tongue, 625, 625f
  tympanic membrane, 525
  ureteric, 209
  visceral sensory, 31
Interarytenoid notch, 598
Interatrial septum, 110–111
  defect in, 117b
Interchondral joints, 74f, 75
Intercondylar area, of tibia, 311–312
Intercondylar eminence, 311
Intercondylar fossa, 310
Intercostal artery, 155
Intercostal muscles, 78, 79f
Intercostal nerve block, 83b

Intercostal nerves, 81, 82f
Intercostal nodes, 80, 82f
Intercostal spaces, 75–81, 77f
  arterial supply of, 77f, 78–80
  innervation of, 81
  lymphatic drainage of, 80, 82f
  muscles of, 78, 79f
  venous drainage of, 80, 81f
Intercostobrachial nerve, 81
Intermediate group of back muscles, 50, 50f,
    50t
Intermediate layer, forearm muscles, 414, 415f,
    415t
Intermediate tarsal bone, 343
Internal carotid arteries, 468, 564
Internal ear, 522, 530–535, 531f
  bony labyrinth, 531–532
  innervation, 534
  membranous labyrinth, 532–534, 532f
  sound transmission, 534–535, 535f
  in temporal bone, 531f
  vessels, 534
Internal iliac artery, 258–260, 258f
  anterior trunk of, 258–260, 259f
  posterior trunk of, 258, 258f
Internal iliac nodes, 274
Internal iliac vein, 274, 274f
Internal intercostal muscle, of thoracic wall,
    78, 78t
Internal jugular vein, 565
Internal laryngeal nerve, 604
Internal oblique, 150, 150t
  inguinal canal and, 158f
Internal os, 246–247, 247f
Internal pudendal artery, 259, 259f, 272–274,
    273f
Internal pudendal veins, 274, 274f
Internal rectal venous plexus, 260–261,
    261f
Internal spermatic fascia, 157–158
Internal thoracic artery, 79, 155
Internal urethral sphincter, 240, 241f
Interossei muscles, 431
Interosseous membrane
  of forearm, 412, 412f
  of leg, 333, 333f
Interosseous talocalcaneal ligament, 348f
Interosseus sacro-iliac ligament, 228, 228f
Interphalangeal joints
  of hand, 426
  of toes, 350f, 351
Interspinales, 52
Interspinous ligaments, 47, 47f
Intertarsal joints, 346–350, 346f
Intertransversarii, 52
Intertrochanteric crest, 291
Intertrochanteric line, 291
Intertubercular plane, of abdomen, 147
Intervertebral discs, 42–43, 45f
  herniation of, 45b–46b
Intervertebral foramina, 40, 42f
Intestine
  large, 173–176, 173f
  small, 169–173
Intracerebral aneurysm, 468b
Intracranial hemorrhage, 473b
Intracranial venous connections, 495

Intramuscular injections, to gluteal region, 307b
Intravenous urogram, of urinary tract, 211b
Intravenous urography, 8
Intrinsic ligaments, of larynx, 596–597
Intrinsic muscles
of auricle, 522
of eye, 522t
of foot, 355–357, 355f, 355t
first layer of, 355, 356f, 356t
fourth layer, 357, 357f, 358t
second layer, 355, 356f, 356t
third layer, 355–357, 357f, 358t
of hand, 431t
of larynx, 600–601, 600t
of orbit, 510
of tongue, 624
Introitus, 247
Investing layer, of neck fascia, 558
Iodine, as contrast agent, 4
Iris, 519–521
Irregular bones, 10
Ischemia, chronic leg, 320b
Ischial spine, 224f–225f, 225–226, 230
Ischial tuberosity, 224f–225f, 225–226, 287, 289f
Ischio-anal fossae, 264–265, 264f
Ischiofemoral ligament, 294
Ischiopubic ramus, 288
Ischium, 225f, 226
Isthmus, 246, 246f

J

Jaundice, 186b
Jejunal arteries, 190–192
Jejunostomy, 182b
Jejunum, 170, 171f, 171b
Joint capsule, 11
elbow joint, 406f
of temporomandibular joint, 539
Joints, 11–13, 11f
atlanto-occipital, 38
costotransverse, 73
costovertebral, 73, 74f
diseases of, 46b
of elbow, 405–406
of foot, 344–351
of forearm, 412–414
of hand, 425–426
of hip, 292–295
interchondral, 74f, 75
laryngeal, 597–598
of leg, 333
of lower limb, 287f
manubriosternal, 74f, 75, 75b
of pelvis, 227–229
of shoulder, 372–376
solid, 11–13, 11f, 13f
sternocostal, 73–74, 74f
synovial, 11–12, 11f
temporomandibular, 538–539, 538f
"uncovertebral", 45, 45f
between vertebrae in back, 42–45
between vertebral arches, 44–45
xiphisternal, 74f, 75
zygapophysial, 44–45, 45f

Jugular notch, 76b
Jugular tubercle, 459
Jugular veins
anterior, 561
external, 560, 573, 574f
superior bulb of, 565
Jugular wall, of middle ear, 526
Jugulodigastric node, 583
Jugulo-omohyoid node, 583

K

Kidneys, 206–208
fat and fascia of, 206–207, 208f
relationships to other structures, 206, 207f
retroperitoneal position of, 206f
structure of, 207, 208f
transplant, 210b
vasculature and lymphatics of, 208, 209f
Knee joint, 323–328, 323f
articular surfaces of, 323, 324f
fibrous membrane, 325f, 326
flexion and extension, 288f
ligaments of, 326–328
locking mechanism of, 327–328, 327f
menisci, 323–324, 324f
synovial membrane, 324, 325f
vascular supply and innervation, 328
Knuckle cracking, 426b
Kyphosis, 44b

L

Labial branches, of facial artery, 493
Labia majora, 267b–268b
Labia minora, 267b–268b
Labyrinthine artery, 534
Labyrinthine vein, 534
Labyrinthine wall, of middle ear, 527–528
Laceration, of scalp, 500b
Lacrimal apparatus, 505–506
Lacrimal artery, 513
Lacrimal gland, 505, 505f
innervation of, 508f, 555
Lacrimal lake, 505–506
Lacrimal nerves, 490, 516–517
Lacrimal sac, 505, 506f
Lacteals, 18
Lactiferous ducts, 64
Lacunar ligament, 150
Lambda, 452, 455f
Lambdoid suture, 448
Laminae, 68
of modiolus, 532
of vertebra, 38
Large intestine, 173–176, 173f
Laryngeal cartilage, 593–595
Laryngopharynx, 590
Laryngoscopy, 593b
Larynx, 569, 592–604, 593f
cartilages, 593–595
cavity of, 598–600
extrinsic ligaments, 595
function of, 601, 602f
intrinsic ligaments, 596–597
intrinsic muscles, 600–601, 600t

Larynx (Continued)
laryngeal joints, 597–598
nerve, 603–604, 604f
vessels, 602–603
Lateral aortic nodes, 216–217
Lateral arcuate ligament, 204
Lateral circumflex femoral artery, 318–319, 319f
Lateral compartment, of leg, 337–338
arteries in, 337, 338f
muscles in, 337, 338f, 338t
nerves in, 337–338, 338f
veins in, 337
Lateral condyle, 311
Lateral cord of brachial plexus, branches of, 394
Lateral costotransverse ligament, 73
Lateral crus, 157
Lateral cutaneous branch, 81
Lateral cutaneous nerve, of thigh, 219t, 221
Lateral, describing anatomical location, 2f, 3
Lateral epicondyle, 310
Lateral ligament, of temporomandibular joint, 539
Lateral malleolus, 342
Lateral masses, atlas and axis, 38
Lateral nasal artery, 614
Lateral pectoral nerve, 394
Lateral plantar artery, 357–358, 357f
Lateral plantar nerve, 360f, 361
Lateral pterygoid muscle, 543, 543f
Lateral rectus, check ligament of, 510
Lateral sacral arteries, 258, 258f
Lateral thoracic artery, 387
Lateral vertebral muscles, 576t, 577f
Lateral wall
of axilla, 384, 385f, 385t
of bony orbit, 502
of infratemporal fossa, 541
of nasal cavities, 605, 605f, 610–611, 610f
Latissimus dorsi, 48f, 49, 49t
Layers
of eyeball, 520–521
of forearm muscles
anterior compartment, deep layer, 414, 416f, 416t
intermediate layer, 414
posterior compartment, deep layer, 418, 420f, 420t
posterior compartment, superficial layers, 418, 419f, 419t
superficial layer, 414, 414f, 414t
of intrinsic muscles of foot, 355–357
first layer of, 355, 356f, 356t
fourth layer, 357, 357f, 358t
second layer, 355, 356f, 356t
third layer, 355–357, 357f, 358t
of scalp, 496–498, 497f
Least splanchnic nerve, 141
Left atrium, 113, 114f
visualizing, 113b
Left brachiocephalic veins, 127, 127f, 129b
Left bundle branch, 123
Left colic artery, 193
Left common carotid artery, 563
Left coronary artery, 118, 119f
Left fibrous trigone, 117

Left gastric artery, 188
Left jugular trunk, 139
Left lung, 90, 91f
Left phrenic nerves, of superior mediastinum, 134
Left pulmonary artery, 96f, 97
Left pulmonary surface, of heart, 105
Left subclavian artery, 131
Left superior intercostal vein, 129, 129f
Left vagus nerves, of superior mediastinum, 133, 133f
Left ventricle, 113–114, 115f
Leg, 286, 331–340, 331f
   anterior compartments of, 338–340
     arteries in, 338–340
     muscles in, 338, 339f, 339t
     nerves in, 340
     veins in, 340
   bones of, 331–333
   compartments of, 331
   joints of, 333
   lateral compartment of, 337–338
     arteries in, 337, 338f
     muscles in, 337, 338f, 338t
     nerves in, 337–338, 338f
     veins in, 337
   posterior compartment of, 333–337
     arteries in, 335–336, 336f
     muscles in, 333–335, 334f–335f, 334t
     nerves in, 336–337, 337f
     veins in, 336
Lens, 520
Leptomeninges, 466b
Lesion
   at and around geniculate ganglion, 496b
   at and around stylomastoid foramen, 496b
   central, 496b
   of cranial nerves, 481b
Lesser occipital nerve, 498, 576
Lesser omentum, 166, 167f
Lesser palatine nerve, 632
Lesser petrosal nerve, 530, 547, 548f
Lesser sciatic foramen, 230–232, 231f–232f
Lesser sciatic notch, 224f–225f, 225
Lesser splanchnic nerve, 141
Lesser trochanter, 290–292, 291f
Lesser tubercle, 372
Lesser wing, of sphenoid bone, 457
Levator anguli oris, 484–486, 485t–486t
Levator ani, 233–234, 233f
   nerves to, 251f
Levatores costarum, 52
Levator labii superioris alaeque nasi, 484–486, 485t–486t
Levator palpebrae superioris, 503–504, 505f
Levator prostatae, 234
Levator scapulae, 48, 48f, 49t, 379
Levator veli palatini, 587, 630t, 631f
Ligamenta flava, 46, 46f, 47b
Ligaments
   associated with
     external oblique, 150, 150f
     liver, 180–181, 180f
   of back, 46–47
   extracapsular, 539
   foot

Ligaments (Continued)
     plantar calcaneocuboid, 349–350, 350f
     support for arches of, 353, 354f
   of hip, 294
   of inguinal region, 151f
   of knee joint, 326–328
   of larynx
     extrinsic, 595, 596f
     intrinsic, 596–597
   of ovary, 250
   of pelvic fascia, 247–248
   of pelvic wall, 230
   peritoneal, 167
   sacro-iliac, 228
   splenic, 187f
Ligamentum arteriosum, 131
Ligamentum nuchae, 46–47, 47f
Linea aspera, 310
Linea terminalis, 224f, 225
Line of attachment, for lateral pharyngeal walls, 585–586, 586f
Lingual artery, 565
Lingual nerve, 546, 625–626
   in floor of oral cavity, 626f
   injury, 546b
Lingual tonsils, 590, 622–624
Lips, 633, 633f
Liver, 180–182
   associated ligaments with, 180–181, 180f
   diaphragmatic surface of, 180, 180f
   lobes of, 181–182
   segmental anatomy of, 182b
   visceral surface of, 180, 181f
Lobar bronchi, 94
Lobes, thyroid gland, 569
Lobule, 522
Locking mechanism, of knee joint, 327–328, 327f
Long bones, 10
Longissimus, 51
Longitudinal arch, of foot, 353, 353f
Longitudinal ligaments, anterior and posterior, 46, 46f
Longitudinal muscles, of pharynx, 586–587, 587t, 588f
Long plantar ligament, 349–350, 350f
Long thoracic nerve, 393, 393f, 393b
Loose connective tissue layers, of scalp, 498
Lordosis, 44b
Lower limb, 285–366
   dermatomes and myotomes in, 362b–363b
   foot, 340–362
   functions of, 286
   gluteal region of, 286, 303–308, 304f
   hip, 287–303
   legs, 331–340, 331f
   regional anatomy of, 286–362, 286f–287f
   thigh, 309–330, 309f
Lumbar arteries, 213, 213t
Lumbar cerebrospinal fluid tap, 59b–60b
Lumbar nodes, 216–217
Lumbar plexus, 219–222, 219f, 297
   branches of, 219t
   cutaneous distribution of nerves from, 221f
   in posterior abdominal region, 220f
Lumbar splanchnic nerves, 198

Lumbar veins, 214, 215f
Lumbar vertebrae, 36f, 37–40, 39f–40f, 201–202
   typical, 37b
Lumbosacral joints, 227, 228f
Lumbosacral plexus, branches of, 297f, 300t
Lumbrical muscles, 355, 356t, 432, 433f
Lunate surface, of acetabulum, 290
Lung cancer, 101b
Lungs, 88–97, 89f
   bronchial arteries and veins in, 96f, 97
   bronchial tree in, 90–94, 94f
   bronchopulmonary segments in, 94–95, 95f
   bronchoscopy, 98b–99b
   high-resolution computed tomography, 98b–99b
   hilum of, 85, 89, 90f
   innervation, 97, 97f
   left, 90, 91f
   lymphatic drainage in, 97, 98f
   plain chest radiograph, 100b
   pulmonary arteries in, 95–97, 96f
   pulmonary veins in, 96f, 97
   right, 89–90, 91f
   root of, 85, 89, 90f
   sounds, 93b
   visualizing, 91b–92b, 98b–99b
Lymph, 18
Lymph nodes, 18–19, 19b
   facial, 495
   inguinal
     deep, 299
     superficial, 299
   level of enlargement, 584b
   in neck
     deep cervical, 583–584
     superficial, 582–583
     superficial cervical, 583
   pre-auricular and parotid, 496, 501f, 582–583
   regions of, 19f
Lymphatic drainage
   of abdominal wall, 155, 155f
   auricle, 524
   of breast, 66
   in esophagus, 136
   eyelids, 504
   of face, 495–496, 496f
   of gastrointestinal tract, 196, 196f
   of intercostal spaces, 80, 82f
   of larynx, 603
   of lungs, 97, 98f
   nasal cavities, 616, 616f
   palate, 632, 632f
   of perineum, 275f
   pharynx, 591, 591f
   of scalp, 500–501, 501f
   thyroid gland, 570
   tongue, 626–627
Lymphatic system, 18–19
   lymphatic trunks and ducts, 19, 19f
   lymphatic vessels, 18
   lymph nodes, 18–19, 19b
   structure and function of, 18f

Index

Lymphatics
  of gluteal region, 308
  of hip, 299–300
  of lower limb, 300f
  of teeth and gingivae, 636

M

Macula lutea, 522
Macula of saccule, 533
Macula of utricle, 533
Magnetic resonance imaging (MRI), 5–6
  of ankle joint, 347b
  of elbow joint, 407b
  of glenohumeral joint, 376b
  of head, 461b
  image interpretation, 8
Malabsorption procedures, for obesity, 172b
Malleus, 529, 529f
Malrotation, of gastrointestinal tract, 178b
Mammary glands, 64
  axillary process of, 397
Mandible, 447–448
  lateral and medial view of, 537
  ramus of, 537–538
Mandibular foramen, 538
Mandibular nerve (V_3), 479, 543, 544f–545f
  branches, 543–546
  innervation, 491–492
Manubriosternal joints, 74f, 75, 75b
Manubrium, of sternum, 72, 73f
Marginal artery, 193b
Margins
  of heart, 106
    visualizing, 110b
  of perineum, 264b
Masseter muscle, 540, 540f
Masseteric nerve, 544
Mastoid area, of middle ear, 527f, 528
Mastoid nodes, 500, 582
Mastoid notch, 451
Mastoid part, of temporal bone, 454
Mastoid wall, of middle ear, 526
Mastoiditis, 528b
Maxillae, 447, 537, 617–618
Maxillary artery, 547–549, 549f, 555–557,
    565, 565t
  branches of, 494, 494f
  in pterygopalatine fossa, 556f
  second part of, 547
Maxillary nerves, 477f, 479, 490, 552–557
  branches of, 553–554, 553f
Maxillary sinuses, 609
Meckel's diverticulum, 172b
Medial arcuate ligament, 203–204
Medial brachial cutaneous nerve, branches of,
    394–395
Medial calcaneal nerve, 337, 337f
Medial circumflex femoral artery, 319–320,
    319f
Medial compartment, of muscles of thigh,
    316, 316f, 317t
Medial condyle, 311
Medial crus, 157
Medial cutaneous nerve, of arm, 393f
Medial, describing anatomical location, 2f, 3
Medial epicondyle, 310

Medial ligament, ankle joint, 345–346, 345f
Medial palpebral artery, 514
Medial pectoral nerve, 394
Medial plantar artery, 357f, 358
Medial plantar nerve, 360, 360f
Medial pterygoid muscle, 543, 543f
Medial rectus, check ligament of, 510
Medial umbilical fold, 258–259
Medial umbilical ligament, 258–259, 259f
Medial wall
  of axilla, 383, 384f, 384t
  of bony orbit, 501–502
  of infratemporal fossa, 541
  of middle ear, 527–528
  of nasal cavity, 608f, 609
Median arcuate ligament, 82–83
Median cubital vein, 408f, 409
Median labial frenulum, 633
Median nerve, 395, 401f, 402, 417, 417f
  of hand, 437f, 438
  recurrent branch of, 426–427
Median sacral artery, 213, 213t, 259f–260f,
    260
Median sacral veins, 261f, 262
Median sagittal plane, 3
Median umbilical ligament, 237, 239f
Mediastinal part, of parietal pleura, 85
Mediastinum, 97–141
  anterior, 102
  lateral view of, 102f
  middle, 102
  posterior, 135–141
  sagittal section of, 103f
  subdivisions of, 102f
  superior, 126–135, 127f, 128b
  visualizing, in axial plane, 141b
Mediastinum testis, 242–243, 242f
Medulla oblongata, 467
Membranous labyrinth, 532–534, 532f
  cross-section, 533f
  organs of balance, 533
  organs of hearing, 533–534
Membranous part of urethra, 240, 241f
Men
  breast in, 66
  heart attack, symptoms of, 125b
  pelvic fascia in, 248, 248f
  reproductive system in, 241–244, 242f
  urethra of, anatomy of, 240, 241f
Meningeal branch, of mandibular nerve,
    544
Meningeal layer, of dura mater, 462
Meningeal spaces, 465–466, 465f
Meninges, 20–21, 57–58, 57f
  arachnoid mater, 465
  arrangement of, 20f
  cranial dura mater, 462–465, 462f
  meningeal spaces, 465–466, 465f
  pia mater, 465
Meningitis, 466b
Meningocele, 43b
Menisci, of knee joint, 323–324, 324f
Mental artery, 494
Mental foramen, 448
Mental nerve, 491, 546, 637
Mentalis, 484, 485t–486t
Mesencephalon, 467

Mesenteric artery
  inferior, 192–193, 192f
  superior, 190–192, 191f
Mesenteries, 166, 167f
Mesoappendix, 174, 174f
Mesometrium, 249f, 250
Mesosalpinx, 249f, 250
Mesovarium, 245, 249f, 250
Metacarpals, 424–425
Metacarpophalangeal joints, 425–426, 425f
Metatarsals, 343–344, 344f, 344b
Metatarsophalangeal joints, 350, 350f
Metencephalon, 467
Midbrain, 467
Middle cardiac vein, 120
Middle cervical ganglion, 581
Middle colic artery, 192
Middle cranial fossa, 457–458, 457f
  fissures and foramina, 458
  sella turcica, 457–458
  sphenoid, 457
  temporal bone, 458
Middle ear, 522, 526–530
  auditory ossicles, 528–529, 529f
  boundaries, 526–528, 527f
  innervation, 530, 530f
  mastoid area, 528
  muscles of, 529t
  parts of, 526f
  pharyngotympanic tube, 528, 528f
  vessels, 529–530
Middle mediastinum, 102
  ascending aorta in, 125, 126f
  heart in, 105–124
  pericardium in, 102–104, 103f
  pulmonary trunk in, 124–125, 126f
  vasculature in, 126, 126f
Middle meningeal artery, 461f, 461b, 549,
    550b
Middle part, of laryngeal cavity, 599
Middle rectal artery, 259, 259f
Middle temporal artery, 541
Midgut, 188, 188f
Mid-thigh, transverse section through, 314f
Mitral valve, 114
Mitral valve disease, 116b
Modiolus, 531–532
Molar teeth, 634
Mons pubis, 267b–268b
Morton's neuroma, 361b
Motor function of median and ulnar nerves
    in hand, 438b
Motor innervation, of face, 491–492
Motor neurons, 21, 21f
  visceral, 24
Movements
  of crico-arytenoid joints, 598f
  of cricothyroid joint, 598f
  of eyeball, 511f, 513
  of forearm, 369f
  of hand at wrist joint, 369f
  of scapula, 368f
  of synovial joints, 12
  of temporomandibular joints, 539, 539f
  of thoracic wall and diaphragm, during
    breathing, 84, 85f
  of thumb, 369f

Multifidus, 51–52
Multinodular goiter, 572b
Muscles
  of anal triangle, 265t
  in anterior compartment of leg, 338, 339f, 339t
  in anterior triangle of neck, 562t
  in anterior wall of axilla, 383t
  of arm, 401
  atrophy, 16b
  auditory ossicles, associated with, 529, 530f
  auricle, 522–524, 523f
  within deep perineal pouch, 235t
  epaxial, 21
  eyeball, 512f–513f, 512b
  facial, 484–487, 485t–486t, 486f
    nasal group of, 487f
    orbital group of, 487f
  in floor of oral cavity, 622t
  of forearm
    anterior compartment, 414
    posterior compartment, 418
  of gluteal region, 303–305, 304f–305f, 306t
  of hand, 430–432, 431t
  hypaxial, 21
  injuries and strains, 16b
  of lateral and posterior wall of axilla, 385t
  in lateral compartment of leg, 337, 338f, 338t
  of mastication, 540t
  of medial wall of axilla, 384t
  of middle ear, 529t
  within orbit, 510–522
  paralysis, 16b
  of pectoral region, 66, 68f, 69t
  of pelvic diaphragm, 233t
  of pelvic wall, 230, 231t, 232f
  of pharynx, 586–587
  of posterior compartment of leg, 333–335, 334f–335f, 334t
  of posterior scapular region, 379t
  of posterior triangle of neck, 572–573, 574f, 574t
  of shoulder, 378t
  of soft palate, 630, 630t
  of superficial perineal pouch, 267, 267f, 267t
  support for arches of foot, 353, 354f
  of thigh, 313–317
  of tongue, 624, 624t, 625f
  types of, 15
Muscular artery, 514
Muscular branches, of cervical plexus, 576
Muscular system, 15–16
Muscular triangle, 561
Musculature, of back, 48–55
  deep group of muscles, 51–53, 51f
  intermediate group of muscles, 50, 50f, 50t
  superficial groups of muscles, 48–50, 48f, 49t
  thoracolumbar fascia, 53–55, 54f
Musculi pectinati, 110
Musculocutaneous nerve, 394, 401, 401f
Musculophrenic artery, 79
Musculus uvulae, 630, 630t, 631f
Myelencephalon, 467
Myelomeningocele, 43b

Mylohyoid groove, 538
Mylohyoid muscle, 562, 622f
Myotomes, 23, 23f, 23b
  in lower limb, 362b–363b
  in upper limb, 439b

N

Nares, 497b, 611
Nasal bones, 446
Nasal cavities, 604–616, 605f
  arteries, 613–614, 614f
  choanae, 611, 612f
  external nose, 606–607, 607f
  floor, 609, 609f
  gateways, 611–613, 613f
  innervation, 614–616, 615f
  lateral wall, 605, 605f, 610–611, 610f
  lymphatics, 616, 616f
  medial wall, 608f, 609
  regions of, 605, 606f
  roof, 609–610, 610f
  skeletal framework, 606
  veins, 614, 615f
  visualizing, 608b
  walls of, 609–611
Nasal group, of facial muscles, 484, 487f
Nasalis, 484
Nasal nerves, 553
Nasal vestibule, 605
Nasociliary nerve, 517–518, 518f
Nasolacrimal duct, 505, 605f, 611
Nasopalatine nerve, 553, 616, 632
Nasopharynx, 588–590
Navicular fossa, 240, 241f
Neck, 443–640
  anterior triangle of, 557, 558f, 558b, 561–571
  of bladder, 238–239, 239f
  compartments of, 445, 445f, 557f
  fascia, 558–560, 559f
  lymphatics, 582–584, 583f
  of mandible, 538
  overall design of, 445f
  posterior triangle of, 557–558, 557f, 558b, 572–577
  of ribs, 69
  root of, 577–584, 577f
  superficial veins of, 560f
  superficial venous drainage, 560–561
  surgical neck of humerus, 372
Nerve injury
  affecting superficial back muscles, 49b
  brachial plexus, 402
  lingual nerve, in infratemporal fossa, 546b
  median nerve, in arm, 402b
  radial nerve, 439b
    in arm, 403f, 403b
  ulnar nerve, 436b–437b
    at elbow, 408b
Nerve plexuses, 32, 32f
Nerves
  in anterior compartment of leg, 340
  of arm, 401–403
  associated with posterior scapular region, 380f
  cranial, 475–484, 475t–476t, 477f

Nerves (Continued)
  in foot, 359–362
  of forearm
    anterior compartment, 417–418
    posterior compartment, 421
  of gluteal region, 305–308, 306f
  of hip, 297, 297f
  larynx, 603–604, 604f
  in lateral compartment of legs, 337–338, 338f
  to lateral pterygoid, 544
  to medial pterygoid, 544
  mylohyoid, 546
  of neck, 565–568
    root of neck, 580, 580f
  to obturator internus, 305
  palatine, 632f
  of parasympathetic system, 29–31
  of pelvis, 251–255
  of pericardium, 104
  peripheral, regions of skin innervated by, 363b
  of pharynx, 591–592
  in posterior compartment of leg, 336–337, 337f
  posterior scapular region, 380–381
  of posterior triangle of neck, 575–577
  pterygoid canal, 506, 554–555, 554f
  to quadratus femoris, 305
  somatic, of perineum, 271
  to stapedius and chorda tympani, 534
  in superior mediastinum, 131–134
    phrenic, 133–134
    vagus, 131–133
  of temporal fossa, 542f
  of thigh, 321–323
  tongue, 625f
Nervous system, 20–32
  CNS, 20–21, 20f
  dermatomes, 22–23, 22f, 23b
  enteric system, 31–32, 31f
  myotomes, 23, 23f, 23b
  nerve plexuses, 32
  parasympathetic system, 25, 29–31, 30f
  in posterior abdominal region, 217
  somatic part of, 21–22, 21f
  somatic plexuses, 32
  sympathetic system, 25–29, 25f–26f
  visceral part of, 21, 23–25, 24f
  visceral plexuses, 32
Neural layer, of retina, 522
Neuralgia, trigeminal, 491b
Nine-region pattern, of abdomen, 146–147, 146f, 147b
Nipple, 64
Noncoronary cusp, 114
Noncoronary sinus, 114
Nuchal lines, 451, 453f
Nuclear medicine imaging, 6–7
  image interpretation, 8
  of urinary tract, 211b
Nucleus pulposus, 43

O

Obesity, surgery for, 172b
Obliquus capitis inferior, 52, 53f, 54t
Obliquus capitis superior, 52, 53f, 54t

Index

Obturator artery, 259, 259f, 297–298, 320, 320f
Obturator canal, 231, 232f, 295
Obturator externus, 316, 316f
Obturator foramen, 224f, 225
Obturator groove, 225f, 226
Obturator internus, 230, 231t, 232f, 303
   nerve to, 251f, 254, 305
Obturator membrane, 224f, 225
Obturator nerve, 222, 321–322, 322f, 363b
Obtuse margin, of heart, 106
Occipital artery, 565
Occipital bone, 451, 454
   squamous part, 459
Occipital nodes, 582
Occipitofrontalis, 487, 498f
Occipitomastoid suture, 448
Oculomotor nerve (III), 477–478, 477f, 478t, 515–516, 516f
Olecranon fossa, 400
Olfactory nerves (I), 475, 477f
Olfactory region, of nasal cavity, 605
Omenta, 165–166
Omental appendices, 173
Omental bursa, 164
Omental (epiploic) foramen, 164, 165f
Ophthalmic artery, branches, 495, 499
Ophthalmic nerves (V), 477f, 478, 490, 516–518
   branches from, 615–616
   divisions of, 517f
   relationship in divisions to the muscles of the eyeball, 517f
Ophthalmoscopy, 519f, 519b
Optic canal, 507–508, 509f
Optic disc, 522
Optic nerves (II), 475, 477f, 515
Ora serrata, 521
Oral cancer, 617b
Oral cavity, 616–638, 617f
   cheeks, 620
   floor, 621–627
   oral fissure and lips, 633–634, 633f
   oropharyngeal isthmus, 634
   roof (palate), 629–632, 630f
   salivary glands, 627–629
   skeletal framework, 617–620
   teeth and gingivae, 634–638
   tongue, 621–627
   walls of, 620
Oral cavity proper, 617
Oral fissures, 616, 633–634, 633f
Oral group, of facial muscles, 484–486
Oral vestibule, 617
Orbicularis oculi, 502–503, 503f
Orbit
   bony, 501–502, 508f
   eyeball, 519–522
   eyelid, 502–505
   fascial specializations, 509–510
   fissures and foramina, 507–508
   innervation, 506, 515–519
   lacrimal apparatus, 505–506
   muscles, 510–522
   sensory innervation, 506–507
   vessels, 513–515

Orbital group, of facial muscles, 484, 487f
Orbital septum, 503, 503f
Orientation, of pelvis, 229, 229f
Oropharyngeal isthmus, 634, 634f
Oropharynx, 590
Osteoporosis, 11b, 44b
Ostomies, 182b
Oval window, 528
Ovarian arteries, 213, 213t, 260, 260f
Ovarian cancer, 245b
Ovarian veins, 262
Ovaries, 245, 245f

P
Pain
   back, 45b
   referred, 33b, 125b
Palate, 629–632, 630f
   innervation of, 632, 633f
Palatine aponeurosis, 631f
Palatine bones, 618–619
Palatine branch, of ascending palatine artery, 4510
Palatine canal, 551
Palatine processes, 452
Palatoglossus muscle, 624t, 630t, 631f
Palatopharyngeal sphincter, 588
Palatopharyngeus muscle, 586, 587t, 630t, 631f
Palatovaginal canal, 551
Palmar aponeurosis, 427–428, 428f
Palmar digital artery, 434
Palmar digital nerves, 438
Palmar interossei, 431, 432f
Palmar metacarpal arteries, 435
Palmaris longus tendon, 421b–422b
Palpebral fissure, 497b, 502
Palsy
   facial nerve, 496b
   recurrent laryngeal nerve, 580b
Pancreas, 183–184, 183f, 184b
   arterial supply to, 184, 185f
   visualizing, 184b
Pancreatic cancer, 185b
Pancreatic duct, 183f, 184
Pancreaticoduodenal artery, inferior, 190
Papilla, 621–622
Papillary muscles, 111
Para-aortic nodes, 216–217
Paracolic gutters, 176
Paralysis, muscle, 16b
Paranasal sinuses, 605f, 607–609, 607f
   visualizing, 608b
Parasternal nodes, 80, 82f, 155
Parasympathetic fibers, 255, 256f–257f
Parasympathetic innervation, 124
   of gastrointestinal tract, 199–200, 200f
   of glands in head, 628f
   lacrimal gland, 506–507
   nasal cavity, 616
   salivary glands, 628–629
Parasympathetic root to ciliary ganglion, 518
Parasympathetic system, 25, 29–31, 30f
   visceral sensory fibers in, 31
Parathyroid glands, 570–571

Para-urethral mucous glands (Skene's glands), 240, 241f
Paravertebral sympathetic chain, 255, 256f–257f
Paravertebral sympathetic trunk, 28
Parietal pelvic fascia, 151
Parietal pleura, 85, 87f
   innervation of, 86b
   reflections and recesses, 88f
Parietomastoid part, of temporal bone, 449
Parotid glands, 487–489, 489f
   stones in, 490b
   tumors in, 490f, 490b
Parotid nodes, 500, 582–583
Pars interarticularis fractures, 48b
Patella, 311, 311f
Patellar ligament, 314f, 315, 326
Pecten pubis (pectineal line), 150, 225f, 226, 229f
Pectinate line, 237, 238f
Pectinate muscles, 110
Pectoral region, of thorax, 64–66
   breast in, 64–66, 65f, 65b
   muscles of, 66, 68f, 69t
Pectoralis major, 382, 383f, 383t
Pectoralis minor, 66, 68f, 69t, 382, 383f, 383t
Pedicle, of vertebra, 38
Pelvic bone, 202, 224–226, 224f
   components of, 225–226, 225f
   linea terminalis of, 224f, 225
Pelvic cavity, 224, 224f
Pelvic diaphragm, 232–234, 233f, 233t
Pelvic extensions, of prevertebral plexus, 255, 256f–257f
Pelvic floor, 232–235
   pelvic diaphragm and, 233–234, 233f, 233t
   perineal membrane and deep perineal pouch and, 234–235, 235f, 235t
Pelvic fracture, 230b
Pelvic inlet, 230, 230f
Pelvic nerves
   somatic plexus in, 251–255
   visceral plexuses in, 255
Pelvic outlet, 224, 232, 232f
Pelvic plexuses (inferior hypogastric plexuses), 255, 256f–257f
Pelvic splanchnic nerves, 29–30, 198, 200, 251, 251f, 256f–257f
Pelvic veins, 260–262, 261f
Pelvic viscera, 236–247
   gastrointestinal system and, 236–237, 238f
   MRI in sagittal plane, 6f
   reproductive system and, 241–247, 244f
   sympathetic innervation of, 28–29, 29f
   urinary system and, 237–240, 239f
Pelvic wall, 230–232
   apertures in, 230–232, 232f
   ligaments of, 230
   muscles of, 230, 231t, 232f
Pelvis, 223–284
   blood vessels of, 258–262
   bones, 224–227
   fascia, 247–248, 248f
   fracture, 230b, 290b
   gender differences in, 229–230, 229f
   imaging app for, 276b, 279b, 281b

Pelvis (Continued)
 joints, 227–229
 lymphatics of, 262, 262f
 measurements, in obstetrics, 232b
 nerves, 251–255
 orientation of, 229, 229f
 peritoneum, 248–250, 249f
 regional anatomy of, 224–262, 224f
 true, 230–236, 230f
Penis, 265f, 266–267
 corona of glans, 269b–270b
 deep dorsal vein of, 274
 dorsal nerve of, 271
 erectile tissues of, 265f
 erection of, 267
 fundiform ligament of, 149, 266, 267f
Percutaneous coronary intervention, 124b
Perforated bowel, 165b
Perforating arteries, of deep femoral artery,
  319f, 320
Perforating cutaneous nerve, 251f, 254,
  307–308
Perforation, of tympanic membrane,
  525b–526b
Pericardiacophrenic vessels, 103
Pericardial effusion, 105b
Pericarditis, 104b
Pericardium, 102–104, 103f
 fibrous, 103, 103f
 innervation of, 104b
 nerves of, 104
 sagittal section of, 103f
 serous, 103–104, 104f
 vessels of, 104
Pericranium, 498
Perilymph, 530
Perineal artery, 273, 273f
Perineal body, 235–236, 236f
Perineal flexure, 234
Perineal membrane, 232, 234–235, 235f–236f,
  235t, 244, 263–264, 263f
Perineal nerve, 271–272, 272f
Perinephric fat, 206
Perineum, 223–284, 224f, 263f
 anal triangle and, 265, 265f, 265t
 blood vessels of, 272–274
 borders and ceiling of, 263–264, 263f
 imaging app for, 276b, 279b, 281b
 ischio-anal fossae in, anterior recesses of,
  264–265, 264f
 lymphatics of, 274–275, 275f
 regional anatomy of, 224–275, 224f
 somatic nerves of, 271
 surface anatomy of, 264b
 urogenital triangle and, 263f, 265–270
 veins of, 274, 274f
 visceral nerves of, 271–272
Periorbita, 509, 509f
Periosteal layer, of dura mater, 462
Peripheral artery pulses, in upper limb, 441b
Peripheral nervous system, 20, 20f
 parasympathetic system, 25, 29–31, 30f
 sympathetic system, 25–29, 25f–26f
Peripheral reflections, 86–87, 87f–88f
Peripheral sympathetic innervation, 26–28,
  27f
Peripheral vascular disease, 320b

Perirenal fat, 206
Peritoneal cavity, 164–167, 165f
Peritoneal dialysis, 164b
Peritoneum
 of abdominal viscera, 163–164, 163f, 164b
 of abdominal wall, 153
 in men, 249f, 250
 in women, 249–250, 249f
Persistent ductus arteriosus (PDA), 117b
Petrosal nerve, 458, 530, 534, 555, 628–629
 grooves and hiatuses for, 530f
Petrosal sinuses, 471–472
Petrotympanic fissure, 534, 536
Petrous part, of temporal bone, 454
Phalanges, 344, 344f, 344b
 of hand, 425
Pharyngeal branch, of maxillary artery, 556
Pharyngeal fascia, 587
Pharyngeal nerves, 553
Pharyngeal recess, 590
Pharyngeal tonsil, 590
Pharyngeal tubercle, 454
Pharyngeal wall
 lateral, line of attachment for, 585–586,
  586f
 muscles, 586–587
Pharyngobasilar fascia, 587
Pharyngotympanic tube, 528, 528f
 cartilaginous part of, 619
Pharynx, 569, 584–592, 584f
 fascia, 587
 innervation, 592f
 laryngopharynx, 590
 mucosal features of, 589f
 nasopharynx, 588–590
 nerve, 591–592
 oropharynx, 590
 pharyngeal wall, 586–587
  structures passing through gaps in,
   587–588
 skeletal framework, 585–586
 vessels, 590–591
Philtrum, 497b, 633
Phonation, larynx role in, 601, 602f
Phrenic arteries, inferior, 213, 213t
Phrenic nerves, 579
 of diaphragm, 83, 205
 of superior mediastinum, 133–134
Pia mater, 21, 57f, 58, 465
Pigmented layer, of retina, 521
Piriform aperture, 446
Piriformis, 230, 231t, 232f, 303–304
 nerve to, 251f, 254
Pisiform, 423
Pituitary gland, surgical approach to, 609b
Pivot joints, 12, 13f
Plain chest radiograph, in lungs, 100b
Plain radiography, 3–5
 image interpretation, 7–8
Plane joints, 12
Plantar aponeurosis, 353, 354f
Plantar arch, 357–358
Plantar calcaneocuboid ligament, 349, 350f
Plantar calcaneonavicular ligament, 349
Plantar interossei, 358t
Plaques, atheromatous, 468b
Platysma, 486–487

Pleura, 84–87, 86f
 parietal, 85–87, 87f
 visceral, 85, 87
Pleural cavities, 84–97, 86f
 lungs, 88–97, 89f
 visualizing, 91b–92b
Pleural effusion, 88b
Pleural recesses, 87b
 visualizing, 91b–92b
Plexuses
 brachial, 577
 cervical, 576–577, 576f
 myenteric and submucous nerve, 31
 nerve, 32
 of pelvis
  somatic, 251–255
  visceral, 255
 pterygoid, 549–550, 550f
 somatic, 32
 visceral, 32, 32f
Pneumonia, 101b
Pneumothorax, 88b
Polyhydramnios, 184b
Popliteal artery, 329–330, 335–336, 336f
Popliteal fossa, 329–330, 330f
 contents of, 329–330, 330f
 roof of, 330
Popliteal nodes, 300
Popliteal pulse, 365b
Porta hepatis, 180
Portal vein, 193–196, 194f
Portosystemic anastomosis, 195b
Positron emission tomography, 7
Posterior abdominal region, 201–222, 201f
 abdominal wall of, 201–205, 201f
 lymphatic system in, 216–217, 216f, 216t
 nervous system in, 217
 sympathetic trunks and splanchnic nerves
  in, 217–222
 vasculature of, 212–215
 viscera of, 206–212
Posterior arch, atlas and axis, 38
Posterior auricular artery, 565
Posterior auricular nerve, 491
Posterior auricular vein, 500, 560
Posterior cardiac vein, 120
Posterior chamber, of eyeball, 519–520
Posterior ciliary artery, 514, 520
Posterior circumflex humeral artery, 381,
  388–389
Posterior commissure, 267b–268b
Posterior compartment
 of forearm
  arteries and veins, 418–419
  muscles, 418
  radial nerve, 421
 of leg, 333–337
  arteries in, 335–336, 336f
  muscles in, 333–335, 334f–335f, 334t
  nerves in, 336–337, 337f
  veins in, 336
 of muscles of thigh, 316–317, 318f, 318t
Posterior cord of brachial plexus, branches
 of, 396
Posterior cranial fossa, 456t, 458, 459f
 boundaries, 458
 foramen magnum, 458–459

Posterior cranial fossa (Continued)
grooves and foramina, 459
squamous part of occipital bone, 459
Posterior cutaneous nerve
of arm, 396
of thigh, 307
Posterior (dorsal), describing anatomical
location, 2f, 3
Posterior divisions of brachial plexus, 390
Posterior drawer test, 328b
Posterior femoral cutaneous nerve, 251f, 254
Posterior inferior iliac spine, 225f, 226
Posterior intercostal arteries, 78–79, 80f
Posterior interosseous artery, 418–419, 420f
Posterior interventricular sulci, 106
Posterior interventricular vein, 120
Posterior median sulcus, 55, 55f
Posterior mediastinum, 135–141
azygos system of veins, 137–139, 139f
esophagus in, 135–137, 135f
sympathetic trunks in, 140–141
thoracic aorta in, 137, 138f, 138t
thoracic duct in, 139–140, 140f
Posterior nasal spine, 619
Posterior papillary muscles, 112
Posterior rami, 59
Posterior root, of spinal nerves, 58–59
Posterior sacro-iliac ligament, 228, 228f
Posterior scapular region
arteries and veins, 381
gateways to, 380f
nerves, 380–381
Posterior spinal artery, 56, 56f, 467
Posterior superior alveolar artery, 635
Posterior superior alveolar nerve, 554
Posterior superior iliac spine, 225f, 226
Posterior talofibular ligament, 346
Posterior tibial artery, 335–336, 357–358, 357f
Posterior tibial pulse, 365b
Posterior triangle, of neck, 557–558, 557f,
558b, 572–577
Posterior trunk
of internal iliac artery, 258, 258f
mandibular nerve, 545f
Posterior vagal trunk, 137, 167
Posterior view, of skull, 451, 451f
occipital bone, 451
temporal bone, 451
Posterior wall
of axilla, 384–386, 385t
of middle ear, 526
Posterolateral sulcus, 55, 55f
Postganglionic fibers, 24
Postganglionic sympathetic fibers, 516
Pouch of Douglas, 249, 249f
Pre-aortic nodes, 216–217
Pre-auricular nodes, 496, 501f, 582–583
Preganglionic fibers, 24
parasympathetic, 30–31
peripheral sympathetic innervation, 26–28, 27f
Preganglionic parasympathetic fibers, 30–31
Premolar teeth, 634
Preperitoneal fascia, 153b
Preprostatic part of urethra, 240, 241f
Prepuce
of clitoris, 267b–268b
of penis, 269b–270b

Pretracheal layer, of neck fascia, 559
Pretracheal space, 560b
Prevertebral layer, of neck fascia, 558–559
Prevertebral muscles, 576t, 577f
Prevertebral plexus
abdominal, 198–199, 199f, 217–219, 218f
pelvic extensions of, 255, 256f–257f
Princeps pollicis artery, 435
Procerus, 484
Profunda brachii artery, 404
Prominence of facial canal, 528
Promontory, 226–227, 227f
Pronation
elbow joint, 405f
in forearm, 412–414, 413f
Pronator quadratus, 416t
Prostate, 242f, 243–244
problems, 244b
Prostatectomy, impotence and, 258b
Prostatic fascia, 248, 248f
Prostatic part of urethra, 240, 241f
Prostatic sinus, 240, 241f
Prostatic utricle, 240, 241f
Proximal, describing anatomical location, 3
Proximal end
of fibula, 313, 313f
of radius, 400, 400f
of tibia, 311–313, 312f
shaft, 312–313, 312f
tibial condyles and intercondylar areas,
311–312
tibial tuberosity, 312
of ulna, 400–401, 400f
Proximal femur, 290–292, 291f
greater and lesser trochanters, 290–292
Proximal group of tarsal bones, 341–343
calcaneus, 342–343, 343f
talus, 341–342, 341f
Proximal humerus, 371–372, 372f, 372b
Proximal row, of carpal bones, 423
Psoas major, 202, 315f
Psoas minor, 202
Psoas muscle abscess, 205b
Pterion, 448, 449f
fractures, 461b
Pterygoid canal, 551
artery of, 557
nerve of, 554, 554f
Pterygoid muscles, 543
lateral, 543f
medial, 543f
Pterygoid plexus, 549–550, 550f
Pterygoid processes, 453, 619
Pterygomandibular raphe, 585
Pterygopalatine fossa, 550–557, 551f
fossa, 551
gateways, 551–552, 552f
maxillary artery in, 556f
maxillary nerve, 552–557
pterygopalatine ganglion, 555
skeletal framework, 551
Pterygopalatine ganglion, 555
Ptosis, 505b
Pubic bone, 288
Pubic crest, 225f, 226
Pubic symphysis, 226, 228–229, 229f
Pubic tubercle, 224f–225f, 225–226

Pubis, 225f, 226
Puboanalis muscles, 234
Pubocervical ligament, 247–248, 248f
Pubococcygeus, 233f, 234
Pubofemoral ligament, 294
Puboprostatic ligaments, 239, 239f
Puboprostaticus, 234
Puborectalis, 233f, 234
Pubovaginalis, 234
Pubovesical ligaments, 238, 239f
Pudendal block anesthesia, 254b
Pudendal nerve, 250f–251f, 252t–253t, 254,
271, 272f, 307
Pulled elbow, 407b
Pulmonary artery, 95–97, 96f
left, 97
right, 95
Pulmonary ligament, 89, 90f
Pulmonary trunk, 124–125, 126f
Pulmonary valve, 113, 113f
Pulmonary veins, 96f, 97
visualizing, 113b
Pulse points, 365b
head and neck, 639b
upper limb, 441b
Pyloric sphincter, 168–169
Pylorus, 168–169
Pyramidalis, 150t, 152, 152f

Q

Quadrangular membrane, 596–597, 597f
Quadrangular space
posterior scapular region, 380, 380f
posterior wall of axilla, 386
Quadrangular space syndrome, 380b
Quadrants
abdominal, 147b
of gluteal region, 307b
Quadrate lobe, of liver, 181
Quadratus femoris, nerve to, 251f,
254, 305
Quadratus lumborum, 202
Quadratus plantae, 355, 356t
Quadriceps, injury to, 315b

R

Radial artery, 415, 419
Radial fossa, 399
Radial nerve, 402, 418, 421
in arm, 402f
superficial branch of, 438, 438f
Radialis indicis artery, 435
Radiation exposure dosages, 8t
Radicular arteries, superior and inferior, 56,
56f
Radiography
of foot bones, 344b
of head, 461b
of knee joint, 328b
of normal glenohumeral joint, 375b
of normal right acromioclavicular joint,
374b, 376b–377b
plain, 3–5
image interpretation, 7–8
Radioisotope, 7
Radionuclide, 7

Radius
   head, fracture of, 407b
   proximal end of, 400, 400f
   shaft and distal end, 410–411, 411f
Ramus
   ischiopubic, 288
   of mandible, 537–538
   superior pubic, 225f, 226
Raphe of penis, 269b–270b
Rectal ampulla, 237, 238f
Recto-uterine fold, 249, 249f
Recto-uterine pouch, 249, 249f, 250b
Rectovaginal septum, 247–248, 248f
Rectovesical pouch, 250
Rectovesical septum, 248, 248f
Rectum, 176, 177f, 236–237, 238f
Rectus abdominis, 150t, 151–152, 152f
Rectus capitis posterior major, 52–53, 53f, 54t
Rectus capitis posterior minor, 52, 53f, 54t
Rectus sheath, 152, 152f
Recurrent laryngeal nerve, 133, 134b–135b
Referred pain, 33b, 125b, 175f
Reflexes, tendon taps
   in lower limb, 364b
   in upper limb, 439b
Regional anatomy
   abdomen, 146–222, 146f
   of back, 36–60
   thorax, 64–141, 64f
Regional approach, to anatomy study, 2
Regional vertebrae, 39f–40f
Renal arteries, 213, 213t
Renal cortex, 207
Renal fascia, 206–207, 208f
Renal pelvis, 207
Reproductive system
   in men, 241–244, 242f
   in women, 244–247, 244f
Respiration, larynx role in, 601, 602f
Respiratory group, of back muscles, 50, 50t
Respiratory region, of nasal cavity, 605
Respiratory system, elements in neck,
   568–569
Restrictive procedures, for obesity, 172b
Rete testis, 242–243, 242f
Retina, optic part of, 521–522
Retinacula, of foot, 352, 353f
Retromammary space, 65
Retromandibular vein, 489, 560
Retroperitoneal fascia, 152–153, 153b
Retroperitoneal lymph node surgery, 217b
Retropharyngeal space, 560b
Rheumatoid arthritis, 46b
Rhomboid major, 48, 48f, 49t
Rhomboid minor, 48, 48f, 49t
Rib I, 69–70
Rib II, 70
Rib X, 72
Rib XI, 72
Rib XII, 72
Ribs, 66, 69–72, 71f
   cervical, 72b
   fractures in, 72b
      rib I, 389b
   thoracic vertebrae in, articulation of, 68–69
   upper and lower, distinct features of, 69–72,
      72f

Right atrium, 109–111, 111f
Right auricle, 110
Right brachiocephalic veins, 127, 127f
Right bundle branch, 122–123
Right colic artery, 192
Right common carotid artery, 563
Right coronary artery, 117–118, 119f
Right ear, 523f
Right fibrous trigone, 117
Right lung, 89–90, 91f
Right marginal vein, 120
Right phrenic nerves, of superior
   mediastinum, 133–134
Right pulmonary artery, 95, 96f
Right pulmonary surface, of heart, 105
Right vagus nerves, of superior mediastinum,
   132–133, 133f
Right ventricle, 111–112, 112f
Rima glottidis, 599–600
Rima vestibuli, 599–600
Risorius, 484–486
Roof
   of bony orbit, 501
   of cranial cavity, 455, 455f
   of infratemporal fossa, 541
   of middle ear, 526
   of nasal cavity, 609–610, 610f
   of oral cavity, 629–632, 630f
   of popliteal fossa, 330, 330f
Root
   of accessory nerve, 480–484
   of brachial plexus, 389–390
      branches, 390–393
   of clitoris, 265f, 266
   of lungs, 85, 89, 90f
   of neck, 577–584, 577f
      lymphatics, 582
      nerves in, 579–582, 580f
      vessels, 578–579
   of penis, 266
   superior root of ansa cervicalis, 568
Rostral, describing anatomical location, 3
Rotator cuff disorders, 377b
Rotator cuff muscles, 375–376, 376b
Rotatores, 52
Round ligament of uterus, 157, 159f–160f,
   160, 249f, 250
Round window, 528
Rupture
   of Achilles tendon, 343b
   of biceps tendon, 401b
   of spleen, 187b
   urethral, 271b

S

Saccule
   laryngeal, 599
   of membranous labyrinth, 533
Sacral canal, 226–227, 227f
Sacral foramina, 226–227, 227f
Sacral hiatus, 226–227, 227f
Sacral plexus, 251–254, 251f, 252t–253t
Sacral preganglionic parasympathetic fibers,
   29–30
Sacral splanchnic nerves, 198, 255, 256f–257f
Sacro-iliac joints, 228, 228f, 228b

Sacrospinous ligaments, 230, 231f
Sacrotuberous ligaments, 230, 231f
Sacrum, 36f, 37, 39f–40f, 40, 201–202, 224,
   224f, 226–227, 227f
Saddle joints, 12, 13f
Safety, in imaging, 8–9, 8t
Sagittal planes, 2f, 3
   female pelvic cavity and perineum in, 279b
   MRI of pelvic viscera in, 6f
   vertebral column curvatures in, 43b
Sagittal section
   of brain, 467f
   of broad ligament, 249f
Salivary glands, 627–629
Salpingopharyngeal fold, 590
Saphenous nerve, 222, 361f, 362
Saphenous opening, of hip, 301, 301f
Saphenous vein, 298
Scala tympani, 532, 532f
Scala vestibuli, 532, 532f
Scalene tubercle, 69–70
Scalp, 496–501, 497f
   arterial supply, 499
   innervation, 498, 499f
   layers, 496–498, 497f
   lymphatic drainage, 500–501, 501f
   meninges and, 474b
   venous drainage, 499
Scaphoid, 423
   fracture of, 426b
Scaphoid fossa, 619
Scapula, 371f
   borders of, 370
   movements of, 368f
   "winging" of, 384b
Scarpa's fascia, 149, 149f
Sciatic foramen
   greater, 295
   lesser, 295–297
Sciatic nerve, 250f–251f, 251–254, 252t–253t,
   305, 306f, 307b, 322–323, 322f, 363b
Sclera, 504, 520–521
Scleral venous sinus, 520
Scoliosis, 44b
Secretomotor innervation
   of glands in head, 628f
   lacrimal gland, 506
   mucous glands, 614–615
Segmental bronchi, 94
Segmental medullary arteries, 56, 56f
Segmental muscles, of back, 52, 53f, 54t
Segmental spinal arteries, 56, 56f
Sella turcica, 457–458
Semicircular canals, 530–531
Seminal vesicle, 242f, 243
Semispinalis capitis, 52
Semispinalis muscles, 51
Sensory innervation
   of auricle, 524f
   face, 490, 497b
   lacrimal gland, 506
   upper limb, testing of, 440b
Sensory neurons, 21, 21f
   visceral, 24, 31
Sensory receptors, for balance, 533
Sensory root to ciliary ganglion, 518
Septal papillary muscles, 112

Index

Serous pericardium, 103–104, 104f
Serratus anterior muscle, 383, 384t
Serratus posterior muscles, 50, 50f, 50t
Sesamoid bones, 10
Shaft
   of femur, 291–292, 292f, 310, 310f
   of fibula, 332–333, 332f
   of humerus, 398–400, 399f
   of radius, 410–411, 411f
   of tibia, 312–313, 312f, 331–332
   of ulna, 411–412, 411f
Shin splints, 313b
Short bones, 10
Shoulder, 370–379
   bones of, 370–372
   joints, 372–376
   muscles, 377–379
Shunts, ventriculoperitoneal, 164b
Sigmoid arteries, 193
Sigmoid mesocolon, 167
Sigmoid sinuses, 471
Sino-atrial node, 121, 122f
Sinuses
   dural venous, 469–472, 469f, 470t
   paranasal, 605f, 607–609, 607f
   tarsal, 343, 344f
Sinus of venae cavae, 110
Skeletal age, determination of, 10b
Skeletal framework
   of back, 36–41
   nasal cavities, 606
   oral cavity, 617–620
   pharynx, 585–586
   pterygopalatine fossa, 551
   sternum, 72–73, 73f
   of thorax, 68–75
      joints, 73–75
      ribs, 69–72, 71f
      sternum, 72–73, 73f
      thoracic vertebrae, 68–69
Skeletal muscle, 15
Skeletal system, 9–13
   bone, 9–10
   cartilage, 9
   joints, 11–13, 11f
Skene's glands, 267b–268b
Skin, 15
   eyelid, 502
   layers of scalp, 496
Skull, 446–454
   anterior view of, 446–448, 447f
      frontal bone, 446
      mandible, 447–448
      maxillae, 447
      zygomatic and nasal bones, 446
   base and lateral aspects of, 618f
   external foramina, 448t
   fractures of, 461b
   internal foramina, 456t
   lateral view, 448–451, 449f, 449b
      calvaria, 448–449, 452f
      facial skeleton, visible part of, 450–451
      inferior view, 452, 453f
      mandible, 451
      temporal bone, 448–449

Skull (Continued)
   posterior view, 451, 451f
      occipital bone, 451
      temporal bone, 451
      superior view, 451–452, 451f
Small cardiac vein, 120
Small intestine, 169–173
Small saphenous vein, 298, 359
Smooth muscle, 15
Soft palate, 630
   muscles of, 630, 630t
   open mouth with, 634f
Soft tissue injury, to knee, 328b
Sole of foot, muscle layers of, 356t
Solid joints, 11–13, 11f, 13f
Somatic motor efferents, 22
Somatic motor fibers, 22
Somatic part, of nervous system, 21–22, 21f
Somatic plexuses, 32, 32f
Somatic sensory afferents, 22
Somatic sensory fibers, 22
Somites, 21, 21f
Sound
   of heart, 116b
   of lungs, 93b
   transmission of, 534–535, 535f
Spermatic cord, 158–160, 159f–160f, 242, 242f
Sphenoidal sinuses, 609
Sphenoid bone, 452, 537, 551, 552f, 619
   lesser wing of, 457
Sphenomandibular ligament, 539, 542
Sphenopalatine artery, 556, 613
Sphenopalatine foramen, 551, 612–613
Sphenoparietal suture, 448
Sphincter
   within deep perineal pouch, 235
   muscle of face, 497b
   urethral, 235, 236f, 240
Sphincter pupillae, 521
Sphincter urethrovaginalis, 235, 236f
Spigelian hernia, 163b
Spina bifida, 43b
Spinal cord, 20, 55–60, 55f
   features of, 55f
   inferior ends of, 58f, 58b
   meninges, 57–58, 57f
   nerves of, 58–60, 59f
   vasculature, 56–57
Spinal fusion, 48b
Spinal ganglion, 58–59
Spinal nerves, 58–60
   nomenclature of, 60, 61f
   organization of, 59f
Spinal segment, 59
Spinalis, 51
Spine of sphenoid, 537
Spinotransversales muscles, 51, 51f, 51t
Spinous process, 38
Spiral ganglion, 532f, 534
Spiral lamina, 532
Spiral ligament, 533
Spiral organ, 533f, 534
Splanchnic nerves, 28–29, 197, 198f, 217–222
Spleen, 186–187, 186f
Splenic artery, 188–190

Splenic vein, 193–195
Splenius capitis, 51, 51f, 51t
Splenius cervicis, 51, 51f, 51t
Splenomegaly, 187b
Spondylolisthesis, 48b
Spongy bone, 9
Spongy urethra, 240, 241f
Sportsmen's groin/sportsmen's hernia, 163b
Squamous part
   of occipital bone, 459
   of temporal bone, 448, 454
Stapedius, 529t
Stapes, 529, 529f
Stellate ganglion, 581
Stent graft, abdominal aortic, 213b–214b
Sternal angle, 75, 76b
Sternal bone marrow, collection of, 73b
Sternoclavicular joint, 373, 373f, 373b
Sternocostal joints, 73–74, 74f
Sternohyoid muscle, 563
Sternum, 66, 72, 73f
   body of, 72–73
   manubrium of, 72
   xiphoid process in, 73
Stomach, 168–169, 168f
   sympathetic innervation of, 200–201
   visualizing, 169b
Stones
   bladder, 240b
   in parotid gland, 490b
Straight sinus, 469–471
Strangulation, of hernia, 163b
Stroke, 468b
Stylohyoid muscle, 562
Styloid process, 449
   of temporal bone, 618f
Stylomandibular ligament, 539
Stylomastoid foramen lesions, 496b
Subarachnoid hemorrhage, 473f, 473b
Subarachnoid space, 57–58, 465–466
   inferior ends of, 58f, 58b
Subclavian arteries, 467, 573, 578–579
Subclavian vein, 575, 579
Subclavius muscle, 66, 68f, 69t, 382, 383f, 383t
   nerve to, 394
Subcostal muscle, 78, 79f
Subcostal nerve, 81, 153–154
Subcostal plane, of abdomen, 147
Subcutaneous tissue, of eyelid, 502
Subdivisions
   of anterior triangle of neck, 571, 573t
   functional, of central nervous system, 21–32
Subdural hematoma, 473f, 473b
Subdural space, 465
Sublingual glands, 623f, 627–628
Submandibular ganglion, 546
Submandibular glands, 623f, 627
Submandibular nodes, 495, 583
Submandibular triangle, 561
Submental nodes, 495, 583
Submental triangle, 561
Suboccipital muscles, 52–53, 54f, 54t
Suboccipital triangle, 53, 54f
Subphrenic recess, 180
Subpopliteal recess, 324

Subscapular artery, 387–388
Subtalar joint, 348, 348f
Subtraction angiography, 4–5, 5f
Sulci, of heart, 106, 109f
Sulcus tali, 341
Sulcus terminalis cordis, 109–110
Superficial cervical lymph nodes, 583
Superficial, describing anatomical location, 3
Superficial fascia, 15
  abdominal, 148–149, 148f–149f
  of urogenital triangle, 270, 271f
Superficial fibular nerve, 337–338, 338f, 361f, 362
Superficial group of muscles
  in back, 48–50, 48f, 49t
  in posterior compartment of leg, 334, 334f, 334t
Superficial inguinal nodes, 155, 275, 275f, 299
Superficial inguinal ring, 157, 158f
Superficial layer, forearm muscles, 414, 414f
  anterior compartment, 414t
  posterior compartment, 418, 419f, 419t
Superficial lymph nodes, 582–583
Superficial palmar arch, 434, 434f
Superficial perineal pouch, structures in, 266–267, 267f
Superficial temporal artery, 565
Superficial veins, of neck, 560f
Superior articular processes, 68
Superior bulb of jugular vein, 565
Superior cervical ganglion, 28, 516, 581
Superior costal facet, 68
Superior costotransverse ligament, 73
Superior, describing anatomical location, 2f, 3
Superior epigastric artery, 79
Superior gemellus, nerve to, 251f, 254
Superior gluteal artery, 258, 258f, 297–298, 308
Superior gluteal nerve, 251f, 254, 305
Superior hypogastric plexus, 199, 217, 255, 256f–257f
Superior labial artery, 613
Superior laryngeal artery, 602
Superior laryngeal nerves, 603–604
Superior laryngeal veins, 603
Superior mediastinum, 126–135, 127f, 128b
  aorta and its branches, arch of, 130–131
  left superior intercostal vein in, 129, 129f
  nerves of, 131–134
  right and left brachiocephalic veins in, 127
  superior vena cava in, 129
  thoracic duct in, 135
  with thymus and venous channels removed, 130f
  thymus in, 127, 127b, 128f
  with thymus removed, 128f
  trachea and esophagus in, 131, 132f
  visualizing structures in, 128b, 134b
Superior mesenteric artery, 190–192
  branching of, 191f
  distribution of, 191f
Superior mesenteric vein, 195–196
Superior oblique, 511t, 512
Superior ophthalmic vein, 514
Superior orbital fissure, 458, 507, 509f
Superior part, of duodenum, 169

Superior petrosal sinuses, 471–472
Superior phrenic arteries, 83
Superior pubic ligament, 229, 229f
Superior pubic ramus, 225f, 226
Superior rectal artery, 193
Superior sagittal sinus, 469
Superior subscapular nerve, 396
Superior thoracic aperture, 67, 68f–69f
Superior thoracic artery, 387
Superior thyroid artery, 565, 565t, 569
Superior vena cava, 129, 130b
Superior vesical artery, 259, 259f
Superior view, of skull, 451–452, 451f
Supination
  elbow joint, 405f
  in forearm, 412–414, 413f
Supraclavicular cervical nerve, 577
Supracondylar fracture, of humerus, 407b
Supracondylar lines, 310
Suprahyoid muscle, 562, 563f
Supra-orbital artery, 514
Supra-orbital nerve, 490, 498
Suprapatellar bursa, 324
Suprapleural membrane, 85
Suprapubic catheterization, 240b
Suprarenal glands, 210–212
Suprascapular artery, 381
Suprascapular foramen, 379–380
Suprascapular nerve, 380–381, 393
Supraspinatus tendon, 377b
Supraspinous ligament, 46–47, 47f
Suprasternal notch, 72
Supratrochlear artery, 514
Supratrochlear nerve, 490, 498
Supreme intercostal artery, 78, 579
Sural nerve, 336–337, 337f, 361f, 362
Surfaces
  of heart, 105, 107f–108f
  inferolateral, of bladder, 238, 239f
  of tongue, 621
    inferior, 622
    pharyngeal, 622–624
Surfer's ear, 524b
Surgery
  approach to pituitary gland, 609b
  for obesity, 172b
Surgical neck of humerus, 372, 372f
Suspensory ligament
  of clitoris, 266, 267f
  of eyeball, 510
  of lens, 521
  of ovary, 249f, 250, 260
  of penis, 266, 267f
Suspensory muscle, of duodenum, 169
Sustentaculum tali, 342
Sutural ligament, 13
Sutures, 13, 14f
  skull, 448, 451f
Swallowing, larynx role in, 601, 602f
Swimmer's ear, 524b
Sympathetic fibers, 255, 256f–257f
Sympathetic innervation, 124
  of glands in head, 629f
  lacrimal gland, 507
  nasal cavity, 616

Sympathetic nervous system
  cervical part of the sympathetic trunk, 581, 581f
  ganglia, 581–582
Sympathetic root to ciliary ganglion, 518–519
Sympathetic system, 25–29, 25f–26f
  visceral sensory fibers in, 31
Sympathetic trunks, 197–198, 197f, 217–222
  of pelvis, 251f, 256f–257f
  in posterior mediastinum, 140–141, 141f
Symphyses, 13, 14f
  between vertebral bodies, 42–43, 45f
Synchondroses, 13, 14f
Syndesmoses, 13, 14f
Synovial joints, 11–12, 11f
  descriptions based on shape and movement, 12
  types of, 12, 13f
Synovial membrane, 11, 294, 294f, 324, 325f
  of elbow joint, 405, 405f
  of glenohumeral joint, 375f
Synovial sheaths, of hand, 429f
Systemic approach, to anatomy study, 2

T

Tail, of epididymis, 242f
Talocalcaneonavicular joint, 348–349, 349f
Talus, 341–342, 341f
  fracture of, 342b
Tarsal bones, 340–343
  distal group of, 341f, 343
  intermediate, 343
  proximal group, 341–343
    calcaneus, 342–343, 343f
    talus, 341–342, 341f
Tarsal glands, 504
Tarsal plates, 503f, 504
Tarsal sinus, 343, 344f
Tarsal tunnel, 351–352, 351f, 352b
Tarsometatarsal joint, 350, 350f
Tarsus, 503–504, 503f
Tears
  in cruciate ligaments, 328b
  in supraspinatus tendon, 377b
Technetium-99m, 7
Tectorial membrane, 46
Teeth, 634–638
  innervation, 637–638
  successive sets of, 634
  vessels, 635–636
Tegmental wall, of middle ear, 526
Telencephalon, 466
Temporal and infratemporal fossae, 535–550, 535f
  bony framework, 536–538, 536f
  infratemporal fossa, 541–550, 542f
  masseter muscle, 540, 540f
  temporal fossa, 540–541, 541f
  temporomandibular joints, 538–539, 538f
Temporal bone, 448–449, 536–537, 619
  facial nerve, 534, 535f
  lateral view, 448–449
  middle cranial fossa, 458
  petrous part, 454
  posterior view, 451
  styloid process of, 618f

Index

Temporal pulse, 639b
Temporalis, 540–541, 541f
Temporomandibular joints, 538–539, 538f
  disorders, 539b
  extracapsular ligaments, 539
  joint capsule, 539
  ligaments associated, 539f
  movements of, 539, 539f
Tendinous arch, 233f, 234
Tendinous intersections, 151–152
Tendons, 12
  in distal forearm, 421b–422b
  identifying, 421b–422b
  of rotator cuff muscles, 375–376
  of wrist, 426
Tendon taps, 364b
Tennis elbow, 407b
Tenosynovitis, 429b
Tensor fasciae latae, 301
Tensor tympani, 529t
Tensor veli palatini muscles, 630, 630t, 631f
Tentorium cerebelli, 457, 463
Testes, 242–243, 242f
  descent of, 156f
Testicular arteries, 213, 213t, 274
Testicular tumors, 243b
Testosterone, exogenous, 601b
Thenar muscles, 431, 433f
Thigh, 286, 309–330, 309f
  arteries of, 317–320
  bones of, 309–313, 310f
  deep artery of, 317–320, 319f
  knee joint, 323–328, 323f
  lateral cutaneous nerve of, 219t, 221
  muscles of, 313–317
    anterior compartment, 313–315, 314f,
      315t
    medial compartment, 316, 316f, 317t
    posterior compartment, 316–317, 318f,
      318t
  nerves of, 321–323
  posterior cutaneous nerve of, 307
  tibiofibular joint, 329, 329f
  veins of, 321
Third occipital nerve, 498
Third space within prevertebral layer of neck,
  560b
Thoracic aorta, in posterior mediastinum,
  137, 138f, 138t
Thoracic duct
  in posterior mediastinum, 139–140, 140f
  in root of neck, 582, 582f
  in superior mediastinum, 135
Thoracic outlet syndrome, 67
Thoracic spinal nerve, 25f
Thoracic splanchnic nerves, 197–198
Thoracic vertebrae, 36, 36f, 38, 39f–40f,
  68–69, 71f
  articulation with ribs, 68–69
  typical, 37b, 68, 70f
  variations in number of, 44b
Thoracic viscera, sympathetic innervation of,
  28, 28f
Thoracic wall, 64f, 66–81
  arteries of, 80f
  inferior thoracic aperture in, 67, 70f
  intercostal spaces of, 77f, 78

Thoracic wall (Continued)
  lymphatic vessels and nodes of, 82f
  movement of, during breathing, 84, 85f
  muscles of, 78t
  skeletal framework of, 68–75
  superior thoracic aperture, 67, 68f–69f
  veins of, 81f
Thoracoacromial artery, 387
Thoracolumbar fascia, 53–55, 54f
Thoracostomy, 82b
Thorax, 64, 64f
  diaphragm, 81–84
  mediastinum, 97–141
  pectoral region, 64–66
  pleural cavities, 84–97
  regional anatomy, 64–141, 64f
  thoracic wall, 66–81
Thrombosis, deep vein, 298b
Thumb
  hyperextension and abduction, 421b–422b
  movements of, 369f
Thymus, 127, 128f
  ectopic parathyroid glands in, 127b
Thyro-arytenoid muscle, 600t, 601f
Thyrocervical trunk, 579
Thyrohyoid membrane, 595
Thyrohyoid muscle, 563
Thyroid cartilage, 594, 594f
  inferior tubercle, 586
Thyroid gland, 569–570
  how to find, 572f, 572b
Thyroid ima artery, 131
Thyroidectomy, 571b
Tibia, 332f
  condyles and intercondylar areas of,
    311–312
  popliteal fossa, 329–330
  proximal end of, 311–313, 312f
  shaft and distal end of, 331–332
  shaft of, 312–313, 312f
Tibial nerve, 329, 336–337, 337f, 360–361, 360f
Tibial part, sciatic nerve to, 251f
Tibial tuberosity, 312
Tibialis anterior, 339t
Tibiofibular joint, 329, 329f
Tic douloureux, 491b
TIV vertebral level, visualizing structures at,
  132b
TIV/V vertebral level, 75, 75f
  visualizing structures at, 76b
Toes, fibrous sheaths of, 353–354, 354f
Tongue, 621–627, 623f
  innervation, 625, 625f
  lymphatics, 626–627
  muscles, 624, 624t, 625f
  papillae, 621–622
  surfaces of, 621–624
  vessels, 624–625
Tonsils, 590
  lingual, 590, 622–624
  palatine, 590
  pharyngeal, 590
Torus levatorius, 590
Torus tubarius, 590
Total hip replacement, 14f
Trabeculae, arachnoid, 57
Trabeculae carneae, 111

Trachea, 90–94
  in superior mediastinum, 131, 132f
Tracheobronchial injury, 569b
Tracheostomy, 603b
Tragus, 522
Trans/non-binary anatomical terminology, 3
Transmission of sound, 534–535, 535f
Transplantation, bone marrow, 10b
Transpyloric plane, of abdomen, 147
Transversalis fascia, 15, 151
Transverse arch, of foot, 353, 353f
Transverse cervical artery, 573–575, 579
Transverse cervical nerve, 567–568, 568f, 577
Transverse cervical or cardinal ligament,
  247–248, 248f
Transverse costal facet, 38, 68
Transverse facial artery, 488, 493–494
Transverse facial vein, 495
Transverse ligament, of atlas, 38
Transverse mesocolon, 167
Transverse pericardial sinus, 104
Transverse perineal muscle, deep, 235, 236f
Transverse plane, 2f, 3
Transverse process, 38, 68
Transverse sinuses, 471
Transversospinales muscles, 51–52, 53f, 53t
Transversus abdominis, 150t, 151
  aponeurosis and, 151f
  inguinal canal and, 159f
Transversus thoracis muscle, 78, 79f
Trapezium, 423
Trapezius, 48–49, 49t, 377, 378f
  innervation and blood supply of, 49f
Trendelenburg's sign, 305b
Triangular interval, posterior wall of axilla,
  386
Triangular space
  posterior scapular region, 380
  posterior wall of axilla, 386
Triceps brachii, 402t
Tricuspid valve, 112–113
Trigeminal innervation, of scalp, 498
Trigeminal nerves (V), 476t, 477f, 478
  cutaneous distribution of, 492f
  leaving the skull, 491f
Trigeminal neuralgia, 491b
Trigger finger, 429b
Trigone, 237–238, 239f
Trochanters, 290–292, 291f
Trochlea of humerus, 399
Trochlear nerves, 476t, 477f, 478, 481b, 516,
  516f
True epididymis, 242f
True pelvis (lesser pelvis), 224, 224f, 230–236,
  230f
  pelvic floor, 232–235
  pelvic inlet, 230, 230f
  pelvic outlet, 232, 232f
  pelvic wall, 230–232
  perineal body, 235–236, 236f
True ribs, 69
Trunks
  brachial plexus, 390
    branches, 393–394
  costocervical, 579
  internal iliac artery and, 258–260, 258f
  lymphatic, 19, 19f, 583f

Trunks *(Continued)*
  paravertebral sympathetic, 28
  sympathetic, 251f, 256f–257f
  thyrocervical, 579
Tubal ligation, 246b
Tubercle, of ribs, 69
Tuberculum of iliac crest, 225f, 226
Tuberosity, tibial, 312
Tubes, uterine, 246, 246f
Tumors
  in parotid gland, 490f, 490b
  testicular, 243b
Tunica
  albuginea, 242–243, 242f
  vaginalis, 242, 242f
Tunica externa (adventitia), 16
Tunica intima, 16
Tunica media, 16
Tunicae, of blood vessels, 16
Tympanic membrane, 524–525, 525f
  perforation of, 525b–526b
Tympanic nerve, 480
Tympanic part, of temporal bone, 449, 536

U
Ulceration, duodenal, 172b
Ulna
  abduction during pronation, 413–414, 413f
  proximal end of, 400–401, 400f
  shaft and distal end, 411–412, 411f
Ulnar artery, 415–417, 426
Ulnar nerve, 395, 401f, 402, 417–418, 436, 436f
Ultrasonography, of head, 461b
Ultrasound, 5
  abdominal, 5f
  Doppler, 5
  of urinary tract, 211b
Umbilical artery, 258–259, 259f
Umbilical hernias, 163b
Umbo of tympanic membrane, 524
Uncovertebral joints, 45, 45f
Undescended testes, 242b
Upper limb, 367–442
  anterior view of, 368f
  arm, 398–404, 398f
  axilla, 381–397, 382f
  cubital fossa, 408–409, 408f–409f
  dermatomes and myotomes, 439b
  elbow joint, 405–406
  forearm, 410–414, 410f
    anterior compartment of, 414–418
    posterior compartment of, 418–421
  hand, 422–438
  posterior scapular region, 379–381, 379f
  regional anatomy of, 368–438
Ureteropelvic junction, 209
Ureters, 208–209, 209f, 237, 239f
  innervation of, 209
  vasculature and lymphatics of, 209
Urethra, 239f, 240, 241f
  in men, 240
  in women, 240
Urethral artery, 273, 273f
Urethral catheterization, 241b
Urethral crest, 240, 241f

Urethral rupture, 271b
Urethral sphincter, external, 235, 236f
Urinary system, pelvic viscera and, 237–240, 239f
Urinary tract cancer, 210b
Urinary tract stones, 210b
Urogenital hiatus, 233f, 234, 263
Urogenital triangle, 263, 263f
  superficial fascia of, 270, 271f
Urological contrast studies, 8
Uterine artery, 259–260, 259f–260f
Uterine tubes, 246, 246f
Uterosacral ligament, 247–248, 248f
Uterus, 245–246, 246f
Utricle, 533

V
Vagal trunks, 167
Vagina, 247, 247f–248f
Vaginal artery, 259, 260f
Vaginal fornix, 247, 247f–248f
Vaginal vault, 247, 248f
Vagus nerve (X), 200, 480, 566, 566f, 580
  pharyngeal branch, 591
  of superior mediastinum, 131–133, 134b–135b
Vallate papillae, 622
Valve disease, 116b
Valves, anal, 237, 238f
Varicose veins, 17b, 298b
Vas deferens, 242
Vascular compartments, of neck, 445f, 446
Vascular layer, of eyeball, 521
Vascular supply, of knee joint, 328
Vasculature
  eyelids, 504f
  facial, 494f
  of posterior abdominal region, 212–215
  renal, 208, 209f
  of root of neck, 578f
  scalp, 500f
  suprarenal, 211–212, 211f
  thyroid gland, 571f
  ureteric, 209
Vasectomy, 243b
Veins, 16, 381, 417, 419
  in anterior compartment of leg, 340
  of arm, 404
  azygos system of, in posterior mediastinum, 137–139, 139f
  emissary, 472b
  facial, 495
  in foot, 359, 360f
  of gluteal region, 308
  of hand, 435
  harvesting for grafts, 299b
  in lateral compartment of leg, 336
  of lower limb, 298f
  of neck, 565
  of orbit, 514–515
  pelvic, 260–262, 261f
  of perineum, 274, 274f
  in posterior compartment of leg, 336
  pterygoid plexus of, 550f
  of pterygopalatine fossa, 557, 557f

Veins *(Continued)*
  in root of neck, 579
  of spinal cord, 57, 57f
  of teeth and gingivae, 636
  of thigh, 321
  of tongue, 625
Veins of Thebesius, 120
Venae cordis minimae, 120
Venous access
  for central and dialysis lines, 130b
  central, via subclavian/axillary vein, 389b
Venous drainage
  of abdominal viscera, 193–196
  of abdominal wall, 155
  of auricle, 524
  of brain, 469–472
  of breast, 66
  of diaphragm, 83
  of esophagus, 136
  of eyeball, 515f, 520
  of eyelid, 504
  of gastrointestinal tract, 194f
  of intercostal spaces, 80, 81f
  of internal ear, 534
  of larynx, 603, 604f
  of nasal cavities, 614, 615f
  of palate, 631–632, 632f
  of pharynx, 591, 591f
  of scalp, 499
  superficial, of neck, 560–561
  of thyroid gland, 570
Ventricles
  cerebral, 20
  laryngeal, 599
Ventricular septal defect (VSD), 117b
Ventriculoperitoneal shunts, 164b
Vertebrae
  cancer and, 44b
  cervical, 36, 36f, 36b, 38
  fractures of, 47b
  joints of, 42–45
  lumbar, 36f, 37–40, 39f–40f, 201–202
  thoracic, 36, 36f, 38, 39f–40f
  variations in number of, 44b
Vertebral arch, 38
  posterior spaces between, 41, 42f
Vertebral arteries, 467, 468b, 578
Vertebral body, 37
Vertebral canal, 38
  anesthesia within, 60b
  arrangement of structures in, 58, 59f
  spinal nerves in, 60f
Vertebral column
  anterior and posterior longitudinal ligaments of, 46f
  cervical region of, 36b
  clinical, 47b
  curvatures of, 41, 43f
Vertebral compartments, of neck, 445, 445f
Vertebral foramen, 68
Vertebral notches, superior and inferior, 38
Vertebroplasty, 43b–44b
Vertex
  innervation of scalp anterior to, 498
  innervation of scalp posterior to, 498
Vertical muscles, of abdomen, 151–152
Vesico-uterine pouch, 249, 249f

Index

Vessels, of pericardium, 104
Vestibular aqueduct, 531
Vestibule, 267b–268b, 530–531, 599
    of laryngeal cavity, 599
Vestibulocochlear nerves (VIII), 479–480
Visceral afferent fibers, 255
Visceral afferents, 31, 124
Visceral compartments, of neck, 445f, 446
Visceral nerves, of perineum, 271–272
Visceral part, of nervous system, 21, 23–25, 24f
Visceral pleura, 85, 86f, 87
    innervation of, 86b
Visceral plexuses, 32, 32f
    of pelvis, 255, 256f–257f
Visceral sensory innervation, 31
Vitreous humor, 520
Vocal cord mass, 601b
Vocalis muscle, 600t, 601f
Vomer, 452
Vorticose veins, 520
Vulva, 267b–268b

W

Walls
    of eyeball, 520
    lateral pharyngeal, line of attachment for,
        585–586, 586f
    of nasal cavity, 609–611
    oral cavity, 620
White matter, 20, 55f, 56
White ramus communicans, 25
"Winging," of scapula, 384b
Women
    heart attack, symptoms of, 125b
    pelvic fascia in, 247–248, 248f
    peritoneum in, pelvic, 249–250, 249f
    reproductive system in, 244–247, 244f
    urethra of, anatomy of, 240, 241f
Wrist, carpal tunnel and structures at,
    426–427, 427f
Wrist drop, 439b
Wrist joint, 424b, 425

X

Xiphisternal joints, 74f, 75
Xiphoid process, 73, 73f
X-rays, cathode ray tube for production of,
    3, 4f

Z

Zonular fibers, 521
Zygapophyseal joints, 44–45, 45f, 227, 228f
Zygomatic bones, 446, 450, 537
Zygomatic nerve, 553–554
Zygomatic process, 446–449
Zygomaticofacial branch, 490
    of zygomatic nerve, 554
Zygomaticotemporal branch, 490
    of zygomatic nerve, 553–554
Zygomaticotemporal nerve, 498, 541
Zygomaticus major, 484–486
Zygomaticus minor, 484–486